D0998933

A History of Nursing Ideas

Linda C. Andrist, PhD, RNC
Associate Professor and Coordinator,
Women's Health Nurse Practitioner Specialty
MGH Institute of Health Professions
Graduate Program in Nursing

Patrice K. Nicholas, DNSC, MPH, APRN, BC
Professor and Chair of Advanced Practice Nursing
MGH Institute of Health Professions
Graduate Program in Nursing

Karen A. Wolf, PhD, APRN, BC
Clinical Associate Professor and Chair of Generalist Level Nursing
MGH Institute of Health Professions
Graduate Program in Nursing

JONES AND BARTLETT PUBLISHERS
Sudbury, Massachusetts
BOSTON   TORONTO   LONDON   SINGAPORE

World Headquarters
Jones and Bartlett Publishers
40 Tall Pine Drive
Sudbury, MA 01776
978-443-5000
info@jbpub.com
www.jbpub.com

Jones and Bartlett Publishers Canada
6339 Ormindale Way
Mississauga, Ontario L5V 1J2
Canada

Jones and Bartlett Publishers International
Barb House, Barb Mews
London W6 7PA
United Kingdom

Jones and Bartlett's books and products are available through most bookstores and online booksellers. To contact Jones and Bartlett Publishers directly, call 800-832-0034, fax 978-443-8000, or visit our website www.jbpub.com.

Substantial discounts on bulk quantities of Jones and Bartlett's publications are available to corporations, professional associations, and other qualified organizations. For details and specific discount information, contact the special sales department at Jones and Bartlett via the above contact information or send an email to specialsales@jbpub.com.

Copyright © 2006 by Jones and Bartlett Publishers, Inc.

All rights reserved. No part of the material protected by this copyright may be reproduced or utilized in any form, electronic or mechanical, including photocopying, recording, or by any information storage and retrieval system, without written permission from the copyright owner.

Production Credits
Acquisitions Editor: Kevin Sullivan
Production Director: Amy Rose
Production Editor: Jenny L. McIsaac
Associate Editor: Amy Sibley
Marketing Manager: Emily Ekle
Cover Design: Timothy Dziewit
Composition: Auburn Associates, Inc.
Printing and Binding: Malloy
Cover Printing: Malloy

ISBN-13: 978-0-7637-2289-0
ISBN-10: 0-7637-2289-8

Library of Congress Cataloging-in-Publication Data

History of nursing ideas / [edited by] Linda C. Andrist, Patrice K. Nicholas, Karen A. Wolf.
  p. ; cm.
    Includes bibliographical references and index.
    ISBN-13: 978-0-7637-2289-8 (pbk.)
  1. Nursing—History. 2. Nursing—Philosophy—History.
  [DNLM: 1. History of Nursing. 2. Nurse's Role—history. WY 11.1 H5576 2006] I. Andrist, Linda C.
II. Nicholas, Patrice K. III. Wolf, Karen.
  RT31.H575 2006
  610.73′09—dc22
                                                                              2005011493
6048

Printed in the United States of America
10 09 08 07 06   10 9 8 7 6 5 4 3 2

Dedication and Acknowledgments

We dedicate this book to the memory of Christine Bridges, DNSc, RN who conceived this book. All of us were deeply saddened at the loss of Chris in June, 2004. She was a boundless source of energy and inspiration to us all in her roles as nursing educator, wife and mother of five children, tireless community activist, and friend. Chris was a passionate teacher who loved to share her fervor for nursing theory and nursing ideas. Her excitement about theory development and the potential to guide nursing practice was integral to her teaching and our faculty community. Chris truly inspired her nursing students, mentoring them in their first courses—The History of Nursing Ideas, Biobehavioral Principles and Theories, Community Health, and later guiding them in writing their Scholarly Projects to complete requirements for their MSN. Her spirit lives on through the ideas in this book.

We wish to thank Arlene Lowenstein, PhD, RN, Former Director of the Graduate Program in Nursing and Professor Emerita at the MGH Institute of Health Professions. Dr. Lowenstein also taught The History of Nursing Ideas course and supported our efforts in birthing this text. Her enthusiasm and knowledge about nursing history and the social forces that impacted the profession were invaluable in developing the themes herein.

We would like to thank our individual families:

Linda C. Andrist:

To my husband, Russ Hereford, for giving me the love, support, and time to write;

To Erin Hereford, for sharing her experiences in the global village;

To Nathan Hereford, for his spirit of adventure and love of indigenous music;

To Clio, our Airedale puppy, named for the Muse of History, who always knows how to inspire me with a walk on the beach; and

To my mother, Millicent Andrist, and my sister, Kim Andrist, for their love and support through thick and thin.

Karen Anne Wolf:

To my husband, Edward Oberholtzer and children Josiah and Jenny for their embrace of creativity and intellectual pursuits; and willingness to support me with food, love, and humor through this project.

Patrice Kenneally Nicholas:

To my husband, Tom, for his inspiration and for sparking the ideas;

To Thomas, for his love and contributions to the music of our family's soul;

To Gregory – brilliant, loyal, loving, generous, and true blue;

To Seven, who helps our family relish each day; and

To my parents, George and Carole Kenneally for believing that the profession of nursing would bring me a sense of lifelong joy.

We would like to acknowledge the following people who helped bring this book to publication: Susan Rich, MEd, for typing transcripts, Katherine Simmonds, MSN, MPH, WHNP and Patricia Lussier-Duynstee, PhD, RN for editing chapters, Kevin Sullivan, Amy Sibley, and Jenny McIsaac at Jones and Bartlett for their patience and support. And finally, to all of our students past and present, who continue to inspire us and challenge our profession to move forward.

Contents

SECTION 3   ADVANCING THE PROFESSION   301

Preface

"A History of Nursing Ideas" evolved from our experience teaching a course by the same title to graduate students at the MGH Institute of Health Professions. Our goal has been to guide students in their appreciation and understanding of the contextual nature of nursing knowledge and practice. In tracing the history of nursing, we find voices echoing from the past that are heard in the winds of the present. This legacy of knowledge development in nursing will challenge future generations of scholars to continue to extend our body of knowledge in the care of persons and their families, communities, and the environment.

Nursing ideas do not exist in isolation, but in the context from which they arise, and while nursing does hold some unique ideas and ideals, it is generally reflective of the social context and knowledge paradigms of the times. Nursing's intellectual inheritance includes long-standing ideals about human needs, nursing caring, and service. That heritage also illustrates that inherent biases about gender, class, race, and the persistence of paternalism in health care, have created barriers to nursing development. Despite such barriers, nurses have generated an impressive effort in theory development, professional growth, research, and education.

As the world around nursing has changed so too has the profession been challenged to grow, evolve, and yes—sometimes rebel. Common beliefs have given way to new perspectives and new conceptions of nursing education and practice have emerged from the turmoil of social change. While nurses have struggled to build a common knowledge base and culture, the reality is that there is great diversity in the theory and praxis of nursing. We celebrate the history and diversity of nursing ideas with this book.

Contributors

Linda C. Andrist, PhD, RNC
Associate Professor and Coordinator,
Women's Health Nurse Practitioner Specialty
MGH Institute of Health Professions
Graduate Program in Nursing
Boston, MA

Deva-Marie Beck, PhD, RN
International Director
Nightingale Initiative for Global Health
   (NIGH)
Ottawa, Canada

Michael Carter, DNSc, APRN, BC, FAAN
Dean Emeritus
College of Nursing
The University of Tennessee-Memphis
Memphis, TN

Peggy L. Chinn, PhD, RN, FAAN
Professor Emeritus
School of Nursing
University of Connecticut
Storrs, CT

Inge Corless, PhD, RN, FAAN
Professor
Graduate Program in Nursing
MGH Institute of Health Professions
Boston, MA

Denise J. Drevdahl, RN, PhD
Associate Professor
Nursing Program
University of Washington, Tacoma
Tacoma, WA

Jeanette Ives Erickson, RN, MS, CNA
Senior Vice President for Patient Care
   Services & Chief Nurse
Massachusetts General Hospital
Boston, MA

Joan Evans PhD, RN
Associate Professor
School of Nursing
Dalhousie University
Halifax, Nova Scotia
Canada

Annette Flanagin, MA, RN, FAAN
Managing Senior Editor
Journal of the American Medical
   Association
Chicago, IL

Noreen Cavan Frisch, PhD, RN, FAAN
Professor and Director
School of Nursing
Cleveland State University
Cleveland, Ohio

Susan R. Gortner, MN, PhD, FAAN
Professor Emeritus
University of California San Francisco
San Francisco, CA

Tamara S. Hammer, MSN, APRN, BC
Fellow, Department of Behavioral Health
Harvard Vanguard Medical Associates
Boston, MA

Melinda L. Jenkins, PhD, APRN, BC
Assistant Professor
School of Nursing
Columbia University
New York, NY

Lucille A. Joel, EdD, RN, FAAN
Professor
College of Nursing
Rutgers-the State University of New Jersey
   College of Nursing
Newark, NJ

Lea Johnson, RN, MSN
Assistant Dean
Northeastern University
Boston, MA

Ursula Kelly, PhD, APRN, BC
Assistant Professor
MGH Institute of Health Professions
Boston, MA

Maureen Shawn Kennedy, MA, RN
News Director
American Journal of Nursing
New York, NY

Dorothy Kleffel RN, MPH, DNSc
Adjunct Faculty
University of San Diego
San Diego, CA

Jean D. Leuner, PhD, RN
Director
School of Nursing
College of Health and Public Affairs
University of Central Florida
Orlando, FL

Rozzano C. Locsin, RN, PhD
Professor
Christine E. Lynn College of Nursing
Florida Atlantic University
Boca Raton, FL

Patricia Maher, RN, MS, RNCS
Nurse Practitioner—Health Care for the
  Homeless Program
Cambridge Health Alliance
Cambridge, MA

Diana J. Mason, RN, PhD, FAAN
Editor in Chief
American Journal of Nursing
New York, NY

Sr. Sharon McGuire, OP, PhD, APRN, BC
Assistant Professor
Hahn School of Nursing and Health Science
University of San Diego
San Diego, CA

Janice Bell Meisenhelder, DNSc, RN
Associate Professor
MGH Institute of Health Professions
Boston, MA

Brenda Nevidjon, MSN, RN
Associate Clinical Professor
School of Nursing
Duke University
Durham, NC

Margaret A. Newman, PhD, RN, FAAN
Professor Emeritus
University of Minnesota
School of Nursing
Minneapolis, MN

Patrice Nicholas, DNSc, MPH, APRN, BC
Professor and Chair of Advanced Practice
  Nursing
MGH Institute of Health Professions
Graduate Program in Nursing
Boston, MA

Hollie Noveletsky, PhD, RNC
Private Practice
Greenland, NH

Angela Pizzo, RN, MSN, ANP
Adult Nurse Practitioner
Maine Center for Diabetes
Scarborough, ME

Joyce Pulcini, PhD, RNCS, PNP, FAAN
Associate Professor
School of Nursing
Boston College
Chestnut Hill, MA

Evelyn D. Quigley, RN, MN
Senior Executive and
Chief Nursing Officer and CO-Clinical
Patient Safety Officer
MeritCare Health System
Fargo, ND

Susan Jo Roberts, DNSc, ANP, FAAN
Associate Professor
School of Nursing
Bouvé College of Health Sciences
Northeastern University
Boston, MA

Deborah A. Rosenbloom-Brunto, MSN, RN,
  ACNP
Clinical Instructor
MGH Institute of Health Professions
Boston, MA

Margarete Sandelowski, PhD, RN, FAAN
Cary C. Boshamer Professor
School of Nursing
University of North Carolina at Chapel Hill
Chapel Hill, NC

Rozella M. Schlotfeldt, PhD, APRN, BC,
  FNP
Professor Emeritus
School of Nursing
Columbia University
New York, NY

Thelma M. Schorr, RN, Hon-CNNFC,
  FAAN
Former Editor in Chief and Publisher
American Journal of Nursing Company
New York, NY

Elizabeth Speakman, EdD, RN
Associate Professor
College of Health Professions
Thomas Jefferson University
Philadelphia, PA

Patricia St. Hill, PhD, RN, MPH
Associate Professor
Hunter-Bellevue School of Nursing
Hunter College of the City University of
  New York (CUNY)
New York, NY

Debra Sylvester, RN, MSN, GNP
Geriatric Nurse Practitioner
Boston University Division of Geriatrics
Boston Medical Center
Boston, MA

Nancy Terres, PhD, RNCS
Assistant Professor
Graduate Program in Nursing
MGH Institute of Health Professions
Boston, MA

John Twomey, PhD, RN
Associate Professor
MGH Institute of Health Professions
Boston, MA

Deborah Washington, RN, MSN
Director, Diversity, Patient Care Service
Massachusetts General Hospital
Boston, MA

Jill White, RN, RM, MEd, PhD
Dean, Faculty of Nursing, Midwifery
  and Health
University of Technology
Sydney, Australia

Karen Anne Wolf, PhD, APRN, BC
Clinical Associate Professor and
Chair of Generalist Level Nursing
MGH Institute of Health Professions
Graduate Program in Nursing
Boston, MA

SECTION 1

WEAVING CRITICAL THREADS
THROUGH NURSING IDEAS

Linda C. Andrist

The term *critical threads* is used to identify issues that are central to every situation in nursing and that we believe should be addressed in education, practice, research, and theory development. Gender, culture, race, community, environment, and the dialectic between technology and caring all impact the profession as well as the individual nurse who provides nursing care. Examining the historical context of these issues can help us to understand the nature and progression of nursing as a movement. Each author in this section situates a critical thread in a historical context and discusses its impact on nursing ideas.

The growth of Western nursing, and American nursing in particular, has been shaped by complex social, economic, and political forces. Historically, nursing has been largely a women's profession. Given this, examination of gender issues and the effect of gender discrimination is critical in order to understand the societal constraints on the development of the profession over the past 150 years. Questions that can be considered include: As a profession that provides critical services to the public, why has nursing not utilized our potential power in creating change in the healthcare system? Why has nursing not achieved the same status as other professions? Why has nursing long been considered secondary to medicine?

Women's movements have addressed many of women's concerns—the right to vote, equal pay for equal work, improved working conditions—and yet, as history demonstrates, nursing has been slow to join these movements. In Chapter 1, Andrist examines the historical relationship between nursing and feminism and how feminism has influenced nursing since the beginnings of the modern nursing movement in the late 1800s. Like many before her, Andrist links women's issues with nursing's issues. She discusses the progress that nursing has achieved in its alliance with feminist thought and practice as the profession continues to mature as a respected healthcare profession.

Roberts (1983) has previously argued that the reason nursing has long been subordinate to organized medicine and hospital administration is because nurses are viewed as an oppressed group. Based on the model developed by Freire (1971), oppressed group behavior becomes the dominant method of reacting by those being subordinated. The root of the cycle of oppression is the learned belief by dominated people that they are inferior. Roberts expands her work on oppressed group behavior in Chapter 2. She discusses the oppressed group model, explains its relevance to nursing, and explores ways that nurses can empower themselves by changing self-defeating behaviors. She asserts that this action will benefit nurses and will ultimately improve the healthcare system.

Although the oppressed group model may be one explanation for the historical lack of power of the nursing profession, some writers have argued that the development of the nursing profession has been hampered because it is predominantly female. The expressive roles of femininity (e.g., nurturing, caring, dependence, and submission) stand in marked contrast to the instrumental roles of masculinity (e.g., aggression, self-control, competitiveness, and dominance). Although this dualism has been used to explain differences between the experiences of men and women, one could use it in a historical context to explain differences among nurses, physicians, and hospital administrators. For cxample, the inclusion of women in medicine and hospital administration is a very recent development. The inclusion of men in nursing also is relatively new. In Chapter 3, Evans explores gendered and sexed relations in nursing and the relations of masculinity and the power they embody. She extends this analysis to women in medicine to illustrate how gendered relations structure unequal opportunities for men and women within and across nursing and medicine.

Although gender is a powerful thread, culture and race are equally critical threads in the development of nursing ideas. The prevailing voices throughout nursing's history have been White Euro-American women. The 1990s brought a wake-up call; both the United States and Canada experienced the largest influx of immigrants in history. In the United States, these immigrants came from North and South America, Asia, and Africa. Hispanics are now the largest minority group in the United States. In Chapter 4, Washington describes the increasing importance of culture and how to incorporate theoretical models of culture into patient care. She stresses the importance of becoming culturally competent.

The profession needs to attract a diverse workforce for two important reasons: (1) to care for our multicultural population, and (2) to increase the number of nurses in the 21st century workforce. As we face the largest nursing shortage in history, the profession needs to attract women and men of all races and ethnic/cultural backgrounds. St. Hill argues that racism is one of the reasons that minorities have not entered the profession in larger numbers. In Chapter 5, she traces the historical roots of race and race relations among Blacks and Whites in American society and its impact on the nursing profession as it transitioned from a task-oriented vocation to a profession in its own right. She highlights several critical periods and turning points in American history and traces their reverberations and influences on the nursing profession.

McGuire extends the analysis of culture and race to issues of migration and health in Chapter 6. She presents an overview of the historical foundations of nursing in immigrant communities and a discussion of contemporary human migration patterns and trends, the causes of immigration, and the health exigencies of immigrants in the context of a postmodern, postcolonial world. She argues that a global environment of rapid social, political, economic, and eclogical upheavals presents formidable challenges to nurses in providing competent and appropriate health care to migrant communities.

McGuire's work connects the threads of culture and race to community, our next critical thread. Drevdahl, in Chapter 7, reviews the concept of community in nursing history, with the goal of stimulating thinking and discussion about community to further social justice. She asserts that community is an important paradigm for nursing practice that has coursed its way through theory and practice, surfacing at different moments in nursing history. Writers of the new millennium bring to light how the concept of community can simultaneously be conceived as a spatial entity as well as a place where relationships are maintained or allowed to perish. We also are reminded that struggles over the meanings of *community* are struggles over power.

Drevdahl impresses upon us that the elements that unite a community also create partitions, especially along class lines, and that nursing needs to attend to issues of social justice. Her idea of community is interlocked with the environmental paradigm.

In Chapter 8, Kleffel analyzes three environmental paradigms: the egocentric, the homocentric, and the ecocentric. The egocentric paradigm is grounded at the individual level, the homocentric at the societal level, and the ecocentric at the cosmos level. The egocentric model is rooted in individual rights, the homocentric model in social justice, and the ecocentric in holism and interconnectedness with the planet and cosmos. She argues that the global conditions of worldwide hunger, water shortages, global warming, emerging and reemerging infectious diseases, wars, and desertification, to name a few issues, are causing indescribable human misery, disease, and death. Kleffel traces the historical evolution of nursing's ideas of environment and leaves us with an intriguing proposition: to expand the environmental paradigm beyond the individual and envelope the larger global, societal, economic, and political arenas through nursing organizations and in partnership with other concerned groups.

The last critical thread, the dialectic between caring and technology, poses the greatest challenge to nursing: If caring is the essence of nursing, how do nurses practice caring in an increasingly technological environment? In Chapter 9, Sandelowski explores the notion that the "body ultimately will be of no material consequence in cyberspace or the virtual worlds created by existing and yet to be developed telecommunications and computer-mediated technologies" and the potential problems this may bring to nursing. She raises the point that virtual environments, such as the Visible Human Project and the Human Genome Project, are creating new views of humans that are at odds with the humanistic views that nurses and physicians cherish. Virtual environments offer nurses an opportunity to celebrate the body work of nursing and reunite it with the information work of nursing. In Chapter 10, Locsin carries this theme to the bedside and explores the dichotomy between machine technology and caring. He argues that nurses recognize that technologic proficiency is a desirable attribute—that can enhance, but not substitute, caring.

CHAPTER 1

The History of the Relationship between Feminism and Nursing

Linda C. Andrist

Nursing history, as a piece of women's history, has faced the paradox of being women's work—invisible, devalued, underpaid—and yet a critical necessity to society. Reverby (1987) posed the dilemma that nurses have been ordered to care in a society that devalues caring. Conversely, at the turn of the 19th century, Lavinia L. Dock argued that "nursing represented women's first emancipated step after a century and a half of subjugation" (Baer, 1992, p. 459). Despite Dock's assertion, nursing's professional status has been in limbo for over 100 years; some believe it is because of its gender-specific association (Baer, 1992).

While feminist activists of the late 18th and early 19th centuries worked for suffrage, accessible birth control, and other women's rights, most nurses and nursing leaders shied away from joining their sisters. During the second wave of the women's movement in the late 20th century, nursing once again resisted the feminist call to action. If circumstances had been different, would nurses have struggled for over a century to attain professional status, autonomy, and control over their practice? This chapter will explore this tenuous relationship and how historical events have shaped 21st-century nursing.

NURSING: THE INVISIBLE PROFESSION

The contributions of prominent nurses and the profession of nursing have remained hidden from the collective consciousness of most Americans. The lay public may not know that the well-known women who participated in the antislavery movements and the Civil War were also nurses. Although the Civil War preceded formal training for nurses, over 10,000 women took up nursing duties during the war (Kalisch & Kalisch, 1986). Dorothea Dix was the Union Supervisor of Female Nurses; she and Clara Barton were instrumental in organizing the Union's nursing corps. Louisa May Alcott, Walt Whitman (although not a woman!), Jane Stuart Woolsey, and Mary Ann Bickerdyke all nursed during the war. In the South, Kate Cummings chronicled her experiences as a nurse. Harriet Tubman and Sojourner Truth, in addition to leading the abolitionist movement, also offered their services as nurses during the war. Other prominent nurses of the 19th and early 20th centuries who made significant contributions to the nation include Margaret Sanger, Emma Goldman, and Lillian Wald.

Even with the emergence of women's studies and the historical examination of the role of women in the United States, nursing has been invisible. In the 1970s, with the surfacing of the second wave of the women's movement, feminist activists belittled traditional women's roles and occupations, including nursing, rallying behind the move into male-dominated professions. As Janet Muff (1988) stated,

> . . . for in the eagerness of some women to embrace new roles has come a denigration of old ones. No one, these women say, *should* want to be *just a* housewife; no one with brains should want to be just a nurse. Have a career! Be a doctor! (p. 178)

Baer (1992) asserted that feminist researchers avoided nursing because it was too painful to examine an occupation that represented women's "inherently unvalued place in American society" (p. 467) and that to thoroughly understand nursing is to comprehend the "deeply negative status of women in this society" (p. 467). The disparagement of nursing by feminists is a prime example of the horizontal violence that Roberts discusses in Chapter 2. In their attempt to become more like the oppressor, the oppressed "turn" on each other and denigrate the values of their own group. It took the third wave of the women's movement[1] to come to this realization.

Nursing did not step forward as an active player in women's movements, but maintained an "uneasy alliance" (Vance, McBride, & Mason, 1985) with the organized women's movements of the 19th and 20th centuries. As an example, the American Nurses' Association did not support women's right to vote until 1915 and did not support the Equal Rights Amendment until 1971. It has taken nursing over 100 years to understand that women's issues are nurses' issues and that the "personal" struggles of nursing are indeed "political" issues. Lavinia Dock, considered the most radical nursing leader during the first wave of the women's movement, tried to convince nursing leaders of the critical need to join the woman movement,[2] because without the vote, and later the Equal Rights Amendment, nursing would not easily achieve professional status. In order to place the 19th-century women's movement in its social context, we need to take a look back at the status of women.

WOMEN'S RIGHTS IN THE 19TH CENTURY

From the vantage point of the 21st century, it is difficult to comprehend the status of women during the past two centuries. After the American Revolution, New Jersey was the only state that enfranchised women and Blacks. Although they were given the right to vote in 1790, it was rescinded 17 years later (Maier, Smith, Keyssar, & Kevles, 2003). A woman's legal status was tied to her marital status; once married, a woman became the property of her husband, along with any estate or wages she brought to the union. She could not sue, execute a will, or vote. In addition, she had no legal rights to her children and was excluded from higher education. Single women over 18 and widows could own property but could not vote (Zinn, 1995).

The period from 1780 to 1830 was characterized by vast transformations in the United States. The major changes included intense economic growth, sustained urbanization, social stratification, growing inequality in the distribution of wealth, and the birth of domesticity (Cott, 1977). Prior to this period, because husbands and wives typically farmed together, both played a role in the economy; however, once the nation began the transition from an agrarian to an industrialized economy, men went out to earn their wages, while women remained behind and tended the household. A married woman was thus left economically dependent on her husband and relied on his beneficence (Cott, 1977). Women were "robbed of the kind of social space that makes it possible to think and act on one's own behalf, the first step in acting on behalf of women collectively" (Barry, 1988, p. 17). This "cult of domesticity" consigned women to silence for the first third of the 19th century (Cott, 1977).

Of course, this applied primarily to upper-class women. Women of the working class comprised a significant part of the workforce, largely employed in the burgeoning textile factories. The invention of the cotton gin and then the power loom in 1815 contributed to the rise of industrialization. By 1822, mills began to operate in New England, with farm girls between the ages of 14 and 18 years old hired to work at meager wages. By the 1830s, women made up 68% of workers in the cotton mills (Cott, 1977).

By the mid-1800s, middle- and upper-class women grew increasingly dissatisfied with the cult of domesticity and became interested in expanding their roles outside the home. They were particularly concerned about access to higher education and family planning. Social commentators were concerned about the influx of immigrants and posited a theory of "race suicide" in which "traditional" Americans would be outnumbered by people of other races and cultures. Middle- and upper-class women were being convinced of their delicate nature. Physicians and contemporary scientists began to describe the relationship between the nervous system and the reproductive system, arguing that the brain and ovary could not develop simultaneously (Smith-Rosenberg & Rosenberg, 1984). Smith-Rosenberg and Rosenberg assert that the threat of immigration to the dominant social structure influenced the science of the day:

> Society, mid-century physicians warned, must protect the higher good of racial health by avoiding situations in which adolescent girls taxed their intellectual faculties in academic competition . . . One gynecologist complained as late as 1901, "the nervous force, so necessary at puberty, for the establishment of the menstrual function, is wasted on what may be compared as trifles to perfect health" . . . "our great grandmothers got their schooling during the winter months and let their brains lie fallow for the rest of the year." (pp. 15, 16)

Thus began the movement toward denying women access to higher education. In addition to being denied education, married women of the upper classes had very restricted roles, accentuating the Victorian ideals of femininity, docility, fragility, and asexuality. The forced idleness of these women began to spark demands for female emancipation. One of the first movements that White women became involved in was the antislavery movement, but the woman movement of the day also concentrated on other areas.

The Woman Movement

The woman movement concentrated on three issues. The first issue—service and social action—spawned the reformation of almshouses and the development of training schools for nurses. The second issue was the campaign for women's rights, initially in the form of temperance unions and abolition, and gradually to calls for access to birth control and suffrage. According to Cott (1987), the third issue was more amorphous and included emancipation from structures, conventions, and attitudes reinforced by law and custom. The underlying theme of the woman movement was that women were human beings too and had similar intellectual and spiritual properties as men, and, therefore, they deserved similar rights and opportunities to develop their potential as human beings. By the time the Seneca Falls Convention was held in 1848, women were ready for a sea of change.

By 1858, the woman movement was well underway. Susan B. Anthony was already positioning herself as a leader in the woman and antislavery movements; Sojourner Truth had made her infamous speech "Ain't I a Woman" in 1851. However, the Civil War interrupted women's rights campaigns. Despite Anthony's attempts to mobilize people to work for suffrage, the public was more concerned about slavery, and efforts were concentrated on the antislavery movement. Following the Civil War, the 14th Amendment to the Constitution was ratified, granting voting rights to *male* U.S. citizens. Anthony and Elizabeth Cady Stanton resurrected the suffrage campaign on behalf of women; however, it would be 55 years before full woman's suffrage was the law of the land.

National Growth and Rebellion

During the last two decades of the 19th century, the United States experienced unprecedented growth. This expansion was the outcome of intense urbanization, the Industrial Revolution, the consolidation of capitalism, and a second wave of massive immigration. These were to be important years for women with regards to educational opportunities, occupations, and professional careers (Cott, 1987). Earlier in the century, jobs for women consisted of factory work or teaching; however, now more and more jobs for the middle class were being created. The typewriter, invented in 1868, created secretarial occupations for women. By the late 1800s, most state universities were open to White women and all-female colleges such as Vassar, Smith, and Wellesley had been founded. By 1882, New York passed legislation granting women wider property rights and the right to sue their husbands for brutality. Gradually, other states granted women the right to sue, own property, retain their earnings, and make contracts (Kalisch & Kalisch, 1986).

The consolidation of industrial capitalism produced significant shifts in the economy and class structure in the United States. One of the largest immigrations in American history brought large numbers of Russians, Italians, Greeks, Jews, and Chinese to the United States. These newcomers looked more "alien" to native-born Anglos than had previous immigrant groups from northern Europe. This growing ethnic diversity contributed to discrimination and racism and fueled debate over "race suicide" of the native Anglo population (Smith-Rosenberg & Rosenberg, 1984). The large number of new immigrants in the 1880s and 1890s created a labor surplus that kept wages low. Racism spawned Jim Crow laws, and African Americans had fewer opportunities than did immigrants. These events stirred the workforce and fueled the largest labor movement in history. Americans began to question the split between capital and labor, forming the Socialist Party in 1877 (Zinn, 1995).

Rebellion accelerated. The Women's Assemblies of Textile Workers and Hatmakers went on strike in 1884; the movement for the 8-hour workday began in 1886. On May 1, 1886, the American Federation of Labor called for nationwide strikes. Over 350,000 workers in more than 11,000 establishments went on strike, leading to the Haymarket Massacre on May 4. The year 1886 became known as the great uprising of labor (Zinn, 1995). The question is, where was nursing in all of this?

THE BIRTH OF MODERN AMERICAN NURSING

Organized American nursing was in its infancy in 1878 when Mary Eliza Mahoney entered the New England Training School at the New England Hospital for Women and Children (NEHWC) for her training. Under the supervision of Dr. Marie Zakrzewska, the hospital was the first in the United States to offer formal nurse training, although it was not located in a general hospital and was not modeled on the Nightingale plan. It also was the first program to foster cultural diversity in nursing. According to Davis (1999), "This institution demonstrated the first evidence of pride in a racially, culturally, and socially diverse patient population, and was the first to open its educational opportunities to a Black woman and encourage males to enter nursing" (p. 43). Not only did America's first trained nurse, Linda Richards, graduate from the school, but Mary Eliza Mahoney graduated as the first trained Black nurse in the United States. Both women would play major roles in the development of nursing. Mahoney pioneered civil rights in nursing, working for the acceptance of Black women in nursing and elevating the status of Black nurses (Davis, 1999).

Lavinia Dock went to Bellevue Hospital in New York City for her training in 1884. Bellevue was the first of a trio of training programs to open in the United States in 1873; all three were modeled on the Nightingale plan. By 1880, there were 15 schools in the United States and by 1900 there were 432; most only admitted White women. The immense growth in the number of training schools was directly related to the growth of hospitals; administrators learned quickly that student nurses were a cheap labor force. The training schools evolved into the departments of nursing, perhaps the most critical mistake for the future of the profession. Without substantial endowments and independent budgets, training schools were totally dependent on private donations and hospital administrators for their financial support (Kalisch & Kalisch, 1986).

Training schools differed in their content and length of training. When Dock entered the Bellevue program, it consisted of one year of training and one year of work in the hospital. Students worked 7 day weeks and between 70 and 90 hours per week (Kalisch & Kalisch, 1986). Much has been written about the strict discipline of nurse training. Barbara Melosh (1982) described an environment that fits Erving Goffman's (1961) concept of a total institution, "a place where the usual social boundaries between public and private life collapse" (p. 49):

> "Inmates" of total institutions sleep, work, and play under a single pervasive authority. Subordinated to this authority, they lose or surrender many of their normal prerogatives. Their most mundane activities are closely controlled; their most intimate actions are open to surveillance. Total institutions deliberately construct a separate social world, marked off by systematic and routine violations of "outside" expectations. (Melosh, 1983, p. 49)

The benefit to the institution was total loyalty; students who did not conform either left or were dismissed. Hospitals were thus able to create a culture of nurse training that produced a docile, loyal, dedicated, submissive, and cheap workforce. Student nurses had no advocates in a hierarchical system that was perpetuated by the lack of a professional nursing staff that could have provided diversity in training and traditions, thereby preventing the strong inbreeding of customs so entrenched in hospital-training programs. The superintendents had little interest in reform; physicians had less. Physicians repeatedly argued against teaching nurses theory, and one declared in 1896:

. . . a tendency of the trained nurse to interfere excessively in the conduct of medical and surgical cases. They hint . . . that doctors' prescriptions and treatment might be a little amended. They make suggestions of their own as to diagnosis and prognosis. They elevate themselves in a measure to the order of the medical practitioner himself. Their smattering of knowledge of anatomy and physiology leads them to suggest to their patients diseases which never could, by any possibility, have entered the heads of the patients themselves. (Kalisch & Kalisch, 1986, p.183)

Prior to the development of training schools, men had worked as "untrained nurses." However, men were not admitted to the female training schools until after the Korean War. The American model of nursing, based on Nightingale's ideals, had "no place" (Kalisch & Kalisch, 2004, p. 100) for men; men were used in hospitals to care for insane and violent patients, alcoholics, and men with genitourinary diseases. Bellevue Hospital opened the Mills School of Nursing for men in 1888 with a training program similar to other schools, but this option was not widely replicated (Kalisch & Kalisch, 2004).

New graduates of the female training schools were not employed by hospitals, except for positions as nurse superintendents. Instead they were employed as private duty nurses and later in public health roles. Private duty nurses were isolated because they worked in their employers' homes; even though they did have some autonomy over their work, estrangement from other nurses insulated them from sharing their labor concerns. The culture of the training programs, the separation of students from professional colleagues, and the isolation of private duty nurses prohibited nurses from fully understanding the nature of their oppression and prevented them from joining forces with the labor movement. The national movement for an 8-hour workday provides an example of this dilemma.

By the mid-1890s the length of the nurse-training course was increased to 3 years. Isabel Hampton, a pioneer in nursing education, warned that if schools increased the training period, they had to limit the workday to 8 hours. Her words fell on deaf ears. Physicians, hospital administrators, and nurse superintendents argued that the 8-hour workday would be the demise of hospitals. In 1896, a decade after the national movement for the 8-hour workday, Massachusetts introduced a bill to limit the hours that nurses in training could work. It was adamantly opposed by nurse superintendents. The move to shorten the workday would not be settled until the report of The Committee on the Grading of Nursing Schools was published in 1928. The publication, *Nurses, Patients, and Pocketbooks,* written by May Ayers Burgess, was the first organized analysis of nursing education. It revealed many inequities, not the least of which was the finding that the vast majority of schools still required students to work more than 40 hours a week (Kalisch & Kalisch, 2004).

Early Professional Organizations

The fact that nursing superintendents opposed the legislation was due in part to the inevitable conflicts that arose from the formation of two nursing organizations. When nursing leaders from several countries around the world met at the Chicago World's Fair in 1893, they discussed the need to organize the leadership. Nurses from Canada and the United States formed the American Society of Superintendents of Training Schools for Nurses of the United States and Canada (also known as the Superintendents Society, it was renamed the National League of Nursing Education in 1912). They held their first meeting the following year. Although the group's main focus was standardizing training-school curricula, the Superintendents Society also was concerned about the lack of legal status of nurses and the consequent problems of regulating practicing nurses. This led to the formation of a second organization, the Nurses' Associated Alumnae of the United States and Canada (also called the Associated Alumnae, it was renamed the American Nurses' Association in 1911), with the purpose of obtaining legal status for nurses. Although one organization emphasized nursing education and the other obtaining legal status, both organizations sought to further the advancement of nursing as a profession (Lewenson, 1996).

As Joann Ashley (1977) so aptly noted:

> With the control of education in the hands of one organization and the control of practice in the hands of another, gaps in communication were inevitable. The lack of concerted action by both educators and practitioners created serious problems, as future decades were to prove. With this separation of functions, the foundation was laid for continuing lack of unity accompanied by conflicts and misunderstandings. The two separate organizations still exist today, and so do the conflicts and the misunderstandings. (p. 96)

In addition to this problem, none of the nursing leaders had the foresight to know that organized medicine and hospital administrators, both more powerful and male dominated than nursing, would attempt to stop the growth of nursing, much less allow nursing to become an autonomous profession. Nursing leaders particularly did not appreciate the extent to which their mission would be thwarted because women had "no political freedom, little legal status, and no right to become professional people" (Ashley, 1977, p. 101).

Black nurses had little opportunity to join either organization because of racial discrimination. Martha Minerva Franklin, a colleague of Mary Mahoney, organized the National Association of Colored Graduate Nurses (NACGN) in 1907. The first meeting was hosted by Adah Belle Samuels Thoms, Acting Superintendent of Lincoln Hospital and Home in New York City. Franklin, Mahoney, and Thoms were friends and colleagues who worked tirelessly to improve Black women's access to education and nursing practice (Davis, 1999).

Relations between Black nurses and Black physicians were very different from those between White nurses and White doctors. The National Medical Association (NMA), the Black physicians' organization, took an early interest in the NACGN and invited the members to have their conventions simultaneously in the same cities, published nurses' articles in their journal, and were generally supportive of nurses' efforts to enhance their professional image (Davis, 1999).

Radical Reformers

Powerful women in a society where they have few legal rights soon learn that they must win over the power brokers in order to achieve anything. Many nurse leaders did not support the woman movement, or did so only in the shadows. Others left nursing to work for radical change in society. Emma Goldman and Margaret Sanger were two such reformers who began their careers in nursing; it was nursing the poor and downtrodden that led them to work for fundamental social change. Goldman was an anarchist. Sanger, a socialist and radical reformer, believed vehemently that until women could control their own bodies and have access to birth control, legislation for suffrage, working conditions, and equal property rights would not free women

(Roberts & Group, 1995). Both women felt strongly that nursing was palliative at best, and that until poverty was resolved and the masses were in charge of their destinies, merely keeping people alive was worthless. They recognized that nursing at the individual level was not enough and devoted their lives to social and political change (Roberts & Group, 1995).

Sojourner Truth and Harriet Tubman were also radical feminists; they understood the importance of elevating Blacks and women in society, which would elevate the status of nursing as well. In this respect, they were among the few to share Lavinia Dock's political ideology.

The Henry Street Settlement

Lillian Wald was another prominent nurse leader and progressive activist. She founded the Henry Street Settlement House in New York City in 1895. Her commitment to improving the lives and health of the immigrant poor is renowned. Wald had to temper her activism with her philanthropy in order to secure funding for the many projects she supported (Siegel, 1988). Henry Street was to become a center for many activist nurses, including Lavinia Dock, who arrived there in 1896. Already involved in the labor movement, Dock found herself in the midst of a supportive network of independent-thinking women. Her work with settlement nurses who were virtually independent practitioners was fundamental to her later vision of nursing as an autonomous profession, distinct and not subservient to medicine.

Dock eventually came to the realization that until women had equal rights with men, which began with the vote, nurses could not be masters of their professional lives. Her journey toward activism in the suffrage movement was kindled once she began to see similar labor issues between nurses and other workers. Like Emma Goldman and Margaret Sanger, she was ready to work for fundamental social change.

Labor: Nurses' Issues Equal Women's Issues

Lavinia Dock understood that for nursing to be autonomous and control its own practice, basic changes had to be made: Nurses needed shorter working hours and improved working conditions. It was clear to Dock that nurses needed to work with the labor movement for change. Alongside the workday-hours limit, another critical topic was begging to be addressed—the case of nurse licensing—yet another fundamental issue for autonomy.

As nurses began to strive for passage of legislation for control of the nursing practice at the turn of the century, Dock (1900) wrote the classic article for the first issue of *The American Journal of Nursing,* "What we may expect from the law." She advocated that nurses must act to control their own practice and not allow outside agencies, such as medicine or the state, to control nursing. She asserted that nursing must first set standards for education and licensure and then seek legislation to support the standards (Dock, 1900). As she traveled around the country, Dock became aware of the opposition by both legislators and physicians to nurse registration. In a letter to Adelaide Nutting, she said:

> The doctors movement against training is a movement of men against women. I am certain of that—the devils—they have been getting frightened for a long time. It is also a protection movement for their own unrestricted rights of exploiting women as nurses (Dock, September 12, most likely between 1899–1907[3])

Dock concluded in that letter that until women had the vote, nursing's voice would never be heard in the legislatures.

Labor Issues for Women

Just a fraction of women workers were unionized during the early years of the first decade of the 20th century. Similar to nurses, women were valued as factory workers because they were unorganized and accepted low wages, and employers used many tactics to prevent women from organizing (Cott, 1987). However, the biggest difference between nurses and factory workers was the fact that women in factories worked side by side, without the rigid socialization that nurses had. This gave them more exposure to the public sphere, where they could discuss their problems after work. Henry Street was clearly an exception.

In 1903, settlement house workers and trade unionists organized the National Women's Trade Union League to urge women workers to join unions. Lavinia Dock was an early member. The connection between women's economic roles and the justification for the ballot was becoming critical; however, organized nursing had yet to see this as a critical link to the future of the profession. The Equity League of Self-Supporting Women was formed in 1907; this organization joined both working women and wealthier women as allies. Members immediately prepared to testify before the New York State Legislature on full suffrage for women.

Activists in the suffrage movement were now impassioned and began using techniques of the political left and the more radical methods of the British suffrage movement. The 1910s saw a massive movement for suffrage in which women from virtually all walks of life were united (Cott, 1987).

LAVINIA DOCK: NURSE ACTIVIST

Lavinia Dock was clearly committed to the suffrage movement, and she felt it was her duty to share this vision with her nurse colleagues. She needed to convince them that nursing, because it was largely a woman's profession, had to join forces with suffragists. Dock addressed the 10th annual convention of the Nurses' Associated Alumnae of the United States. In perhaps her most famous speech, and most likely one of the first political speeches addressed to a nursing organization, Dock challenged nurses to join with other women to obtain the vote:

> . . . As the modern nursing movement is emphatically an outcome of the original and general woman movement and as nurses are no longer a dull, uneducated class, but an intelligent army of workers, capable of continuous progress, and titled to comprehend the idea of social responsibility, it would be a pity for them to allow one of the most remarkable movements of the day to go on under their eyes without comprehending it . . . What is to be our attitude toward full citizenship? Shall we be an intelligent and enlightened body of citizens, or an inert mass of indifference? (Dock, 1907, pp. 896–897)

Dock went on to discuss how women's equality was an issue for nurses as well and that there were women's issues in the profession, not only as workers, but also in areas of educational reform, the ability to control one's own labor, and in equal pay for equal work. She ended her speech with: "Until we possess the ballot we shall not know when we may get up in the morning to find that all we had gained had been taken from us" (Dock, 1907, p. 901).

The furor that this speech raised is at first surprising. That Dock was asking nurses to become politically active on their own behalf, as a large body of women, and forcing nurses to look at their own oppression, was obviously very difficult. Miss Davis, one of the officers of the Association who was asked to lead the discussion of the paper, was taken aback. Although Davis supported the franchise for women and stated that "many thinking people believe in giving the vote to women . . . [however] we are striving in a small way to gain legislation in our profession, and to take hold of this question might injure us, and probably would" (Nurses' Associated Alumnae of the United States, 1908, p. 901), there was a general lack of support for Dock at that meeting. The following year at the annual convention, a resolution calling for the Association's support of suffrage was made and defeated by a large majority.

Lavinia Dock's outrage was published in *The American Journal of Nursing* in a letter to the editor in September 1908. She said she had never been disappointed in the actions of the body since she had helped found the organization in 1896, until she had read, "with humiliation, I must frankly say" (Dock, 1908, p. 925), that the resolution had been defeated. She added that she did not expect nurses to be actively engaged in the suffrage movement, but that it took little time to give moral support and endorsement. She then went on to give specific examples of why nurses must support suffrage. She cited men's control of affairs that belonged to women and to nurses, such as the almshouses and issues of child health (Dock, 1908).

In the same issue of the journal, an editorial warned of the necessity of neutrality on the part of the editors concerning the suffrage issue: "This magazine is a professional journal, devoted to the interests of nursing. On every subject, nursing has a definite policy. On all other broad questions its attitude is neutral" (Nurses' Associated Alumnae of the United States, 1908, p. 956). The editors cited the diversity of opinion amongst the nursing body at large on the suffrage issue, with the editor-in-chief claiming only a moderate ground on the subject of suffrage. This is a prime example of nursing leaders being internally focused to the exclusion of an external lens to help them appreciate the commonality of issues among all working women (Roberts & Group, 1995).

Letters to the editor in subsequent issues reinforced the editor's position that the suffrage question was not an issue that should be discussed in a nursing journal nor in a convention assembled to "strengthen the union of nursing organizations, to elevate nursing and to promote ethical standards in all the relations of the nursing profession" (Eastern Delegate, 1908, p. 203). This woman further claimed that the "suffrage question takes rank with social hygiene, moral prophylaxis, almshouse reforms, does not hold water. . . the matter of woman suffrage is one in which as members of our profession we should have no opinion whatsoever" (p. 204).

There is little mention of the suffrage question again in *The American Journal of Nursing* until six years later, in July 1915. The minutes from the 15th Annual Convention reported the passage of the Susan B. Anthony Amendment and urged its passage by the 64th Congress. Ashley's analysis of this period in nursing history reflects the culture of nursing discussed earlier:

> Nurses were among the most conservative of the conservatives. With rare exceptions they were non-feminists . . . The failure of nurses to identify with radical feminists seeking to change the social order led to the failure of the nursing profession to liberate both education and practice. (Ashley, 1975, p. 68)

Given the socialization of nurses, perhaps it is little wonder they were such a conservative group.

Lavinia Dock continued to work for suffrage. She picketed the White House on many occasions and was among the first group of women to be jailed for "obstructing sidewalk traffic" around the White House. In 1920, with the passage of the 19th Amendment, Dock, as a member of the National Advisory Council of the National Women's Party, joined in pressing for the Equal Rights Amendment (ERA). She wrote a four-page Letter to Nurses dated December 22, 1923, urging nurses to work for passage of the ERA. She asked nurses to understand that the right to vote alone was not enough to guarantee equality with men. The ERA was introduced into Congress every year from 1923 to 1973, when it was finally passed. However, it failed to be ratified by enough states to make it law. The ANA voted to endorse the ERA in 1971.

RETURN OF THE CULT OF DOMESTICITY[4]

Between the 1930s and 1960s, the United States was caught up in the aftermath of the Great Depression, World War II (WWII), and the Korean War. During the war years, the urgent need for women workers, particularly nurses, emphasized the importance of women in the workforce (Group & Roberts, 2001). After WWII, soldiers returned from their assignments and resumed jobs, many of which had been filled by women during the war. Group and Roberts point out that nurses, like other women, were indispensable during wartime and subservient during peacetime.

Conservative gender stereotypes prevailed in the postwar period, and nurses were targeted as distancing themselves from "traditional" female roles. The print media was particularly adept at resocializing nurses. Even nursing manuals asserted the need for nurses to be feminine. During the 1950s, a genre of nurse romance novels reflected the prevailing cultural stereotypes of women's work and status (Melosh, 1983). Although Cherry Ames and Sue Barton were dedicated nurses, romance was a major part of their nursing adventures. Women's magazines ran countless stories reassuring young women that one of the greatest rewards of nursing was to find physician husbands. Nursing was clearly viewed as a stopgap to marriage (Hughes, 1988).

There was little change regarding nurses' roles in the hospital. During this time of economic prosperity and growth, nursing failed to attract women who wanted or needed to work. The meager salaries, combined with the rigid and subordinated roles, prompted as many as 75% of nurses in one survey to admit they were leaving nursing or were working part-time to supplement their husbands' salaries (Group & Roberts, 2001). In 1946, the average salary for a staff nurse was 74 cents an hour. In the same year, the average typist wage was 97 cents an hour, a librarian made around $1.11, and a seamstress averaged an hourly rate of $1.33 (Kalisch & Kalisch, 2004). Nurses averaged a 48-hour work week, which more often then not included nights and weekends. Under these conditions, it was impossible for hospitals to retain or attract nurses. The profession had few activist leaders to argue for better working conditions. Because of this, nursing had difficulty unifying and organizing after the war. To make matters more complicated, new subsidiary workers were being created, often by hospitals and administrators, in response to the nursing shortage. Ironically, hospital administrators continue to create new categories of cheaply paid workers rather than meet registered nurses' demands for better working conditions and higher salaries (Group & Roberts, 2001).

In the early 1900s, nurses had pressed for collegiate education to increase their status and eliminate the abuses of hospital-based training; however, by the 1950s, licensed practical nurse training programs had increased substantially. Organized medicine and hospital administrators were increasingly resistant to nursings' professional and economic goals, as witnessed by the attack on the 1948 paper, "Nursing for the future," by Lucille Brown. Brown had recommended a move toward collegiate nursing education based on her study of hospital-based training schools, in which she rated 46% of the 602 schools as poor or very poor. Physicians at the 1948 American Medical Association (AMA) convention criticized the report, dismissing Brown because she was not a nurse. This move lead the NLN, the ANA, and the National Organization for Public Health Nursing to join forces and create the National Committee for the Improvement of Nursing Services (NCINS), which coordinated the accreditation of training schools across the country (Group & Roberts, 2001; Kalisch & Kalisch, 2004).

Higher education was not the only threat to medical and hospital organizations, collective bargaining was potentially even more dangerous. The Taft-Hartley Act, passed in 1947, excluded nurses from the right to unionize, despite the efforts of the ANA; both the AMA and the American Hospital Association (AHA) lobbied against nurses having the right to unionize. Group and Roberts (2001) stated that "the Taft-Hartley Act is a textbook example of gender discriminatory legislation that effectively stalled women's unification against sexist treatment in salaries and work conditions" (p. 184). By 1960, university-educated registered nurses were earning little more than hospital-trained nurses, providing disincentives to advance their education.

THE SECOND WAVE

The second wave of the women's movement began in the early 1960s with the report of President John F. Kennedy's Commission on the Status of Women (1963), and the publication of the *Feminine Mystique* (1963) by Betty Friedan. But it was not until the early 1970s, 62 years after Lavinia Dock urged nurses to support suffrage, that feminist nurses began speaking out for reform in the profession. Nurses became radicalized to their subordinate roles, the call for professional unity was heard, and several nurse scholars began a critical analysis of the historical impediments to nursing. Wilma Scott Heide, then President of the National Organization of Women (NOW), voiced a clear connection between nurses' issues and women's issues. Heide (1971) wrote passionate and caustic analyses on the problems in nursing and how nurses needed to play the doctor–nurse game in order to survive:

> Heide believed that physicians were over trained for cure and undereducated for care and nurturance, usually provided by nurses who, as an oppressed group, identify with and accommodate to their oppressors for survival, economic support, and career advancement. Thus, nurses become mired in the doctor–nurse game, the transactional neurosis that allows the physician to appear to be in complete authority. (Roberts & Group, 1995, p. 191)

Heide was confident that nurses could lead in the revolution for social change that would bring about equal rights for women and improve the human race by liberating one-half of the population. She called the women's movement, "the most profound social movement the world has ever known" (Heide, 1971, p. 16). Nursing scholar Virginia Cleland (1971), writing in the *American Journal of Nursing,* noted that sex discrimination was nursing's most pervasive problem. She chastised a system in which nursing administration had no control over its budget and where women faculty members in schools of nursing were paid far less than men.

The first hint of discordance between nurses and feminist activists came in early 1971, when activists began encouraging women to go into traditional male occupations. Nursing was not seen as an emancipatory career path, but rather an occupation in which nurses "perpetuate their inferior status as women" (Roberts & Group, 1995, p. 194). Edelstein, a nurse, wrote that:

> . . . rather than admonishing women to stay out of nursing, feminists would be well advised to encourage creative and talented people to enter the field, for the status of pervasively female nursing profession with its massive membership has a major impact on the status of women. (Edelstein, 1971, p. 294)

Nurses were dismayed by the activists' presumed devaluation of the nursing profession. Although Roberts and Group found few published attacks on nursing by activists in the women's movement, they asserted that feminists' emphasis that women should go into male-dominated occupations implied a devaluation of nursing. The rift between nurses and feminists lasted for a long time, despite the many nurse leaders who supported the women's movement.

Teresa Christy was one of the first nurses to place feminism in a historical perspective by tracing early feminist leaders' work in the early 1900s. She wrote about the lack of nurses' support for the current women's movement and agreed with others before her that nursing needed to pay attention to the sexist discrimination in the workplace. For example, in one legal case the defendants were arguing for higher pay for male orderlies because they did more lifting than females. Christy asserted that nurses must pay attention to discrimination in pay and job opportunities (Roberts & Group, 1995). Rosamond Gabrielson investigated the subordinate role that nurses had with physicians. She studied nurses' actions with regard to verbal orders for medications and found that 21 out of 22 nurses followed doctor's orders to give a medication that did not exist. Nurses were blindly following orders without questioning. Gabrielson urged nurses to challenge these relationships and strive for collaborative practice (Roberts & Group, 1995).

These two issues—pay and job equity and the nurse–physician relationship—were paramount in arguing that nurses needed to join the women's movement. Both were framed as women's issues—the inherent discrimination of women in the workforce and the socialization of women as subordinate to men. Most nurses did not make this connection because of the strong socialization they received in nursing school.

Joann Ashley captured the socialization issue in 1976 with the publication of *Hospitals, Paternalism, and the Role of the Nurse.* Ashley, an ardent feminist, was perhaps the strongest critical spokeswoman for nursing since Lavinia Dock (Roberts & Group, 1995). Her untimely death in 1980 robbed the profession of one of its most profound thinkers. Ashley pointed out that the apprenticeship model of nursing education that was implemented in the 1870s differed from the Nightingale model in that the American schools were not independently funded. She argued that this lack of financial backing was perhaps one of the most important reasons that set the stage for nursing's problems with autonomy and independence. Because the schools had agreed to give nursing service to the hospital in return for lowered tuition for students, hospital administrators quickly realized that opening a school would provide inexpensive nursing care. As apprentices, nurses were therefore at the mercy of the hospital administration as well as the supervising physicians—both groups that were predominantly male.

As more and more nurses began to write about the connection between women's and nurses' labor issues, feminism became a valuable lens in which to view practice, education, and scholarship (Chinn, 1995). Roberts (1983) argued that nursing was an oppressed group, and that like other oppressed peoples throughout history—such as people of color—nursing was controlled by "societal forces that have determined its leadership behavior" (p. 21). Roberts' model of oppressed group behavior provided a tool to critique power relationships and the behaviors that arise from oppression. She asserted that once nurses were able to understand these dynamics, they would be able to liberate themselves and create an autonomous profession.

The now classic text on women's issues in nursing, *Socialization, Sexism, and Stereotyping in Nursing* (1982), edited by Janet Muff, was the first nursing book that examined developmental and discrimination issues for women and linked them to nursing's dilemmas of professionalization. Muff argued that "nurses are affected both by their female socialization and by the social, political, and psychological issues inherent in nursing and the health care system" (p. 349). Not only did the book raise the consciousness of many nurses, but it offered solutions to challenge and change the system.

In the same vein, Chinn and Wheeler (1985) challenged that nurses could not afford to "remain aloof from the women's movement" (p. 74) and argued that an understanding of feminist theory would provide a frame of reference for historical, political, and personal issues in nursing. This article was among the first in nursing to outline the contemporary feminist theories: liberal, Marxist, socialist, and radical. They defined feminism as "a world view that values women and that confronts systematic injustices based on gender" (p. 74). Sampselle (1990) extended the importance of feminist philosophy on nursing practice. She wrote that gender equity, a critical tenet of feminist philosophy, advocates a partnership model of human interaction, rather than a dominance model. A second tenet is that one's value to society should be determined, not by gender, but by one's capacity to contribute to society. Together with her third principle—that women have personal sovereignty over their bodies—Sampselle challenged nurses to embrace feminist philosophy in nursing practice.

Bunting and Campbell (1990) reviewed the conflicts and contradictions between nurses and feminism from a historical perspective. They captured the historical relationship between differing feminist epistemologies and their relevance to nursing, stating that:

> History can be viewed as a series of movements (always having their resistors) and retreats (backlashes) that are probably accelerating in their frequency, forming complex patterns. Feminism and nursing have both nurtured one another and formed opposing patterns that have led to new syntheses. (p. 23)

Bunting and Campbell urged nurses to move beyond playing the victim and blaming themselves for the lack of feminism in nursing and toward an understanding and a valuing of the complex history of nursing, "celebrating this new and exciting version of their synthesis" (p. 23).

In 1991, Mason and colleagues questioned whether the profession was ready to critique the healthcare system and its "hierarchical model of inequality" (Heide, 1971, as cited in Mason, Backer, & Georges, 1991, p. 72) in order to create alternative models of power or whether nurses would continue to perpetuate the male-dominated model of power. In a new model, the traditional power-holders—administrators and educators—would be willing to share power with staff nurses in a collaborative relationship. Their feminist model of political empowerment was defined as:

> . . . the enabling of individuals and groups to participate in actions and decision-making within a context that supports an equitable distribution of power. Empowerment

requires a commitment to connection between self and others, enabling individuals and groups to recognize their own strengths, resources, and abilities to make changes in their personal and public lives. It is a process of confirming one's self and/or one's group. (Mason et al., 1991, pp. 72–73)

This model included three dimensions that would move the profession forward: raising nurses' consciousness of sociopolitical realities, formulating positive self-esteem, and developing the political skills necessary to both negotiate and change the healthcare system.

Since the mid-1980s, nurses have incorporated feminist theory and philosophy in scholarship, practice, and education. MacPherson (1983) first described feminist methods as a model for research in nursing, followed by Chinn's (1985) challenge to debunk myths related to the dominance of the positivist scientific method in nursing research. These two articles birthed a reconceptualization of scholarly inquiry, which led to a multitude of theoretical frameworks and methodologies for research, as well as approaches to knowledge development.

Liberal feminism, although popular in the 1970s, was eventually recognized as insufficient for transforming society. Two schools of thought developed. Cultural feminism embraced radical, social, and poststructural feminism, which ". . . celebrates rather than denigrates that which has been associated with being female in patriarchal cultures, and offers visions of transformation rooted in a concern for the social and psychological liberation of women that will ultimately benefit all" (Chinn, 1995, p. 269). Critical social feminism, another school of thought, examines fundamental social change with specific attention toward the class and gender issues that maintain oppression. It emphasizes empowerment strategies such as grass-roots activism to bring about social change (Chinn, 1995).

TOWARDS THE FUTURE OF FEMINISM AND NURSING

Just as the third wave of feminism is celebrating women's difference and the feminine traits of women, so, too, has nursing reclaimed its essential nature—caring. The explosion of clinical narratives, reflective practice, and theoretical work on caring in the past 10 years exemplifies this move toward valuing what nurses do. Publishing narratives and telling our stories about real nursing work can only increase the image of nursing in the public's eye. This being said, there also are inherent dangers in claiming caring as nursing's core. Perhaps the solution is for society to value women's work as well as nurses' supremacy at caring.

Falk Rafael (1998) discusses three forms of power: ordered caring, assimilated caring, and empowered caring. *Ordered caring,* such as Reverby (1987) discussed, polarizes caring and power as opposites. *Assimilated caring* changes the power relationship as nurses assimilate to the dominant values; however, it is still power *over. Empowered caring* involves embracing caring and the intrinsic power it holds; caring "encompasses the social, economic, and political determinants of health" (Falk Rafael, p. 30). Only under these conditions can nurses create changes in the healthcare system and in the lives of their patients.

Conditions for nurses at the dawn of the new millennium have thus far provided disincentives to work for social change. Managed care, the looming nursing shortage, downsizing, caring for increasingly acutely ill patients, and long and irregular hours are all burdensome issues for nurses (Letvak, 2001). The United American Nurses (2003) conducted a survey of 600 nurses in 2003 and found a resounding call for increased salaries (82%), reduced nurse–patient ratio

(85%), greater autonomy and control for staff nurses (66%), and safer working conditions (65%). Professional nursing is beginning to combat these problems.

Falk Rafael (1998) envisioned empowered caring as a tool, not to obtain power as an end, but as a means of creating social and cultural change. In this respect, nurses should grab onto this concept with gusto! The public has already rated nurses as the most trusted professionals in the United States (Gallup News Service, 1999). Johnson & Johnson have an unprecedented campaign to recruit people into nursing (http://www.discovernursing.com). *U.S. News and World Reports* ("Who Needs Doctors?", 2005) featured nursing and other nonphysician health-care providers as leading the way in health care. As nurses, we must continue to demonstrate our power and take our place in the complex healthcare system. As history shows us, women's issues and nurses' issues are intertwined—empowering nursing empowers women and, eventually, all people.

ACKNOWLEDGMENTS

I want to acknowledge Bianca Passarelli for her help in researching this topic.

REFERENCES

Ashley, J. (1975). Nurses in American history: Nursing and early feminism. *American Journal of Nursing, 75*(9), 1465–1467.

Ashley, J. (1977). *Hospitals, paternalism, and the role of the nurse.* New York, NY: Teachers College Press.

Baer, E. D. (1992). Nurses. In R. D. Apple (Ed.), *Women, health and medicine in America: A historical handbook* (pp. 451–467). New Brunswick, NJ: Rutgers University Press.

Barry, K. (1988). *Susan B. Anthony: A biography.* New York, NY: New York University Press.

Brown, E. L. (1948). *Nursing for the future.* New York, NY: Russell Sage Foundation.

Bunting, S., & Campbell, J. C. (1990). Feminism and nursing: Historical perspectives. *Advances in Nursing Science, 12*(4), 11–24.

Chinn, P. L. (1985). Debunking myths in nursing theory and research. *Image: Journal of Nursing Scholarship, 17*(2), 45–49.

Chinn, P. L. (1995). Feminism and nursing. *Annual Review of Nursing Research, 13,* 267–289.

Chinn, P. L., & Wheeler, C. E. (1985). Can nursing afford to remain aloof from the women's movement? *Nursing Outlook, 33,* 74–77.

Cleland, V. S. (1971). Sex discrimination: Nursing's most pervasive problem. *American Journal of Nursing, 71*(8), 1542–1547.

Cott, N. F. (1977). *The bonds of womanhood: Women's sphere in New England.* New Haven, CT: Yale University Press.

Cott, N. F. (1987). *The grounding of modern feminism.* New Haven, CT: Yale University Press.

Christy, T. E. (1971). Equal rights for women: Voices from the past. *American Journal of Nursing, 71*(2), 288–293.

Davis, A. T. (1999). *Early Black American leaders in nursing: Architects for integration and equality.* Boston: Jones and Bartlett.

Dock, L. L. (1900). What we may expect from the law. *American Journal of Nursing, 1,* 8–12.

Dock, L. L. (1907). Some urgent social claims. *American Journal of Nursing, 7,* 895–901.

Dock, L. L. (1908). The suffrage movement [Letter to the Editor]. *American Journal of Nursing, 8,* 925–926.

Dock, L. L. (September 12, no year). [Letter to Adelaide Nutting]. Mary Adelaide Nutting Collection, The History of Nursing, The Archives of the Department of Nursing Education, Teachers College, Columbia University.

Eastern Delegate (1908). [Letter to the Editor]. *American Journal of Nursing, 8,* 203–204.

Edelstein, R. G. (1971). Equal rights for women: Perspectives. *American Journal of Nursing, 71*(2), 294–298.

Falk Rafael, A. R. (1998). Nurses who run with the wolves: The power and caring dialectic revisited. *Advances in Nursing Science, 21*(1), 29–42.

Freidan, B. (1963). *The feminine mystique.* New York, NY: W.W. Norton.

Gallup News Service (1999). Medical practitioner's top list of most trusted professions. Retrieved January 26, 2005, from http://www.globalethics.org/newsline/members/issue.tmpl?articleid=11219922225391

Goffman, E. (1961). *Asylums: Essays on the social situation of mental patients and other inmates.* Garden City, NY: Doubleday Anchor.

Group, T. M., & Roberts, J. I. (2001). *Nursing, physician control and the medical monopoly: Historical perspectives on gendered inequality in roles, rights, and range of practice.* Bloomington: University of Indiana Press.

Heide, W. S. (1971). Women's liberation means putting nurses and nursing in its place! *Imprint, 18,* 824–827.

Hughes, L. (1988). Little girls grow up to be wives and mommies: Nursing as a stopgap to marriage. In J. Muff (Ed.), *Women's issues in nursing: Socialization, sexism, and stereotyping* (Rev. ed., pp. 157–168). Prospect Heights, IL: Waveland Press.

Kalisch, P. A., & Kalisch, B. J. (1986). *The advance of American nursing* (2nd ed.). Boston: Little, Brown and Company.

Kalisch, P. A., & Kalisch, B. J. (2004). *American nursing: A history.* (4th ed.). Philadelphia: Lippincott, Williams & Wilkins.

Letvak, S. (2001). Nurses as working women. *AORN On Line, 73*(3), 675–676, 678, 680–682.

Lewenson, S. B. (1996). *Taking charge: Nursing, suffrage, & feminism in America 1873–1920.* New York, NY: NLN Press.

MacPherson, K. I. (1983). Feminist methods: A new paradigm for nursing research. *Advances in Nursing Science, 5*(2), 17–25.

Maier, P., Smith, M. R., Keyssar, A., & Kevles, D. J. (2003). *A history of the United States: Inventing America.* New York, NY: W.W. Norton.

Mason, D. J., Backer, B. A., & Georges, A. (1991). Toward a feminist model for the political empowerment of nurses. *Image: Journal of Nursing Scholarship, 23*(2), 72–77.

Melosh, B. (1982). *"The physician's hand": Work culture and conflict in American nursing.* Philadelphia: Temple University Press.

Melosh, B. (1983). Doctors, patients, and "big nurse": Work and gender in the postwar hospital. In E. C. Lagemann (Ed.), *Nursing history: New perspectives, new possibilities* (pp. 164–179). New York, NY: Teachers College Press.

Muff, J. (Ed.) (1982). *Women's issues in nursing: Socialization, sexism, and stereotyping.* Prospect Heights, IL: Waveland Press.

Muff, J. (1988). Why doesn't a smart girl like you go to medical school? The women's movement takes a slap at nursing. In J. Muff (Ed.), *Women's issues in nursing: Socialization, sexism, and sterotyping* (Rev. ed., pp. 178–185). Prospect Heights, IL: Waveland Press.

Nurses' Associated Alumnae of the United States (1908, September). The Journal's attitude on the suffrage question [Editorial]. *American Journal of Nursing, 8,* 956–957.

Report of the President's Commission on the status of women. (October 11, 1963). American women. *Journal of Reprints of Documents Affecting Women, 1,* 24.

Reverby, S. M. (1987). *Ordered to care: The dilemma of American nursing, 1850–1945.* Cambridge, England: Cambridge University Press.

Roberts, J. I., & Group, T. M. (1995). *Feminism and nursing: An historical perspective on power, status, and political activism in the nursing profession.* Westport, CT: Praeger.

Roberts, S. J. (1983). Oppressed group behavior: Implications for nursing. *Advances in Nursing Science, 5*(4), 21–30.

Sampselle, C. M. (1990). The influence of feminist philosophy on nursing practice. *Image: Journal of Nursing Scholarship, 22*(4), 243–247.

Siegel, B. (1988). *Lillian Wald of Henry Street.* New York, NY: MacMillan.

Smith-Rosenberg, C., & Rosenberg, C. (1984). The female animal: Medical and biologic views of woman and her role in 19th century America. In J. W. Leavitt (Ed.), *Women and health in America* (pp. 12–27). Madison: University of Wisconsin Press.

United American Nurses, AFL-CIO (2003). Poll of Registered Nurses conducted by Lake Snell Perry and Associates, pp. 1–3 (press release).

Vance, C., McBride, A., & Mason, D. (1985). An uneasy alliance: Nursing and the women's movement. *Nursing Outlook, 33*(6), 281–285.

Who needs doctors? (2005, January 31). [Special health issue]. *U.S. News and World Report,* 44–74.

Zinn, H. (1995). *A people's history of the United States 1492–present* (2nd ed., Rev.). New York, NY: New York University Press.

ENDNOTES

[1]Although there are many interpretations of first-, second-, and third-wave feminisms, *first* generally refers to the suffrage movement, *second* to the 1960s and 1970s, and *third* to the new millennium.

[2]The 19th-century women's movement was called the *woman movement,* and according to Cott (1987) symbolized the unity of the female sex.

[3]The letters from Dock to Nutting were not dated with the year. Mary Ann Burnam's research showed many factual errors—some of the letters were dated years later. With this in mind, Dr. Burnam suggests reading for context, rather than specific time frames (personal communication, June 1999).

[4]Thanks to Joan I. Roberts and Thetis M. Group for their comprehensive work on feminism and nursing that provided the outline for this section (see references).

CHAPTER 2

Oppressed Group Behavior and Nursing

Susan Jo Roberts

Over the past 20 years, the oppressed group behavior model has been used to explain the behavior of nurses. This model explains not only how powerless groups have behaved in response to domination, but also lends insight into changing the cycle of oppression and enhancing empowerment. This chapter will discuss oppressed group behavior, explain its relevance to nursing, and explore ways that nurses can empower themselves by changing self-defeating behaviors. These changes can benefit not only nurses, but also the healthcare systems in which they work.

OPPRESSED GROUP BEHAVIOR

Oppressed group behaviors were first described in writings about colonized Africans (Fanon, 1963, 1967; Memmi, 1965, 1968), South Americans (Freire, 1971), African Americans (Carmichael & Hamilton, 1967), Jews (Lewin, 1948), and American women (Miller, 1986). Freire (1971) developed a model of oppressed group behavior and instruction for liberation based on his work with Brazilians who had been dominated by Europeans. He explained that the root of the cycle of oppression is a learned belief by dominated people that they are inferior. Although this belief is not accurate, the belief occurs because the dominant group creates norms and values for the culture in its own image, and the group initially has the power to enforce it. Subordinate groups learn to hate their own attributes (e.g., skin color, food, language, clothing), because they are not valued and they are made to feel that who they are is not the "right" way to be. Over time, the origins of this process are lost, and the culture accepts the system as truth. This belief by the oppressed in their own inferiority, their powerlessness in the system, and their lack of pride in their own culture leads to feelings of low self-esteem and a lack of respect for their attributes and each other.

Memmi (1965) explained that natives who want to get ahead in the culture feel that they need to change and look more like the oppressor. He notes that this assimilation is easy when it means learning a different language or changing dress or food, but the ability to "pass" is impossible when it involves skin color or gender (Memmi, 1968). Lewin (1948) explained the difficulty for American Jews who desired success in a society dominated by non-Jewish culture and values: "The individual has certain expectations and goals for the future. Belonging to his group is seen as an impediment to reaching these goals" (p. 189). People who are successful at this assimilation are known as "marginal," because they are on the fringes of their own culture, but are not really full members of the dominant group either. Marginality leaves one without a clear cultural identity. Carmichael and Hamilton (1967) have argued that many African Americans became marginal by adopting the cultural characteristics of White America and abandoning their African roots.

Internalization of inferiority, a lack of pride in one's own culture or group, and powerlessness create certain characteristics that continue the cycle of subordination. This cycle allows for the power differential to exist even after physical domination is no longer a factor. Low self-esteem and lack of confidence in one's ability leaves individuals without the belief that they could/should have control over their own lives. One behavior observed in the powerless is the "submission–aggression syndrome." This means that although the oppressed feel aggression toward the powerful, their fear and low self-esteem make them submissive when confronted by authority and power (Carmichael & Hamilton, 1976). This fear and insecurity also leads to an inability to express clearly their own needs when they might be able to be heard because the power differential no longer exists. Similarly, Fanon (1963) noted that aggression and anger toward the powerful often is turned inward toward one's own group because of the same fear and low self-esteem. He called this internal conflict "horizontal violence" and felt that it functioned as a way of maintaining the status quo by limiting revolt. This behavior keeps the group from organizing and from developing the sense of unity and cohesiveness necessary to revolt.

A similar process has been described in American women who developed poor self-esteem and lack of pride because they were not like the valued persons in society—men (Miller, 1986). Miller noted that oppression was maintained by denying access to opportunities in the culture, such as to education and jobs. The dominant group defines "one or more acceptable roles for the subordinant . . . which typically involves providing services that no dominant group wants to perform" (Miller, 1986, p. 6). Even though women were intelligent and capable, they were denied access to education and roles in which they could utilize these abilities. This helped to maintain the cycle of powerlessness.

Freire (1971) observed that oppression is also maintained by an educational system that perpetuates the myth of inferiority and by rewards to those who help keep the status quo. Jobs, financial support, and positions of relative power are given to those oppressed members who support the dominant view. Members of the oppressed group who are capable and eager to succeed often are rewarded in this way and therefore become the leaders of the group. These members are often the most "marginal" and are not interested in developing pride or esteem in their group members because that might change the status quo and end their personal privilege. Leaders in oppressed groups are therefore skeptical of their own group and are controlling and rigid in their management approach (Kanter, 1977). As Freire (1971) has noted, "it is the rare peasant who, if promoted to landowner, does not become the tyrant of the peasant" (p. 29).

LIBERATION FROM OPPRESSION

In most cases, liberation from oppression cannot come from the leadership of the group or from the dominant group. Empowerment comes from unveiling the cycle of oppression and the myths developed in the system (Freire, 1971). Freedom comes from rejecting the negative images of one's own culture and replacing it with a sense of pride in the group's characteristics and abilities. Analyses of the process of liberation suggest that this change involves several stages of personal insight and development before the group is ready to become actively involved in change (Cross, 1971; Cross, Parham, & Helms, 1991; Downing & Roush, 1985). Freire has argued that the leadership for this process must come from the larger group and not be dependent on an elite leadership that has traditionally represented the goals of the oppressor. Similarly, emancipatory education of the oppressed involves critical reflection on processes accepted as routine to detect the myths in the system.

NURSING AS AN OPPRESSED GROUP

Nursing, because of its lack of power and control in the workplace, and because health care has primarily occurred in the hospital, has been viewed as an oppressed group (Cleland, 1971; Clifford, 1992; DeMarco & Roberts, 2003; Glass, 1997, 1998; Hedin, 1992; McCall, 1996; Roberts, 1983, 1996, 1997, 2000; Torres, 1981). Sociologists trace the beginning of the domination (colonization) of nursing to the early 1900s, when medicine became a dominant force and care of the sick became institutionalized (Twaddle & Hessler, 1977). Other authors have documented nursing's lack of control and autonomy in hospitals and argue that hospitals and physicians have benefited from this exploitation of nurses (Ashley, 1979; Lovell, 1981). A recent study documented that nurses in the 1990s still felt that they were devalued and viewed as "handmaidens" as a result of their domination by others (McCall, 1996). Torres (1981) explained that nursing education was originally autonomous, but became controlled by physicians in the 1890s. This explanation may be difficult to believe because nursing has become so acculturated to its subordinate position that it seems natural. As Cleland (1971) suggested: "Nursing in its utter isolation from all vestiges of power except in its own group, can be likened to the exploitation of American Negroes. . . . With women, as with Negroes, dominance is most complete when it is not even recognized" (p. 1543).

Allen and Hall (1988) explained that the values of nursing are rarely recognizable in patient care because the values of medicine and the medical model have been accepted as the norm. A nursing identity has been subsumed under medicine, which claims all of health care as its legitimate domain. This difficulty in defining *nursing* is symptomatic of its marginality (Greenleaf, 1978). Medicine controls the environment and hands to nursing the tasks that physicians do not want to do. Nursing is constantly compared with medicine and made to feel inferior. Nurses are often greeted with "disbelief that one would prefer to be a nurse rather than a physician" (LeRoux, 1978, p. 26). The term *bicultural* became popular in describing the process that nurses who were educated in a nursing school culture needed to go through to be accepted in the hospital workplace (Kramer & Schmalenberg, 1978). Even in academia, nurses have been rewarded for looking more like other academics than like nurses (Benoliel, 1975; Torres, 1981). Advanced practice nurses are especially at risk for becoming "marginal" because they are rewarded for looking and acting like doctors although they never truly obtain the full privilege (Roberts, 1996).

Characteristics of oppressed groups frequently have been found in nurses. Lack of self-esteem has been observed in nurses (Bush & Kjervik, 1978; Greenleaf, 1978; Grissum & Spengler, 1976). Horizontal violence, intergroup rivalry, and inward aggression have frequently been described in the workplace and in the nursing academy (Cox, 1991; Glass, 1997, 1998; Farrell, 1997, 1999; Freshwater, 2000; Griffin, 2004; McCall, 1996; McKenna, Smith, Poole, & Coverdale, 2003; Thomas, 2003). Gordon, a journalist who writes frequently about nurses, stated that she is "struck by the negative messages nurses broadcast to one another" (Gordon, 1998). Bowman and Culpepper (1974) felt that lack of unity and pride in professional nursing organizations was symptomatic of lack of esteem and the presence of intergroup hostility. The constant battle of nurses with each other allows other groups to maintain control and remain unchallenged.

Ineffective communication, both passive aggressiveness and silencing, has been an ongoing pattern within nursing. Stein (1967), in his now classic observations of communication between nurses and doctors, described nurses making recommendations to physicians, but doing so in a way that made the doctor think it was his idea. This submission may no longer be needed, but it continues as a learned response. Chandler (1995) observed that nurses lack a "public voice" that describes their contributions to patient care; they are silent about their importance to patient care. DeMarco (1997; 2002) found that nurses silence themselves as a strategy to avoid conflict and to maintain the status quo in the workplace. This behavior was also found in their private lives and is felt to be embedded in what they have learned in their socialization as women. Glass (1998) found that traditionally nurses have thought that being a "good nurse" meant not challenging the system. As female journalists who have great respect for nurses, Buresh and Gordon (2000) expressed surprise at the silence of nurses and their reluctance to explain the benefits of nursing to patients and to the public. A recent study found that "avoiding and compromising" were the most common conflict management strategies utilized by nurses (Valentine, 2001). This style of communication is part of the cycle of oppression because it discourages dissent and positive expressions about nursing.

Nursing leaders often have not been helpful in changing the balance of power. Cleland (1971) noted that many nursing leaders are "Aunt Jane," the nursing equivalent of the Black "Uncle Tom" and the feminist "Queen Bee" leaders. These leaders are marginalized because they are usually chosen with the approval of powerful physicians and administrators in the institution. Often it is men, although a minority in nursing, who are promoted to leadership positions, adding gender to the power dynamic (Glass, 1998). As one nurse sarcastically observed, "I forget there are male (nurses) around. I don't look high enough up the hierarchy to see them" (Glass, p. 128). Nursing administrators need to possess extraordinary insight, ability, and skill to be able to empower their staff and at the same time remain loyal to the agenda of administration and medicine. Nursing leaders and administrators who understand and work from an appreciation of oppressed group behavior support and communicate with their staff in different ways. They publicly acknowledge and support the work of the nurses as well as advocate for their success within the organization. They publicly and privately describe the importance of the nurse to the care of patients and support the need for resources to deliver it. They support nurses who report problems with other team members. They develop a climate where the staff feel listened to and respected, which then leads to increased reporting and discussion of successes, problems, and conflicts in patient care. They reward staff and leaders for supporting each other and creating new and innovative approaches to improving care. These leaders recognize that empowering the staff is the most important way to improve patient care (Roberts, 1997).

Another problem is that nurses who leave clinical work for administration and education often feel "better than" other nurses and are proud of their elite status (Grissum & Spengler, 1976; Roberts, 1997). These leaders may hide their nursing roots when they reach these positions because they feel that "being a nurse" makes them less credible. Educators and administrators also may pass their negative feelings about nursing to their students and to others, thus continuing the cycle of low self-esteem. This dynamic creates a loss of many accomplished nurses who could be useful in changing the power structure, but have essentially lost a positive connection to their profession.

LIBERATION FOR NURSING

The first step in altering the oppression of nurses is to understand the cycle that has helped to continue it. Awareness alone is often liberating for nurses who have felt inferior and have been blamed for their own inability to make change (Freshwater, 2000; Roberts, 2000). Lynaugh and Fagin (1988) have pointed out that nurses have much to be proud of when they learn the history of nursing:

> This confluence of paradoxes, problems, and characteristics of nursing development can be responded to in two ways. One is to bewail our failures and accept the inevitability in the face of an historically hostile environment. The other is to wonder at and celebrate the accomplishments of nurses, mostly of the wrong sex and class, who have the wrong history and education, who persist and achieve in spite of being held back by some of the most powerful forces in our society. (p. 184)

Convincing nurses that they are gifted human beings who have struggled against great odds and accomplished much is not an easy task. Challenging the myths that underlie their beliefs that they are inferior is the first step: ". . . one of the first tasks in nursing is to motivate nurses not only to image the unimagined but also to become aware of how their social conditioning has affected them (LeRoux, 1978, p. 26). Understanding the power structure of health care and the benefits to it of keeping nurses powerless is a start. As Gordon has suggested, "To build community, self-esteem and to truly understand the past and change the present, I think nurses have to jettison the old mantras, and reexamine reality, and reaffirm their considerable strengths" (Gordon, 1998). Her book with Bernice Buresh, *From Silence to Voice*, is a valuable manual for nurses on how to develop their voices and have them heard (Buresh & Gordon, 2000).

Nursing leaders and educators who understand oppressed group behavior can assist their staff by providing opportunities to critically reflect on the dynamics of the workplace (Freshwater, 2000). This reflection allows for analysis of the workplace through the lens of oppressed group dynamics, often leading nurses to a new appreciation of themselves and their nursing colleagues and of their previously "unspoken" and unrecognized contributions to the care of patients. It also allows nurses to recognize and applaud their own efforts at working under and resisting oppression in the workplace. This open discussion improves individual and collective self-esteem and communication and develops a work environment in which they can be better supported by their colleagues and leaders.

The use of writing groups has been found to develop support, connection, and "voice" in nurses (DeMarco, Roberts, & Chandler, 2005). Another project sensitized beginning staff nurses to horizontal violence in their interactions with more experienced staff and taught them strategies to confront and change the cycle of negative feedback (Griffin, 2004). These novices have found that more experienced staff members can be helpful and supportive to them if they can react in ways that change the dynamics of the interaction. These efforts not only help to change behaviors, but also provide support and change the dynamics of the workplace. It is probable that education and support can increase retention. Support also is needed for nursing administrators and leaders as they face the difficult task of increasing self-esteem and empowering a powerless group. They often lack a peer support group because of their small numbers and the competition that exists between agencies (Roberts, 1997).

The development of personal and professional self-esteem is not an easy process, especially in a group that works long hours and often has multiple commitments in and outside of work. Also, most nurses are action oriented and rarely have time to reflect. Many nurses are women and have been taught from their earliest years how to behave as women. The merger of their socialization as a woman and as a nurse creates assumptions and beliefs that are not understood but are acted out in their behavior (DeMarco, 1997, 2002; Roberts, 2000). It is likely that many nurses have left the profession or have abandoned clinical work for academia or related businesses because they are unwilling to tolerate the oppression experienced in working as a staff nurse.

Literature from other oppressed groups suggests that the development of positive self-esteem is a slow process that occurs over time (Cross, 1971; Cross, Parham, & Helms, 1991; Downing & Rousch, 1985; Tatum, 1992, 1998). The process involves an understanding of the external system of oppression and the internal belief system that has helped to maintain it. As Lorde (1984) reminds us, "The true focus of revolutionary change is never merely the oppressive situation which we seek to escape, but that piece of the oppressor which is planted deep within each of us" (p. 123). Analysis of change in other groups suggests that identity development for nursing can be conceptualized as five stages (Table 2.1) (Roberts, 2000).

The first stage, *unexamined acceptance*, represents the passive acceptance of oppression without any thought to there being another way. Nurses in this phase may complain about but accept their role as subservient and not question the dominance of the medical system. They talk about other nurses in a demeaning way (e.g., "nurses are their own worst enemies," "nurses eat their young," and "I just hate being around a group of nurses"). They discourage young women and their own daughters from becoming nurses, making statements such as, "I wouldn't want my worst enemy to be a nurse, much less my daughter." And yet they often have been nurses for many years and have no plans to leave. They express a lot of negativity and when given the opportunity for change, they dismiss it as impossible. When challenged to change the divisiveness, the response often heard is, "Nurses could change things if they would just take charge and get things done, but they never do." They accept blame in clinical situations in which multiple disciplines are responsible.

Table 2.1 Identity Development for Nursing

Unexamined Acceptance	Awareness	Connection	Synthesis	Political Action
Acceptance of roles of nurses Unquestioned belief in the power structure Belief that physicians should control system Internalized negative view of nursing	Awakening to a sense of injustice Nurses are always right, others are wrong Overwhelmed by a sense of having been wronged Seeks out other nurses for support	Affiliation with nursing groups Dependent on support of other nurses for new ideas Viewed as strident and rigid Affirmation of positive identity as a nurse	Internalizes new positive view of nursing Evaluates others on an individual basis Increase in interdisciplinary involvement Strategic approach to problem Nurses are different but equal	Commitment to change Actively involved Broad scope of activities to further social justice

Source: S.J. Roberts, Development of a positive professional identity: Liberating oneself from the oppressor within, *Advances in Nursing Science*, Vol. 22, no 4, page 75. Copyright Aspen Publications, 2000. Reprinted with permission.

The second stage, *awareness*, involves a beginning understanding of the dynamics of the dominant power structure and the myths that support it. Women who become nurses after working in social justice work or the feminist or civil rights movements often understand the oppression of nursing immediately. They become frustrated by the lack of awareness and unwillingness to change in other nurses. Women who have worked in other fields prior to becoming nurses often are mystified by the inequity in the medical system and nurses' lack of response to it. For nurses with more traditional nursing backgrounds, the awareness often occurs when they return to school or have an opportunity outside of the workplace to analyze and reflect on the profession with other nurses. This change may also occur through work with collective bargaining or other professional group activity. Or, an injustice in the workplace may occur that is so unfair that the dynamics of the power structure become clear. Whether it is the firing or disciplining of a nurse when others were responsible for a problem or when a physician is repeatedly ill behaved and nothing is done, the nurse suddenly is acutely aware that she is not the problem. In this stage, the nurse often feels anger and rage at everything. She begins to feel a greater connection to other nurses and a dislike for physicians, administrators, and the system. The view is often dualistic and extreme, with no room for middle-of-the-road opinions—nurses are right and everyone else is wrong.

In the next stage, *connection*, nurses find a group to explore their evolving positive identity. This is a time of reflection and commitment to change, supported by other like-minded people. Respect and support develop from this connection with other nurses. Nurses in this phase seem strident and overly critical of the system, which helps to consolidate their movement away from the old. Slowly, a new view emerges that is more complex and allows for more strategic action. If this change occurs in an academic setting, their work life becomes unsettled and uncomfortable because they see things differently than the nurses with whom they work.

In the fourth stage, *synthesis*, the change feels more authentic as it becomes internalized. The positive identity becomes a real part of life and allows for a less reactive stance with others. The nurse moderates her stance and begins to be able to analyze situations and plan strategically without the anger that she felt earlier. The commitment to work with other nurses continues and expands to include others who have not changed their views. The nurse is now able to appreciate and work with an array of nurses and other professionals without feeling that her new beliefs are being challenged. She is able to express her own changes to others.

In the last stage, *political action*, a commitment to social change becomes a part of life. The nurse is not only involved in helping to change the system for nurses, but also for patients, and is involved in broader social justice activities. This phase involves a broader understanding of the interrelationships between systems and the broader power structure that controls them. The nurse becomes interested in and often active in a wide range of issues and activities.

This model of change is theoretical. It is based on the experiences of other oppressed groups, and it has not been tested. It is probably not linear, but rather involves movement back and forth between stages over time. Stress, personal changes, and insights may cause the nurse to revert back to another phase or through the whole cycle. As noted in research on the development of voice in women, the process requires trust, support, and safety (Belenky et al., 1986). This model suggests that reflection, support, insight, and connection are necessary ingredients for nurses to develop the positive professional identity and voice needed to change the cycle of oppression (Roberts, 2000).

One study of a group of nurses who had returned to school after many years offers glimpses into the emancipation process (Glass, 1998). According to Glass, "Whilst empowerment was emerging, though being valued and performing well at university, reflecting upon and being part of an oppressive cycle at work was distressing, and feeling 'up' and 'down' simultaneously reflected a dialectical relationship regarding forces within themselves" (p. 128). Glass observed that the nurses' survival was dependent on sharing with other nurses. These nurses also noted that similar changes happened within their families as in the workplace. Glass found that "once nurses have recognized the value of their own voice they can then effectively listen to other nurses and value each other in their own right" (p. 134). She found that once women felt "safe to speak" they experienced "empowered states." She noted that these feelings of empowerment were not always the same, but were altered by circumstances and waxed and waned over time.

CHANGE IN THE HEALTH CARE SYSTEM

This chapter has focused on the individual behavior of nurses as it has been formed by their socialization as women and as nurses. Nurses have been molded by a system that has often devalued and oppressed them. This analysis does not intend to blame nurses for their behavior, nor does it ignore the fact that many have resisted and fought against the power inequality. Discussion and recognition of the ongoing efforts of nursing to shape and contribute to the healthcare system are most important and need to be encouraged. The purpose of analyzing oppressed group behavior is to explain how nurses can avoid the cycle that can contribute to the continuation of powerlessness. Awareness of their own behavior can enhance nurses' efforts to improve their work life as well as patient care.

Some nurses have been critical of this focus, because they feel that it keeps nurses from taking responsibility for their own behavior and for changing the system. Farrell (2001) appears to agree with this critique when he states: "We have to acknowledge that it is possible to combat conflict within nursing without first having to dismantle the prevailing hegemony of the alleged oppressors" (p. 32). He argues, "It is contended that it is not the alleged misogyny intrinsic to oppression theory that shackles and impedes nurses, but nurses themselves, who in their everyday work and interpersonal interactions act as insidious gatekeepers to an iniquitous status quo" (Farrell, p. 26). This analysis of oppression theory would appear to miss the point. An understanding and use of it does not await a change in the power structure, but, in fact, is an integral part of insight into changing nurses' behavior and the system.

West (1993), writing about empowerment of African Americans, has noted that change must involve both the person and the system because environmental conditions are so intertwined with the individuals: "First we must acknowledge that structure and behavior are inseparable, that institutions and values go hand in hand. How people act and lives are shaped—though in no way dictated or determined—by the larger circumstances in which they find themselves" (p. 12). He understands that, although positive identity development is important for African Americans, it is not all that is necessary for change to occur: "The quest for Black identity involves self-respect and self-regard, realms inseparable from, but not identical to, political power and economic status" (West, 1993, p. 66). He warns against social policies that only focus blame for the problems of African Americans on poor self-esteem, thereby avoiding change in the inequities that led to them. He supports attacking both. For nursing as well, the focus needs to be on enhancing the considerable impact that nurses have on the system already, understanding the cycle of oppressed group behaviors that inhibit potential and developing strategies to change inequities that limit the contributions and the benefits of their work.

CONCLUSION

This chapter has reviewed the theory of oppressed group behavior and its implications for the empowerment of nurses. The theory explains that powerless groups develop certain characteristics (i.e., low self-esteem, intergroup conflict, poor communication, and lack of group pride and cohesion) as a way of survival under domination. These behaviors can develop into a self-defeating cycle that continues the oppression even when less overt dominance exists. Nurses have been theorized to be an oppressed group. Despite their many contributions, nurses exhibit oppressed group behaviors that have not allowed them to reach their optimal potential in the healthcare system. Understanding oppressed group behavior is a first step in changing the cycle and empowering nurses. The theory suggests that a process of reflection, support, insight, and connection can help nurses to change the cycle that keeps them powerless. Nursing leaders, as well, can benefit from an understanding of their role in the continuation of oppression and seek support for change. This change can create the positive personal and professional identity needed to improve the workplace for nurses and the healthcare system for patients.

REFERENCES

Allen, J., & Hall, B. (1988). Challenging the focus on technology: A critique of the medical model in a changing health care system. *Advances in Nursing Science, 71*, 1542–1547.

Ashley, J. (1979). *Hospitals, paternalism, and the role of the nurse.* New York: Teachers College Press.

Belenky, M. F., Clinchy, B., Golderger, N. R., & Tarule, J. M. (1986). *Women's ways of knowing, the development of self, voice, and mind.* New York: Basic Books.

Benoliel, J. (1975). Scholarship—A woman's perspective. *Image, 1*(2), 22–27.

Bowman, R., & Culpepper, R. (1974). Power: Rx for change. *American Journal of Nursing, 74*, 1054–1056.

Buresh, B., & Gordon, S. (2000). *From silence to voice.* Ithaca, NY: Cornell University Press.

Bush, M., & Kjervik, D. (1978). The nurse's self-image. In D. I. Kjervik & I. Martinson (Eds.), *Women in stress: A nursing perspective* (pp. 46–58). New York: Appleton-Century Crofts.

Carmichael, S., & Hamilton, C. (1967). *Black power.* New York: Random House.

Chandler, G. (1995). Taking the private voice public—sharing nursing knowledge. *Revolution, 5*(1), 80–83.

Cleland, V. (1971). Sex discrimination: Nursing's most pervasive problem. *American Journal of Nursing, 71*, 1542–1547.

Clifford, P. G. (1992). The myth of empowerment. *Nursing Administration, 16*(31), 1–5.

Cox, H. (1991). Verbal abuse nationwide, Part I: Oppressed group behavior. *Nursing Management, 22*, 32–35.

Cross, W. E. (1971). The negro to black conversion experience: Toward a psychology of black liberation. *Black World, 20*(9), 13–27.

Cross, W. E., Parham, T. A., & Helms, J. E. (1991). The stages of black identity development: Nigrescence models. In R. Jones (Ed.), *Black psychology* (3rd ed.), (pp. 319–338). San Francisco: Cobb & Henry.

DeMarco, R. (1997). The relationship between family life and workplace behaviors: Exploring the gendered perceptions of staff nurses through the Framework of Systemic Organization (dissertation). Detroit: Wayne State University.

DeMarco, R. (2002). Two theories/a sharper lens: The staff nurse in the workplace. *Journal of Advanced Nursing, 38*(6), 549–556.

DeMarco, R., & Roberts, S. J. (2003). Negative behaviors in nursing. *The American Journal of Nursing, 103*(3), 113–116.

DeMarco, R., Roberts, S. J., & Chandler, G. (2005). The use of a writing group to enhance voice and connection among staff nurses. *Journal for Nurses in Staff Development, 21*(3), 1–6.

Downing, N. E., & Roush, K. L. (1985). From passive acceptance to active commitment: A model of feminist identity development for women. *Counseling Psychology, 13*(4), 695–709.

Fanon, F. (1963). *The wretched of the earth.* New York: Grove Press.

Fanon, F. (1967). *Black skins, white masks.* New York: Grove Press.

Farrell, G. A. (1997). Aggression in clinical settings: Nurses' views. *Journal of Advanced Nursing, 25*(3), 501–508.

Farrell, G. A. (1999). Aggression in clinical settings: Nurses' views—A follow-up study. *Journal of Advanced Nursing, 29*(3), 532–541.

Farrell, G. A. (2001). From tall poppies to squashed weeds: Why don't nurses pull together more? *Journal of Advanced Nursing, 35*(1), 26–33.

Freire, P. (1971). *Pedagogy of the oppressed.* New York: Herder & Herder.

Freshwater, D. (2000). Crosscurrents: Against cultural narration in nursing. *Journal of Advanced Nursing, 32*(2), 461–384.

Glass, N. (1997). Horizontal violence in nursing. *The Australian Journal of Holistic Nursing, 4*(1), 15–23.

Glass, N. (1998). Becoming de-silenced and reclaiming voice: Women nurses speak out. In H. Keleher & F. McNerney (Eds.), *Nursing matters: Critical sociological perspective* (pp. 121–138). Australia: Churchill Livingstone.

Gordon, S. (1998). No, you are not your own worst enemy. *Revolution, 8*(1), 60–65.

Greenleaf, N. (1978). The politics of self-esteem. *Nursing Digest, 6*(3), 1–7.

Griffin, M. (2004). Teaching cognitive rehearsal as a shield for lateral violence: An Intervention for newly licensed nurses. *Journal of Continuing Education in Nursing, 35*(6), 257–263.

Grissum, M., & Spengler, C. (1976). *Women power and health care.* Boston: Little, Brown & Co.

Hedin, B. (1992). A case study of oppressed group behavior in nursing. *Image, 18*(2), 53–57.

Kanter, R. (1977). *Men and women of the corporation.* New York: Basic Books.

Kramer, M., & Schmalenberg, C. (1978). *Path to biculturalism.* Wakefield, MA: Nursing Resources.

LeRoux, R. (1978). Power, powerlessness and potential—Nurse's role within the health care delivery system. *Image, 10*(3), 75–83.

Lewin, K. (1948). *Resolving social conflicts.* New York: Harper & Row.

Lorde, A. (1984). *Sister outsider.* Trumansburg, NY: The Crossing Press.

Lovell, M. (1981). Silent but perfect "partners": Medicine's use and abuse of women. *Advances in Nursing Science, 3*(2), 25–40.

Lynaugh, J., & Fagin, C. (1988). Nursing comes of age. *Image, 20*(4), 184–189.

McCall, E. (1996). Horizontal violence in nursing. *The Lamp, 53*(3), 28–29, 31.

McKenna, B. G., Smith, N. A., Poole, S. J., & Coverdale, J. H. (2003). Horizontal violence experiences of Registered Nurses in their first year of practice. *Journal of Advanced Nursing, 42*(1), 90–96.

Memmi, A. (1965). *The colonizer and the colonized.* New York: Orion Press.

Memmi, A. (1968). *Dominated man.* New York: Orion Press.

Miller, J. B. (1986). *Toward a new psychology of women* (2d ed.). Boston: Beacon Press.

Roberts, S. J. (1983). Oppressed group behavior: Implications for nursing. *Advances in Nursing Science, 5*(3), 21–30.

Roberts, S. J. (1996). Breaking the cycle of oppression: Lessons for nurse practitioners. *Journal of the American Academy of Nurse Practitioners, 8*(5), 209–214.

Roberts, S. J. (1997). Nurse executives in the 1990s: Empowered or oppressed? *Nursing Administration Quarterly, 22*(1), 64–71.

Roberts, S. J. (2000). Development of a positive professional identity: Liberating oneself from the oppressor within. *Advances in Nursing Science, 22*(4), 71–82.

Stein, L. (1967). The nurse–doctor game. *Archives of General Psychiatry, 16,* 699–703.

Tatum, B. D. (1998). *Why do all the Black students sit together in the cafeteria?* New York: Basic Books.

Tatum, B. D. (1992). Talking about race, learning about racism: The application of racial identity development theory in the classroom. *Harvard Education Review, 62*(1), 1–24.

Thomas, S. P. (2003). Horizontal hostility. *American Journal of Nursing, 103*(10), 87–91.

Torres, G. (1981). The nursing education administrator: Accountable, vulnerable, and oppressed. *Advances in Nursing Science, 3*, 1–16.

Twaddle, A., & Hessler, M. (1977). *A sociology of health.* St. Louis: CV Mosby Co.

Valentine, P. E. B. (2001). Gender perspectives on conflict management strategies of nurses. *Journal of Nursing Scholarship, 33*(1), 69–74.

West, C. (1993). *Race matters.* Boston: Beacon Press.

CHAPTER 3

Men Nurses and Women Physicians: Exploring Masculinities and Gendered and Sexed Relations in Nursing and Medicine

Joan Evans

Although women have made inroads into traditionally male occupations, such as medicine, the reverse has not been the case of men entering nursing (Jacobs, 1993; Wootton, 1997). Despite major changes in healthcare delivery in the last century, nursing has remained a quintessential feminine occupation. This situation has significant implications for both men and women nurses and the profession of nursing itself. This chapter explores the gendered and sexed relations in nursing and, more specifically, the relations of masculinity and power they embody. The situation of women in medicine also is presented to illustrate how such relations structure unequal opportunities for women and men within and across nursing and medicine. Qualitative data gathered from eight male registered nurses in Nova Scotia, Canada, are integrated into the discussion and offer insight into how men and women's practices of masculinity reflect and perpetuate the patriarchal gender regime of health care.

This paper begins with a discussion of assumptions that inform my interpretations of the experience of men in nursing and women in medicine. They offer the advantage of allowing us to question established norms and break out of increasingly inadequate category systems to create theory that is capable of grasping the complexities of people's lives and the cultures they create (Lather, 1991).

MOVING BEYOND SEX ROLE THEORY

The methodology employed in my research with men nurses was grounded in feminist, postmodernist, and masculinity theories. This perspective rejects the sex role paradigm, which has been, and continues to be, the major framework for analyses of gender and men's participation in nursing. Within the sex role paradigm, "expressive" feminine sex role traits of nurturing, caring, dependence, and submission exist in marked contrast to "instrumental" masculine traits of aggression, self-control, competitiveness, and dominance (Carrigan, Connell, & Lee, 1987; Kimmel & Messner, 1992). This dualism, based on "natural" differences between women and men, has been used to explain differences between the experiences of men and women.

Gaps in our understanding of the experience of men in nursing become increasingly apparent as limitations of sex role theory are identified. One limitation is that when men's practices do not conform to prescribed sex roles, nonconformity is conceptualized as a problem with individuals, not with sex role theory itself (Carrigan et al., 1987; Connell, 1993). The labeling of men nurses as "gay" can be understood as an example of nonconformity in relation to prescribed sex role identity. Heikes (1991) suggests that men nurses are trapped in a homosexual role that is imposed on them from outside nursing. He adds that the homosexual generalization is applied to all men who deviate from traditional expressions of masculinity, and that because it is a highly stigmatized role, both inside and outside nursing, the homosexual trap results in a "spoiled identity" for men nurses.

An additional limitation of sex role theory is its inability to address relations of power and the ways in which men as a group exert power over women (Connell, 1993; Kimmel & Messner, 1992). The conclusion that men generally live many aspects of their lives in and through power relationships over women is accepted fact among feminists and many researchers and scholars exploring masculinities (e.g., Carrigan et al., 1987; Connell, 1993, 1995; Kenway, 1995; Messner, 1990). Within nursing, this situation has received extensive attention in relation to the subordinate status of women nurses to men physicians. Because gender relations themselves, as pointed out by Connell (1993), produce large-scale collective advantages for men and disadvantages for women, masculinity itself has now become problematic.

Multiple Masculinities

Masculinity theorist Connell (1987) defines *masculinity* as a social construction about what it means to be male in a certain time and place. This definition captures the complexity and multiplicity of men's lives and moves us away from the essentialist notion that a stable, uniform masculine essence exists. When theorizing about men and masculinity, the concept of multiplicity is reflected in the pluralizing of the term, such that we now talk of *masculinities* (Connell, 1987, 1995; Hearn & Morgan, 1990). The experience of masculinity is not a uniform one, and the concept of hegemonic masculinities addresses itself to this issue by pointing to the dominance in society of certain forms and practices of masculinity that are historically constructed. Today's model of hegemonic masculinity, which is White, heterosexist, middle/upper class, and associated with stereotypical sex role traits, implies that not all men can, or do, measure up to the ideal. Thus, hegemony implies that men may experience subordination and marginalization as a consequence of not measuring up to the standard against which all men are judged (Connell, 1995). Men who represent alternative or nonhegemonic masculinities include poor men, non-White men, gay men, and perhaps those men suspected of being gay due to their association with women's work.

CROSSING OVER INTO NONTRADITIONAL OCCUPATIONS

In Canada and the United States, only 5.3 to 5.4% of nurses are men (CNA, 2003; Minority Nurse Statistics, 2004). This trend is significantly different from the situation of women entering medicine. In 1960, only 6% of physicians were women; in 2000, they comprised about a third of the physician population; at present, they represent approximately half of all students in medical schools (Gautam, 2001).

Several reasons for the low numbers of men crossing over into nursing are cited in the nursing literature. These include men's fear of being subordinate to women (Fottler, 1976); nursing's threat to men's self-esteem and masculinity (Egeland & Brown, 1989; Lewis, 1981); and nursing's low salary and lack of occupational prestige (Egeland & Brown, 1989; Galbraith, 1991; McCloskey & Grace, 1994). Each of these reasons provides insight into the consequences or penalties men experience in relation to masculinity as a result of their participation in women's work. As pointed out by the men nurses in my research, powerlessness or feelings of powerlessness characterize the experience of being affiliated with a low-status, feminine-identified occupation: "When you come into nursing as a man, you're also taking on the weakness of the profession" (Evans, 2001, p. 187). Men who defy prevailing gender norms are well aware of the risks associated with not measuring up to the hegemonic standard. The fear that they will be perceived to be gay consequently poses a significant barrier to men entering and remaining in the profession (Evans & Frank, 2003; Kelly, Shoemaker, & Steele, 1996).

Gender as Status Contradiction

Work signifies our social status; what we do for a living influences how others evaluate and rank us and how we feel about ourselves. Because masculinity is defined by the work men perform, men's labor holds additional meaning as a demonstration of masculinity (Levine, 1992). Segal (1962) suggests that the stigmatizing label of gayness associated with men who do women's work provides a basis for a lack of personal and professional status. In support of this statement, England and Herbert (1993) point out that men nurses, regardless of their status in nursing, lack the power and prestige that normally accrues to men in patriarchal society. Despite some status being regained by men nurses who assume leadership positions, they still continue to be disadvantaged in terms of salary in comparison to men outside the profession.

In addition to using income as a measure of masculinity and status, Segal (1962) points out that the low status of men in nursing leadership positions is also a reflection of the masculine character of competition. He suggests that the situation of women being subordinate to men is the expected norm, but is never quite normal for men nurses because they compete with women. Masculinity theorist Pleck (1992) adds that women reduce the stress of male competition by serving as an underclass. He points out that under patriarchy, women represent the lowest status to which men can fall, and then only in the most exceptional circumstances, if at all. This notion was illustrated in a 1963 study in Detroit of 19 low socioeconomic status, unemployed Black men who entered a 52-week retraining program for practical nurses (Rutledge & Gass, 1967). The researchers reported that the men experienced a "battered sense of maleness" (p. 54) due to the tensions and status contradiction associated with their participation in nursing. An interesting observation, however, was that the men bolstered their compromised sense of masculinity by (re)affirming their superior status to women. This was illustrated in the statement made by one man that "I may not be much, but at least I am not a woman" (p. 57).

That women represent the lowest level to which any man can fall provides some insight into the gender-based class regime of the healthcare system. Within this system, women as nurses represent a lower class relative to men physicians. This class system based on gender also is supported by class and race relations within the broader society, because traditionally nurses have been from working- or middle-class families (Darbyshire, 1987; Murray & Chambers, 1990; Salvage, 2000), and physicians, regardless of gender, race, or ethnicity, have been from the upper-middle or upper classes (Darbyshire, 1987; More, 1999). More (1999) points out that the economic ramifications of medical education have not resulted in major changes in the gendered and classed structure of health care because many of the women "joining their brothers" in medicine are also from the middle and upper classes.

Within patriarchal culture, the situation of men entering nursing presents a status contradiction, because high-status men enter an occupation numerically dominated by lower-status women doing lesser-valued work. This situation is different from that of women in medicine. In this context, lower-status women enter an occupation dominated by high-status men performing highly valued work. Indeed, in the case of medicine, the status contradiction presented by increasing numbers of women is often explained by the faltering social status of that occupation. As pointed out by Wegar (1993), as the status of an occupation decreases, the percentage of women in the occupation is expected to increase.

Reconciling the Status Contradiction: Men Nurses and Women Physicians

Despite the fact that men are crossing over into nursing and women into medicine, patriarchal gender relations remain largely intact, as evidenced by the gendered division of labor and the inequitable distribution of power and privilege within and across these professions. In nursing, men occupy a disproportionate number of elite specialty (e.g., psychiatry, critical care, emergency care, operating room) and leadership positions (Squires, 1995; Trudeau, 1996; Williams, 1989). This situation is attributed, in part, to the preferential treatment afforded men nurses by women nurses and men physicians—a situation that ultimately results in men being tracked or pushed into masculine-congruent, high-status positions (Heikes, 1991; Williams, 1989).

That men expect and are expected to achieve positions of status and privilege in the profession points to the powerful ideology of gender and the division of labor based on gender in patriarchal culture. Not all of the participants in the research study I conducted aspired to leadership positions, yet all, to varying degrees, acknowledged being pressured by women colleagues to do just this because they were men. They were offered transfers, encouraged to assume more responsibility, asked to represent nursing in professional associations and unions, and repeatedly called upon for advice. One participant commented that it was not easy for men nurses to remain at the bedside in the face of such pressure (Evans, 2001). Similar findings are reported by Soerlie, Talseth, and Norberg (1997) based on a qualitative study of the experiences of 13 men nurses. The researchers concluded that weak men nurses are not able to resist the pressure to become leaders and that it takes strength to stay at the bedside and do the *mothering* work of nursing. I would add that because masculinity itself confers benefits, expecting men *not* to take up privilege is unreasonable, if not impossible, given that existing institutional power structures merely reproduce the male sex role and the privilege associated with it (Brod, 1992). Thus, the situation of men nurses taking up privilege and women nurses helping or pushing men to do this can be understood as women and men engaging in complex practices of masculinity that support patriarchal gender relations.

Fottler (1976) suggested that the situation of women nurses supporting and nurturing the careers of men nurses can be conceptualized in terms of women nurses experiencing a status contradiction due to men's presence in the profession. Practices by women nurses that privilege men colleagues are consequently understood as attempts to restore status to men as a means of reconciling this contradiction. Kenway and Fitzclarence (1997) added to the complexity of this situation by suggesting that femininities that involve compliance, service, subservience, self-sacrifice, and the accommodation of the needs and desires of men support hegemonic masculinity.

In medicine, where women represent the lower-status group, the status contradiction experienced by men physicians due to women's presence appears to be reconciled in a similar way, but with a significantly different outcome. In this situation, women medical students and women physicians are channeled away from high-status specialties (More, 1999), such as general surgery, orthopedics, and neurosurgery, and into feminine-identified, lower-status specialties, such as pediatrics, family practice, and obstetrics–gynecology (Baxter, Cohen, & McLeod, 1996; More, 1999). That women expect and are expected to assume these positions is illustrated by Chidambaram (1993), who reported that women physicians from different countries, such as India and Finland, saw their vocation as an extension of their domestic roles as wives, mothers, and caregivers. A negative consequence of working in low-status specialties, according to the author, is that the career patterns of women physicians are likely to afford them fewer opportunities to exercise or regulate their professional privileges. Thus, their low status in the profession is perpetuated.

GENDERED AND SEXED RELATIONS AND THE GENDER REGIME OF HEALTH CARE

A significant challenge for men in nursing is the adjustment to working with women as a peer group. Nurse Porter-O'Grady (1995) suggested that men make a serious mistake when they assume that the quality and nature of relationships they previously established in male-dominated fields can prevail in a woman-oriented field such as nursing. The notion that men nurses "can't work with women like men" (Streubert, 1994, p. 30) is one that underpins much of the nursing literature written about relations between men nurses and women nurses. This situation has added significance within the context of masculinity theory if, as suggested by Berger, Wallis, and Watson (1995), masculinity is performatively constituted, primarily in the company of other men. Assuming this to be the case, a major challenge faced by men nurses is the struggle to maintain a positive sense of self and masculine identity in the absence of other men (Evans & Frank, 2003).

The participants in my study described their relationships with other men nurses in terms of comradery and kinship, and they gravitated to other men nurses because they shared common interests, experiences, and hardships. In contrast, relationships with women colleagues were characterized as distant. This situation was deemed acceptable due to the perception that natural differences between men and women meant that men and women just did not talk the same language. A second factor that participants described as contributing to the distance between themselves and their women colleagues was the perception that men were vulnerable in man–woman interactions due to sexualization of such interactions. The men nurses in my study were well aware that joking around and engaging in on-the-job banter with women exposed them to the risk of misunderstandings and accusations of sexual harassment (Evans & Frank, 2003). They attributed this situation to factors such as their highly visible status; the unpredictable "treacherous" nature of women; the sexually explicit or "impoverished" nature of women nurses' small talk; and a double standard that disadvantaged men, not women, in social interactions (Evans, 2001).

The perception that women nurses' interactions with men nurses are not constrained by concerns of sexual harassment reflects the patriarchal and heterosexist culture of nursing that fuels the stereotype that men, not women, are sexual aggressors (Evans & Frank, 2003). This conclusion moves our thinking about the quality of interactions between men and women in nursing beyond a limited and limiting consideration of sexual harassment to a broader consideration of the social practices of institutions and the particular forms of sexuality and masculinity they endorse. To illustrate this point and to highlight the complexity of sexed relations in nursing and medicine, Bradley (1993) suggested that sexual innuendo and flirting between doctors and nurses is an important and generally accepted part of hospital culture. Hazel (1981) supported this conclusion and added that women operating room nurses are not harassed when they are subjected to sexually explicit jokes or asked to give back rubs to surgeons because these actions are considered to be part of the culture of nursing. That this culture is one of subordination and oppression is not articulated. This is a troubling omission given that harassment is acknowledged in thought, policy, and statute to be an exercise of power (Frank, Brogan, & Schiffman, 1998). The differences in women nurses' perceptions as to what constitutes acceptable behavior on the part of men nurses, as compared to men physicians, points to the need for alternative analyses of nurse–physician and nurse–nurse interactions that make explicit the ways in which women's and men's practices support heterosexism, hegemonic masculinity, and patriarchal gender/power relations that maintain the subordinate status of women to men.

The masculinist and heterosexist culture of health care also is evidenced by the gendered and sexed relations in medicine. In the medical literature, this is often discussed in relation to practices of gender-based and sex-based harassment, both of which are acknowledged to be significant and long-standing barriers to women physicians' psychological well-being and satisfaction with medicine as a career (Frank, McMurray, Linzer, & Elon, 1999; Komaromy, Bindman, Haber, & Sande, 1993). *Gender-based harassment*, which is characterized by discriminatory events attributed to women being in a male-dominated environment, is distinguished from *sexual harassment*, which is understood as harassment with a sexual or physical component (Frank, Brogan, & Schiffman, 1998). It is not surprising that more women than men in medicine report experiencing gender-based discrimination (Cook, Liutkus, Risdon, Griffith, Guyatt, & Walter, 1996)—a situation that reflects the power imbalance between men and women in patriarchal culture.

An interesting finding reported by Cook and colleagues (1996) was that women residents were significantly more likely to have experienced gender-based discrimination by both men and women nurses and other healthcare workers. The situation of women nurses sexually harassing women physicians initially appears to be contradictory. However, given that harassment is an exercise of power, such practices may also be conceptualized as attempts by women nurses to reconcile the superior status of women in medicine and the status contradiction this presents for them. That women participate in practices of hegemonic masculinity that reinforce men's power over women illustrates the complexity of gender relations and the role they play in supporting the gender regime of institutions such as nursing and medicine.

THE NURSE–PHYSICIAN RELATIONSHIP

The traditional doctor–nurse relationship described by Stein (1967) captures the hierarchical structure of authority in health care and the subordinate role of women nurses to physicians. The nursing literature suggests, however, that the nurse–physician relationship is changing, a situation that Svensson (1996) attributed to the feminization of medicine, changing ideas about nursing and nurses' autonomy, and nursing students being socialized to assume a more independent professional role. Each of these factors point to changes in traditional gender/power relations, and they suggest that femininities, other than those that underwrite hegemonic masculinity, are increasingly evident in nursing.

The traditional physician–nurse power dynamic is also changing due to the presence of men in nursing. Murray and Chambers (1990) reported that men nurses, as compared to women nurses, are significantly less sympathetic to the dominant role of the physician. The disruption of the subservient nurse, dominant physician dynamic also was described by the men nurses in my research. Participants commented that they were treated with greater respect, listened to more, and taken more seriously by men physicians than were their women colleagues. They were also more likely than their women colleagues to be on a first-name basis with physicians, engage in on-the-job banter, and socialize with them outside of work (Evans, 2001).

Particularly problematic were reports by participants that women nurses were often subjected to verbal abuse by men physicians—a situation that participants reacted to with embarrassment, frustration, and anger. This reaction was directed not just at men physicians but at women nurses themselves for allowing the abuse. Participants commented that men nurses were not verbally abused by physicians simply because they "wouldn't take it" (Evans & Frank, 2003, p. 284). Such a statement glosses over complex gender/power relations alluded to in one participant's observation that "there's a certain fear element there. . . I think nurses are conditioned to be afraid all the time, afraid of doctors, afraid of the head nurse, afraid of management or any authority" (Evans, 2001, p. 165). The fact that women as a group lack the power that accrues to men in patriarchal society is attributed not to societal gender inequalities that are imported into the work environment, but rather to a deficiency with women themselves. The practice of blaming women contributes to the perception that women are undeserving and/or incapable of assuming positions of leadership in the profession. This situation illustrates how men physicians' practices of abuse, women nurses' practices of tolerating abuse, and men nurses' practices of blaming women colleagues constitute practices of hegemonic masculinity that maintain masculine privilege and the patriarchal gender regime of nursing and medicine.

When the nurse is a man and the physician a women, the traditional gender dynamic is further disrupted. The men nurses in my research described women physicians as more collegial with both men and women nurses. Nevertheless, the power and status associated with the physician role was conferred on those women who occupied that role. As one participant aptly noted, "if you regard them [women physicians] as a female and not a physician, then I suspect you're looking for trouble—understandably so" (Evans, 2001, p. 168). The notion that women physicians subscribe to practices of hegemonic masculinity may be evidenced by research that found that women physicians in the United States and Mexico do not express more positive attitudes toward physician–nurse collaboration than do their men colleagues (Mohammadreza et al., 2001). The researchers concluded that role theory, social learning, and cultural factors prescribed professional roles. An alternative explanation is that women physicians' practices of allying themselves with men maintains their own status and privilege relative to other women—particularly women nurses. In this way, practices by women physicians are revealed to support hegemonic masculinity and masculine privilege.

CONCLUSION

Men take up the offer of gender privilege in diverse ways, and within any workplace or peer group there are likely to be different understandings of masculinity and different ways of "doing" masculinity (Connell, 1996). This notion has significant implications for men and women in nursing and medicine, because practices of masculinity play a major role in structuring the heterosexist and patriarchal culture of health care. That women in nursing and medicine also subscribe to practices that support hegemonic masculinity reveals the reciprocal nature of masculinity and femininity and the notion that hegemonic masculinity requires that women play their prescribed role of doing things to make men feel more manly (Pleck, 1992). In this way, women's practices of hegemonic femininity, knowingly or otherwise, reinforce their own subjugated status in the healthcare hierarchy. This situation points to the power and pervasiveness of gender relations and illustrates how stereotypical attitudes inform how men and women make sense of their lives. The challenge in nursing and medicine, if women and men are to enjoy equal access to power and privilege and fulfilling, professional relationships, is to begin to explicate the gendered and sexed relations and those practices of hegemonic masculinity that support the current gender regime.

REFERENCES

Baxter, N., Cohen, R., & McLeod, R. (1996). The impact of gender on the choice of surgery as a career. *Medical Journal of Surgery, 172*, 373–376.

Berger, M., Wallis, B., & Watson, S. (1995). Introduction. In M. Berger, B. Wallis, & S. Watson (Eds.), *Constituting masculinities* (pp. 1–7). New York: Routledge.

Bradley, H. (1993). Across the great divide. The entry of men into "women's jobs." In C. Williams (Ed.), *Doing "women's work." Men in nontraditional occupations* (pp. 10–28). London: Sage.

Brod, H. (1992). Fraternity, equality, liberty. In M. Kimmel & M. Messner (Eds.), *Men's lives* (2nd ed.) (pp. 554–560). Toronto: Maxwell MacMillan Canada.

Carrigan, T., Connell, B., & Lee, J. (1987). Hard and heavy: Toward a new sociology of masculinity. In M. Kaufman (Ed.), *Beyond patriarchy: Essays by men on pleasure, power, and change* (pp. 139–192). Toronto: Oxford University Press.

Chidambaram, S. M. (1993). Sex stereotypes in women's contributions to medicine. In E. Riska & K. Wegar (Eds.), *Gender work and medicine: Women and the medical division of labor* (pp. 13–27). London: Sage.

CNA (Canadian Nurses Association) statistics (2003). Retrieved April 2004 from http://www.cna-aiic.ca/cna/documents/pdf/publications/2003_NursingStatisticalHighlights-e.pdf.

Connell, R. W. (1987). *Gender and power. Society, the person, and sexual politics*. Stanford, CA: Stanford University Press.

Connell, R. W. (1993). The big picture: Masculinities in recent world history. *Theory and Society, 22*, 597–623.

Connell, R. W. (1995). *Masculinities*. Cambridge: Polity.

Connell, R. W. (1996). Teaching the boys: New research on masculinity, and gender strategies for schools. *Teachers College Record, 98*(2), 206–235.

Cook, D., Liutkus, J., Risdon, C., Griffith, L., Guyatt, G., & Walter, S. (1996). Residents' experiences of abuse, discrimination and sexual harassment during residency training. *Canadian Medical Association Journal, 154*(11), 1657–1665.

Darbyshire, P. (1987). The burden of history. *Nursing Times, 83*(4), 32–34.

Egeland, J., & Brown, J. (1989). Men in nursing: Their fields of employment, preferred fields of practice and role strain. *Health Services Research, 24*(5), 693–707.

England, P., & Herbert, M. (1993). The pay of men in "female occupations." Is comparable worth only for women? In C. Williams (Ed.), *Doing "women's work." Men in nontraditional occupations* (pp. 28–48). London: Sage.

Evans, J. (2001). *Men in nursing: Exploring the gendered and sexed relations in nursing.* Unpublished doctoral dissertation, Dalhousie University, Halifax, Nova Scotia, Canada.

Evans, J., & Frank, B. (2003). Contradictions and tensions: Exploring relations of masculinities in the numerically female-dominated nursing profession. *The Journal of Men's Studies, 11*(3), 277–292.

Fottler, M. D. (1976). Attitudes of female nurses toward the male nurse: A study of occupational segregation. *Journal of Health and Social Behaviour, 17*(2), 99–110.

Frank, E., Brogan, D., & Schiffman, M. (1998). Prevalence and correlates of harassment among U.S. women physicians. *Archives of Internal Medicine, 158*(4), 352–358.

Frank, E., McMurray, J., Linzer, M., & Elon, L. (1999). Career satisfaction of women physicians. *Archives of Internal Medicine, 159*(13), 1417–1426.

Galbraith, M. (1991). Attracting men to nursing: What will they find important in their career? *Journal of Nursing Education, 30*(4), 182–186.

Gautam, M. (2001). Women in medicine: stresses and solutions. *Western Journal of Medicine, 174*(1), 37–41.

Hazel, H. (1981). Sexual harassment and nurse anaesthetists. *American Association of Nurse Anaesthetists Journal, 49*, 277–279.

Hearn, J., & Morgan, D. (1990). Men, masculinities and social theory. In J. Hearn & D. Morgan (Eds.), *Men, masculinities, and social theory* (pp. 1–18). Boston: Unwin Hyman.

Heikes, E. J. (1991). When men are the minority: The case of men in nursing. *The Sociological Quarterly, 32*(3), 389–401.

Jacobs, J. (1993). Men in female-dominated fields. Trends and turnover. In C. Williams (Ed.), *Doing "women's work." Men in nontraditional occupations* (pp. 49–63). London: Sage.

Kelly, N., Shoemaker, M., & Steele, T. (1996). The experience of being a male student nurse. *Journal of Nursing Education, 35*(4), 170–174,

Kenway, J. (1995). Masculinities in schools: Under siege, on the defensive and under reconstruction? *Discourse: Studies in the Cultural Politics of Education, 16*(1), 59–79.

Kenway, J., & Fitzclarence, L. (1997). Masculinity, violence and schooling: Challenging 'poisonous pedagogies.' *Gender and Education, 9*(1), 117–133.

Kimmel, M., & Messner, M. (1992). Introduction. In M. Kimmel & M. Messner (Eds.), *Men's lives* (2nd ed.) (pp. 1–11). Toronto: Maxwell MacMillan Canada.

Komaromy, M., Bindman, A., Haber, R., & Sande, M. (1993). Sexual harassment in medical training. *The New England Journal of Medicine, 328*(5), 322–326.

Lather, P. (1991). *Getting smart.* New York: Routledge.

Levine, M. (1992). The status of gay men in the workplace. In M. Kimmel & M. Messner (Eds.), *Men's lives* (2nd ed.) (pp. 251–266). Toronto: Maxwell MacMillan Canada.

Lewis, M. C. (1981). A black perspective: Afro-American men in nursing. *Nursing Leadership, 4*(3), 31–33.

McCloskey, J. C., & Grace, H. K. (1994). Addressing the imbalances. In J. McCloskey & H. Grace (Eds.), *Current issues in nursing* (4th ed.) (pp. 656–657). Toronto: Mosby.

Messner, M. (1990). Men studying masculinity: Some epistemological issues in sport sociology. *Sociology of Sport Journal, 7*, 136–153.

Minority Nurse Statistics, USA (2004). Retrieved April 2005 from http://www.minoritynurse.com/statistics.html.

Mohammadreza, H., Nasca, T., Cohen, M., Fields, S., Rattner, S., Griffiths, M., et al. (2001). Attitudes toward physician–nurse collaboration: A cross-cultural study of male and female physicians and nurses in the United States and Mexico. *Nursing Research, 50*(2), 123–128.

More, E. (1999). *Restoring the balance. Women physicians and the profession of medicine, 1850–1995.* Cambridge, MA: Cambridge University Press.

Murray, M., & Chambers, M. (1990). Characteristics of students entering different forms of nurse training. *Journal of Advanced Nursing, 15*(9), 1099–1105.

Pleck, J. (1992). Men's power with women, other men, and society. A men's movement analysis. In M. Kimmel & M. Messner (Eds.), *Men's lives* (2nd ed.) (pp. 19–27). Toronto: Maxwell Macmillan Canada.

Porter-O'Grady, T. (1995). Reverse discrimination in nursing leadership: Hitting the concrete ceiling. *Nursing Administration Quarterly, 19*(2), 56–62.

Rutledge, A. L., & Gass, G. Z. (1967). *Nineteen negro men. Personality and manpower retraining.* San Francisco: Jossey-Bass.

Salvage, J. (2000). In a class of their own. *Nursing Times, 96*(23), 26.

Segal, B. (1962). Male nurses: A case study in status contradiction and prestige loss. *Social Forces, 41*(1), 32–38.

Soerlie, V., Talseth, A., & Norberg, A. (1997). Male nurses—reasons for entering and experiences of being in the profession. *Scandinavian Journal of Caring Sciences, 11*(2), 113–118.

Stein, L. (1967). The doctor–nurse game. *Archives of General Psychiatry, 16*(6), 699–703.

Streubert, H. (1994). Male nursing students' perceptions of clinical experience. *Nurse Educator, 19*(5), 28–32.

Squires, T. (1995). Men in nursing. *RN, 58*(7), 26–28.

Svensson, R. (1996). The interplay between doctors and nurses—a negotiated order perspective. *Sociology of Health and Illness, 18*(3) 379–398.

Trudeau, R. (1996). Male registered nurses, 1995. *Health Reports, 8*(2), 21–27.

Wegar, K. (1993). Part IV conclusions. In E. Riska & K. Wegar (Eds.), *Gender, work, and medicine. Women and the medical division of labour* (pp. 173–188). London: Sage.

Williams, C. (1989). *Gender differences at work: Women and men in nontraditional occupations.* Los Angeles: University of California Press.

Wootton, B. (1997). Gender differences in occupational employment. *Monthly Labour Review, 120*(4), 15–24.

CHAPTER 4

Moving Towards a Culturally Competent Profession

Deborah Washington

> *You will find as a general rule that the constitutions and the habits of a people follow the nature of the land where they live.*
>
> —Hippocrates

Historically, nursing has put great effort into establishing itself as a separate and unique discipline. This has meant overcoming challenges to boundaries and functions of practice as well as defining illness and wellness phenomena appropriate to the scope of practice. Over time, the domain of nursing has been clarified through a series of steps, resulting in a recognizable profession with a distinct approach to the delivery of health care.

The 21st century brings a new set of challenges to the ongoing evolution of the nursing profession. In the United States, for example, Census data reflect an unprecedented situation in that non-Western cultures are reshaping the national population. The dominant Euro-American culture has shifted to a more pluralistic one. As a consequence, nursing is confronted with a new and provocative undertaking—to explore the professional tenets of nursing as well as to critique whether the United States has a serviceable healthcare system for the current social order. In this chapter, I will describe the increasing importance of culture as a direction for growth in clinical practice and discuss how to incorporate theoretical models into patient care. Culture is large in scope and content and has the potential to influence the domain of knowledge unique to nursing as a discipline focused on the phenomenon of care. Although the influence of culture should not change the basic tenets of practice, a determining factor in care is the inclusion of a person-centered approach to the restoration and maintenance of health.

BACKGROUND

The healthcare setting of the 20th century was the result of conventions that no longer reflect the reality of the new millennium. The original healthcare model was designed primarily to serve patients who spoke English, were able to read and write that language, typically had the resources to pay for care, believed in the germ theory of disease, valued biomedical preventative health practices, and acquiesced to the authoritarian model of the patient–healthcare provider relationship. The typical user of health services today no longer matches this image. The current patient population includes a wide array of lifestyles and is multicultural, multiethnic, and multilingual. More specifically, patients may not speak English, much less be able to read or write in their native language. They may be employed, but frequently do not have health insurance. Patients may be refugees, recently arrived immigrants, undocumented workers, or residents not yet acculturated to Western life because of indigenous pride or as a consequence of social isolation.

Human migration continues to be an all-embracing phenomenon. Few countries are unaffected by its trends. In the United States, the foreign-born population increased from 7.90% in 1990 to 11.70% in 2003. Information on immigration in 2003 documents that 305,973 people emigrated from the Americas, 251,296 from Asian nations, and 48,738 from African nations (Global Data Center, 2005). Hispanics surpassed African Americans in the 2000 Census and are now the largest minority group in the United States. Non-Hispanic Whites are the slowest-growing group, and some predict they will constitute a smaller percentage of the U.S. population in the future (Day, 2005).

THE DIASPORA

The diaspora (Greek for "to scatter") of new populations presents challenges to the host culture. Historically, host communities have the unstated expectation that the new arrivals will assimilate into the dominant culture. Adapting to new social norms often requires disengagement from old traditions, customs, and practices and frequently precipitates a loss of heritage-based identity. Culture shock and isolation related to the new environment generate a sense of dislocation, stress, and anxiety. Support services and appropriate resources are necessary to provide for and maintain the mental and physical well-being of groups seeking to establish themselves in new places (Kim, Cho, Klessig, Gerace, & Camilleri, 2002).

Immigrants familiar with health systems and practices in their country of origin face obstacles that can hinder access to care (Leduc & Proulx, 2004). Therefore, informational resources related to health services are of critical importance for new arrivals. The lack of such information influences decision making and compromises timely contact with needed care. Proficiency with English, an understanding of bureaucratic systems, and the ability to acquire health insurance are determining factors with consequences for the clinical encounter. The complexities of providing care to individuals who are unable to cope with these factors can result in culturally insensitive encounters and result in care that is inappropriate and, in some cases, even dangerous.

The inability to communicate and the negative consequences to quality of care have generated both research and awareness among practitioners. Within the paradigm of healthcare disparities, language and communication have been identified as critical additions to a culturally competent healthcare system. In 1999, the U.S. Department of Health and Human Services, Office of Minority Health, proposed national standards for culturally and linguistically appropriate services in order to establish the importance of these criteria as benchmarks for consumers, providers, and health systems. Fourteen recommendations were formulated, five of which explicitly address the need for language support (Table 4.1).

Table 4.1 Culturally and Linguistically Appropriate Standards (CLAS)

1. Provide all clients with limited English proficiency access to interpreter services.
2. Provide oral and written notices and signage to clients in their primary language, including the right to an interpreter at no cost.
3. Make available patient education and other materials in the language of the predominate group in the relevant service area.
4. Ensure the language proficiency and skills of the interpreter.
5. Ensure that the language preference and self-identified race/ethnicity of the client is included in the organization's information systems.

Source: http://www.omhrc.gov/omh/programs/2pgprograms/finalreport.pdf.

These recommendations are unprecedented. Ramifications for the practice of nursing in all healthcare settings are still to be determined. Safe practice and effective approaches to care are the anticipated outcomes. To include the consumer in full clinical decision making, it is incumbent on the clinician to understand the resource needs of patients from different cultural backgrounds.

Limitations of Multiculturalism

Becoming fluent in cultural mores is not easy and can be compromised by assumptions that all people from one geographic area are the same. Separating a culture into its component parts as a guide for understanding the whole culture risks reducing complex meanings into formulas. It also is critical to understand people's perceptions of being marginalized as the "Other." Canales and Bowers (2001) described the "Other" as:

> . . . Someone who is perceived as different from self. Historically, persons labelled as Other, as them, are categorized primarily according to how their differences from the societal norm are perceived. Their Otherness is signified by their relational differences; when compared to the 'ordinary,' 'usual' and 'familiar' attributes of persons, they appear 'different,' as Other. It is persons categorized as Other who often reside at the margins of society. (p. 103)

Additionally, variables such as class, education, gender, and religion significantly influence individuals. Although these factors can be generalized as themes of personhood, care must be exercised to prevent their use as a basis for stereotypes. The importance of identifying this information strongly affects the course of events that establish quality of care. Access to the best information available as it relates to the patient has significance for length of stay, appropriate discharge planning, and patient satisfaction.

Health Disparities

The constitution of the World Health Organization (WHO) states:

> Health is a state of complete physical, mental and social well-being and not merely the absence of disease or infirmity. The enjoyment of the highest attainable standard of health is one of the fundamental rights of every human being without distinction of race, religion, political belief, economic or social condition. (http://www.who.int/ governance/en/)

Decisive evidence of disparities in health care is attracting attention in the literature. The information provided is focused on comparative data that describe a statistical picture of morbidity and mortality, as well as increased awareness of problems of access to care and quality of care. For example, health status and utilization of services by diverse groups have become familiar parts of the discourse on equity in health care. Access and documented health outcomes illustrate a lack of parity between defined populations. However, the lack of national standards in service delivery and the paucity of evaluative research hamper explanations of the causes (Horowitz, Davis, Palermo, & Vladek, 2000). Disparities as an area of concern for healthcare providers is supported by studies that underscore inconsistencies between length of life and quality of life associated with specific cultural groups. The number of excess deaths and the difference between rates of death for minority groups as compared with a reference group reveal a situation in health care that warrants attention (LaVeist, Bowie, & Cooley-Quille, 2000). It is possible to extract issues from current research that indicate the need for close and careful observation of extant conditions. The ability to corroborate the implications of these studies with the daily conventions of clinical practice creates the conditions for strategies to address this dilemma.

Coleman-Miller (2000) emphasized the importance of cultural sensitivity training for healthcare providers to counteract the effects of cultural disregard in the form of poor interpersonal relationships, language with culture-based meanings, and ineffective services. Nontraditional health system designs that serve to improve or advance respectful attention to the needs of a multicultural population must be substantiated with more evaluative research. The significance of this is clear when due consideration is given to the need to delineate the function of factors such as racism and discrimination on health outcomes, despite an inherent discomfort with the concept. A restructuring of the healthcare delivery system driven by budgetary constraints has mobilized entrants into environments where previously they may not have been encountered in great numbers (Williams & Rucker, 2000). This can result in personal and professional challenges for any clinician.

CULTURE AND WESTERN HEALTH CARE

Culture can be a facilitator or a barrier to health care (Searight, 2003), and belief systems can sway an individual's use of information (IOM, 2002). Western biomedicine tends to dismiss non-Western approaches to healing because many of them do not base disease causality in germ theory or practice the scientific method. Many non-Western societies find the Western emphasis on pathophysiology and biomedicine to be problematic. The biomedical definition *absence of disease* fails to acknowledge the interrelationship of body, mind, *and* spirit. In *The Spirit Catches You and You Fall Down*, Fadiman (1997) captures this cultural clash. The lack of understanding between doctors and a Hmong family led to tragedy. Lia, a child diagnosed with severe epilepsy, eventually died from complications; her parents did not understand how important the medication was, and the healthcare team did not understand the complex cultural customs of the Hmong.

Cultural interpretations of the value of abandoning natal beliefs in favor of more dominant customs can be life-altering. For instance, in Haitian culture, the power of a spirit that rides or possesses a believer is used to explain changes in personality (Holcomb, Parsons, Giger, & Davidhizar, 1996). In Western culture, the ability to medicalize behavior considered outside the norm endows professional experts with civil power (Reddy, 2002).

These differences in belief practices beg several questions:

- ☐ What culturally relevant treatments maintain health and well-being?
- ☐ Is the definition of health and well-being a moving target—does it mean different things to different cultures?
- ☐ Is quality care based on the Western biomedical model? What is the role of the traditional healer?
- ☐ What frame of reference does a culturally competent clinician use to answer these questions?

The answers have the potential to place the clinician in a ethical dilemma. The ability to offer a proven best treatment is not simply a function of perspective or worldview. Scientific facts exist and are the basis for evidenced-based practice. However, biomedicine does have the capacity to coexist with other belief systems. Therefore, a plan of care can be negotiated that coordinates treatment options, taking into consideration cultural values and customs.

Nursing Lens of the Multicultural Professional

The impact of culture on nursing must be considered from another perspective if the topic and the profession are to be examined with new vision. The Western model dominates nursing identity and definition (Herdman, 2001). This has evolved into describing the field as science as well as art. In spite of this dual interpretation, however, science and its methods are explicitly positioned as the most desired path to knowledge within the discipline. Observation and experiments are the foundation used to develop tenets of practice, and a knowledge base framed as unique to the profession is the goal of what has become a prolonged endeavor.

Nevertheless, there is also a non-Western perspective on the discipline. From this aspect, nursing can be a formal or an informal concept. This specific differentiation is determined by the infrastructure that validates the role function. When tasks and activities in a particular society are solely the result of an apprenticed experience accepted by the general community, cultural rituals and traditions often dominate. However, when the role is the consequence of an educational regimen controlled by a professional body that confers the status of licensure, there are accustomed methods and procedures resulting from discipline-specific conventions that must be followed. Historically, the scientific approach has carried the designation of *modern*, and consequently is more highly valued. This has essentially negated the usefulness and importance of learning accessed through the customs, rituals, and traditions of other cultures and societies. These paths to knowledge should be explored for the value they offer to the complementary part of nursing customarily known as its *art*. The nursing lens of the multicultural professional has much to offer to this part of nursing, which has been deemphasized in the pursuit of its scientific identity.

Ethnic identity influences all of the domains of nursing: person, health, environment, and nursing. In exploring ethnicity as culture, Phinney (1996) suggested that such factors as values and attitudes were assumed to describe the cultural characteristics of a specific group. This perspective was portrayed in a study conducted by Struthers (2001) that explored nursing from a Native American point of view. Here, caring and holism, among other dimensions, were delineated culturally. Caring involved the elements of humor and partnership; holism included balance and the use of nonverbal interaction. Pang and colleagues (2004) compared Chinese, American, and Japanese nurses' understanding of ethical responsibilities. Interestingly, there were different degrees of value placed on statements related to respect. Chinese nurses gave higher marks to language related to respect for nurses, Japanese nurses gave higher marks to respect for patients, and American nurses gave higher value to statements related to respect for individual rights. Pang and colleagues also examined the experience of nursing practice in Chinese culture. The concept of nursing was rooted in the philosophical principles of the society and the nuances of the associated language. For example, Chinese terms that describe good practice include *truthfulness, responsibility*, and *service*, along with *understanding* and *knowledge* in conjunction with the actions of *protect* and *interact*. Chen (2000) points out that cultural values influenced by relevant philosophical and religious beliefs are by their nature embedded in attitudes related to health in Chinese culture. To merge these cultural ideologies into a universal understanding of the concept "to nurse" or "to be a nurse" holds great promise for the next steps as the profession continues to develop.

CULTURALLY COMPETENT CARE

An overall definition of *culture* and a description of its basic elements outline the basis for group identity. Leininger and McFarland (2002) offer a broad-based definition that describes culture as a "way of life belonging to an individual or a group that reflects values and customs taught and learned generationally" (p. 9). In her transcultural nursing model, Leininger (2001) includes religious, kinship, social, political and legal, economic, educational, technologic, and cultural values as components of culture.

The individual with a distinct cultural viewpoint has a dynamic and integral relationship with the nurse who provides culturally congruent care. *Cultural competence* has many definitions in the literature. However, in essence, it is a compilation of the clinical skills and professional behaviors of a healthcare provider focused on the cultural values, beliefs, and perceptions of the consumer while both are engaged in the therapeutic relationship. Cultural competence is an aspect of nursing that will move the profession to its next developmental phase.

Leininger (2001) defines *culture care preservation* or *maintenance* as:

> . . . those assistive, supporting, facilitative, or enabling professional actions and decisions that help people of a particular culture to retain and or preserve relevant care values so that they can maintain their well-being, recover from illness, or face handicaps and/or death. (p. 48)

Nursing has continuously acknowledged the status of the individual. Recognition of the cultural life, values, and beliefs of persons is simply an expansion of that attention. The nursing assessment, problem list, diagnosis, progress note, or discharge plan can only be effective if cultural influences are addressed. This viewpoint is in deference to the concept of cultural autonomy. The dimension of the individual experience is characterized by such concepts as *acculturation*, the implementation and acceptance of customs different from the primary culture; *assimilation*, the blending of one culture with another; and *cultural autonomy*, the ability to retain principal identity in the presence of one or more dominant groups (see **Figure 4–1**).

Cultural autonomy upholds the importance of the valued presence of customs, conventions, and folkways of all cultures within any given society without the pressure to assimilate. The imperative of one culture should not be the cause for dismissal of another.

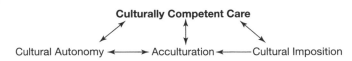

Figure 4.1 Aspects of Culturally Competent Care

In contrast, acculturation denotes an ability to adapt to the rules and conventions of a society different from the country of origin. The newcomer must manage culture shock and develop survival skills that allow for an effective level of function in new and unfamiliar surroundings. Navigating the healthcare system is one of those skills. The culturally competent provider must organize appropriate resources to enable proficient and uncompromising care. Meeting the needs of the unacculturated challenges system design and tests the justification for and the philosophy in support of care delivery. Explanations for professional practice must be grounded in findings more substantive than mere tradition to avoid the entanglements of ethnocentrism. Providing rationale for current methods prompts analysis and objective application of practice principles.

Cultural imposition imposes the way of life of one culture on that of another. It necessitates a belief in the superiority of the prevailing manner of living and conveys compulsory adherence to accepted norms. However, if any culture and its way of life are to endure, the cultural imposition of one group must be offset by the cultural autonomy of the other. This is the point that underpins the complexities associated with multiculturalism in a pluralistic society. It can be especially problematic in a healthcare situation. In this context, those recently arrived and unaccustomed to the attitudes and values of the culture to which they are not yet accustomed initially present as a problem-solving task in the clinical encounter. Under these circumstances, culturally-controlled values and norms can become the focus of intervention as a first step in managing treatment.

THE SUBSTANCE OF NURSING: THEORY AND CULTURE

Nursing theory is the source of discipline-specific concepts. Theory suggests explanations for what nursing does that differentiate it from other branches of knowledge. Theory explains why nurses act as they do and describes how nurses should use those explanations to assist maintenance or restoration of health and well-being. The influence of culture in this schema deserves exploration.

Transcultural Nursing

Cultural diversity, or multiculturalism, is a social construct of increasing importance to the understanding of healthcare quality. Clarification of the influence of culture on the domains of nursing will be a sign of the next evolutionary stage of the profession. Issues that will move nursing forward include the influence of culture in defining excellence in patient care and the significance of culture as an applied intervention for the improvement of health.

When the concept of transcultural nursing was introduced in the 1950s, it was not viewed as relevant to nursing practice (Leininger, 1978), perhaps because nursing theory was young or because of the hegemonic views of the Euro-American culture of the time. Because the nursing profession is dynamic, it reflects the social needs and conscience of any given era (Henderson, 1966), thus the profession has come to embrace the pioneering efforts of Madeleine Leininger and her conceptualization of transcultural nursing.

Leininger defined *transcultural nursing* as "a formal area of study and practice focused on comparative human-care differences and similarities of the beliefs, values and patterned lifeways of cultures to provide culturally congruent, meaningful, and beneficial health care to people" (Leininger & McFarland, 2002, p. 6). Culture is the facilitator through which the nurse can understand and support individual needs. The full range of anthropological constructs (for example, language, group history, religion, and politics) are used as reference for a more fully developed understanding of every person and the circumstances of each individual life.

Transcultural nursing provides a holistic approach to understanding each individual within the context of the various influences on that unique life. The sunrise model includes information on the following factors: education, economic, political and legal, kinship and social, religious and philosophical, and technological. This biographical history captures the important details of a patient's life. These details provide a comprehensive depiction of the individual that serves to enhance care based in knowledge with both depth and abundant detail. Such detail implements a process for increasing familiarity with those who are dissimilar and decreases anxiety related to contact with the unknown for the healthcare provider and patient alike.

Transcultural nursing also possesses an implicit advantage. Many of the concepts that identify a holistic approach to care enable the building of an authentic relationship between patient and provider. In the practice domain, socially sensitive issues related to bias, prejudice, cultural imposition, cultural blindness, and cultural pain become part of the definition of culturally congruent care. Cultural conflict is an expected development when dissimilar groups who have minimal contact find it necessary to interact. Transcultural nursing supplies a knowledge base by which disharmony can effectively be addressed. For example, Leininger (2001) formulated a concept to describe the psychological and emotional distress experienced by patients when healthcare providers demonstrate a lack of concern for the cultural beliefs and customs of others.

As defined by Leininger and McFarland (2002), "cultural pain refers to suffering, discomfort, or being greatly offended by an individual or group who shows a great lack of sensitivity toward another's cultural experience" (p. 52). Understanding an individual within the context of their worldview is the crux of the presence or absence of cultural pain. As an example of emotional distress, cultural pain is associated with hurtful memories, damaging words that evoke those memories, insults, and indignities. It must be acknowledged that what is considered hurtful from one standpoint may not be understood as such from another. Although inflicting cultural pain is not always intentional or conscious, insensitivity can be enmeshed in a lack of awareness. Concomitant understanding and social blunders often are associated with inadequate knowledge related to cultural *triggers* that are well known to the insider but less so to the outsider. The resulting distress should not be dismissed by the person hurt simply because the deed was not intended. The prevention of a recurrence is more important and requires an exploration of context and meaning from all relevant perspectives. For example, it is a particular affront to an African American to have his or her smile described as a "big, toothy grin." This can be understood within the context of racist caricatures from the pre-civil rights era. Or the individual who speaks accented English can become sensitized to questions about citizenship status.

Understanding the elements of culture in an approach to care that is holistic is a demonstration of cultural competence. As nursing continues to refine the relevance of culturally competent care to its domain of knowledge, an understanding of cultural pain will contribute to an understanding of the impact of diversity on the healthcare system and the clinical encounters that are part of the environment of care.

Elements of culture are a route of communication to generate collaboration between a patient, family, or community and their chosen provider. Separating a culture into its component parts to guide the understanding of a particular people is a more complex process than simple fact-finding. Insight that assigns meaning is necessary if the nature and significance of culture is to have value in the care experience.

Purnell's Model for Cultural Competence

The incorporation of cultural skills and knowledge into clinical practice is facilitated by a well-grounded reference, making the gathering of information more manageable. Many culturally-based assessment tools for gathering information are very detailed. A busy practitioner would not attempt to collate, at one time, all the information suggested by the instrument. However, the culturally-prepared clinician would be mindful of important specifics suggested by these tools that would enhance the quality and usefulness of the information collected.

Larry Purnell developed a conceptual model for the culturally competent provider in 1995 that was originally intended as a nursing assessment tool (Purnell, 2002). His 12 domains of culture (2000) are relevant guideposts for the initial health history (see Table 4.2).

A guide of this nature helps to focus the interview process and draws attention to key elements of each unique cultural perspective. When information is clustered in this way, a useful care plan can be formulated from synthesized information. If this framework is used, some fore-knowledge of the cultural group is required to support a focused interview process that remains timely and is not haphazard. Not all questions need to be asked. Clinical judgment should guide the clinician. For example, once the issue of communication has been resolved, for the African American patient with a chief complaint of chest pain the initial assessment would most likely include the domains of healthcare practices and practitioners, high-risk behaviors, biocultural ecology (i.e., physical features), and nutrition to determine the most essential information for this complaint. The culturally prepared practitioner would be aware of the following:

☐ Prominence of cardiovascular disease among African Americans
☐ Possibility of traditional practices and self-adjusted dosage of medication
☐ Ability to metabolize medications
☐ "Soul" food
☐ Social history of African Americans as context for clinical encounter

CONCLUSION

Cultural diversity, or multiculturalism, is a social construct of increasing importance in understanding healthcare quality. Clarification of the influence of culture on the domains of nursing will be an indication of the next evolutionary stage of the profession. What is the influence of culture in defining excellence in patient care? What is the significance of culture as an applied intervention for the improvement of health? What is the impact of culture on interpersonal and therapeutic relationships?

Culture can be a paradigm for worldviews. In transcultural nursing, these paradigms utilize anthropological concepts to inform a nursing perspective on health and illness beliefs that orig-

Table 4.2 Purnell's Model of Cultural Domains

Heritage	Communication
Family roles	Workforce issues
Biocultural ecology	High-risk behaviors
Nutrition	Pregnancy
Death rituals	Spirituality
Healthcare practices	Healthcare practitioners

inate in the cultural life of a given society. Culture is the facilitator through which nurses can understand and support individual needs. The full range of anthropological constructs (e.g., language, group history) is used as a reference for a more fully developed understanding of every person and the context of each individual life and worldview.

Leininger and McFarland (2002) give an orientational definition of worldview as "the way an individual or group looks out on and understands their world about them as a value, stance, picture, or perspective about life or the world" (p. 83). Blacks, Hispanics, Asians, American Indians, and Caucasians have had vastly divergent social experiences in the United States. These experiences are so disparate that perspectives often are polarized. Empathy and increased cultural knowledge of other ethnic heritages are essential to the promotion of positive and more trusting clinical encounters. However, active questions stimulate discourse on Western definitions of what constitutes good care. For example, the Western philosophies of *self-care* and *out-of-bed activity* are representative of differing perspectives on wellness behavior.

As a topic of research, the value of culturally competent care to the patient remains unclear and undefined. For example, some practitioners contend that it is possible to generate a sense of well-being for a patient without undue attention to issues of culture. Also, long-established practices reframed as issues of culture (e.g., referrals to spiritual care givers or dietary consults) can be viewed as standard procedure as opposed to culture-specific care. However, cultural customs that conflict with policy and procedures (e.g., newborn-naming customs of Cambodians call for a wait of one week and the naming is done by grandparents) are clear illustrations that cultural knowledge does indicate the need for new precedents.

Culture is a form of identity. Identity is a complex concept that involves the explication of factors that, among other things, characterize cultural heritage. The ongoing exploration of the meaning of cultural identity is poised to enhance the functioning of our pluralistic society. History has shown cultural heritage can be a highly charged domain of inquiry when it involves race and ethnicity. However, knowledge-based methods of care underpin the type of practice competence that includes awareness of the human dimensions of diversity. The proficient healthcare provider is sensitive to the distinctions of difference and models a nursing process that promotes the reciprocal relationship between culture and quality care.

REFERENCES

Canales, M., & Bowers, B. (2001). Expanding conceptualizations of culturally competent care. *Journal of Advanced Nursing, 36*(1), 102–111.

Chen, Y. (2000). Chinese values, health and nursing. *Journal of Advanced Nursing, 36*(2), 270–273.

Coleman-Miller, B. (2000). A physician's perspective on minority health. *Health Care Financing Review, 21*(4), 45–56.

Day, J. C. (2005). National population projections. Retrieved February 2, 2005, from http://www.census.gov/population/www/pop-profile/natproj.html.

Fadiman, A. (1997). *The spirit catches you and you fall down*. New York, NY: Farrar, Straus, Giroux.

Global Data Center (2005). United States: Inflow of foreign-born population by country of birth, 1986 to 2003. Retrieved May 9, 2005, from http://www.migrationinformation.org/GlobalData/countrydata/data.cfm.

Henderson, V. (1966). *The nature of nursing: A definition and its implications for practice, research, and education*. New York, NY: Macmillan.

Herdman, E. (2001). The illusion of progress in nursing. *Nursing Philosophy, 2*(1), 4–13.

Holcomb, L. O., Parsons, L. C., Giger, J. N., & Davidhizar, R. (1996). Haitian Americans: Implications for nursing care. *Journal of Community Health Nursing, 13*(4), 249–460.

Horowitz, C. R., Davis, M. H., Palermo, A. G., & Vladek, B. C. (2000). Approaches to eliminating socio-cultural disparities in health. *Health Care Financing Review, (21)*4, 57–74.

Institute of Medicine (IOM) (2002). Speaking of health: Assessing health communication strategies for diverse populations. Washington, DC: Institute of Medicine.

Kim, M. J., Cho, H., Klessig, Y., Gerace, L., & Camilleri, D. (2002). Primary health care for Korean immigrants: Sustaining a culturally sensitive model. *Public Health Nursing, 19*(3), 191–200.

LaVeist, T. A., Bowie, J. V., & Cooley-Quille, M. (2000). Minority health status in adulthood: The middle years of life. *Health Care Financing Review, 21*(4), 9–21.

Leduc, N., & Proulx, M. (2004). Patterns of health services utilization by recent immigrants. *Journal of Immigrant Health, 6*(1), 15–27.

Leininger, M. (1978). *Transcultural nursing: Concepts, theories, and practices.* New York: Wiley.

Leininger, M. (2001). The theory. In M. Leininger (Ed.), *Culture care diversity and universality* (pp. 5–68). Boston: Jones and Bartlett.

Leininger, M., & McFarland, M. (2002). *Transcultural nursing: Concepts, theories, research, practice.* New York: McGraw-Hill.

Pang, S., Wong, T., Wang, C., Sheng, Z., Zhi Jun, C., Helen, Y., Lam, C., & Chan, K. (2004). Towards a Chinese definition of nursing. *Journal of Advanced Nursing, 46*(6), 657–670.

Phinney, J. (1996). When we talk about American ethnic groups, what do we mean? *American Psychologist, 31*(9), 918–927.

Purnell, L. (2000). A description of the Purnell model of cultural competence. *Journal of Transcultural Nursing, 11*(1), 40–46.

Purnell, L. (2002). The Purnell model of cultural competence. *Journal of Transcultural Nursing, 13*(13), 193–196.

Reddy, S. (2002). Temporarily insane: Pathologising cultural difference in American criminal courts. *Sociology of Health and Illness, 24*(5) 667–687.

Searight, H. (2003). Bosnian immigrants' perceptions of the United States health care system: A qualitative interview study. *Journal of Immigrant Health, 5*(2), 87–93.

Struthers, R. (2001). A conceptual framework of nursing in Native American culture. *Journal of Nursing Scholarship.* Retrieved August 5, 2004 from the HighBeam Research Database.

Williams, D. R., & Rucker, T. D. (2000). Understanding and addressing racial disparities in health care. *Health Care Financing Review, 21*(4), 75–90.

World Health Organization. Governance. Retrieved September 2, 2004, from http://www.who.int/governance/en/.

CHAPTER 5

Race, Race Relations, and the Emergence of Professional Nursing, 1870–2004

Patricia St. Hill

It is widely known that racial and ethnic minorities experience higher rates of illness and disability and die earlier than Whites. The Institute of Medicine, in its 2003 report titled *Unequal Treatment: Confronting Racial and Ethnic Disparities in Healthcare,* stated the obvious—that minorities receive inferior health care. The current national mandate is to end racial and ethnic discrimination in health care by 2010 and to increase the number of minority healthcare providers.

Barriers to ending racial discrimination can best be understood by examining the social history of the United States. Even though health disparities and minority representation in nursing span many races and ethnic cultures, history best documents this for African Americans (Sullivan Commission, 2004). This chapter examines the influence of race and race relations among Blacks and Whites in American society on the developing nursing profession as it emerged from a task-oriented vocation to a profession in its own right. In doing so, the chapter highlights several critical periods and turning points in American history and traces their reverberations and influences on the emerging nursing profession. In closing, the chapter looks to the future and attempts to predict the challenges and rewards faced by professional nursing.

THE CIVIL WAR ERA

A retrospective view of the nursing profession in the United States mirrors the country's existing sociocultural norms, beliefs, and values. Historical documentation of the social climate prior to and during the 1800s explicates the social inequities, unjust laws, and discriminatory practices that Black nurses were subjected to at the dawning of the profession. The works of Carnegie (1986), Staupers (1961), and Hine (1989) make direct linkages between the difficulties and hardships faced by Black nurses in the early years and the prevailing segregationist views of the nursing leadership, nursing organizations, and large segments of American society.

Elmore (1976), speaking to this issue, noted that there are no special records about Blacks from the earliest days of this country and argued that it was difficult to believe that the slave nursemaid did not become the nurse of the time, in "her" family at least. Similarly, George, Bradford, and Battle (1995) pointed out that a review of nursing history texts showed that "Negro" nurses were rarely mentioned as contributors to the development of the profession.

With the onset of the Civil War, some minor changes occurred, and the historical record, according to Elmore (1976), becomes clearer. During this period, the names of several early Black nurses surface. Among them are Harriet Tubman and Sojourner Truth, both of whom are well known for activities other than nursing, but they also are credited with having cared for wounded soldiers during the Civil War.

Even more widely recognized is Namahyoke Sockum Curtis, who volunteered her services during the Spanish American War and was assigned as a contract nurse by the War Department. History also shows that she later served as a Red Cross volunteer during the Galveston Flood and the San Francisco Earthquake. The ultimate recognition of her work was a government pension and burial at Arlington Cemetery (Elmore, 1976).

Despite the seeming gains and inroads made by this select group of Black nurses, American society remained very much divided along racial lines. In general, the environment for Blacks throughout the 1800s was hostile. In fact, Massey (1934), recounting the sacrifices, struggles, lack of recognition, and adversities faced by Blacks in America, parallels the history of Black nurses in America.

THE SEGREGATION LAWS AND NURSING

Nineteenth-century America was by all measures a hostile, suppressive, and dangerous place for Blacks. The indelible need to dominate and control a perceived inferior group persisted under the guise of the Jim Crow laws, a series of discriminatory laws in the Southern states that called for the separation of the races. Under Jim Crow, segregation of the races was the order of the day. This social custom prevailed and was supported legally in the 1896 Supreme Court ruling of *Plessy vs. Ferguson*. Furthermore, under these laws, the notion of separate but equal was contrived and promulgated to justify the rigid segregation laws that imposed legal punishment on people for consorting with members of another race and that served to divide all of American society, as well as the emerging nursing profession, along racial lines.

The healthcare system post-Civil War to the late 1960s was composed of two separate and unequal systems—one for Whites and a considerably more inferior one for Blacks. As one woman put it:

> Dr. Bailey on Main Street in Greenville was our family physician. There was a separate waiting room for Blacks and you had to wait 'til all the White patients were seen before he'd see the blacks. As long as White patients kept coming in, you kept being pushed further and further back. (Smith, 1999, as cited in Sullivan Commission, 2004, p. 32)

Black nursing students, for the most part, were excluded from White hospital-based nursing programs and were relegated to Black-operated schools, whose curricula and programs have been described as deplorable (Pitts-Mosley, 1995). A select few Blacks were provided limited access to White schools in accordance with strictly enforced institutional quotas. It should also be pointed out that educational barriers and challenges existed in both the Northern and the Southern states for Black women interested in pursuing a nursing career. Pitts-Mosley (1995) noted that although Black codes limiting access to practice opportunities and to institutions of learning were legislated and enforced by law in the Southern states, they also were observed and enforced unofficially in the North, a phenomenon frequently referred to as *de facto segregation*.

For example, The New England Hospital for Women and Children in Boston, Massachusetts, although renowned for having graduated America's first Black trained nurse, Mary Mahoney, in 1879, nonetheless employed the quota system, limiting the number of Blacks admitted each year to two. This number was later altered to include one Black and one Jewish student (Carnegie, 1986).

Between 1886 and 1977, 77 schools for "Negroes" had been established in 20 states and the District of Columbia (Carnegie, 1986). For the women attending Black-operated programs, many of which were, in actuality, lead by white superintendents, curricula and programs were less than adequate. Documented evidence points to curricula deficiencies, lack of resources, and inadequately trained teachers. Admittedly, the majority of nursing schools (both Black and White) operating during the late 1800s and early 1900s were plagued by inadequacies, including poorly designed or nonexistent curricula. This prompted the establishment of the American Society of Superintendents of Training Schools of Nurses (The Superintendents' Society) in 1893, which later became the National League for Nursing Education (NLNE), and then the National League for Nursing (NLN).

The purpose of The Superintendents' Society was to improve nursing curricula and develop standards of admissions to schools of nursing (Bullough & Bullough, 1978). These actions contributed to the advancement and professionalization of nursing; however, they were of no benefit to Black nurses. For Black, or "Negro," schools, the lack of support and recognition from professional nursing organizations such as the NLNE and the American Nurses Association (ANA) undermined their legitimacy and called into question their professional standing. It was not until 1942 that the NLNE offered individual membership to Black nurses, whose many previous attempts to gain membership had been systematically denied (Champinha-Bacote, 1988). In 1948, six years later, the ANA finally extended its membership to Black nurses.

Nursing Practice Under the Segregation Laws

Upon graduating from nurse training programs, Black nurses faced the challenges of limited practice opportunities and lower wages than their White counterparts. As a general rule, the practice of Black nurses was limited to caring for Black clients either in the home, as private-duty nurses, or in the hospital. The prevailing sentiment was that "Colored" or "Negro" nurses were best suited to care for "Colored" patients (Carnegie, 1986; Staupers, 1961). It was common practice for Black student nurses to care for Black patients in the home, as private duty nurses, without supervision. This practice, although inarguably dangerous and unsafe for both clients and nursing students, was, nonetheless, routine with Black schools that relied on the monies paid to the students (Pitts-Mosley, 1996).

With the establishment of public health nursing at the Henry Street Settlement in 1893, the few Black nurses hired by Lillian Wald, founder and director of the Henry Street Settlement Visiting Nursing Service, were afforded the opportunity to extend their practice into this arena of nursing (Pitts-Mosley, 1996). Still, the pervasive inequities that haunted the profession persisted and were intimately tied to three issues. The first was the educational structure in place for training Black and White nurses separately, which prevented disadvantaged Black nurses from receiving a high-quality education. The second was the administration of separate licensing examinations for Black and White nurses, which served only to further divide the profession along racial lines. The third issue was the exclusion of Black nurses from membership and representation in professional organizations, such as the ANA and the NLNE, hence denying Black nurses and Black nursing practice legitimacy within a system that already had preconceived notions about the competence of Black nursing programs and their graduates.

Racial Quotas and the Wars (1901–1951)

The 20th century was witness to two major world wars, World War I (1914–1918) and World War II (1939–1945), both of which created additional demands for nurses to care for wounded soldiers. Typically, under conditions of a reasonably normal nursing supply, race is one of several characteristics, along with age, education, sex, and marital status, that are taken into account in the hiring and acceptance of nurses. In the face of necessity, such as war, however, the characteristics least relevant to professional performance are dropped, and individuals who can fulfill minimum standards, such as having a license as a professional nurse, get their chance (Goldstein, 1960). In the case of the U.S. military, however, despite its desperate need for nurses to care for wounded soldiers during World War I, the use of Black nurses was not an option. It took the flu epidemic of 1918 to see the first 18 Black nurses accepted and assigned to army camps in Ohio and Illinois, with other assignments to follow (Elmore, 1976).

In 1943, the Cadet Nurse Corps was established to address the acute nursing shortage caused by World War II. Students who signed on would receive reimbursement for tuition, books, uniforms, and a monthly stipend if they agreed to complete one year of military or civilian nursing for the remainder of the war. By 1944, the Corps was recruiting both Black and White nursing students, and 2000 Black nursing students were enrolled. However, even though the National Nursing Council for War Service urged that all qualified nurses—regardless of race—be appointed to military service, most Black nurses were still denied service. The army set a small quota for the number of Black nurses it was willing to accept; by the end of the war in 1945, there were only 479 Black nurses out of 50,000 members of the Army Nurse Corps (Bellafaire, 2000). Notably, all of them were confined to segregated areas of the South or sent overseas to care for Black troops (Kalisch & Kalisch, 2004). Because the War Department set a quota of 10% for Black troops, recruiting more nurses was problematic, as illustrated by this statement in a rejection letter sent to an applicant for the Army: "colored nurses are authorized for assignment only to those stations where colored troops predominate" (Kalisch & Kalisch, 2004, p. 369). The Navy did not accept Black nurses until 1945. Kalisch and Kalisch (2004) note that, had both military branches taken advantage of the numbers of Black nurses in the Cadet Nurse Corps, each would have enlisted at least 1520 nurses.

Organizing for Strength

Barred from professional affiliation or membership, especially in the Southern states, Black nurses as early as 1901 realized that the problems of discrimination and segregation they faced could only be overcome through collective action. In 1901, Black graduates of established schools in New York, Washington, D.C., and Chicago organized alumnae associations. By 1908, under the leadership of Martha Franklin, Black nurses organized at the national level (Carnegie, 1992). The organization, which came to be known as the National Association of Colored Graduate Nurses (NACGN), lasted from 1908 until 1951. The organization's goals were to (Pitts-Mosley, 1995):

☐ Achieve higher professional standards for Black nurses
☐ Breakdown discriminatory practices in schools of nursing, in jobs, and in nursing organizations
☐ Develop leadership among "Negro" nurses

By the time the NACGN was dissolved in 1951, because its leaders felt that the organization had accomplished its mission and there was no justification for its continued existence, its members had fought discrimination on all fronts. It had fought especially hard for the integration of Black nurses into the ANA (Carnegie, 1992).

Another recognizable strength of the NACGN, although little recognized by prominent White nursing leaders during its early years, was its ability to form alliances with and gain the support of powerful groups and individuals able to further the cause of the Black nurse. For example, Lillian Wald displayed her faith in Black nurses by hiring three Black nurses in the Visiting Nursing Service in New York (Staupers, 1961). Other support for the NACGN came from the National Medical Association (NMA), the Black physicians' professional organization. The NMA invited the NACGN to hold meetings simultaneously in the same cities and published nurses' articles in its journals (Davis, 1999).

LOWERING THE RACIAL BARRIERS

The 1950s through the early 1970s was one of the most turbulent periods in American history. Hallmarked by the enactment of antidiscrimination and civil rights legislation, beginning with the Eisenhower administration in the 1950s and the Civil Rights Movement in the 1960s, parts of American society were ready and willing to embrace desegregation and observe antidiscriminatory laws. The South, however, remained highly resistant to change. The Civil Rights Act of 1964, passed by the Johnson administration, which prohibited racial discrimination in institutions receiving federal funding, dealt a blow to the segregationists.

Within nursing, the winds of change sweeping the nation also were being felt. The gains that had been achieved by Black nurses up to this point, such as the establishment of the NACGN, collaboration with the NMA, acceptance into the military, and integration into the ANA, were about to be expanded. These gains were consistent with the steady and purposeful strides nursing was making toward establishing itself as a profession. This included the initiation of nursing research and nursing theory development (Schultz, 1990). The profession not only backed away from its previous separatist policies, but took decisive action to lower racial barriers and integrate Black nurses into hospitals. Unprecedented studies on the integration of "Negro" nurses into the workforce were undertaken. Several research articles and editorials addressing civil rights and integration issues were published in some of nursing's most prestigious journals (Goldstein, 1960). In an *American Journal of Nursing* article, for example, Goldstein studied how the services of Negro nurses were being utilized on the nursing staffs of several hospitals. The study findings suggested that technological know-how and specialized skills were more of a determinant for employment in hospitals than race. Goldstein went on to note that as educational standards in professional nursing were raised, the "Negro" nurse with special preparation could qualify for a position for which preferred personnel (White nurses) were scarce. As such, the technical competence stressed in all nursing jobs became almost the sole criterion for acceptability in highly skilled specialties.

Goldstein made clear, however, that the "Negro" nurse, as a less-preferred type, would lose out on promotions. She went on to assert that the trend toward specific educational requirements for particular positions, such as head nurse, would work to the ultimate advantage of those "Negro" nurses who take advantage of training. Yet in the hospitals studied, Negro nurses still faced a status dilemma that needed to be solved in order for the hospitals to function smoothly. Goldstein urged a deemphasis on race and a greater focus on professional status and skills.

A July 1964 article appearing in the *American Journal of Nursing* entitled, "Problems of Integration" reported on the difficulty of the ANA to get certain districts, such as the New Orleans district, to comply with the ANA's admission policy and practices. The New Orleans district still barred "Negro" nurses from membership. Issuing an ultimatum, the ANA warned the Louisiana State Nurses Association that the state would be disqualified as an ANA constituent if its practices in the New Orleans district were not corrected by January 1, 1965 (Staupers, 1961). Further, advocating on behalf of the "Negro" nurse, a delegate from Michigan called on the ANA to help districts not only to admit "Negro" nurses, but to help them participate. Staupers also examined the integration of "Negro" nursing in the United States. The April 1965 copy of the *American Journal of Nursing* ran an article on how two nurses had integrated a nursing staff that had long been completely segregated.

From the 1950s to the 1970s, there was a significant shift in nursing's race and race relations policies, which had once intentionally erected barriers that excluded Black nurses from membership in professional nursing organizations, from participation in the mainstream of nursing, and from equal access to hospital-based employment.

THE NURSING SHORTAGE AND MINORITY CONSIDERATIONS

The new millennium has brought with it a tremendous shift in the demographics of the nursing workforce. In addition, a nursing shortage is looming in the distance. Just as nursing has seemed to be emerging as a true science- and research-based profession, evidenced by the successful integration of nursing theory, research, and practice (Schultz, 1990), it is experiencing one of the largest and most serious nursing shortages ever.

In 2002, the Health Resources and Services Administration estimated that 30 states had shortages of Registered Nurses in 2000. It predicted that these shortages will intensify over the next 20 years. In February 2004, the U.S. Bureau of Labor Statistics predicted that more than 1 million new and replacement nurses will be needed by the year 2012. In a similar vein, reports from the American Association of Colleges of Nursing (AACN) have predicted a 20% shortage of Registered Nurses by the year 2020, translating into a shortage of over 400,000 Registered Nurses nationwide (AACN, 2004).

Factors contributing to this gloomy outlook include: (1) lower enrollments in schools of nursing (enrollments in 2001 were 17% lower than in 1995); (2) a shortage of faculty in schools of nursing, which is expected to increase dramatically in the next decade; (3) the increasing age of nurses due to the aging baby boom generation and the lowered numbers of people entering the profession; and (4) burnout and dissatisfaction, as reported in several studies (AACN, 2004).

Evidence shows that staffing shortages contribute to increased mortality. A landmark study by Aiken and colleagues (2003) found that nurses reported greater job dissatisfaction and emotional exhaustion when they were responsible for more patients than they could care for safely. They also found that burnout and job dissatisfaction predicted nurses' intentions to leave their jobs within a year. Similarly, Goodin (2003) conducted an integrative review of the literature and found that, in addition to the reasons for the shortage presented earlier, the lingering poor image of nursing and the wide range of professional occupations now open to women also contribute to the nursing shortage. Substantiation of Goodin's findings came from the National Sample Survey of Registered Nurses (U.S. Department of Health and Human Services, 2001). The National Sample Survey showed that in March 2000, a total of 135,696 Registered Nurses were not employed in nursing, with a total of 72,568, or 53%, employed in non–health-related occupations. This survey found that the two most important reasons for the prevailing nursing shortage were inconvenient working hours (44.9%) and poor salaries (35.4%).

To fill the nursing gap, the recruitment of minorities into the profession seems a logical step. However, because of the many career options now available to women and the public's unfavorable perception of nursing as a career choice, particularly in minority communities, few minority youngsters are choosing nursing as a career. In fact, statistical data emanating from the U.S. Department of Health and Human Services (US DHHS, 2003) show that members of minority groups, although accounting for about 30% of the U.S. population, make up a mere 12% of the current nursing workforce. These dismal minority statistics, viewed in light of existing nurse shortages and the recognition of minorities as viable additions to the nursing workforce, has prompted legislative action at several governmental levels aimed at narrowing the remaining racial disparities in professional nursing.

Government Intervention

Corrective actions aimed at increasing the number of minorities choosing to pursue nursing as a career came in the form of 16 Nursing Workforce Diversity grant awards from the DHHS in June 2003, totaling nearly $3.5 million to support nursing education opportunities for individuals from disadvantaged backgrounds. The grants were slated to fund scholarships or stipends and pre-entry preparation and retention activities for disadvantaged students, including students from racial and ethnic minority groups that are underrepresented among registered nurses. Minority enrollment in the nursing schools that received the grants averaged 38%, about double the national average of 19%. According to US DHHS Secretary Tommy G. Thompson, "these schools and programs have proven their ability to enroll and graduate competent, skilled health care workers, which is important in expanding access to health care for all Americans" (US DHHS, 2003, p. 1). He went on to note that the grants would encourage minority students to enter the field of nursing and help alleviate the critical shortage. In July 2004, DHHS announced an additional $15.5 million to expand and strengthen the nursing workforce, with $5.4 million earmarked for the Nursing Workforce Diversity Program (US DHHS, 2004).

Nursing Intervention

Several prominent nursing organizations are at the forefront of this move toward increasing minority recruitment into professional nursing. The AACN declared that as the United States struggles to find solutions to the current nursing shortage, nursing schools need to strengthen their efforts to attract more men and minority students (AACN Bulletin, 2001). To these ends, the NLN also has been very active by way of its legislative agenda. One element of its legislative package has been asking for increased funding for minority and disadvantaged students.

In an April 26, 2001 testimonial before the National Advisory Council on Nurse Education and Practice (NACNEP), Ruth D. Corcoran, Chief Executive Officer of the NLN pointed to the NLN's joint and dedicated effort in concert with that of the NACNEP in awakening health care stakeholders in academia, the industry, and government to the long-term effects of leaving major portions of our population substantially out of nursing—primarily, ethnic/racial minorities as well as males (Corcoran, 2001).

Further, statistical data emanating from DHHS, Health Resources and Service Administration Bureau of Health Professions shows that even when these underrepresented groups (minorities and men) pursue a nursing education, Associate degree programs attract a great percentage of them (US DHHS, HRSA, 2000). Accordingly, Corcoran proposed several recommendations for improving access to nursing education programs for groups traditionally underrepresented in nursing. Among these were:

1. Creating partnerships among colleges and universities, pre-college and college institutions, industry, professional societies, and communities that formulate and maintain effective grassroots career awareness activities for K–12 and re-entry students, as well as their teachers, parents, and professional mentors.
2. Commitment in resources and the will to establish the networks and academic enrichment services, which have proven to be labor-and-time intensive, for successful academic advising, tutoring, and general nurturing of the student.
3. Financial assistance to enable disadvantaged students to pursue nursing studies (Corcoran, 2001).

The Importation of Foreign Nurses

One solution to nursing shortages in the United States has historically been the importation of foreign nurses, the majority of whom are people of color coming from underdeveloped and developing countries, such as India, the Philippines, and the Caribbean. Concordant with these recruitment efforts, Congress has passed needed legislation to facilitate the immigration of foreign nurses. For example, the Immigration Nursing Relief Acts of 1986, 1989, and 1990 provided nonimmigrant visas (H-1A) to international nurses hired to fill vacancies in U.S. hospitals (Flynn & Aiken, 2002). Also, the Nursing Relief to Disadvantaged Areas Act of 1999 addressed the nursing shortage in underserved rural and urban areas that are generally difficult to staff. This piece of legislation allowed for the issuance of a maximum of 500 nonimmigrant visas (H-1C) per year to international nurses employed in designated health professional shortage areas, as defined by the US DHHS. Unlike this legislative action, which was viewed as essential and needed, the Immigration Nursing Relief Act, because of political pressure, was allowed to "sunset" (Flynn & Aiken, 2002).

Admittedly, the importation of foreign nurses is a short-term solution to a much larger problem inherent in the U.S. healthcare system (Joel, 1996). Critics, such as the ANA, also question the ethics of importing nurses from other countries during a global nursing shortage. Luring skilled nurses from other countries robs their native countries of talented nurses and increases the global nursing shortage. Additionally, the ANA is concerned about exploiting workers once they begin working in substandard conditions, because many of them are hired to replace American nurses who leave due to deteriorating working conditions (Trossman, 2003).

FACING THE CHALLENGES OF TOMORROW

Gone are the days of Jim Crow and state-mandated segregation laws that curtailed the professional training, practice, and earnings of Black nurses. The major challenge confronting professional nursing today and tomorrow is the disappearance of a qualified replacement nursing workforce to replace the aging baby-boom generation of nurses, the majority of whom are at, or rapidly approaching, retirement age.

Today more than ever before the doors of opportunity are open to African Americans and other minorities interested in pursuing a nursing career or advanced preparation in nursing. However, the question that remains is whether White nurses and the power structure within nursing are committed and/or prepared to share the power base in professional nursing with African Americans and other minority nurses. The Cleveland Council of Black Nurses (CCBN) believes that old habits and racial stereotypes are hard to kill. Pointing to the high attrition rates among African American nursing students around the country, the CCBN describes a "revolving door syndrome," and notes that the growing body of literature documents the difficulties of African American nursing students. They report feelings of estrangement and isolation on campus; pressure to conform to stereotypes; less equitable treatment by faculty, staff, and teaching assistants; and more faculty racism than other students of color. The CCBN noted a parallel between the occurrences of "today" and those of "yesterday," when White nurse educators and administrators took no responsibility for negative attitudes and discriminatory practices that excluded "Negroes" from admission into nursing programs and limited their employment opportunities (George, Bradford, & Battle, 1995).

Many predict that the appearance of the future nursing workforce will look quite different. In the final analysis, this may indeed be true. George, Bradford, and Battle (1995) remind us that our "tomorrow" rests in the minds, hearts, commitments, motivation, and achievements of African American nursing students and nurses, along with the commitment of all nurses, to the values and ideals of the nursing profession.

REFERENCES

AACN Bulletin (2001). Effective strategies for increasing diversity in nursing programs. Retrieved October 7, 2004 from www.aacn.ncheedu/publications/issues/dec01.

AACN (2004). Nursing shortage resources. Retrieved January 12, 2005, from www.aacn.nche.edu/Media/shortageresource.htm#about.

Aiken, L. H., Clarke, S. P., Cheung, R. B., Sloane, D. M., & Silber, J. H. (2003). Educational levels of hospital nurses and surgical patient mortality. *JAMA, 290*(12), 1617–1623.

Bellafaire, J. A. (2000). Black nurses in WWII. Retrieved January 12, 2005, from www.ww2medicine.org/black.html.

Bullough, V. L., & Bullough, B. (1978). *The emergence of modern nursing.* New York: MacMillan.

Carnegie, M. E. (1986). *The path we thread: Blacks in nursing, 1854–1984.* New York: J.B. Lippincott Company.

Carnegie, M. E. (1992). Black nurses in the United States: 1879–1992. *Journal of National Black Nurses' Association, 6*(1), 13–18.

Champinha-Bacote, J. (1988). The Black nurses' struggle toward equality: An historical account of the National Association of Colored Graduate Nurses. *Journal of National Black Nurses' Association, 2*(2), 15–25.

Corcoran, R. E. (2001). Testimony of the NLN before the National Advisory Council on Nurse Education and Practice. April 26, 2001. Silver Spring, MD.

Davis, A. T. (1999). *Early Black American leaders in nursing: Architects for integration and equality.* Boston: Jones and Bartlett.

Elmore, J. A. (1976). Black nurses: Their service and their struggle. *American Journal of Nursing, 76*(3), 435–437.

Flynn, L., & Aiken, L. H. (2002). Does international nurse recruitment influence practice values in U.S. hospitals? *American Journal of Nursing Scholarship, 34*(1), 67–72.

George, V. D., Bradford, D. M., & Battle, A. (1995).Yesterday, today & tomorrow. *Nursing and Health Care Perspectives, 21*(5), 219–227.

Goldstein, R. L. (1960). Negro nurses in hospitals. *American Journal of Nursing, 60*(2), 215–218.

Goodin, H. J. (2003). The nursing shortage in the United States of America: An integrative review of the literature. *Journal of Advanced Nursing, 43*(4), 335–343.

Hine, D. C. (1989). *Black women in white: Racial conflict and cooperation in the nursing profession, 1890–1950.* Bloomington: Indiana University Press.

Institute of Medicine (2003). *Unequal treatment: Confronting racial and ethnic disparities in healthcare.* Washington, DC: Institute of Medicine.

Joel, L. A. (1996). Immigration: Why is it still up for discussion? *American Journal of Nursing, 96*(1), 7–8.

Kalisch, P. A., & Kalisch, B. J. (2004). *American nursing, A history (*4th ed.). Philadelphia: Lippincott, Williams, & Wilkins.

Massey, E. (1934). The Negro nurse student. *American Journal of Nursing, 34*, 608–610.

Pitts-Mosley, M. O. (1995). Despite all odds: A three-part history of the professionalization of Black nurses through two professional nursing organizations, 1908–1995. *Journal of National Black Nurses' Association, 7*(2), 10–19.

Schultz, P. R. (1990). Milestones in the success of nursing as an emerging discipline. *American Journal of Pharmaceutical Education, 54* (Winter), 370–373.

Smith, D. B. (1999). *Health care divided: Race and healing a nation.* Ann Arbor: University of Michigan Press.

Staupers, M. K. (1961). *No time for prejudice: A story of the integration of Negroes in nursing in the United States.* New York: MacMillian.

Sullivan Commission (2004). *Missing persons: Minorities in the Health Professions.* Washington, DC: The Sullivan Commission.

Trossman, S. (2003). The global reach of the nursing shortage: The American Nurses' Association questions the ethics of luring foreign-educated nurses to the United States. *Nevada RNformation, 12*(1), 25.

US DHHS, HRSA (2000). The registered nurse population: Findings from the national sample survey of registered nurses. Retrieved October 4, 2004, from http://bhpr.hrsa.gov/healthworkforce/reports/rnsurvey/rnss1.htm.

US DHHS (2001). The registered nurse population: Findings from the 2000 National Sample Survey. Retrieved January 12, 2005, from http://bhpr.hrsa.gov/healthworkforce/reports/rnsurvey/default.htm.

US DHHS (2003). HHS Awards nearly $3.5 million to promote diversity in the nursing workforce. Retrieved October 7, 2004, from http://www.os.hhs.gov/news/press/2003pres/20030602.html.

US DHHS (2004). HHS Awards $15.5 Million to Expand, Strengthen Nursing Workforce. Retrieved October 7, 2004, from http://www.hhs.gov/news/press/2004pres/20040722.html.

CHAPTER 6

Exploring Migration and Health

Sharon McGuire

Both popular and professional literature attest to the significance of migration as one of the most critical issues of the 21st century (Hovy, 2002; Matthei, 1999; Parfit, 1998; Sussex Center for Migration Research, 2004). It has become a topic for scholarly research among the social science disciplines and a focus of conferences, seminars, and academic majors. The topic of migration also sparks debate within various governments around the world. The prestigious Worldwatch Institute associates increasing human migration with both population increases and economic globalization, noting that the free movement of capital and goods is not commensurately accompanied by the free movement of labor (Daly, 2004). These trends will dramatically change the world as we know it, as more persons find their regional economies in shambles and therefore will be forced to leave home to find work, often without authorization from the country of destination. Since the latter part of the 20th century, international migration has expanded in historically unprecedented ways. Today, an estimated 175,000,000 to 185,000,000 people live outside their country of natal origin, doubling the number of international migrants in the last 35 years. By the year 2050, the number of non-nationals living abroad will equal or surpass 250,000,000 (Deen, 2003; IOM, 2003).

Rapidly shifting demographics due to migration have profound implications for both sending and receiving countries and will likely contribute to high-priority policy formulations directed to migrant flows in receiving countries. Migrant advocates contend that the root causes of migration and widening economic disparities must be the focus of attention and action to address the phenomenon, rather than establishing prescriptive measures targeted at migrants and immigrants (BBC, 2000).

The stresses associated with migration have significant implications for health. Because roughly half of all migrants and immigrants are women who generally are responsible for the health of their families, this topic is critical for nursing.

NURSING AND MIGRATION

Organized nursing has recognized that global migration is salient to the profession by issuing a formal declaration. In 1995, the American Academy of Nursing (AAN) focused its annual conference on human population movements and their implications for the health of the world's migrants and refugees (AAN, 1995). Although Western nursing has a long history of caring for the health and well-being of immigrants, this document represented the first official acknowledgment within professional nursing of the nature, scope, and critical health issues inherent in world population movements.

This chapter presents an overview of the historical foundations of nursing with immigrant communities and a discussion of contemporary human migration patterns and trends, their roots, and their health exigencies in the context of a postmodern, postcolonial world. A global environment of rapid social, political, economic, and ecological upheavals presents formidable challenges to nurses in providing competent and appropriate health care to migrant populations. Nurses must also develop an understanding of how complex, interrelated power relations operate to produce migrants tearing people away from their roots and communities. Such an understanding can lead nurses engaged in clinical practice, education, and research to participate in the transforming actions of an emancipatory nursing praxis that influences migration policies and politics, and ultimately the health of migrant, immigrant, and refugee communities in positive ways.

An emancipatory nursing praxis apropos to health care with new diasporas of immigrants would be adapted to 21st-century realities, yet be anchored solidly in the historical tradition of Lillian Wald, who is acknowledged as the founder of public health nursing in the United States, and the work of nurses with immigrants during earlier periods of U.S. history (Daniels, 1989; Davis, 1984; Davis & Haasis, 1920; Silverstein, 1985; Wald, 1991). Because migration is a worldwide phenomenon, I will employ both a global view and a regional view from a North American, particularly U.S., perspective.

HISTORICAL FOUNDATIONS OF
U.S. NURSING AND IMMIGRANT HEALTH

Nursing in the United States has a long history of dedication to the health and well-being of immigrants, who bring with them health beliefs, practices, and behaviors that may clash with predominant biomedical thought, theory, and healthcare delivery models typical of Western societies. Migrants also bring with them personal and collective political, economic, and ecological histories that have exerted influences on their health and well-being, either in positive or negative ways. Some arrive as survivors of torture, bearing the scars and trauma of horrific persecution, in addition to other losses of great magnitude (Moreno & Grodin, 2000). Impoverished immigrants might end up in squalid living conditions and in working conditions that are inimical to health and potentially threatening in terms of morbidity and mortality. The work done by many poor immigrants has been described as the "3Ds"—dirty, dangerous, and difficult (Stalker, 2001; Walter, 2002).

From the era of Lillian Wald, Mary Brewster, and their colleagues more than a century ago to the present, nurses have searched for ways to appreciate the influence of cultural characteristics on the health of immigrant communities. These early pioneering nurses also struggled to understand the societal influences on immigrant health and pushed for policy changes at the local, regional, and national levels to enhance the health and well-being of immigrant communities. In response to the miserable conditions she witnessed in the tenements where new immigrants from Eastern and Southern Europe lived, Wald founded the Henry Street Settlement in 1895 (http://www.henrystreet.org) on New York's Lower East Side (Eisman, 1976). Wald, Brewster, and their companions took a dual approach to immigrant health. They capitalized on the strengths and abilities they discovered within immigrant women by recognizing their Old World handicrafts, cultures, and customs; teaching them childcare; enhancing their nutritional knowledge and status; and providing the women with a range of other classes and health services at the Henry Street Settlement and through the Visiting Nurse Service.

Lillian Wald also was concerned with the sickening conditions in which many immigrants lived and worked. Together with her colleagues, she sought ways to remedy the social context of immigrants' lives. Wald believed that "the call to the nurse is not only for the bedside care of the sick, but to help in seeking out the deep-lying basic causes of illness and misery, that in the future there may be less sickness to nurse and to cure" (Wald, 1991, p. 65). As a member of the Social Reform Club, she knew how to network with other concerned social activists, such as lawyers, doctors, journalists, and social workers, to understand these conditions, strategize for solutions, and influence government officials to create policies favorable to the daily lives of immigrants. For example, due to the abhorent child labor practices she witnessed, Wald conceived of the idea of a federal children's bureau that would publicize data about the status of children throughout the country. This idea came to fruition when Congress established the Children's Bureau in 1912.

Wald's outstanding reputation as a nurse social activist and a supporter of union organizing led to an official appointment by the governor of New York to study the problem of the exploitation of immigrants in the workplace. This appointment led to New York State's establishment of the Bureau of Industries and Immigration to protect immigrant workers from exploitation. Immigrant women also became social and political activists in the arenas of workers' rights and women's rights, including reproductive rights, children's issues, the abolitionist movement, communitarianism, and other progressive social movements (Schwartz-Seller, 1994).

Wald and her colleagues carried out these activities during the first wave of U.S. feminism—the suffragettes' struggle for women's right to vote. As a public figure, Wald described the intelligence of immigrant women at the first referendum on the women's vote in 1915 as a way to counteract negative stereotypes of immigrants perpetrated by nativists. Ever an impassioned advocate, Wald ensured that people would know of the great contributions immigrants made through their ambition, labor, culture, and creativity to national life and the good of the country (Daniels, 1989; Eisman, 1976; Silverstein, 1985; Wald, 1991).

After Wald

As the 20th century progressed, public health nurses concerned themselves with sensitivity to culture and language issues in order to work effectively among immigrant communities. However, as nursing moved to hospital-based practice, nurses lost their belief in the role of social activism as a valid nursing approach to resolving health problems and enhancing well-being (Davis & Haasis, 1920; Kleffel, 2003). Nursing became more focused on the individual and the family rather than attending to the social roots of disease.

During the latter half of the 20th century, the contributions of nurse anthropologists led to a realization of the role of culture in shaping health beliefs, practices, and behaviors, moving notions of cultural sensitivity and competence along an evolutionary trajectory. Leininger is credited as the founder of transcultural nursing and with fostering an awareness of the importance of cultural consciousness and competence in the discipline (Davis, 1984; Davis & Haasis, 1920; DeSantis, 1990; Dougherty & Tripp-Reimer, 1985; Leininger, 1995; Meleis, 1997; Silverstein, 1985). Nurses with doctorates in anthropology used cultural concepts and anthropological methods to guide the bulk of nursing research on the immigrant health phenomena. The subsequent trend in developing culture concepts, based on principles of Western anthropology, has focused largely on human behavior, practices, and health-belief models, rather than on societal influences on health (Kleffel, 2003; McGuire, 1998).

The Late 20th Century and the New Millennium

Contemporary nurse scholars have conducted health research with numerous immigrant and refugee populations, such as the Hmong (Cheon-Klessig, Camilleri, Elmurry, & Ohlson, 1988; Helsel & Mochel, 2002; Johnson, 2002); Cambodians (Kulig, 1995; Lenart, Clair, & Bell, 1991); Filipinas (Hautman, 1996); Korean women (Elliott, Berman, & Kim, 2002; Im, Lee, & Park, 2002; Park, Yoo, & Chang, 2002; Park, Kim, Kang, & Chun, 2001); Latinas (Juarbe, Turok, & Perez-Stable, 2002; Villarruel, Harlow, Lopez, & Sowers, 2002); Haitians (Santana & Dancy, 2000); and other ethnic and social immigrant groups.

More recently, Meleis (1991) and Lipson with numerous colleagues (Lipson, Hosseini, Kabir, Omidian, et al., 1995; Lipson & Miller, 1994; Lipson & Omidian, 1997) who have conducted studies on Middle Eastern women's immigrant experiences and their influence on health, have advanced theories of transitions and other research frameworks for understanding immigrant women's health. These pioneering scholars have urged nursing to prioritize research on the health concerns and experiences of marginalized immigrant women to develop appropriate nursing interventions that facilitate the health and well-being of immigrant women and their families (Meleis, 1997; Meleis, Arruda, Lane, & Bernal, 1994). Messias (2002) has reported on the transnational health practices and patterns of immigrant Brazilian women in the United States, contributing to knowledge of how immigrant Brazilian women cross borders to take advantage of health assets in other countries. McGuire and Georges (2003) highlight some of the health issues faced by undocumented women from Oaxaca, Mexico.

Nurses are revitalizing nursing's tradition of social activism by understanding historical antecedents to migration, paying attention to environmental contexts for health, and focusing on the health of excluded and marginalized ethnic communities, heavily populated by people of color and the nation's newest immigrants (Butterfield, 1990; Butterfield, 2002; Chopoorian, 1986; Drevdahl, 1995; Hall, Stevens, & Meleis, 1994; Kendall, 1992; Kleffel, 1996; McGuire & Georges, 2003; McGuire, 1998; Meleis, 1996, 1997).

New immigrants are less likely to access health care and have the economic ability to pay for health care and are more likely to be misunderstood by health professionals or receive substandard care from health professionals due to bias, thus contributing to disparities in access and in health status (Kalofonos & Palinkas, 1999; Levin, 2001; Meleis, 1996). Although the United States is a country of immigrants, contemporary migration is a poorly understood phenomenon, making it vulnerable to many negative myths. Migration requires updated theories from both a historical and a nursing perspective to sort out the bewildering array of migration patterns that can lead to a more contextualized understanding of immigrants and their lives.

ANTHROPOLOGICAL PERSPECTIVES AND THE HISTORY OF MIGRATION

Having discovered the use of fire, the first humans, *Homo erectus*, kicked off migration when they left Africa about 1,500,000 years ago and settled in northern climates. By 200,000 years ago, *Homo sapiens* populated most of the Old World in small numbers. By the end of the Ice Age 12,000 years ago, East Asians had discovered and disseminated their numbers from the Arctic region to Tierra del Fuego at the southern tip of Chile (Bancroft, 1998; Westin, 1996). This human penchant to move, seek, and find continues to this day.

By 1900, Europeans had colonized much of the non-European world, beginning with the British colonization of Ireland that started with the invasion of Normandy in 1166. Later, Great Britain, Spain, Portugal, France, Germany, and other Western European countries fanned out across the seas to conquer and colonize much of the non-European world, which was inhabited by native peoples of color, multitudes of cultures and languages, and sustainable economic practices and systems, agricultures, and civilizations. Some 60,000,000 Europeans, including 20,000,000 people from England, participated in this first great tide of migrants, the modern world's first boat people (Castles & Miller, 1998; Crosby, 1986; Metress, 1997; Miller, 1985; Stalker, 2001). Some of the first European migrants also enslaved millions of Africans, dispersing them throughout their colonies in South America, North America, the Caribbean, and the Arabian Peninsula, forming the great African Diaspora. This unspeakable trauma of capture and forced migration, known as the Middle Passage, is remembered as a shameful legacy of humankind (Bancroft, 1998; Castles & Miller, 1998; Clarke, 2003; Kane, 1995).

Both Great Britain and Spain formed vast empires with the riches they expropriated from conquered lands and from the wealth generated from slave labor. Many native peoples were displaced, impoverished, disenfranchised, and oppressed within new colonial structures and colonial legal systems (Cockcroft, 1998; Golden, McConnell, Mueller, Poppen, & Turkovich, 1991; Maiguashca, 1994; Stannard, 1992). Colonization left a legacy of infectious diseases, initiating the "microbial unification" (Berlinguer, 1999, p. 582) of the world with imported communicable diseases that decimated native populations.

Racism was another legacy of colonization. For aboriginal peoples, scores of epidemics constituted a form of early bioterrorism, and early Anglo settlers deliberately infected Indians with smallpox-saturated blankets (Cook, 1998; Stannard, 1992). Smallpox and measles were the two greatest killers, but malaria, yellow fever, diphtheria, cholera, typhus, and typhoid fever also contributed to the deaths of indigenes, who were especially vulnerable because they had not evolved immunities to these diseases. Although indigenous peoples began a slow recovery a century or two after the early traumas of colonization, the experiences of colonization have permanently altered the lives of an estimated three-quarters of the world's population (Crosby, 1986, 1994; Golden et al., 1991; Green & Troup, 1999).

From a postcolonial perspective, European colonial ventures have contributed substantially to the conditions that drive migration today. One of the most salient features of migration from Third World nations, known as Majority Countries, to the rich nations of Europe and the United States is a history of colonization that established links of language, economics, politics, and citizenship in the empire. The historical acquisition of overseas colonies, for example, by Spain, England, Portugal, etc. constituted their respective empires (Ashcroft, Griffiths, & Tiffin, 1998; Gould & Findley, 1994). Two other established links are the recruitment of workers from a country, as between the United States and Mexico or China, or recruitment to help in combats, as happened with the Hmong. Well-established patterns of network migration between these countries, Mexico, China, and Laos, for example, and the United States now exist (Fadiman, 1997; Johnson, 2002; Portes & Borocz, 1989; Stalker, 2001).

Patterns of Migration

Officially, migration is recognized as either a voluntary activity or an involuntary emergent response to a crisis. This narrowly constructed classification appears to ignore a broad unarticulated space between voluntary and involuntary migration that reflects a range of economic need and the role of environmental disasters or famine as a legitimate impetus to relocate. Officially, involuntary migrants are refugees and asylum seekers who cross borders seeking safety from danger. Another larger group of involuntary migrants are internally displaced persons (IDPs) who are the least visible to the world community. Refugees merit formal legal recognition and protections according to the United Nations and the signatories of the 1951 Geneva Convention on Refugees. The Convention excludes economic and environmental refugees and IDPs, who are most often created by civil conflicts that target civilian populations (Lobe, 2002; Mandalakas, 2001).

Migration from rural to urban areas has exploded over the last few decades. Many cities in Majority Countries are unable to keep up with infrastructure development and work opportunities. The resultant squalid conditions and the loss of social support systems breed new diseases and cause mental/emotional health problems (Garrett, 1994; ICN, 2000; Kim, Millen, Irwin, & Gershman, 2000; McGuire, 1998). Transnational migration has increased due to the ease of newer and faster transportation modalities and communication innovations. A combination of population increases and global economic policies, directed principally by the G8 countries (rich countries) and the powerful Bretton Woods Institutes, the World Bank (WB) and the International Monetary Fund (IMF), are implicated in the migration to the cities and across borders. Structural adjustment policies (SAPs) imposed by the WB and IMF undermine the sovereignty of nations by forcing reduced spending for health care and education; the privatization of public- and state-owned enterprises, goods and services; and the opening of these economies to foreign investors and speculators. These practices of neoliberal economic globalization are heightening economic disparities and exacerbating the conditions that fuel migration (Hilton, 2002; McGuire & Georges, 2003; News, 2004; Sassen, 1998; Thompson, 2001).

Trends in Migration

The adequacy of the Geneva Conventions on Refugees for today's world is currently controversial, as are its provisions for the protection of refugees (UNHCR, 2001). Currently, some of the wealthiest countries to which refugees flee are erecting major obstacles to asylum seekers, sometimes incarcerating or detaining them indefinitely, and sometimes deporting them to certain danger or death upon their return to the country of origin (Lawson, 2002). Human rights groups have decried the detention and harsh treatment of refugee children, mainly those from Central American countries and China, in the United States (Alonzo-Zaldivar, 2003). Because many refugees arrive traumatized, possibly from torture, they are in highly vulnerable positions when they are denied asylum hearings (Alibhai-Brown, 2002; Baird, 2002; Moreno & Grodin, 2000). Simultaneously, poor countries have opened their doors to refugees, albeit somewhat reluctantly. For example, Iran, a poor country, harbors 2,550,000 of the world's refugees, or 17%, followed by Pakistan, Jordan, and Tanzania. Asia and Africa receive 80% of the world's total refugees (Nasim, 2002).

Western Europe, by admitting countries of Eastern Europe into the European Union, has in the last few years established a large perimeter of inclusion/exclusion known as Fortress Europe. This model is now being imitated by the United States as it enlists Canada and Mexico as border sentinels to seal off migration from Central and South America and entry points from the north. In 2001, Mexico's President, Vicente Fox, initiated Plan Sur, as this policy is known on the southern perimeter of Mexico, in response to pressures from Washington to harmonize refugee policies and immigration and visa laws. Canada is likewise following suit (Klein, 2003). Despite these new barriers, migrants will continue to arrive in the rich countries where jobs await them. Some will be admitted under current immigration admission annual quotas as legal residents; some will arrive as undocumented persons who occupy that murky space between voluntary and involuntary migrants. A sign of both their desperation and their courage is that they will risk life and health to reach their destination. Many new arrivals, legal or undocumented, are women, who as a group have a long history of migration.

WOMEN AND MIGRATION

Because women are generally the primary caretakers of their children and carry major responsibilities for the health of their families, human migration, especially the migration of women, is salient to nursing research and clinical practice. Today, women and children constitute a slight majority of transnational migrants, comprising about 80% of all refugees (Hune, 1991; Zlotnik, 1994, 2003). Migration in general has become increasingly feminized, although recent scholarship notes that women have historically participated in large numbers during human migrations (Zlotnik, 2003).

Recent genetic evidence suggests that women have far outnumbered men in intercontinental human movements for numerous reasons, and that an understanding of migration would be enhanced by understanding the role of women in migration (Seielstad, Minch, & Cavilli-Sforza, 1998; Stoneking, 1998). Migration scholarship, located principally in the social science disciplines and in history, has tended to depict women migrants narrowly, as dependents of males, thus reducing their visibility and their importance in global demographic shifts. This view ignores female agency, which can be a source of strength for health and well-being, and diminishes attention to the frightful dangers that many women migrants and refugees face before and during their migration journey (Hollifield et al., 2002; McGuire & Georges, 2003; Moreno & Grodin, 2000; Muecke, 1992; Murray, 2002).

Women's roles in migration did not gain prominence in scholarly discourses until feminist scholarship made women more visible. Women as migrants and immigrants are now being recognized for their motivations, risk taking, experiences, and contributions to the societies in which they finally relocated. Simultaneously, and not surprisingly, women and children are at higher risk for violence, rape, and adverse health events than are male migrants. With the tightening of borders between the United States and Mexico, for example, women are even more vulnerable to rape associated with border militarization because of the use of rape as a weapon of war. The U.S. border is treated as a war zone under the auspices of the War on Drugs, and more recently the War on Terror. The rape of women (and some men) is seen as an abuse of power and control designed to degrade and terrify civilians, especially migrant women. Some women heading to the border from Mexico began using oral contraceptives in anticipation of these sexual assaults, suggesting that rape has become acceptable policy within border policing while revealing the desperation of migrant women who anticipate these risks (Falcon, 2001). A migration phenomenon to which nursing has paid scant attention is that of the smuggling of women and children across borders, often as captives of traffickers who force them to work as commercial sex workers or indentured servants (Altink, 1995).

Depending on cultural constraints, sexually traumatized women may be averse to disclosing experiences of sexual assault to family members for fear of rejection, isolation, or banishment from the family. They may conceal this information from health providers if they do not have a sense of trust or if they are not screened for such risks with sensitivity. They are at risk for sequelae such as human immunodeficiency virus (HIV) or sexually transmitted infections (STIs). Women who have been traumatized either before and during migration or flight as refugees may suffer symptoms of depression and anxiety, sleeping and eating problems, intrusive thoughts, or psychic numbing. If they are from regions of the world that practice female genital mutilation (FGM), they may have symptoms associated with this procedure, and girl children may be subject to FGM in a host country even if the practice is prohibited (Martin, 1992). With their continually acquired cultural savvy, nurse clinicians who work with undocumented immigrant women should keep in mind the risks inherent in migration journeys to guide approaches to practice.

UNDOCUMENTEDNESS

One of the fastest growing forms of migration today, undocumented migration has been linked to globalization and includes refugees who have been denied asylum, workers, and visitors who have overstayed their visas. The civil conflict in El Salvador during the 1980s exemplifies the phenomenon of proxy wars in which the host country participates by funding one party in the war and refusing its refugees (Appleyard, 2001; Sussex Center for Migration Research, 2004; Tactaquin, 1992). In the United States, the undocumented have been pejoratively referred to as "illegal aliens" in public media and have been criminalized by contemporary border policies (McGuire, 1998). This designation reflects a contradiction between the categories of inclusion and exclusion set up by the powerful global market economy that has become the new grand narrative of the 21st century and a social discourse that fosters nativist sentiment. Seabrook (1996) defines *economic globalization* as the integration of all of the world's economies into a single economic entity. Another contradiction is embedded in the postmodern cultural rejection of grand narratives that coexist with the grand narrative of a global neoliberal economy imposed by the most powerful nations. Grand narratives, a postmodern term, are those overarching theoretical discourses and ideas, or metatheories, that ignore history and context. They are "one size fits all" explanations of existence that privilege certain groups over others, and maintain hegemonic relations of power. Examples of grand narratives are Western science with its assumptions of objectivity, Freudian psychoanalysis, Marxism, humanism, and White middle-class feminism. This basic understanding can help nursing appreciate undocumented transnational migrants as a consequence and reflection of economic globalization and its propensity to create great economic disparities through the dissolution of local economies and consequent displacement of local communities (Castles, 2000; Sassen, 1998). Without a means of self-support, people move.

Undocumented immigrants are the most vulnerable of all immigrants because they are forced to live in the shadows for fear of deportation. Living a life of constant hypervigilance, always on the lookout for the border patrol, may cause stress-related health problems in the long run. Ironically, the National Immigration Forum has documented that the material contributions of both documented and undocumented immigrants far exceeds their cost in public benefits (Colon & Panuco, 1998). About 70% of undocumented immigrants pay taxes, yet are not eligible for public benefits and tend, even when they procure documents and become eligible after five years, to avoid applying for benefits in order not to jeopardize their legal status.

Undocumented persons are also at risk for exploitation in the workplace and for violations of their human rights. Because of assaults on their rights in the workplace over the last two decades, undocumented workers have suffered disproportionately from "toxic racism" (Tactaquin, 1992) due to exposure to dangerous pesticides, incinerators, and waste dumps. The yield has been higher than normal rates of cancers, anencephalic births and other birth deformities, fertility problems, and psychological changes in undocumented immigrant populations (Huerta, 1993; Tactaquin, 1992). In the 2002 Supreme Court decision known as *Hoffman Plastics*, employers of undocumented workers were given the go ahead to fire workers who try to defend their rights without giving them back pay. This ruling opens up the way for unscrupulous employers to arbitrarily withhold back pay from undocumented workers, adding yet another barrier to their well-being by sanctioning exploitation and the violation of an intrinsic human right to just compensation for work performed.

Undocumented women sometimes arrive without their children, causing intense loneliness and yearnings for reunification, which could take years in the current legal climate. The fracturing of families inherent in the undocumented status of many immigrants coming from Mexico, Central America, or South America raises serious mental and emotional health issues that could be prevented with more family- and worker-friendly immigration policies. Language barriers among non-English-speaking immigrants also exacerbate women immigrants' sense of isolation and hinder their access to health care, in addition to raising fears of being asked for legal documents (McGuire & Georges, 2003). Without documents, women are also more likely to remain with their children in abusive relationships (Tactaquin, 1992).

Because of the militarization of the U.S.–Mexico border, many undocumented migrants feel compelled to remain in the United States and endure prolonged separations from their family members and places of origin. Yet, an estimated 500,000 to 700,000 of undocumented immigrants arrive annually in the United States and approximately 8 to 9 million undocumented persons live in the United States as a result of the great difficulty in moving back and forth across borders without supreme effort and risk (Cornelius, 2003; Liddick, 2003). Ironically, undocumentedness is not an ontological state, but a juridical designation effected through the production of "illegality" (DeGenova, 2002, p. 419; McGuire & Georges, 2003).

CHALLENGES FOR NURSING

Today's world demands analysis, critique, and new scholarly approaches to understanding global migration and health and their historic and contemporary roots in a nexus of international economic, political, cultural, and militaristic relationships between countries of vastly different economic and political strengths. Although colonial histories carry their own specificities of experience and cannot be universalized, employing a postcolonial lens is useful when considering the lasting historical influences of colonial legacies, relationships, and discourses that reinforce ongoing power imbalances affecting people in source countries.

Simultaneously, we must acknowledge human agency as a response to these conditions, especially in an age of globalization and the effects of mandated SAPs. The outcome of these policies has been an increase in poverty and suffering, thus creating new diasporas of migrants (Sassen, 1998; Stalker, 2001; Thompson, 2001). It makes sense then, that nursing grows its awareness and understanding of economic globalization not as a *defacto* historical accident, but as a consequence of deliberate human decision-making within powerful institutions in powerful countries. This understanding can then empower nursing to link with groups trying to change these economic policies. An emancipatory praxis can take many creative expressions at all levels of context, and is directed to transforming action to enhance health possibilities.

Although excellent models exist for assessing cultural preferences (Giger & Davidhizar, 2004; Purnell & Paulanka, 2003), advancing the notion of culture in nursing with immigrants also requires an acknowledgment of the roles of gender, race, class, and legal status as political flashpoints. Providing culturally competent care to immigrants necessitates resisting the tendency to "other" those who are different, embracing difference as a value, and allowing room to learn from and to negotiate nonharmful healthcare practices. Although the position of migrants is contentious (Melanie Dreher, personal communication), Dreher and McNaughton (2002) contend that it is nursing competence that matters and remind us that it is crucial to avoid "ecological fallacy" (p. 181) or assume universal health beliefs and practices within ethnic groups.

Cultural competence might mean assuming intelligence in immigrants who might be preliterate or who have little formal education and assessing needs for and providing intelligible health information in a spirit of respect (McGuire, 2001). Analyzing who has and uses power to erect barriers to health care in order to expose and remedy injustice is an example of emancipatory praxis. Providing venues for migrants' and immigrants' voices to be heard regarding their own health experiences, especially those who have been marginalized because of their color, languages, economic or legal status, gender, or culture will contribute to substantive scholarship and inspire innovative approaches to health care with new populations. An exemplar of creative responses is seen in the work of nurses and other health professionals with Sudanese refugees in Omaha, Nebraska (Hall, Stevens, & Meleis, 1994; Kirkham, 2002; Lainof & Elsea, 2004; McGuire & Georges, 2003; Meleis, 1996, 1997). For nurses so disposed, it may also mean making the effort to learn another's language to enhance communication and to counteract the hegemonic notion of a country in which non–English-speaking peoples are not welcomed.

A caveat is in order: Not all migration can be attributed to the influence of colonial ties, labor recruitment ties, or to economic globalization, and some groups of immigrants enjoyed wealth and privilege in their home countries before leaving, arriving with assets that assist in their transition. However, noted Latino essayist Richard Rodriguez (1998), strikes a deep chord when he says, "The movement of the poor has become the most revolutionary force on earth today, unsettling borders and troubling governments, angering the citizens of the world's wealthy economies."

I hope that our response is compassion and commitment, and that we dare to show a different response in keeping with the healing mandate of our profession and with the memory kindled of our own ancestral histories of migration. Certainly the challenge ahead is clear, and it will last into the unforeseeable future.

REFERENCES

American Academy of Nurses (AAN) (Ed.). (1995). *Global migration: The health care implications of immigration and population movements*. Washington, DC: AAN.

Alibhai-Brown, Y. (2002, October). No room at the inn. *New Internationalist*, 16–17.

Alonzo-Zaldivar, R. (2003, June 18). *Rights group slams U.S. treatment of refugee children*. Retrieved June 18, 2003, from http://www.latimes.com/news/nationworld/world/la-refugee-timjun18,1,5511205.story?coll=la-home-leftrail.

Altink, S. (1995). *Stolen lives: Trading women into sex and slavery*. New York: Harrington Park Press.

Appleyard, R. (2001). International migration policies. *International Migration, 39*(6), 7–18.

Ashcroft, B., Griffiths, G., & Tiffin, H. (1998). *Key concepts in post-colonial studies*. New York, NY: Routledge.

Baird, V. (2002, October). Fear eats the soul. *New Internationalist, 350*, 9–12.

Bancroft, S. (1998). Migration: A journey through time. *New Internationalist.* Retrieved April 5, 2003, from www.newint.org/journey.issue305/htm.

Berlinguer, G. (1999). Globalization and global health. *International Journal of Health Services, 29*(3), 579–595.

British Broadcasting Corporation (BBC). (2000). *Global migration reaches record high.* Retrieved April 9, 2003, from http://news.bbc.co.uk/1/hi/world/europe/1003324.stm.

Butterfield, P. (1990). Thinking upstream: Nurturing a conceptual understanding of the societal context of health behavior. *Advances in Nursing Science, 13*(3), 1–15.

Butterfield, P. G. (2002). Upstream reflections on environmental health: An abbreviated history and framework for action. *Advances in Nursing Science, 25*(1), 32–49.

Castles, S. (2000). *Ethnicity and globalization.* Thousand Oaks, CA: Sage.

Castles, S., & Miller, M. (1998). *The age of migration* (2nd ed.). London: Macmillan Press Ltd.

Cheon-Klessig, Y., Camilleri, D., Elmurry, B. M., & Ohlson, V. (1988). Folk medicine in the health practice of Hmong refugees. *Western Journal of Nursing Research, 10*(5), 647–660.

Chopoorian, T. (1986). Reconceptualizing the environment. In P. Moccia (Ed.), *New approaches to theory development* (pp. 39–54). New York: NLN.

Clarke, J. (2003). *The middle passage.* Retrieved June 26, 2003, from http://www.juneteenth.com/middlep.htm.

Cockcroft, J. (1998). *Mexico's hope: An encounter with politics and history.* New York: Monthly Review Press.

Colon, V., & Panuco, R. (1998). *Say it again: Immigrants give more than they receive.* Hispanic Link News Service. Retrieved November 1, 1998, from http://www.mercado.com/news/html/immigrants.html.

Cook, N. (1998). *Born to die.* Cambridge: Cambridge University Press.

Cornelius, W. (2003, June 8). An immoral policy on illegal entry. *Los Angeles Times,* p. M5.

Crosby, A. (1986). *Ecological imperialism: The biological expansion of Europe, 900–1900.* Cambridge: Cambridge University Press.

Crosby, A. (1994). *Germs, seeds & animals: Studies in ecological history.* Armonk, NY: M.E. Sharpe.

Daly, H. (2004). Population, migration, and globalization. *Worldwatch, 17*(5), 41–49.

Daniels, D. (1989). *Always a sister: The feminism of Lillian Wald.* New York: The Feminist Press at The City University of New York.

Davis, A. (1984). *Spearheads for reform: The social settlement movement and the progressive movement 1890–1914* (2nd ed.). New Brunswick, NJ: Rutgers University Press.

Davis, M., & Haasis, B. (1920). The visiting nurse and the immigrant. *The Public Health Nurse, 12,* 823–834.

Deen, T. (2003). *Law to protect migrant workers awaits one more nation.* Retrieved January 31, 2003, from http://www.ips.org.

DeGenova, N. (2002). Migrant "illegality" and deportability in everyday life. *Annual Review of Anthropology, 31,* 419–447.

DeSantis, L. (1990). Nursing faces imperative challenge: Cultural competence. *The Florida Nurse, 38*(2), 1, 19.

Dougherty, M., & Tripp-Reimer, T. (1985). The interface of nursing and anthropology. *Annual Review of Anthropology, 14,* 219–241.

Dreher, M., & MacNaughton, N. (2002). Cultural competence in nursing: Foundation or fallacy? *Nursing Outlook, 50,* 181–186.

Drevdahl, D. (1995). Coming to voice: The power of emancipatory community interventions. *Advances in Nursing Science, 18*(2), 13–24.

Eisman, A. (1976). *Rebels and reformers.* Garden City, NJ: Zenith Books.

Elliott, J., Berman, H., & Kim, S. (2002). A critical ethnography of Korean Canadian women's menopause experience. *Health Care for Women International, 23*(4), 377–388.

Fadiman, A. (1997). *The spirit catches you and you fall down*. New York: The Noonday Press.

Falcon, S. (2001). Rape as a weapon of war: Advancing human rights for women at the U.S.–Mexico Border. *Social Justice, 28*(2), 31–50.

Garrett, L. (1994). *The coming plague*. New York: Penguin Books.

Giger, J., & Davidhizar, R. (Eds.). (2004). *Transcultural nursing: Assessment and intervention* (4th ed.). St. Louis: Mosby.

Golden, R., McConnell, M., Mueller, P., Poppen, C., & Turkovich, M. (Eds.). (1991). *Dangerous memories: Invasion and resistance since 1492*. Chicago: Chicago Religious Task Force on Central America.

Gould, W. T. S., & Findley, A. M. (Eds.). (1994). *Population movements from the Third World to the developed world: Recent trends and current issues*. New York: John Wiley & Sons Ltd.

Green, A., & Troup, K. (1999). *The houses of history: A critical reader in twentieth-century history and theory*. New York: New York University Press.

Hall, J., Stevens, P., & Meleis, A. (1994). Marginalization: A guiding concept for valuing diversity in nursing knowledge development. *Advances in Nursing Science, 16*(4), 23–41.

Hautman, M. (1996). Changing womanhood: Perimenopause among Filipina-Americans. *Journal of Obstetric, Gynecologic, & Neonatal Nursing, 25*(8), 667–673.

Helsel, D. G., & Mochel, M. (2002). Afterbirths in the afterlife: Cultural meaning of placental disposal in a Hmong American community. *Journal of Transcultural Nursing, 13*(4), 282–286.

Hilton, I. (2002, July 23). Free markets have failed a continent: Latin America is gagging on the prescriptions of the Bush family. *Guardian of London*. Retrieved July 23, 2002, from http://www.commondreams.org/views02/0723-05.htm.

Hollifield, M., Warner, T., Lian, N., Krakow, B., Jenkins, J. H., Kesler, J., Stevenson, J., & Westermeyer, J. (2002). Measuring trauma and health status in refugees: A critical review. *JAMA, 288*(5), 611–621.

Hovy, B. (2002). *Statistics on forced migration*. Migration Policy Institute. Retrieved April 2, 2003, from http://www.migrationinformation.org.

Huerta, D. (Ed.). (1993). *The impact of poverty and environmental degradation on women migrant workers*. In Filomena Chioma Steady (Ed.), *Women and children first* (pp. 223–235). Rochester, VT: Schenkman Books.

Hune, S. (1991). Migrant women in the context of the international convention on the protection of the rights of all migrant workers and members of their families. *International Migration Review, 25*, 800–817.

Im, E., Lee, E., & Park, Y. (2002). Korean women's breast cancer experience. *Western Journal of Nursing Research, 24*(7), 751–771.

International Council of Nurses (ICN) (2000). *The health of indigenous people: A concern for nursing*. Retrieved February 17, 2000, from http://www.nursingworld.org/news/ananews.htm and http://www.icn.ch/matters_indigenous.htm.

International Organization of Migration (IOM) (2003, March). *Facts and figures on international migration*. Retrieved June 8, 2003, from http://www.iom.org.

Johnson, S. (2002). Hmong health beliefs and experiences in the Western health care system. *Journal of Transcultural Nursing, 13*, 126–132.

Juarbe, T., Turok, X., & Perez-Stable, E. (2002). Perceived benefits and barriers to physical activity among older Latina women. *Western Journal of Nursing Research, 24*(8), 868–886.

Kalofonos, I., & Palinkas, L. (1999). Barriers to prenatal care for Mexican and Mexican American women. *Journal of Gender Culture and Health, 4*(2), 1135–1152.

Kane, H. (1995). *The hour of departure: Forces that create refugees and migrants*. Washington, DC: Worldwatch Press.

Kendall, J. (1992). Fighting back: Promoting emancipatory nursing actions. *Advances in Nursing Science, 15*(2), 1–15.

Kim, J. Y., Millen, J. V., Irwin, A., & Gershman, J. (Eds.). (2000). *Dying for growth: Global inequality and the health of the poor*. Monroe, ME: Common Courage Press.

Kirkham, S. (2002). Postcolonial nursing scholarship: From epistemology to method. *Advances in Nursing Science, 25*(1), 1–17.

Kleffel, D. (1996). Environmental paradigms: Moving toward an ecocentric perspective. *Advances in Nursing Science, 18*(4), 1–10.

Kleffel, D. (2003). In L. Andrist, C. Bridges, K. Wolf, P. Nicholas, & A. Lowenstein (Eds.). *The history of nursing ideas* (pp. 97–108). Sudbury, MA: Jones and Bartlett.

Klein, N. (2003, January 16). The rise of the fortress continent. *The Nation*. Retrieved June 13, 2005 from http://thenation.com/doc.mhtml?i=20030203&s=klein.

Kulig, C. (1995). Cambodian refugees' family planning knowledge and use. *Journal of Advanced Nursing, 22*(1), 150–157.

Lainof, C., & Elsea, S. (2004). From Sudan to Omaha. *American Journal of Nursing, 104*(7), 58–61.

Lawson, D. (2002, October). Refugee! Terrorist! Criminal! *New Internationalist, 350*, 24–25.

Leininger, M. (1995). *Transcultural nursing: Concepts, theories, research and practice* (2nd ed.). New York: McGraw-Hill.

Lenart, J., Clair, P. S., & Bell, M. (1991). Childrearing knowledge, beliefs, and practices of Cambodian refugees. *Journal of Pediatric Health Care, 5*(6), 299–305.

Levin, A. (2001). Physicians for human rights. *Annals of Internal Medicine, 134*(6), 537–540.

Liddick, S. (2003, July 7). The border: Need for policy reform gets lost in emotional immigration debate. *San Diego City Beat, 46*, 13.

Lipson, J., Hosseini, T., Kabir, S., Omidian, P., et al. (1995). Health issues among Afghan women in California. *Health Care for Women International, 16*(4), 279–286.

Lipson, J., & Miller, S. (1994). Changing roles of Afghan refugee women in the United States. *Image: Journal of Nursing Scholarship, 15*(3), 171–180.

Lipson, J., & Omidian, P. (1997). Afghan refugee issues in the U.S. social environment. *Western Journal of Nursing Research, 19*(1), 110–126.

Lobe, J. (2002, September 23). *Internally displaced people now outnumber refugees two to one*. OneWorld.net. Retrieved September 23, 2002, from http://www.commondreams.org/headlines02/ 0923-02.htm.

Maiguashca, B. (1994). The transnational indigenous movement in a changing world order. In Y. Sakamoto (Ed.), *Global transformation: Challenges to the state system* (pp. 356–382). New York: United Nations University Press.

Mandalakas, A. M. (2001). The greatest impact of war and conflict. *Ambulatory Child Health, 7*, 97–103.

Martin, S. (1992). *Refugee women*. Atlantic Highlands, NJ: Zed Books.

Matthei, L. (1999). Gender and international labor migration: A network approach. In S. Jonas & S. Thomas (Eds.), *Immigration: A civil rights issue for the Americas* (pp. 69–84). Wilmington, DE: Scholarly Resources, Inc.

McGuire, S. (2001). *Crossing myriad borders: A dimensional analysis of the migration and health experiences of indigenous oaxacan women*. San Diego: University of San Diego Press.

McGuire, S., & Georges, J. (2003). Undocumentedness and liminality as health variables. *Advances in Nursing Science, 26*(3), 185–195.

McGuire, S. S. (1998). Global migration and health: Ecofeminist perspectives. *Advances in Nursing Science, 21*(2), 1–17.

Meleis, A. (1991). Between two cultures: Identity, roles and health. *Health Care for Women International, 12*, 365–377.

Meleis, A. (1996). Culturally competent scholarship: Substance and rigor. *Advances in Nursing Science, 19*(2), 1–16.

Meleis, A. (1997). Immigrant transitions and health care: An action plan. *Nursing Outlook, 45*(1), 42.

Meleis, A., Arruda, E., Lane, S., & Bernal, P. (1994). Veiled, voluminous, and devalued: Narrative stories about low-income women from Brazil, Egypt, and Colombia. *Advances in Nursing Science, 17*(2), 1–15.

Messias, D. (2002). Transnational health resources, practices, and perspectives: Brazilian immigrant women's narratives. *Journal of Immigrant Health, 4*(4), 183–200.

Metress, S. (1997). The great starvation, 1845–1852: A biocultural perspective. *The Review of the Ohio Council for the Social Studies, 33*(1), 39–51.

Miller, K. (1985). *Emigrants and exiles.* New York: Oxford University Press.

Moreno, A., & Grodin, M. (2000). The not-so-silent marks of torture. *JAMA, 284*(5), 538.

Muecke, M. (1992). New paradigms for refugee health problems. *Social Sciences and Medicine, 35*(4), 515–523.

Murray, K. (2002). Torture and rape victims fearful of healthcare staff. *Nursing Standard, 16*(26), 9.

Nasim, K. (2002, October). *Road to freedom.* Retrieved June 6, 2003, from http://www.newint.org/index4.html.

News, M. (2004). *Latin America.* Retrieved June 25, 2004, from http://migration.ucdavis.edu/mn.

Parfit, M. (1998, October). Human migration. *National Geographic, 194*(4), 6–35.

Park, S., Yoo, I., & Chang, S. (2002). Relationship between the intention to repeat a Papanicolaou smear test and affective response to a previous test among Korean women. *Cancer Nursing, 25*(5), 385–390.

Park, Y., Kim, H. K. P., Kang, Y., & Chun, S. (2001). A survey on the climacteric symptoms in Korean women. *Women and Health, 34*(1), 17–28.

Portes, A., & Borocz, J. (1989). Contemporary immigrations: Theoretical perspectives on its determinants and modes of incorporation. *International Migration Review, 23*(4), 606–629.

Purnell, L., & Paulanka, B. (Eds.). (2003). *Transcultural health care: A culturallly competent approach* (2nd ed.). Philadelphia: F.A. Davis Company.

Rodriguez, R. (1998). *For the poor, movement is the only answer to natural disasters.* Retrieved June 3, 2003, from http://www.pacificnews.org/jinn/stories/4.23/981116-nature.html.

Santana, M., & Dancy, B. (2000). The stigma of being named "AIDS carriers" on Haitian-American women. *Health Care for Women International, 21*(3), 161–171.

Sassen, S. (1998). *Globalization and its discontents: Essays on the new mobility of people and money.* New York: New Press.

Schwartz-Seller, M. (1994). *Immigrant women.* Albany: SUNY Press.

Seabrook, J. (1996, August). Internationalism versus globalization. *Around Africa*, 3–4.

Seielstad, M., Minch, E., & Cavilli-Sforza, L. (1998). Genetic evidence for a higher female migration rate in humans. *Nature America Inc, 20*(20), 278–280.

Silverstein, N. (1985). Lillian Wald at Henry Street, 1893–1895. *Advances in Nursing Science, 7*(2), 1–12.

Stalker, P. (2001). *The no-nonsense guide to international migration.* Toronto: New Internationalist Publications Ltd.

Stannard, D. (1992). *American holocaust: The conquest of the new world.* New York: Oxford University Press.

Stoneking, M. (1998). Women on the move. *Nature America Inc, 20*, 219–220.

Sussex Center for Migration Research. (2004). University of Sussex. Retrieved July 8, 2004, from http://www.migrationdrc.org/index.html.

Tactaquin, C. (1992). What rights for the undocumented? *NACLA Report on the Americas, XXVI*(1), 25–28.

Thompson, J. (2001). Diaspora and nursing praxis. *Nursing Philosophy, 2*, 83–86.

United Nations High Commission on Refugees (UNHCR) (2001). Refugees (Vol. 2, pp. 1–31). Retrieved March 14, 2002, from http://www.un.org.

Villarruel, A., Harlow, S., Lopez, M., & Sowers, M. (2002). El Cambio de Vida: Conceptualizations of menopause and midlife among urban Latina women. *Research and Theory for Nursing Practice, 16*(2), 91–102.

Wald, L. (1991). *The house on Henry Street* (2nd ed.). New Brunswick: Transaction Publishers.

Walter, N. (2002). Social context of work injury among undocumented day laborers in San Francisco. *Journal of General Internal Medicine, 17*(3), 221–229.

Westin, C. (1996). Migration patterns. In M. Haour-Knipe & R. Rector (Eds.), *Crossing borders* (pp. 15–30). London: Taylor & Francis.

Zlotnik, H. (1994). The South-to-North migration of women. *International Migration Review, 29*(1), 229–253.

Zlotnik, H. (2003). *The global dimensions of female migration.* Migration Information Source. Retrieved July 8, 2004, from http://www.migrationinformation.org/Feature/display.cfm?ID=109.

CHAPTER 7

The Concept of Community in Nursing History: Its Narrative Stream

Denise J. Drevdahl

The difficulty of writing history is making the account of an event, or in this case a concept, appear coordinated and coherent. Yet, history is complex and dialectical; the best one can hope for is a somewhat fragmented narrative. Although I make no claim to offer an accurate representation of the history of the concept of *community* in nursing, I can provide one path along its stream. In this chapter, I consider the history of the concept of community in nursing literature over the past century and a half with the goal of stimulating thinking and discussion about community to further social justice actions.

Much as the leaf falling into the forest stream, drifting along for some distance, becoming submerged beneath turbulent waters, and then reemerging at some point farther downstream, so, too, has community, as an important paradigm for nursing practice, coursed its way through nursing theory and practice, surfacing at different moments in nursing's history. The concept—visible at the onset of modern-day nursing—faded away. Only recently has it reappeared as a predominant element of nursing, particularly in community/public[1] health nursing theory and practice. The flow of interest in community mirrors the flow of interest in the term in Western society. As the West has advanced technologically, there emerged a sense of loss of what was thought to be "real" community, and much effort has been exerted recently to understand and, perhaps, to nurture its return.

Community is a noun from the Latin word *communis*, meaning fellowship or community of relations or feelings or referring concretely to a body of fellows (Oxford English Dictionary online). Today, phrases such as *Hispanic community*, *lesbian community*, or *nursing community* are common in the nursing profession. Community is coincidentally considered a single entity *and* a collection of unique individuals, producing tensions often reflected within nursing theory and practice. As Hamilton and Keyser (1992) pointed out, "the discipline swings back and forth between sets of opposing ideas and values: community-centered care versus individual- and family-centered care; health promotion versus treatment of illness; client autonomy versus the good of the community" (p. 143). Defining groups of individuals with nongender-, nonethnic-, and nonclass-specific terms, such as *the people* or *the community*, runs the risk of leaving out historically marginalized and oppressed groups. Although as a discipline we struggle with what community means and what community work entails, because ideas about community abound, we often have the impression that little is left to be learned about the concept. Yet, as Boswell

(1990) reminded us, "community calls for investigation in its own right . . . [and needs] intellectual effort" (p. 5). That effort has varied greatly over nursing's history.

Although absent from nursing literature during the periods in which Florence Nightingale and Lillian Wald were conducting their work, by the mid-20th century much intellectual effort encasing exploration of community's definition and meaning was taking place in sociology, anthropology, political science, psychology, theology, and philosophy—disciplines from which nursing draws much of its own understanding about community. Some of the most important work on the concept is attributed to sociologist Robert Park. In 1936, he identified the crucial components of a community as populations, organized in geographic locales, with individuals living in mutual interdependence of other members (as cited in Lyon, 1987). Nineteen years later, Hillery's (1955) examination of the definitions of community in the sociology literature uncovered 94 separate definitions, ranging from community as locale to a totality of attitudes. These definitions largely agreed with Park's core criteria (Lyon, 1987). Clearly, given the number of definitions, the concept has played a central role in many disciplines.

Discussions about community often begin with Tonnies' (1887/1963) concepts of *Geimenischaft* and *Gesellschaft*. For Tonnies, these were ideal community types, with *Geimenischaft* seen as common to families and rural settlements, carrying ideas of strong community identity, emotional attachment, and traditions. *Gesellschaft*, in contrast, was viewed as existing in urban, capitalist societies in which there was little identification with the community, a lack of emotional attachment, and authority based in law rather than in tradition (Lyon, 1987). Tonnies, and later sociologists, such as Durkheim (1893/1964) and Weber (1958), believed that Europe, as well as the United States, were becoming more *Gesellschaft*-like. Attempts to improve the health and well-being of individuals in these societies often addressed the "loss of," "decline in," or "search for" community.

Towards the close of the 20th century, the importance of relationships was stressed in discussions about the concept, although the notion of community as physical space never completely dissipated. For example, Gusfield (1975) believed that the word *community* did not describe any actually existing entity—"[communities] are products of human imagination and not descriptions of a real world" (Gusfield, 1975, p. 11)—but was an analytic term that helped human beings think about and talk about human relationships. The concept of community, for Gusfield, was useful in explaining or justifying a community member's actions, such that "it is the criteria of action that we emphasize rather than the physical arena within which the action occurs" (p. 33). He did point out, however, that there undoubtedly seemed to be a relationship between territorial size and the ability to function as a community, such that the larger the size of the geographic area the less ability there was to maintain a community image.

Today, for most disciplines, including nursing, community remains an indicator of some real physical space. Often that space is linked to a romanticized past in which individuals were in "comfortable proximity of secure neighborhoods and the supportive bonds of friendships and front-porch conversations" (Felkins, 2002, p. 13). This common conceptualization in which community serves as a generic term for a tangible geographic locale had its origins in the

> tendency to identify the local, small, territorial unit with communal relationships and the large urban and regional units with societal characteristics. Thus village, neighborhood and town appear as seats of community, and interest in their appearance and/or disappearance has been generalized to the wider scope of urban communities, since these constitute the context for the discussion of community change in contemporary societies. (Gusfield, 1975, p. 32–33)

The idea that the *Geimenischaft* sense of community has evaporated and in its place is a world in which connections to other human beings are more likely to occur through technological interfaces rather than face-to-face leaves many with a sense of loss and longing for the "good old days" of block parties and chats with neighbors over backyard fences. The nostalgic perspective has left us anxious, unsure, and isolated (Felkins, 2002). Media and academic attention given to Robert Putnam's 2000 tome *Bowling Alone: The Collapse and Revival of American Community* underscored this national feeling of anxiety and evoked larger conversations about the importance of community to the U.S. psyche. For Felkins, "the search for security and significance in daily life and work reflects the need for meaningful participation in a caring community" (p. 14). Felkins' words are notable in that they identify two concepts seen as essential to nursing: community and caring. Community conveys the notion of shared values and norms, an emotional commitment, and personal connection with others in a geographic region. The concept becomes the place and method for actualizing caring. Whether, in fact, this idealized community ever existed is disputed, because for many it was only imagined. The course the concept has taken through nursing's history reflects both its critical role in the profession and the difficulties encountered in understanding and enacting community.

COMMUNITY UPSTREAM

An important step in understanding current meanings of community is to identify the concept's historical source. That is, to appreciate upstream events that have influenced downstream theory and practice. Texts on the history of nursing and, specifically, community/public health nursing, recognized work conducted by deaconesses, widows, nuns, and sisters as early nursing caregivers followed, in turn, by advances Florence Nightingale made in the mid-1800s (Brainard, 1922). Not surprisingly, as noted by several authors in this book, many if not all of nursing's metaparadigms had their origins in the work of Nightingale. The concept of community, like the history of other concepts vital to the discipline, has been an essential element of nursing practice since the profession's founding.

Although Nightingale (1860/1969) never used the term *community* in her seminal work *Notes on Nursing*, she did refer to ideas that are now clearly associated with community. In particular, she recognized the importance of understanding and addressing the contexts of locales in which people lived, particularly if those contexts contributed to ill health through such means as "badly constructed houses," impure water, and lack of adequate waste disposal (p. 24). Nightingale focused on the neighborhoods and communities of the poor and destitute, thus emphasizing the idea of community as a general term for physical space and environment. This conceptualization of community was carried forward into the developing field of community/public health nursing. For example, when describing communities in which public health nurses worked at the turn of the 20th century, Gardner (1917) explained that the public health nurse was "to be found in the juvenile courts and public play grounds, in the department stores and big hotels, in the schools and factories, in the houses of small wage earners and in the swarming tenements of the very poor" (p. 29). Using community to signify a physical space remained an integral aspect of nursing theory and practice over the succeeding decades. Importantly, this use of the concept disregarded Tonnies' ideas about the relational aspects of community.

Dolan noted in her 1973 text on nursing history that the importance of geographic communities as targets for nursing actions was recognized early in public health nursing in the United States. These pioneer nurses realized that paying attention to the health and well-being of individuals residing within geographically bounded communities ultimately contributed to the health and well-being of the greater community. Unmistakably, community now was being conceptualized beyond mere spatial boundaries to include the quality of life within those boundaries. An early nursing "superintendent" commented on the importance of having nurses out in the community:

> The power of keeping a home together, when the alternative is the workhouse, is a social question with far-reaching consequences . . . to save mothers of families from lifelong effects of ignorance and neglect, to teach the proper management of infants and children, are gains to the community at large. (as cited in Dolan, 1973, p. 292)

Although primarily understood as a geographic entity, the importance of a larger view of community for community/public health nursing practice was starting to take shape. The primary impetus for this broader conceptualization of community in nursing was Lillian Wald.

Following in the footsteps of Nightingale and her focus on community as place, Lillian Wald worked to establish nursing as a profession connected to the community and its members, focusing on their social welfare. Mirroring Nightingale's concern about the growth of poverty with increasing urbanization, Wald was drawn to addressing the social conditions of New York City's poor. Rising numbers in the city's overall population, dramatically swollen due to mass immigration, exacerbated the glaring inequities between rich and poor. As with the impoverished inhabiting Nightingale's inner-city London, New York City's poor faced living conditions that were overcrowded, violent, filthy, and lacked "privacy, fresh air, and light"—conditions that contributed to development of disease (Silverstein, 1994, p. 109). Toiling to improve the health and well-being of tenement residents, Wald created the Henry Street Settlement in the midst of the community, noting "We were to live in the neighborhood as nurses, identify ourselves with it socially, and, in brief, contribute to it our citizenship" (Wald, 1915/1991, p. 8–9). Thus, community as a place for creating social connections with the community's individual members was recognized as an important ideal. Silverstein's (1994) assertion that "as the settlement supported the community, the community began to support the settlement" (p. 112) highlighted the newly created reciprocal relationships between community members and the nurses who provided needed care.

Changes in the meaning of community were apparent as nursing transitioned from Nightingale's vision, in which community was a purely physical space, to Wald's conceptualization of community as also containing elements of relationships that needed to be nurtured and new relationships that needed to be developed. Plainly, community was a concept that informed nursing practice. For Nightingale, community as place provided her with direction in how to not only care for the sick, but also to educate women who wanted to be nurses. But, as Wald moved into developing relationships with community members—that is, enhancing relationships between nursing and community members—a fuller picture of the lives experienced by the people for whom Henry Street Settlement nurses were caring came into view. Community members' poverty and their tenement conditions again informed Wald's practice such that social activism became an integral part of her nursing activities. In her book *The House on Henry Street*, Wald included two chapters that emphasized community relationships and the growing importance of social action: "The Nurse and the Community" and "Social Forces." As the concept of community gained depth and breadth, nursing practice, too, gained complexity and fullness—moving from care for the individual to care for the community. In this setting, Lillian Wald and her group at the Henry Street Settlement created a community/public health nursing tradition that enacted a philosophy of social justice to improve community conditions.

Wheeler's (1994) analysis of articles published in the *American Journal of Nursing* (*AJN*) noted that by the beginning of the 20th century, the profession was involved with societal issues such that nurses were advised that they had a duty to safeguard the health of individuals as well as that of the general community. An example of this is early nursing leaders' concern with issues of morality (e.g., preventing the spread of gonorrhea and syphilis). Teaching sex hygiene to community members was a popular topic in *AJN*. However, other nurses, like Wald, were moving beyond using only educational activities to improve the health of individuals to taking political action to ensure that women, especially poor women, were treated fairly and not unjustly targeted for punishment.

The influence of the women's suffrage movement is evident in the activities undertaken by Wald and her colleagues. Nurses argued against legislation that would authorize the jailing of women suspected of prostitution, detaining the women until their venereal disease reports were available, and then charging them with having a social disease. These social activist nurses understood what this bill meant in terms of the complexities of women's lives, noting that poor women were more likely to suffer from undernourishment and infectious diseases such as tuberculosis, making them more susceptible to other pathogens. Nursing leaders believed that focusing on prostitutes and venereal disease ensured that men of higher socioeconomic status did not get infected, while the majority of poor women were left to suffer the consequences of the diseases and poverty. As Wheeler (1994) noted, editorials about the legislation "confirm[ed] that early nursing leaders were not isolated from their community and were leaders in the women's movement" (p. 101). But social activism and practicing in the homes and tenements of the poor were not sustained. "In retrospect, it is unfortunately clear that the growth and promise of public health nursing at that time was little more than a false dawn" (Buhler-Wilkerson, 1983, p. 101). With the rise of modern medicine, further development of the concept of community as both geographic locales and relationships ended, as did the social justice activities of community/public health nursing.

COMMUNITY SUBMERGED

As the Wald era closed and hospitals came more into the foreground, community/public health nursing shifted its focus from the health issues of communities to the health of individuals. Pressures exerted by the external environment changed community/public health nursing, and the "community mother," as Winslow described the community/public health nurse, was no longer seen as vital (as cited in Buhler-Wilkerson, 1983, p. 99). Morbidity and mortality rates in the cities were diminishing, and chronic diseases were exchanging places with infectious diseases as leading causes of death. Medical and health services became concentrated in hospitals. Voluntary nursing organizations' "once clear purpose and vision had become increasingly elusive and financial support was becoming difficult to obtain" (Buhler-Wilkerson, 1983, p. 99). Rather than determining the nursing outcomes they wanted to achieve, community/public health nurses responded to externally applied forces. With the closing of new possibilities for community/public health nursing, additional conceptualizations of the concept of community vanished from nursing literature and practice.

During this time, community, and therefore community/public health practice, ceased to focus on community as physical space and relationships and became more about monitoring individual behavior. This was particularly evident in the great attention given to sexually transmitted diseases and with activities undertaken to acculturate newly arrived immigrants to U.S. customs and culture. Community, no longer the place in which concerns of social justice were predominant, was transformed to the targeting of individuals, who were viewed through the perspective of policies and laws.

All hope was not lost, though, because some recognized that community/public health nursing practice did indeed need to see the community as its focus. In 1944, Goodnow went so far as to say, "the development of the feeling of *community* responsibility in health matters makes public health nursing the most important future development in nursing" (p. 269). With the implementation of the polio vaccine, it seemed her words were prophetic. However, other than Nancy Milio's (1970) work in Michigan, the relational aspect of community, particularly in terms of social activism, largely was absent. It would not be until the end of the 20th century before community/public health nursing would undertake again, in earnest, Wald's earlier vision of nursing and community.

By the 1980s, nursing discussion and study of concepts now considered essential to nursing were in full swing. Key writings, such as Flaskerud and Halloran's (1980) examination of defining nursing concepts and the American Nurses' Association's *Social Policy Statement* (1980), launched a decade of inquiry by nursing scholars about important nursing concepts and philosophies. These authors included Chinn (1983), Meleis (1985), and Moccia (1986). Although there was some disagreement about including *nursing* as an essential concept in the profession, most agreed that *person*, *environment*, and *health* were critical elements of nursing.

Around the same time, other nursing scholars were reflecting on community health nursing and elements critical to that specialty. Williams (1977, 1984, 1985), in asking "What is community health nursing?" directed attention toward the population-focused aspect of the field. Anderson, McFarlane, and Helton (1984) and Goeppinger (1984) argued that for community health nurses, the community was the nurse's client. One element of these discussions was broadening the understanding of the concept of *person* such that it went from encompassing the individual to encompassing the community.

Schultz (1987) clarified the concept of person in the context of community health nursing. In 1985, Williams had suggested that community health nursing was focused on aggregates. From Schultz's perspective, however, the term *aggregate* carried with it statistical meaning rather than meaning in relation to the various dimensions of being human. Based on Meleis' (1986) conclusion that interactions were an integral component of all nursing actions, Schultz argued that the concept of person—and, ultimately, the concept of community—needed to be understood as "interactional units with a plurality of persons as components" (p. 79). Thus, when the client of nursing action was the community, the "plurality of persons" who constituted the community could be described in terms of their geographical/political locations or in terms of their shared bonds, purposes, or values.

In 1989, Chalmers and Kristajanson, arguing that there was lack of clarity regarding what constituted nursing practice at the community level, suggested three models for practice at the community level. These models—public health, community participation, and community change—were offered as approaches to move community health nursing towards improving the health of whole populations rather than only individuals or families.

Further elucidation was accomplished by Hamilton and Keyser in their 1992 study of community health educators' beliefs about ideologies specific to community health nursing. Analysis of data collected from 154 members of the Association of Community Health Nursing Educators revealed that the educators held parallel, separate, and often oppositional ideologies: one focused on the individual and the other focused on society. The study's authors believed this dichotomy was related to several factors: (1) the false division between health and disease; (2) the view of human needs as individual events; (3) reductionistic approaches to science; and (4) nursing theory that centered on the individual without taking into account the relationship between the individual and his/her environment. Hamilton and Keyser suggested that a dialectic ideology of community health nursing could be developed in which individuals and society were of equal importance. Without such a model, the current two-pronged ideologies could lead to bifurcation in nursing practice itself. For the authors, home health was, for example, a case in which an ideology focused on individuals had contributed to an ideologically distinct practice that was viewed as separate from community/public health nursing.

As Hamilton and Keyser's (1992) example illustrated, how community is conceptualized has implications for how practice is carried out and how services are delivered (Chalmers & Kristajanson, 1989). If, as Schultz (1991) argued, communities are more than an extension of individual or family behavior and more than the environment in which they are located, then communities have the ability to act: "They are a human enactment of collective agency" (p. 228). Such conceptualization carries with it notions of power and empowerment, collaboration, and partnership. One example of such community conceptualization is the *De Madres a Madres* program (McFarlane & Fehir, 1994). The program, based on concepts of empowerment and partnership, was initiated in a low-income Hispanic neighborhood in Houston, Texas, to help mothers access prenatal care. Over time, the program has mobilized community members to improve the health of the entire community through the use of lay health volunteers and community coalitions.

By the end of the 20th century, agency, empowerment, and collaboration had come into the fore of community health nursing theory and were seen as foundational to having community involvement in health-directed interventions. Increasingly, community became not only the target for interventions, but also the active participant in creating those interventions rather than the "passive [beneficiary] of health care services" (Watts, 1994, p. 153). Picking up where Wald and her contemporaries left off, the melding of the ideas of community as place and community as relationships and actions was once again emerging. Community health nurses were now articulating the importance of developing relationships with community members, as evident in concepts such as *participation, partnership, community organizing, community development, power,* and *empowerment*. Articles proliferated about integrating these concepts into nursing practice, and textbooks used for community health nursing coursework commonly used one of these principles in their titles, such as Anderson and McFarlane's (2000) text *Community as Partner: Theory and Practice in Nursing*. By linking partners with communities, the language nursing used suggested being in the community and being responsible to the community. Thus, nursing's commitment to social justice for marginalized communities was being re-created.

COMMUNITY RESURFACED

Addressing issues of concern for the poor and marginalized members of society, with a focus on emancipatory interventions, was once more a prime concern in community health nursing (Kendall, 1994). The aim of emancipatory nursing was to "help oppressed and disenfranchised persons gain freedom from the people, ideology, or situation that keeps them oppressed" (Kendall, 1994, p. 222). For Kendall, integral to the impulse toward emancipatory actions was

Katz's (as cited in Kendall, 1994) notion of the synergistic community. Katz took the approach that rather than understanding the world as a place with a limited amount of resources for which individuals must compete, human activities were identified as "intrinsically expanding and renewable and need not be viewed as scarce" (as cited in Kendall, 1994, p. 229). From this perspective, communities could be understood as places and relationships that were sources of vitality, creativity, and possibility.

For nursing, an important ingredient of nursing activities was *caring*. Bent (1999) and Davis (1997) considered the role of caring at the community level. For Bent (1999), community meant entities that "identify with some location, perceive interdependence, and work together to meet community needs" (p. 31). Noting that some conceptualizations of community were limiting, Bent suggested that one way to challenge those limitations was to see the role power, control, and domination played in determining a community's health. For her, any activities initiated as moves toward health could only be achieved through partnerships and collaborations. She introduced a model of eco-caring in which oppositional models of community are joined to create an integrative model that "enfolds ecological dimensions of communities-of-experience, human communities, and more-than-human communities" (p. 34). In this type of model, responsibility for health or illness shifted from the individual and his/her particular behaviors to underlying social, political, and environmental structures and policies that endangered and fostered health. Moving from the individual to the larger societal context provided nurses with the opportunity to practice "an integrated and caring praxis" (p. 35). This integrated, caring approach to practice reflected Butterfield's (1990) idea of upstream thinking—that is, taking into account the role greater economic, political, and cultural conditions play in fostering or inhibiting health and well-being.

Davis (1997) asked, "What kinds of relationships should health care organizations have with their communities? What is a healthy community? What does caring for the community mean?" (p. 92). These questions seemed particularly compelling given the financial and economic considerations governing the practices of many (if not all) healthcare organizations. Although it may be argued that healthcare organizations have a moral obligation to preserve and protect the health of the communities in which they operate, Davis' review of the literature found few authors attending to the linkages between organizations and their respective community's health. Her findings about organizational community care from ethnographic interviews conducted with eight healthcare providers revealed that community had an emotional aspect to it that covered such feelings as *belonging*, *safety*, *comfort*, and *hope*.

Other important themes that emerged from Davis' (1997) study were: developing collaborative relationships with communities to get the work of community care done, offering health promotion/disease prevention education, and having a broad conceptualization of health. Providers believed that the healthcare system needed to be more committed to the community's health. Of significant concern to Davis was that the providers defined their community as those individuals residing in the geographic community who had health insurance. Unanswered was how healthcare providers would build a healthier community for all constituent groups (regardless of insurance status). As issues of power, control, and dominance were highlighted in the community/public health nursing literature, concerns that community created some groups who were inside and others who were outside the community surfaced (Drevdahl, 1998). The closing stages of the 1990s found nursing more closely examining the characteristics and quality of nursing connections to community.

Chalmers, Bramadat, and Andrusyszen (1998) and SmithBattle, Diekemper, and Drake (1999) found that because the definition and use of the concept of community had changed, nurses' roles in and with communities also had changed, such that the nature of the *relationship* between the two now was of prime importance. Community/public health nurses increasingly saw themselves as facilitators of the healthy community process rather than as direct care providers. More and more, community/public health nurses were being influenced by concepts of *partnership, community development, empowerment, dialogue,* and *client participation.* For Chalmers et al., the public health nurse was a resource for communities as they took steps to improve their health, whereas for SmithBattle et al., the physical community was a place of strengths and assets. SmithBattle et al.'s understanding of community serves as an example of Shields and Lindsey's (1998) contention that community was most often conceptualized as *community-as-context* and/or *community-as-resource.* For Shields and Lindsey, community-as-context highlighted the environment in which the nurse's client lived; thus the community encompassed spatial, geographic, and structural elements. With the increasing emphasis on health promotion, community was viewed as ever changing and dynamic, such that rather than a site for deficits, community-as-resource had the assets and capacities needed to build a better and healthier self.

Whether SmithBattle et al.'s and Shields and Lindsey's conceptualization of community-as-resource represents the perception of providers in practice remains unsettled. For example, findings from a study in which I explored meanings of community in a community health clinic revealed that health center staff and administrators described the clinic's community in terms of economic, educational, physical, and psychological deficits (Drevdahl, 1999). In contrast, the women using the clinic depicted it as a place in which they could receive and give each other needed support. In the end, contradictory meanings of community contributed to differing expectations of clinic services.

Beyond understanding community-as-context and/or community-as-resource, Shields and Lindsey (1998) argued that community ought to be understood in terms of being; that is, being within the relationships experienced in day-to-day living:

> Community may be a way of being that permeates people's everyday lives, and thus, people experience themselves as being in community. Just as mind, body, and spirit are inseparable, so are individual and community. Thus, the relational aspects of community encompass people's relational experiences as well as a relational way of being (p. 26).

Echoing Chalmers et al. (1998) and SmithBattle et al. (1999), Shields and Lindsey believed that the meanings given to community informed community/public health nursing practice. Because social justice is the core ethical principle of public health nursing, expanding the meaning of community to include relational aspects, particularly power and political relations, necessitates transforming community/public nursing practice such that the sociopolitical aspects of community care are emphasized (Drevdahl, Kneipp, Canales, & Shannon Dorcy, 2001). Part of transforming practice is moving toward critical reflection, participatory dialogue, and action (Shields & Lindsey, 1998).

Critical reflection on relations of power also was an important aspect in my analysis of the perspectives of the community clinic's personnel and the women who used the clinic. Using critical social and feminist theories to guide the analysis, the use of power was demonstrated in the goals of the clinic, the policies and regulations established by the clinic, and the power relations between clinic personnel and clinic users. Although clinic providers and administrators talked about clinic users as being powerless and having multiple needs, women clinic users fashioned oppositional discourses that resisted the disempowering images conveyed by clinic personnel. Thus, community was a tool through which clinic users challenged the various performances of clinic power.

For Kulbok and her associates (1999), "beliefs about the nature of human beings direct community health nursing practice toward: (a) strengthening agency within groups and communities to co-create health through partnership, and (b) intervening in the environment to support collective agency" (p. 1191). Part of understanding the changing dimensions of community/public health nursing practice for these authors was, again, understanding the shifting meanings of community. Using Reed's (1995) three nursing worldviews (*mechanistic, organismic,* and *developmental-contextual*), the authors described the mechanistic view of community as creating practice that deals with parts (individuals) rather than the whole. The organismic worldview helped form practice in which synthesis of the whole was primary, producing interventions that addressed partnerships and culturally competent care. Finally, in the developmental-contextual worldview, the emphasis was on describing and explaining patterns and relationships between persons and the environment. Parse (1999) echoed the importance of recognizing patterns of community and also called attention to the idea that community patterns are always undergoing transformation. Nursing literature published at the dawn of the new century on the concept of community strengthened Parse's ideas of pattern change.

COMMUNITY TO BE

As the 20th century ended and the 21st commenced, nurses were and are reexamining not only community/public health nursing practice, but also the very concept of community. Much like nursing theorists of the 1990s, those publishing at the beginning of the 21st century have reiterated the belief that restricting the definition of community to geographic space creates a disconnect between meanings of community and intervention frameworks intended to assist with community improvement, such as community development. Kulig (2000), for example, focusing on interactions among community members, required a dynamic conceptualization of community to understand and theorize about community resiliency. She, too, believed that nursing needed a broader conceptualization of community that moved beyond arbitrary boundaries and that examined relationships and interconnections among groups.

Pharris' (2002) work brings to light how the concept of community can simultaneously be conceived as a spatial entity as well as a place where relationships are maintained or allowed to perish. After interviewing 12 adolescent males convicted of murder, analysis of the data revealed that the physical communities in which these young men grew up provided little to help them "identify their unique gifts and find their place in the community" (p. 37). Using Newman's (1994) theory of health as expanding consciousness to guide the study, common patterns and themes were found among the adolescents' support systems. The overwhelming pattern was one of community neglect and lack of nurturance from parents, guardians attained through child protective services, school officials, and/or other community members. There were no significant relationships or connections between the young men and their families, schools, and communities. These youth's experiences help illuminate that the realities of people's experiences in various communities can differ greatly from nostalgic or utopian views of community. In this case, community in the form of gangs, although a source of strength and comfort to an individual community member, was a source of destruction to the larger community, and ultimately to the community member as well. Feeling left out, marginalized, and abandoned by the larger community, it was not surprising the young men had sought the protection of gangs. For these youth, the definition of the community excluded them.

As illustrated in Davis' (1997) and Pharris' (2002) studies, "community, as a device that homogenizes, separates, and divides, automatically carries with it margins and borders; it is a practice that denotes exclusion" (Drevdahl, 2002, p. 11). Community is an unending contradictory process that can mean being home (a place of safety and security) for some, and being on the community's border (a place of danger and difference) for others. One dilemma associated with community is the urge to create unified identities such that differences are subsumed. Consequently, tensions inherent in community call for further analysis and action, including identifying links between community and power, engaging in honest and respectful discourse with community members, and using knowledge gained to inform political action for the purposes of addressing social justice (Drevdahl, 2002).

The move to have community members more actively involved in activities to improve the overall community's health, of course, raises important questions about the nature of the relationship between nursing and the community, because these moves are, in essence, about restructuring how power is positioned and exerted. Do nurses honor the community's priorities or do nurses' priorities take precedence? What form does participation take? Is participation grounded in action or given lip service? For Watts (1994), informing, consulting, and placation—strategies often used in community practice—constitute "tokenism" (p. 157). Can there be a real partnership when there may be vast differences in terms of authority, education, and socioeconomic status between professionals and the community? Others have considered these issues in more depth than is granted here, but it is important to point out that romantic ideas of solving society's ills by partnering with communities are often merely that—romantic—and in fact, have little to do with the redistribution of power.

Struggles over meanings of community are always struggles about power. As Navarro (1984) commented, community "is defined *not* by the individual elements and/or interventions that exist within it but, rather, the structural relationships among these elements and the powers they reproduce" (p. 473). Recognizing the existence of power relations in establishing meanings of community helps us understand that community can serve as an oppressive power and as a form and place of resistance. The dialectical elements of community suggest that in the new century we are called to think more deeply and complexly about community. We are called to deal with issues of social justice.

CONCLUSION

This analysis of the history of community in nursing practice and theory demonstrates that community is an inherently contradictory concept. It is "both pragmatic and ideal, individual and collective, emotional and rational, dispersed and local" (Felkins, 2000, p. 16). Many of the meanings of community used in the discipline throughout its history include the idea that shared values are one element that unite community members. Yet, elements that unite community members also create partitions (e.g., along class lines). Does creating community automatically carry with it divisions and separations such that the ability to foster community is diminished? If shared values are assumed, then what roles do openness and diversity have in creating community norms? These are some of the questions for the new century for community/public health nursing as it strives to "return to its roots of improving the conditions that contribute to poor health and poor quality of life for the whole community" (Smith & Bazini-Barakat, 2003, p. 42).

Because community is ever changing and evolving, nursing needs to continue to reconfigure how it conceptualizes and understands community. From Amit's (2002) perspective,

> The essential contingency of community, its participants' sense that it is fragile, changing, partial and only one of a number of competing attachments or alternative possibilities for affiliation means that it can never be all-enveloping or entirely blinkering. Community is never the world entire, it is only ever one of a number of recognized possibilities (p. 18).

We will never get to the "true" community, and we cannot speak and think our way out of the confusion about community. That is, we can ask questions and develop inquiry around community, but our efforts will not lead us to the irrefutable answer about the meaning of community. This does not mean that we should allow community to disappear below the depths of tumultuous dialogue, but rather use the uncertainty and turmoil to support new ways of thinking about community in the discourse and practice of health, health care, and nursing.

REFERENCES

American Nurses Association (1980). *Nursing: A social policy statement.* Kansas City, MO: American Nurses Association.

Amit, V. (2002). Reconceptualizing community. In V. Amit (Ed.), *Realizing community: Concepts, social relationships and sentiments* (pp. 1–20). London: Routledge.

Anderson, E. T., & McFarlane, J. (2000). *Community as partner: Theory and practice in nursing.* Philadelphia: Lippincott Williams & Wilkins.

Anderson, E., McFarlane, J., & Helton, A. (1984). Community-as-client: A model for practice. *Nursing Outlook, 34,* 220–224.

Bent, K. N. (1999). The ecologies of community caring. *Advances in Nursing Science, 21*(4), 29–36.

Boswell, J. (1990). *Community and the economy.* London: Routledge.

Brainard, A. M. (1922). *The evolution of public health nursing.* Philadelphia: W. B. Saunders Company.

Buhler-Wilkerson, K. (1983). False dawn: The rise and decline of public health nursing in America, 1900–1930. In E. C. Lagemann (Ed.), *Nursing history: New perspectives, new possibilities* (pp. 89–106). New York: Teachers College Press.

Butterfield, P. G. (1990). Thinking upstream: Nurturing a conceptual understanding of the societal context of health behavior. *Advances in Nursing Science, 12*(2), 1–8.

Chalmers, K. I., Bramadat, I. J., & Andursyszen, M. (1998). The changing environment of community health practice and education: Perceptions of staff nurses, administrators, and educators. *Journal of Nursing Education, 37*(3), 109–117.

Chalmers, K., & Kristajanson, L. (1989). The theoretical basis for nursing at the community level: A comparison of three models. *Journal of Advanced Nursing, 14,* 569–5674.

Chinn, P. L. (Ed.). (1983). *Advances in nursing theory development.* Rockville, MD: Aspen Systems Corp.

Davis, R. (1997). Community caring: An ethnographic study within an organizational culture. *Public Health Nursing, 14*(2), 92–100.

Dolan, J. A. (1973). *Nursing in society: A historical perspective.* Philadelphia: W. B. Saunders Company.

Drevdahl, D. (1998). Diamond necklaces: Perspectives on power and the language of "community." *Scholarly Inquiry for Nursing Practice, 12*(4), 303–317.

Drevdahl, D. (1999). Meanings of community in a community health center. *Public Health Nursing, 16*(6), 417–425.

Drevdahl, D. J. (2002). Home and border: The contradictions of community. *Advances in Nursing Science, 24*(3), 8–20.

Drevdahl, D., Kneipp, S., Canales, M., & Shannon Dorcy, K. (2001). Reinvesting in social justice: A capital idea for public health nursing? *Advances in Nursing Science, 24*(2), 19–31.

Durkheim, E. (1893/1964). *The division of labor in society.* New York: The Free Press.

Felkins, P. K. (2002). *Community at work: Creating and celebrating community in organizational life.* Cresskill, NJ: Hampton Press, Inc.

Flaskerud, J. H., & Halloran, E. J. (1980). Areas of agreement in nursing theory development. *Advances in Nursing Science, 3*(1), 1–7.

Gardner, M. S. (1917). *Public health nursing.* New York: The Macmillan Company.

Goeppinger, J. (1984). Community as client: Using the nursing process to promote health. In M. Stanhope & J. Lancaster (Eds.), *Community health nursing: Process and practice for promoting health* (pp. 317–404). St. Louis: Mosby.

Goodnow, M. (1944). *Nursing history.* Philadelphia: W. B. Saunders Company.

Gusfield, J. R. (1975). *Community: A critical response.* New York: Harper & Row Publishers.

Hamilton, P. A., & Keyser, P. K. (1992). The relationship of ideology to developing community health nursing theory. *Public Health Nursing, 9*(3), 142–148.

Hillery, G. A. (1955). Definitions of community: Areas of agreement. *Rural Sociology, 20,* 779–91.

Kendall, J. (1994). Fighting back: Promoting emancipatory nursing actions. In P. L. Chinn (Ed.), *Developing the discipline: Critical studies in nursing history and professional issues* (pp. 222–236). Gaithersburg, MD: Aspen Publishers.

Kulbok, P. A., Gates, M. F., Vicenzi, A. E., & Schultz, P. R. (1999). Focus on community: Directions for nursing knowledge development. *Journal of Advanced Nursing, 29*(5), 1188–1196.

Kulig, J. C. (2000). Community resiliency: The potential for community health nursing theory development. *Public Health Nursing, 17*(5), 374–385.

Lyon, L. (1987). *The community in urban society.* Chicago: The Dorsey Press.

McFarlane, J., & Fehir, J. (1994). De madres a madres: A community, primary health care program based on empowerment. *Health Education Quarterly, 21*(3), 381–394.

Meleis, A. I. (1985). *Theoretical nursing: Development and progress.* Philadelphia: Lippincott.

Meleis, A. I. (1986). Theoretical development and domain concepts. In P. Moccia (Ed.), *New approaches to theory development* (pp. 3–21). New York: National League for Nursing.

Milio, N. (1970). *9226 Kercheval: The storefront that did not burn.* Ann Arbor: University of Michigan Press.

Moccia, P. (Ed.). (1986). *New approaches to theory development.* New York: National League for Nursing.

Navarro, V. (1984). A critique of the ideological and political positions of the Willy Brandt report and the WHO Alma Ata Declaration. *Social Science and Medicine, 18,* 467–474.

Newman, M. (1994). *Health as expanding consciousness* (2nd ed.). Boston: Jones & Bartlett.

Nightingale, F. (1860/1969). *Notes on nursing: What it is, and what it is not.* New York: Dover Publications, Inc.

Oxford English Dictionary. Retrieved July 4, 2003, from http://www.oed.com/.

Parse, R. R. (1999). Community: An alternative view. *Nursing Science Quarterly, 12*(2), 119–124.

Pharris, M. D. (2002). Coming to know ourselves as community through a nursing partnership with adolescents convicted of murder. *Advances in Nursing Science, 24*(3), 21–42.

Putnam, R. D. (2000). *Bowling alone: The collapse and revival of American community.* New York: Simon & Schuster.

Reed, P. (1995). A treatise on nursing knowledge development for the 21st century. *Advances in Nursing Science, 17*(3), 70–84.

Schultz, P. R. (1987). When client means more than one: Extending the foundational concept of person. *Advances in Nursing Science, 10*(1), 71–86.

Schultz, P. R. (1991). Foundations of nursing's perspectives on health education. *Hoitotiede, 3*(5), 223–230.

Shields, L. E., & Lindsey, A. E. (1998). Community health promotion nursing practice. *Advances in Nursing Science, 20*(4), 23–36.

Silverstein, N. G. (1994). *Lillian Wald at Henry Street, 1893–1895*. In P. L. Chinn (Ed.), *Developing the discipline: Critical studies in nursing history and professional issues* (pp. 106–118). Gaithersburg, MD: Aspen Publishers.

Smith, K., & Bazini-Barakat, N. (2003). A public health nursing practice model: Melding public health principles with the nursing process. *Public Health Nursing, 20*(1), 42–48.

SmithBattle, L., Diekemper, M., & Drake, M. A. (1999). Articulating the culture and tradition of community health nursing. *Public Health Nursing, 16*(3), 215–222.

Tonnies, F. (1887/1963). *Community and society*. C. P. Loomis (Ed.). New York: Harper & Row.

Wald, L. D. (1915/1991). *The house on Henry Street*. New Brunswick: Transaction Publishers.

Watts, R. J. (1994). Democratization of health care: Challenge for nursing. In P. L. Chinn (Ed.), *Developing the discipline: Critical studies in nursing history and professional issues* (pp. 153–162). Gaithersburg, MD: Aspen Publishers.

Weber, M. (1958). *The Protestant ethic and the spirit of capitalism*. New York: Charles Scribner's Sons.

Wheeler, C. E. (1994). *The American Journal of Nursing* and the socialization of a profession, 1900–1920. In P. L. Chinn (Ed.), *Developing the discipline: Critical studies in nursing history and professional issues* (pp. 91–105). Gaithersburg, MD: Aspen Publishers.

Williams, C. A. (1977). Community health nursing—what is it? *Nursing Outlook, 25,* 250–255.

Williams, C. A. (1984). Population-focused practice. In M. Stanhope & J. Lancaster (Eds.), *Community health nursing: Process and practice for promoting health* (pp. 805–815). St. Louis: Mosby.

Williams, C. A. (1985). Population-focused community health nursing and nursing administration: A new synthesis. In J. C. McCloskey & H. K. Grace (Eds.), *Current issues in nursing* (2nd ed.) (pp. 386–393). Boston: Blackwell Scientific Publications.

ENDNOTES

[1]Although differences in practice between community and public health nurses may exist, for the purposes of this chapter I am using the terms synonymously.

CHAPTER 8

The Evolution of the Environmental Metaparadigm of Nursing

Dorothy Kleffel

Nurses' views of environment have varied widely over time, ranging from global to individualistic perspectives and back again. In this chapter, I examine the varieties of environmental thought chronologically through three environmental paradigms: egocentric, homocentric, and ecocentric (Merchant, 1990). I also discuss how present trends in environmental thinking may evolve.

The *egocentric* worldview is grounded at the individual level and assumes that what is good for the individual is best for society. It is concerned with liberty, rights, and the independent action of the individual. It is the dominant Western worldview. The *homocentric* worldview is grounded at the social level. Social justice, rather than individual progress, is the key value. It is the utilitarian ethic in which decisions are based on the common good. The *ecocentric* approach is grounded in the cosmos. The entire environment, including rocks and minerals, is assigned intrinsic value. It is rooted in the holistic approach of oneness with a living planet, harmony, balance, interconnectedness, and transcendence (Kleffel, 1996). Nursing's ideas of environment have moved from one paradigm to another, depending on the social context of the day, various political agendas, and nurses' work settings.

ANCIENT TIMES TO THE VICTORIAN ERA

In ancient times, the earth was considered to be a unified living organism and was associated with the image of a wise, nurturing mother. In this view, called *organicism*, this huge organism was considered alive and whole. All parts were connected and related. Any influence on one part mutually affected all others and thus the entire organism (Merchant, 1980). Illness was not viewed separately from other kinds of suffering. When distinctions were made, disease was conceived as a component of suffering. At this time, the majority of healers were women who relied on natural methods. They used herbal remedies, baths, exercise, games, and entertainment to achieve balance. However, they also used purges, bleedings, and perhaps some surgery when necessary (Achterberg, 1991). Their ideas of wholeness, interconnectedness, and harmony place them within the ecocentric paradigm that is reflected in current environmental thinking.

As medicine became more scientific, women healers gave way to male physicians. Hippocrates (460–370 B.C.), the father of scientific medicine, considered disease to be influenced by environmental conditions, such as cold temperatures, the sun, and the winds. Contagious diseases were attributed to *miasmas* (noxious odors), which were inhaled by those living in the affected areas. *Humors*, the four elemental fluids of the body (blood, phlegm, black bile, and yellow bile) determined a person's physical and mental characteristics. Symptoms were expressed in humoral terms that described the temperament of patients as sanguine, phlegmatic, melancholic, or choleric. Treatment was aimed at balancing the humors.

During the Middle Ages and Renaissance (about 400–1600 A.D.), viruses (poison), stains, evil smells, putrescence, and miasmas were associated with infection and contagion. Epidemics were caused by movements in the bowels of the earth that became contaminated with *effluvia* (disagreeable vapors). Infections were caused from the evil smell of slaughterhouses, unpleasant odors hovering over marshes, and bad air. The bubonic plague of 1347 was the impetus for the public health measures of quarantine, street cleaning, and sanctions against the emptying of cesspools. The first statute against nuisances was enacted during this time (Temkin, 1971).

The ideas of what caused infectious diseases did not change very much until the 1800s. However, cleanliness became a moral and aesthetic attribute in the 17th century that merged with the concept of sanitary reform and the idea of health by the end of the 18th century. Filth became known as the cause of disease (Temkin, 1977).

The sanitary movement of the 19th century began in England as a result of a series of cholera epidemics that started in 1831 and that decimated much of the working population that had migrated into the cities. Sanitarians of that time directed their efforts toward the alleviation of squalor and the filthy living conditions that these people endured (Temkin, 1977).

The sanitary movement was part of a larger reform movement that was going on during the Victorian era. The germ theory of disease was controversial during this time, but it became the dominant theory in 1882 with the discovery of the tubercle bacillus by Robert Koch. Pathogenic microorganisms gradually substituted for the ideas of miasmas, effluvia, and evil smells (Eyler, 1979).

EARLY NURSES' COMPREHENSIVE VIEWS

Early nurse leaders had a broad and comprehensive understanding of the environment that later gave way to a more circumscribed view. Florence Nightingale and Lillian Wald's environmental perspectives are discussed in this section.

Florence Nightingale

Born in 1820, Nightingale was profoundly affected by the sanitary reform movement of her day. She maintained an inflexible belief system about sanitation and cleanliness, even though the discovery of bacteria that caused specific diseases occurred during her lifetime (Cook, 1914).

Nightingale maintained that control of the environment was essential for the restoration of health. She introduced scientific administrative methods, systems, and discipline into the healthcare system of the day (Palmer, 1986). She believed that the practical application of all sciences, including politics, administration, education, and the arts, depended on statistics. She was an avid statistician and pioneered the use of statistical methods to achieve social change (Grier & Grier, 1978). She was a close working colleague and personal friend of William Farr, a prominent statistician. He believed that reform could be made scientific through quantitative analysis;

that health was a reflection of broader social and political circumstances; and that disease and death were indices of underlying social pathology (Eyler, 1979). Nightingale shared these views. She considered her model of improved nursing as but one part of the great sanitary movement that she was involved in; the goal of which was the enhanced health of the British soldier (Baly, 1986).

Although best known for her idea of placing the patient in the best possible physical surroundings for the patient to repair her- or himself, Nightingale also had a more comprehensive concept of the environment. Her belief in the importance of environment to health was a central component of all of her work, which included approaches within the egocentric, homocentric, and ecocentric paradigms.

Egocentric Ideas

Nightingale clearly spelled out the physical environmental conditions that were necessary for individual patient healing in her popular book *Notes on Nursing* (1860). She described the need for clean air, pure water, efficient sewage, cleanliness, good nutrition, light, and warmth. She advocated for color, paintings, and views of trees and flowers in the patient's room. In addition, she encouraged a diversity of activities, such as needlepoint, writing, good conversation, and books. She felt that infants and small pets could be enjoyable companions for the sick. She advised caregivers and visitors about sickroom behavior, such as giving patients complete and unhurried attention, showing concern about their dangers and fears, being realistic about their chances of recovery, and not talking about their condition within their range of hearing.

Many of her ideas are the precursors of modern day healing modalities such as nutrition therapy, music therapy, aroma therapy, and pet therapy. Nightingale's ideas of managing the individual patient's surroundings fall into the egocentric paradigm.

Homocentric Ideas

Nightingale (1860) also had great interest in the community surrounding her clients. She shared the community environmental concerns of the sanitarians, including the proper disposal of waste and sewage, the need for irrigation and a clean water supply, the removal of dung heaps, the alleviation of overcrowding, and improved housing. She advocated for the provision of public coffee houses, cooperative stores, and savings banks as a means of improving people's quality of life (Palmer, 1984). In a paper written for the International Congress of Charities (Nightingale, 1884), she explained that nursing was more than giving medicines and treatment. She suggested that health nurses be trained to go into the community and teach sanitary and hygienic principles of health to individuals and families and to report defects in sanitation to the proper authorities. The community would then remove things that caused disease, such as "dirt, drink, diet, damp, draughts, and drains" (p. 451).

Nightingale (1860) used an epidemiological approach to the health of the community, noting increased mortality rates in specific districts and suggesting that sanitary measures be focused in those areas. She suggested that life insurance companies could arrive at a truer estimate of longevity if instead of examining the client, they examined the client's house, street, district, nearness to a river known to cause mortality in children, and ways of life. This community environmental approach falls within the homocentric paradigm of actions that values social justice and promotes the common good.

Ecocentric Ideas

Nightingale understood the necessity of addressing the broader social, economic, and political aspects of the environment to affect the health of individuals. Famine, pauperism, female slavery, prostitution, penitentiary reform, and the protection of wild birds were some of the broad environmental issues with which she concerned herself. Internationally, she spent years gathering statistics and proposing sanitation and educational reform in India. She also made suggestions about colonialism, emigration issues, and aboriginal health (Bishop & Goldie, 1962).

Nightingale used politics to effect social change. She was well born and had influential friends and acquaintances (including the Queen). She was a popular national heroine because of her work in Crimea. However, as a woman limited by the social choices that existed during the Victorian era, she had formidable barriers in carrying out the reforms that were so badly needed. Therefore, she worked behind the scenes and used her powerful contacts in order to achieve social transformations (Palmer, 1982, 1984).

In sum, Nightingale's comprehensive concept of the environment encompassed the egocentric, homocentric, and ecocentric paradigms. She translated her environmental ideas into action within each of these environmental arenas.

Lillian Wald

During Nightingale's lifetime, nearly 30 million immigrants flocked to the United States, resulting in multiple social and economic problems. Cities were plagued by overcrowding and recurring epidemics of typhus, scarlet fever, smallpox, and typhoid fever. Tuberculosis and other contagious diseases were rampant. Because of the large influx of immigrants, huge tenement houses were built without surrounding parks or open space. Cities did not have proper sewage systems and did not dispose of refuse. Rubbish was thrown into gutters, and garbage was allowed to accumulate in alleys and backyards. Dogs ran feral in packs, and rats lived under the wooden sidewalks. Hogs roamed freely and scavenged for food (Kalish & Kalish, 1978).

These were the conditions that existed when Lillian Wald was born in 1867. Wald was raised in comfortable circumstances and attended a private girls' school. She had completed nurses' training and was attending medical school when she was asked to give classes in home nursing in the Lower East Side tenement district of New York City. Appalled at the horrendous social and economic conditions that she found, she quit medical school, moved to the tenement with her friend and colleague, Mary Brewster, and began nursing in the community. In the tenement district, she founded the famous Henry Street Settlement and lived and worked there for 40 years (Christy, 1984).

During that time, the health and social welfare of the family was considered to be the woman's role and responsibility. Wald believed that environmental conditions were the root causes of ill health and poverty, and that the individual was not to blame. She urged her district nurses to direct their actions from the individual client to the larger community. Wald's views were mostly homocentric, although she also acted within the egocentric and ecocentric realms.

Like Nightingale, Wald used statistics to confirm the existence of health problems and to demonstrate the effectiveness of nursing. Like Nightingale, Wald had strong administrative skills and expanded Henry Street to a multiple-service agency that made hundreds of thousands of visits a year. Unlike Nightingale, she accepted the germ theory. Like Nightingale, she had influence and friends in high places and used political action to achieve her goals (Christy, 1984; Frachel, 1988).

Wald's contributions to alleviating the vast environmental problems of her day were substantial. She founded the Henry Street Settlement and directed the Henry Street Visiting Nurse Service; originated the ideas for the United States Children's Bureau, school nursing, and rural nursing in the Red Cross Town and Country Nursing Service; helped to secure changes in child labor laws and improve housing, parks and playgrounds, and pure food laws; upgraded classes for mentally handicapped children; influenced the passage of enlightened immigration laws; and introduced a visiting nurse service for the policy holders of the Metropolitan Life Insurance Company. During this time, Wald actively opposed political and social corruption at all levels (Christy, 1984; Kalish & Kalish, 1978).

Both Nightingale and Wald targeted their nursing actions toward what we understand as the physical, social, political, cultural, and economic environments, although the word *environment* was not in common usage at that time. They functioned within the homocentric and ecocentric as well as the egocentric environmental paradigms. They directed much of their practice to improving the environment as a means of improving the health of individuals. They were in the mainstream of the social reform movements of their times and thus were able to positively affect the lives of millions of people. However, nurses who followed them did not sustain their comprehensive views of the environment.

SHRINKING PERCEPTIONS OF ENVIRONMENT

By the 1930s, immigration had decreased, urban death rates had dramatically declined, and chronic degenerative diseases were replacing infectious diseases. These changes meant that there was less need for public health services. The Great Depression occurred, and community organizations withdrew their funding from public health programs. At the same time, the number of hospital beds increased dramatically. The hospital began its transformation from an institution for the sick poor into the modern technical, scientific, and research institution. As the number of community health nurses decreased, the need for hospital nurses increased. Public health nursing, with its community views of environment, became marginalized as hospital nursing gained ascendancy (Buhler-Wilkerson, 1983). However, by moving to the hospital setting, nurses lost much of their autonomy, and their environmental perspectives narrowed.

In the hospital setting, the concept of environment became limited and circumscribed as nurses focused on assistance with medical regimes organized along biological systems. In most instances, the patient's hospital room was considered to be the patient's environment to be managed and controlled by the nurse for the patient's benefit. The idea of environment was not addressed by most nurse authors except in terms of the patient's immediate milieu. Thus, most nurses' perspectives of environment during that time were within the egocentric paradigm.

However, a small number of public health nurses maintained their more comprehensive views of community environment. As voluntary public health agencies diminished, public health nurses moved into federal, state, and local public health agencies that were controlled by the medical profession. The science of public health is based on epidemiology, which is both a body of knowledge and a method of research. Public health nurses based their practice on the classic epidemiological model of the *host*, which is the individual of concern; the *agent*, the causative factor; and the *environment*, defined as all that is external to the agent and the host. Public health nurses used epidemiology in diagnosing, planning, treating, and evaluating community health problems. Although they worked with individual clients and families, their purpose was to achieve community-level goals (Shortridge & Valanis, 1992). Epidemiology is considered homocentric because of its emphasis on the health of populations rather than individuals. Public health nurses retained the homocentric approach, but their numbers were small and did not significantly influence mainstream nursing.

The profession's lack of consciousness of the broader environment resulted in individual nurses regarding it as outside their domain of action in practice, education, and research. This situation did not substantially change for 40 years.

ENVIRONMENT AS A COMPONENT OF NURSING THEORY

In the 1950s, nursing education began to move from hospitals to the university. Questions about the type of university preparation needed by nurses prompted nurse scholars to develop theoretical views of nursing, and the profession's first nurse theorists were born. Most of these early nurse theorists did not adequately describe the concept of environment and limited it to the immediate surroundings of the patient. Their views of the environment were quite varied and reflected their paradigmatic origins (Meleis, 1997). Little attention was given to the development of the concept, which in most instances was vague and lacked conceptual unity (Kleffel, 1991b).

An exception to the egocentric thinking of the early theorists was Martha Rogers. She developed the *science of unitary human beings*, which focused on human–environment energy fields (Rogers, 1970). She believed that the configuration of events external to humans is a central factor in the definition of environment. Humans and their environment each have energy fields that exchange matter and energy, which is the basis for human's becoming. For the individual, environment is the patterned wholeness of all that is external to the person and is coextensive with the universe.

Rogers has been a significant force in the conceptual understanding of the environment and of human–environmental interactions in nursing. She was one of the few early theorists who transcended her time; however, her theory has been critiqued as too abstract to lend itself readily to practice and research (Meleis, 1997).

Environment became a major metaparadigm of nursing in the late 1970s when Jacqueline Fawcett (1978) articulated four essential concepts of nursing—*person, environment, health,* and *nursing*—which she adapted from those identified by a survey of the curriculum of baccalaureate nursing programs by Helen Yura and Gertrude Torres (1975). These domains have been debated widely within the profession, with nursing scholars discussing, changing, and adding to the domains. Some nurses even argue that there should not be any knowledge domains within nursing, because knowledge should be available to all. However, despite all of the dialogue, there has remained a general consensus that environment is a central construct of nursing. The other concepts of person, health, and nursing have continued to be developed and researched, but environment remained mostly unaddressed until the 1980s when Teresa Chopoorian (1986) challenged nurses to broaden their concept of the environment from the client-oriented paradigm to include sociopolitical and economic contexts.

EXPLORATION OF NEW ENVIRONMENTAL PARADIGMS

Chopoorian (1986) expressed surprise that nurses do not show public outrage about the origins of their client's most serious problems, such as illnesses caused by toxic wastes; water and air pollution; war; malnutrition; and violence against women, children, and the elderly. She suggested that lack of consciousness and theories of environment contribute to the peripheral role of nursing in the social, economic, and political affairs of this country. Her reconceptualization of the environment included social, economic, and political structures; human social relations; and everyday life. Chopoorian's ideas led to an expansion of the concept of environment that had constricted nurses' thinking for so many years.

During the late 1980s and 1990s, nurse scholars began to explore a variety of environmental ideas within the ecocentric framework. Their work was influenced by environmental philosophers who at that time were examining Eastern, traditional Native American, and contemporary Western environmental thinking for possible strategies to guide actions regarding the massive environmental problems confronting the planet. The following is a brief description of a few of these ideas.

Eastern, Native American, and Contemporary Environmental Views

For the most part, Eastern philosophies have themes of a unified, living, conscious, and interacting world. Harmony and balance are emphasized. All aspects of the environment interact with the parts being within the whole and the whole being within the parts (Callicott, 1994). Traditional Native American thought regards all entities as having consciousness and reasoning abilities as intense and complete as humans. This includes the earth itself, the sky, the wind, rocks, streams, and animals, which are part of the Native American's social circle and with which they live in harmony. Although it is difficult to universalize Native American belief systems, because of the large number of different cultures the aforementioned generalizations can be made (Callicott, 1982). The Eastern and Native American worldviews originated in ancient times and resonated with the ancient organicistic ideas. However, there are emerging Western contemporary environmental theories that are reminiscent of these ancient views.

Deep ecology (radical environmentalism) touches on principles of diversity, complexity, autonomy, decentralization, symbiosis, egalitarianism, and classlessness (Devall & Sessions, 1985). Ecofeminism adheres to these general themes but incorporates gender analysis into the discourse. The Gaia hypothesis makes no clear distinctions between living and nonliving material. According to this hypothesis, the planet's organisms act together in unity to regulate the global environment by adjusting the rates at which gases are produced and removed from the atmosphere. This causes a stable state that can be affected by natural or human activity, which could force the climate into a new and different stable state that could result in the elimination of all living organisms (Lovelock, 1988).

Eastern, Native American, and contemporary Western environmental thought are all compatible with the ecocentric paradigm and hold great promise for a unified worldview to which all humans can subscribe. These philosophies have influenced several upstream nursing scholars.

Upstream Nursing Scholars

The middle 1980s and 1990s brought forth a diversity of explorations of environmental thought by nurse scholars. Patricia Butterfield (1990) introduced the idea of upstream thinking to nurses. *Upstream* interventions focus on modifying the broad social, economic, cultural, and political factors that have been shown to be the precursors of poor health. Such actions are aimed at altering environmental conditions for optimum well-being. Society is the locus of change. By contrast, *downstream* interventions are aimed at changing or assisting the individual or group to adapt, rather than altering the system itself.

Barbara Sarter (1988) compared the philosophical perspectives of Rogers and three later theorists—Neuman, Watson, and Parse—and found common shared themes of an evolutionary change of human consciousness: process, self-transcendence, open systems, harmony, relativity of space and time, and holism. Sarter noted that each of these theorists had been influenced, either directly or indirectly, by Eastern philosophies. Sarter's work demonstrated that nursing theory was beginning to evolve into a unitary and transformative metaparadigm that acknowledged the larger environment in many key aspects. She concluded that these common themes form a powerful metaphysical foundation for the further development of nursing theory.

McCarthy, Craig, Bergstrom, Whitley, Stoner, and Magilvy (1991) proposed that the environment itself be considered the nursing client and suggested that nurses consider the environment as an entity to be cared for in order to promote health. They believed that caring limited to individuals, or even the community, as in the case of public health nurses, is inadequate in light of the growing awareness of global interconnectedness and concerns. Some nurse scholars do not agree with the idea of environment as the nursing client, believing that we cannot lose sight of the individual person, and that nursing has a special covenant with society that is oriented toward individuals. However, the idea of environment as the nursing client is gaining acceptance.

Inspired by these and other upstream scholars, I examined current nursing theory and research and noted that almost all are located within the psychosocial, client-oriented nursing paradigm, which does not adequately explain conditions that originate from the environment. I explored models and theories from other disciplines and upstream nursing approaches that address multidimensional environmental characteristics and discussed them in terms of providing direction for making a paradigm shift in nursing's environmental consciousness (Kleffel, 1991b).

I also contended that *ecofeminism* offered a conceptual foundation for developing a new consciousness of the environment. Ecofeminism is a contemporary Western environmental philosophy that synthesizes environmental and feminist theories. Nursing, essentially a woman's profession, and the environment, with its female (mother earth) image, share a long history of domination and oppression. Ecofeminism has potential insights for the liberation of both. I recommended that ecofeminist insights incorporating gender-sensitive and expanded environmental awareness be incorporated into nursing research and theory building as a way to begin to address global health problems (Kleffel, 1991a).

For my qualitative doctoral dissertation research, I selected 17 upstream nursing scholars whose work addressed broad environmental dimensions and asked the participants to describe an ideal environmental domain for nursing. They described an environment that consisted of the entire planet; the plant is alive and whole and made up of interconnected and interacting parts. Within this planetary environment are numerous dynamic patterns, dimensions, and levels that are interconnected and have open boundaries. Because of the interconnections and interactions, any part of the planet that is unhealthy affects the entire planet adversely. The participants made major recommendations, which, if implemented, would change the nature of nursing. Some of the changes were (a) liberating the nursing profession from the patriarchal domination under which it functions; (b) broadening the definition of the nursing client from the individual to the collective client and to the environment itself; and (c) moving the focus of nursing from the egocentric environment of the individual to the ecocentric worldview (Kleffel, 1994).

Theory Revision to Global Arenas

During the 1990s, several of the early theorists revised their ideas of environment to encompass a more global definition. For instance, Roy (1984) originally wrote that the purpose of nursing is to enhance the adaptation of the individual patient to environmental stimuli, which she described as *focal* (immediate), *contextual* (all other), and *residual* (beliefs and attitudes). More recently, she added a philosophy of *cosmic unity*, whereby persons and environment are integrated and achieve a final common destiny (Roy, 2002).

The already farsighted Rogers continued to evolve her ideas. Her final definition was that the environment is "an irreducible, pandimensional energy field identified by pattern and integral with the human field" (Rogers, 1992, p. 29). She wrote that nursing's phenomena of concern were people and their worlds in a pandimensional universe. She believed that her theory also applied to groups, with each group being its own irreducible and indivisible energy field that is integral with its own unique environmental field.

In sum, during the 1980s and through the 1990s, several nurse scholars broadened their environmental thinking from the surroundings of the individual patient and community to a more global realm. Many were influenced by environmental ideas from Eastern, traditional Native American, and contemporary Western ideas. Several of the early theorists revised their theories to incorporate a more holistic cosmology. Nursing's environmental thinking moved from the egocentric paradigm to the ecocentric paradigm, while most public health nurses retained their community homocentric views.

RECLAIMING EARLY NURSES' COMPREHENSIVE VIEWS

Nursing's history of environmental thought began with the comprehensive and broad ideas of Florence Nightingale, Lillian Wald, and other early leaders, who worked within the egocentric, homocentric, and ecocentric environmental paradigms. Changing social conditions caused nursing's environmental thought to be confined, for the most part, to a limited egocentric worldview, where it remained for 40 years. A rising consciousness of the vast global environmental problems that are causing an untold number of diseases, suffering, and death are causing nursing scholars to reclaim their earlier homocentric and ecocentric perspectives and move into the global arenas to solve the health problems of our day.

Writing from a philosophical perspective, Jean Watson (1999) believes that something new is going on that is replacing nursing's conventional theories and practices. She calls this thinking the *transpersonal caring-healing model*. She acknowledges that it is not for all nurses, because many will want to remain in their modern technical milieu. The transpersonal caring-healing model is compatible with the ecocentric approach, but goes beyond a paradigm shift to a more fundamental ontological shift that considers our very essence of being in understanding the symbiotic relationship between humans, technology, nature, and the larger expanding universe. It draws upon the finest of the arts and sciences. It is reclaiming and reintegrating the original tenets of Nightingale at a deeper and higher level to achieve a unity of mind, body, and spirit and to the human oneness of human/environment of being that will transform the worlds of nursing, medicine, and health care.

For the purposes of environmental health research and policy development, Jane and John Dixon (2002) developed an upstream thinking, integrative model. They noted that most environmental health research has focused on the physical causes of environmental processes on health.

However, emphasizing only the physiological domain gives an incomplete picture that is not sufficient for effective environmental health problem solving. They propose four related domains: *physiological*, which concerns the effects of substances in the environment on the health of humans; *vulnerability*, which focuses on who is affected; *epistemological*, which includes personal and social knowledge; and *health protection*, which is concerned with environmental health engagement and action. Each domain reflects an interdisciplinary area of knowledge that is integrated and overlapping. Changes in one domain lead to changes in the other domains. This model provides a framework to support upstream thinking and associated research concerning environment and health.

Building on her earlier ideas of upstream thinking, Patricia Butterfield (2002) developed an upstream framework for practicing nurses that addressed environmental determinants of health. Within the framework, nursing actions are divided into *distributive actions* and *strategic actions*. Distributive actions involve the monitoring of the community for environmental health threats. They focus on the integration of environmental health into the daily work of *all* nurses. These actions include supporting and improving the nation's tracking system for exposures and diseases, improving the reporting of conditions required by state and local health departments, modifying nursing records to include environmental health information and assessment, and translating technical environmental health data into nontechnical language that includes family-specific health actions.

Strategic actions involve the advancement of knowledge of environmental health problems through *discovering* the etiology of environmentally induced diseases, *discovering* strategies for community involvement in addressing local environmental health issues, *advocating* health policies at the population level that are responsive to citizens' concerns, and *reframing* environmental health issues from the consequences of disease to their cause and prevention.

Butterfield's framework challenges the existing boundaries of prevention, cause, and cure. The integration of distributive and strategic actions by nurses will significantly affect both system and health outcomes in a manner that is consistent with the holism of nursing and the voices of clients.

THE 21ST CENTURY AND BEYOND

As we enter the 21st century, many nursing scholars are aware that our environmental problems are worldwide and more complex than ever. They believe that it is simply inadequate for nurses to continue to primarily focus on the individual within the egocentric paradigm, and that we must continue to expand our environmental metaparadigm to include the homocentric and ecocentric approaches to nursing care. World hunger, depletion of water resources, global warming, emerging and reemerging infectious diseases, desertification, Asian and African dust clouds that circle the world, loss of ecosystems resulting in loss of habitat and species extinction, and wars that leave enormous and long lasting environmental devastation—to mention just a few—are all causing indescribable human misery, disease, and death.

If we begin to envision the planet as one enormous whole, interconnected, and living sphere, we will acquire a new consciousness and understanding of our world. We will realize that the client of nursing care must include more than the individual, family, or even community. It is the planet itself that we will have to care for in order to address the enormous environmental degradation that is causing such a huge number of health problems and deaths.

We cannot confront these extremely difficult and widespread problems alone. It becomes obvious that in order to solve global environmental problems, we must act globally and in concert with the rest of the world. We can enter into the larger global, social, economic, and political arenas through nursing organizations and in partnership with other concerned groups. The use of health databases and international communication systems can provide information and networking with other health professions around the world. We can become multidisciplinary and multicultural as we address the environmental problems that affect the health of all living things.

Evolving and expanding our environmental metaparadigm will encourage us to practice, educate, and do research in the global arena in order to affect the widespread major health problems of our present day. We will join forces with those in mainstream society who are addressing the social, economic, and political conditions of the world, just as did Florence Nightingale and Lillian Wald in their day.

REFERENCES

Achterberg, J. (1991). *Woman as healer: A panoramic survey of the healing activities of women from prehistoric times to the present*. Boston: Shambhala.

Baly, M. E. (1986). *Florence Nightingale and the nursing legacy*. London: Crown Helm.

Bishop, W. J., & Goldie, S. (1962). *A bio-bibliography of Florence Nightingale*. London: Dawsons of Pall Mall.

Buhler-Wilkerson, K. (1983). False dawn: The rise and decline of public health nursing in America, 1900–1930. In E. C. Lagemann (Ed.), *Nursing history: New perspectives, new possibilities* (pp. 89–106). New York: Teachers College Press.

Butterfield, P. G. (1990). Thinking upstream: Nurturing a conceptual understanding of the societal context of health behavior. *Advances in Nursing Science, 12*(2), 1–8.

Butterfield, P. G. (2002). Upstream reflections on environmental health: An abbreviated history and framework for action. *Advances in Nursing Science, 25*(1), 32–49.

Callicott, J. B. (1982). Traditional American Indian and Western European attitudes toward nature: An overview. *Environmental Ethics, 4*(4), 293–318.

Callicott, J. B. (1994). Toward a global environmental ethic. In M. E. Tucker & J. A. Grim (Eds.), *Worldviews and ecology: Religion, philosophy, and the environment*. Maryknoll, NY: Orbis Books.

Chopoorian, T. J. (1986). Reconceptualizing the environment. In P. Moccia (Ed.), *New approaches to theory development* (pp. 39–54). New York: National League for Nursing.

Christy, T. E. (1984). Portrait of a leader: Lillian Wald. In L.Y. Kelly (Ed.), *Pages from nursing history: A collection of original articles from the pages of* Nursing Outlook, *the* American Journal of Nursing, *and* Nursing Research (pp. 84–88). New York: American Journal of Nursing Company.

Cook, E. (1914). *The life of Florence Nightingale* (2 vols.). London: Macmillan and Co.

Devall, B., & Sessions, G. (1985). *Deep ecology*. Salt Lake, CO: Perigrine Smith.

Dixon, J. K., & Dixon, J. P. (2002). An integrative model for environmental health research. *Advances in Nursing Research, 24*(3), 43–57.

Eyler, J. M. (1979). *Victorian social medicine: The ideas and methods of William Farr*. Baltimore: Johns Hopkins University Press.

Fawcett, J. (1978). The "What" of theory development. In *Theory development: What, why, how?* (pp. 17–33). New York: National League for Nursing.

Frachel, R. R. (1988). A new profession: The evolution of public health nursing. *Public Health Nursing, 5*(2), 86–90.

Grier, B., & Grier, M. (1978). Contributions of the passionate statistician. *Research in Nursing and Health, 1*(3), 103–109.

Kalish, P. A., & Kalish, B. J. (1978). *The advance of American nursing.* Boston: Little Brown.

Kleffel, D. (1991a). An ecofeminist analysis of nursing knowledge. *Nursing Forum, 26*(4), 5–18.

Kleffel, D. (1991b). Rethinking the environment as a domain of nursing knowledge. *Advances in Nursing Science, 14,* 40–51.

Kleffel, D. (1994). *The environment: Alive, whole, interconnected, and interacting.* (UMI No. 9500795).

Kleffel, D. (1996). Environmental paradigms: Moving toward an ecocentric perspective. *Advances in Nursing Science, 18*(4), 1–10.

Lovelock, J. (1988). *The ages of Gaia: A biography of our living earth.* New York: Norton.

McCarthy, P. M., Craig, C., Bergstrom, L., Whitley, E. M., Stoner, M. H., & Magilvy, J. K. (1991). Caring conceptualized for community health practice: Beyond caring for individuals. In P. L. Chinn (Ed.), *Anthology on caring* (pp. 85–94). New York: National League for Nursing.

Meleis, A. I. (1997). *Theoretical nursing: Development and progress* (3rd ed.). Philadelphia: Lippincott.

Merchant, C. (1980). *The death of nature: Women, ecology and the scientific revolution.* San Francisco: Harper & Row.

Merchant, C. (1990). Environmental ethics and political conflict: A view from California. *Environmental Ethics, 12*(1), 45–68.

Nightingale, F. (1860). *Notes on nursing: What it is and what it is not.* New York: Appleton.

Nightingale, F. (1884). Sick nursing and health nursing. In J. S. Billings (Ed.), *Hospitals, dispensaries and nursing* (pp. 444–463). New York: Garland Publishing.

Palmer, I. S. (1982). *Through a glass darkly—From Nightingale to now.* Washington, DC: American Association of Colleges of Nursing.

Palmer, I. S. (1984). Florence Nightingale: Reformer, reactionary, researcher. In *Pages from nursing history: A collection of original articles from the pages of* Nursing Outlook, *the* American Journal of Nursing, *and* Nursing Research (pp. 13–18). New York: American Journal of Nursing Company.

Palmer, I. S. (1986). A historical perspective on client/environment interaction. *Proceedings of the 1986 National Forum on Doctoral Education in Nursing* (pp. 5–24). San Francisco: School of Nursing, University of California.

Rogers, M. E. (1970). *An introduction to the theoretical basis of nursing.* Philadelphia: F. A. Davis.

Rogers, M. E. (1992). Nursing science and the space age. *Nursing Science Quarterly, 5*(1), 27–34.

Roy, C. (1984). *Introduction to nursing: An adaptation model* (2nd ed.). Englewood Cliffs, NJ: Prentice-Hall.

Roy, C. (2002). *Roy Adaptation Model.* Retrieved December 28, 2002, from http://www2.bc.edu/~royca/htm/faq.htm.

Sarter, B. (1988). Philosophical sources of nursing theory. *Nursing Science Quarterly, 1*(2), 52–59.

Shortridge, L., & Valanis, B. (1992). The epidemiological model applied in community health nursing. In M. Stanhope & J. Lanacaster, *Community health nursing: Process and practice for promoting health* (3rd ed.) (pp. 151–170). Chicago: Mosby/YearBook.

Temkin, O. (1977). *The double face of Janus: And other essays in the history of medicine.* Baltimore: Johns Hopkins.

Watson, J. (1999). *Postmodern nursing and beyond.* New York: Churchill Livingstone.

Yura, H., & Torres, G. (1975). Today's conceptual frameworks within baccalaureate nursing programs. In *Faculty-curriculum development, part III: Conceptual framework—its meaning and function* (pp.17–25). New York: National League for Nursing.

CHAPTER 9

Visible Humans, Vanishing Bodies, and Virtual Nursing: Complications of Life, Presence, Place, and Identity

Margarete Sandelowski

> Visible: The condition of being seen[1]
>
> Vanishing: Disappearing from sight[1]
>
> Virtual: Being something in essence, power, or effect, though not so formally, nominally, or expressly[1]
>
> Virtual = Visible + Vanishing

A frequently cited claim, raised to the level of a "postmodern orthodoxy,"[2] is that the body ultimately will be of no material consequence in cyberspace or the virtual worlds created by existing and yet to be developed telecommunications and computer-mediated technologies. This "conceptual denial of the body"[3] is expressed in the "posthuman"[4] view that the human body is nothing more than "a discursive and informational construction"[2] available for inter-netting with other informational structures like itself. From a posthuman perspective, there are no necessary or "essential differences or absolute demarcations between bodily existence and computer simulation, cybernetic mechanism and biological organism, [and] robot teleology and human goals."[4(p3)] The body is not an "inevitability of life," but rather an "accident of history," or a "prosthesis" that can be replaced.[4,5] While new prosthetic technologies have contributed to the transformation of the body and its organs into "flexible,"[6] fungible, and highly marketable commodities,[7] computer technology has contributed to the reconceptualization of the body as a prosthesis. Bodies are now themselves indistinguishable from other "technological artifacts,"[8] as the donation and transplantation of both human and animal organs, joint replacements and pacemakers, in vitro conception and gamete donation and surrogacy, and genetic and transgenic engineering have made human bodies more "plastic," "bionic," "interchangeable," and "virtual."[9]

Although this posthuman view of the body is anti-body, it is pro-human as it represents a utopian vision for the enhancement of human life. The apparent dispensability of bodies in cyberspace and the ability to create wholly new virtual identities online[10]—that is, to be any body—have engendered the hope that human beings will be able to transcend the gendered, racialized, disabled, disfigured, painful, and mortal bodies that have traditionally served to limit human potential and freedom. The desire for a "body-free environment" is a yearning for an

Source: Reprinted with permission from Lippincott, Williams, & Wilkins. *Advances in Nursing Science, 24*(3), 58–70.

environment free of the constraints and prejudices that "socially and culturally marked bodies" have always implied for human existence.[3]

The posthuman body is at the center of two federally funded and expressly "human" projects of enormous significance to health care and nursing, in particular: the Visible Human Project[11] and the Human Genome Project.[12] The Visible Human Project (VHP) is a digitized archive of anatomic data available over the Internet and is comprised of complete, anatomically detailed, three-dimensional representations of a male and female body achieved via computer tomography, magnetic resonance imaging, and cryosectioning of a male and female corpse. The Human Genome Project (HGP) is a visual archive of genetic data also available over the Internet. Designed to overcome the resistance of the physical body to visual and physical penetration, the VHP and the HGP allow repeated incursions into virtual bodies without actually penetrating any body at all. In contrast to the fleshy body—the one that "eats, drinks, sleeps, gets sick, and dies"—the digitized and "DNA body"[13] in these projects is "infinitely reproducible (without cloning), indefinitely storable (without freezers), almost instantaneously available (without transport), and extremely durable (without preservatives)."[14(p13)] The body in these projects is data come to life on our computer screens. As represented there, these virtual bodies seem less complicated, less immediate, less redolent, and even less lifeless than mortal bodies themselves.[15]

The VHP and HGP exemplify the "vivification of information"[16] and the informaticizing of life that defines the "posthuman,"[4] or "postvital"[17] body. As represented in these "sister" projects, life is the "life of information."[16] Death is, in turn, the "lack of information," and the computer is the "new metatechnology of life."[16] The VHP heralds a "virtual future" in which even the "mysterious materiality of the human body can be hyper-mediated, transported and traversed by the computer,"[16(p4)] and then linked to other information networks. The HGP is, in turn, celebrated as the "informatic equivalents"[15] of the fleshy body. In the HGP, human bodies are also conceived as information databases retrievable via computer and ordered according to the information-processing abilities of the computer.[16] The scientific products of the HGP herald a database of detailed information about the structure, organization, and function of human DNA. As Grady[18] observed, no contemporary information system approaches in content or complexity the amount of data in genomes or in the network governing gene expression. Like the conception of life in the VHP, life in the HGP is "digital information (albeit here) written in DNA."[19(p16)] The HGP is conceived as the book of life or "files of fate,"[20] with 23 chapters (chromosomes), each of which contain several thousand stories (genes), each of which, in turn, contains paragraphs (exons) interrupted by advertisements (introns) and which is made up of words (codons) written in letters A, G, C, T (bases).[19] Life is here the "action of a configuration of molecules . . . represented by (a 4-letter) alphabet."[17(p109)]

In short, the body in the VHP and the HGP is "just another part of an informational network, now machine, now message, always ready for exchange, each for the other."[21(p118)]

Not just the brain, but the entire human body is now conceived as an "information acquisition system" and a "primordial display device"[22] like the computer. Employing the latest techniques in "computed vision"[16] and cryosection, the VHP permits viewers to feel, fly through, and handle the body without the blood and guts of actual anatomical dissection or surgery. The virtual bodies can be made to bleed, though, and they can be repeatedly dissected and deformed without losing either the integrity of the body as a whole or its image quality. Viewers can peel away the skin, internal organs, or skeletal structure[15] in a manner recalling the flayed corpses of classical anatomy. But in a manner unique to computed vision, they can restack and reassemble slices of the body. Haptic feedback systems allow virtual surgery and endoscopy; they allow virtual surgeons and endoscopists to get a feel for the texture, mobility, and resistance of body tissues.

Similarly, the HGP allows viewers to download the "instructions" for the development, functioning, building, and running of a human being.[19] Viewers can access and print out organ data and gene sequences, and they can "interrogate the genome."[23] References to gene replication as photocopying suggest the copying machine. Human beings can now readily be conceived as printouts of their genes.[24] Definitions of heredity as a "modifiable stored program"[19] suggest the equivalence of human genetics to other computer software programs. Indeed, both the VHP and the HGP re-create human anatomy and heredity according to the logic of the computer. Both projects conceive life as information, a transformation that allows information to be conceived, in turn, as life.[25,26]

THE BODY AS RESOURCE AND PROBLEM IN NURSING

The emergence of the posthuman body as a disembodied informational structure with no clearly defined self, and the disappearance of the humanist body, or the flesh-and-blood encasing of a unique and stable self, serve as background for the rediscovery of the flesh-and-blood body as resource and problem in nursing. At the precise moment when this fleshy body is deemed increasingly irrelevant and immaterial in cyberspace come divergent moves in nursing not only toward resurrecting this body, but also toward virtual environments of nursing care, where fleshy bodies never encounter each other.

The fleshy body has been an "absent-presence"[27] in nursing. For much of the history of Western-trained nursing, nurses have been almost exclusively concerned with the corporeal bodies of ailing patients and child-bearing women.[28] While patients' bodies have been the primary "site" of nurses' work, nurses' bodies have been the primary "tools" with which they accomplished it.[29] Nurses offered their bodies as "virtual prostheses for the ailing and inadequate bodies" of their patients.[30(p192)] Yet it is only recently that nursing scholars have turned to the body as an object of study, and toward embodiment as a potential paradigm and explanation for nursing.[31]

Nurses used to be concerned primarily with the "object body" of the patient, ministering to it as a physical entity. More recently, they have turned their attention to the "lived body" as they increasingly adopted more integrated and less fragmented conceptions of the body in relation to the self.[32] Incorporating phenomenological understandings of the body—that is, that lived experience is experience of and through the physical body—nurses now not only attend to the physical body, but also help patients live with and through what happens to those bodies and to themselves as embodied beings: that is, they help patients to "reunite"[33] with their bodies. Nurses have moved away from the "old Cartesian trick"[10] of separating body from mind and toward more integrated and holistic notions of embodiment, whereby the body is seen to be inseparable from mind and self, and as the material and "existential ground"[34] for all human experience, history, and culture. Moving away from an exclusive focus on normative (e.g., anatomical, pathophysiological) concepts of the body, they moved toward an expanded focus on concrete embodiment, or the particularities and variations of individual bodies.[4] As Lawler summarized it, nursing practice remains "essentially and fundamentally about people's experiences of embodied existence, particularly at those times when the body fails to function normally."[32(pvi)] Nursing knowledge is distinctively "somological,"[32] as it is knowledge gained from particular encounters with and between bodies. The most "palpable" feature of nursing work is that pertaining to the bodies of the patients for whom nurses care.[35]

But it is precisely the somological character of nursing that remains both its greatest asset and its greatest liability. Although nursing practice has historically been legitimated and distinguished from other healthcare practices by its body work, it also has been tainted by it. Body work is "sacred" work that has allowed nurses to share intimacies with patients unknown to other healthcare providers, but it is also "profane" work that has compelled nurses to perform functions other healthcare providers will not perform.[36] In Western cultures, body work is conceived as dirty work, and body workers—who are largely women—as dirty workers.[37] The body has thus posed a cultural problem for nursing.[32]

Although it is a problem nurses have not named as a body problem per se, they have nevertheless sought to resolve it by "etherealizing the body"[38] in their philosophies and theories of nursing, and by turning away from traditional body work and toward technology in their practice.[28] These resolutions to the problem of the body in nursing offered a less visceral, less redolent, less dirty, more intellectual, and, most important, more scientific form of nursing practice. Emphasizing the interpersonal and psychosocial, as opposed to the physical, aspects of nursing care—that is, the "troubled psyche" as opposed to the "troubled body" of patients[38]—nurse theorists called attention to the minds of nurses, as opposed to their bodies, and especially their hands. Nurses wanted to be known as something more and/or other than the physician's hand or eyes.[28] By delegating such body work as bathing and toileting to ancillary personnel, nurses could escape the ancillary status of such work. By incorporating the latest information (including surveillance, screening, and diagnostic) technologies into their practice, nurses no longer had to encounter their patients "bare handed."[39] Such technologies permitted nurses both to "scientize and sanitize nursing"[32] (i.e., to replace or, at least, to mitigate the intense body intimacy of nursing with the "technical" and "measured intimacy" of medicine).[40]

By deemphasizing and delegating the traditional body work of nursing, nurses complied with the prevailing cultural practice of denigrating body work and the very "body-knowledge"[41] that is the distinctive forte of the nurse. Nurses' emphasis on the mind of nurses—for example, their ability to think, theorize, diagnose, and, in general, to process information—served only to reify the longstanding Cartesian distinction between mind and body, which has historically served to link nurses subordinately with bodies and doing, and physicians superordinately with minds and thinking. Moreover, in gradually delegating much of their traditional body work to others, nurses lost a "major channel"[42] by which they communicated with and cared for patients; that is, a primary mode of "expressive enactment of some of the cardinal values and meanings of nursing care."[35(p230)] So closely do many patients still connect body care with nursing that they view anyone who gives it as a nurse, thereby further undermining nurses' longstanding efforts to create and preserve a distinctive identity and value in the healthcare arena.

Arguably the new turn in nursing toward a serious consideration of the body signifies, in part, an effort to revalorize the body and recover what nurses lost. For example, Savage[43] found that nurses used their bodies to emphasize their closeness to their patients and thereby to claim a special place for nurses in the hierarchy of health professions. As she concluded from her ethnographic study of the nurse–patient relationship, nurses' bodies were means to establish both intimacy and points of political resistance. Yet ironically, now that nurses have once again turned to bodies—their patients' and their own—as valuable sites of practice, sources of knowledge, and distinctive markers of identity, bodies themselves have come to be seen as immaterial and more uncertain as markers between self and other.

What is especially significant for nursing is that both the human body and the nurse exist as "boundary figures."[44] With continuing advances in computer and prosthetic technologies, there is no longer any certainty about what the human body is,[27] or even where it is; that is, where its "edges" are, where it begins and ends.[45] The same has long been said of nursing. While human bodies are newly conceived as boundary figures, nurses have long served as "ambiguous figures"[46] in health care, located "in between" patients and the illnesses, treatments, and systems that threaten them, and regularly transgressing the borders between the culturally sacred and profane.[47,48] Indeed, the body work nurses do explains much of the ambiguity of nursing care as this work is itself boundary work, in the doing of which nurses "straddle (a host of) classificatory divides," such as between dirty and clean, and sickness and health.[46]

The rediscovery of the body in nursing can be seen as an effort to revive the "traditional culture"[49] of nursing and to defend against what many nurses have seen as the "acidic"[49] effects of new technologies on the "culture of caring" in nursing.[35] At least since World War II and the advent of automation and vital function monitoring, nurses have talked of the potential for new technologies to erode the essence of nursing even as these same technologies were advancing the socioeconomic position of individual nurses.[28] Specifically linking technology with dehumanization, nurses increasingly presented themselves as the boundary workers between two disparate and always potentially irreconcilable forces: technology/touch and humanism/care. Even nurses espousing the existence of a harmony between technology and care depict technology as something nurses must work with and work around in order to make it compatible with nursing care.[50]

The resurrection of the fleshy body in nursing, the simultaneous transformation of the body into information, and the new turn in medicine and nursing toward encountering patients in virtual environments of care[51] challenge nurses once again to address the tension between touch/body and technology/information as paradigms for nursing care,[52] and the "paradox of visibility"[53] that advances in technologically enhanced visibility pose for nursing. As Treichler and colleagues[53] described this paradox, what is newly seen may hide what is not, is no longer, or has never been seen. Like posthuman bodies themselves, nursing is a virtual entity that is at once everywhere and nowhere, in particular. Already "in between" because of the body work they do, nurses are increasingly offering their services in virtual environments of care. No longer simply encountering their patients directly as manifestly physical presences, they now increasingly encounter them indirectly as virtual presences on screen and over telephone lines. The turn to remote and virtual encounters with patients has both resolved and resurfaced the problem of the body and of cultural invisibility in nursing.

PLACE, PRESENCE AND TELENURSING

As nurses move to virtual environments of care, virtual environments are themselves emerging as "empirical-metaphysical testbed(s)" for timeless philosophical inquiries concerning the nature of being and knowing.[54] For nursing, these inquiries must turn on new conceptions of corporeality and "spatiality"[14] in environments of care in which nurses and patients no longer "meet in proximate space."[16]

Nurses have long emphasized and sought to capitalize from a "necessary difference"[39] between nursing and medicine—namely, the spatiotemporal asymmetry between nursing and medical practice.[55] More precisely, nurses have taken pride and advantage from their 24/7, as opposed to episodic, availability to patients and from their always-there and in-between location.

Nurses have derived from this asymmetry a distinctive sense of self, self-esteem, and agency, and a way to differentiate themselves from other healthcare providers.

Defined as "just being there"[56] and as fully available to patients—as opposed to mere spectators of them—presence has generally been conceived as minimally requiring bodily presence.[57] Gardner defined presence as a "core element of nursing" and as an "intervention tool" involving the "physical 'being there' and the psychological 'being with' a patient."[56(p191)] Connoting not only physical, but also "emotional, personal, (and) existential availability" to patients,[58] presence is also a felt perception on the part of embodied and vulnerable patients that they are cared for and safe. Although never conceptually confined to the physical realm, presence has historically connoted physical encounters between nurses and patients in proximate space in which patients can directly sense (see and feel) caring, or the "attentive gaze," "heartfelt listening,"[59] comforting touch, and inclined bodies of their nurses.[60] Physical closeness and use of the body are conceived to be embodiments of caring in nursing.[56] Especially dramatized in touch, physical encounters let neither nurse nor patient "forget that I am my body."[61(p39)] Moreover, "knowing the patient"—a nursing imperative that presence accomplishes and toward which presence is partly directed—has always been seen minimally to require carnal knowledge of the "particularity of a body"[59] occupying a defined physical space.

Yet the new virtual geography of nursing practice challenges nurses' traditional ideas of place and presence, as it calls into question how essential bodily presence is to being there and to patients' feeling that their nurse is there for them. A nurse can be physically but not wholly present to a patient. She or he can be focused on self, task, past, or future, instead of outwardly focused in the present and on the patient.[57] In short, she or he can be there but not here. Over the last century, the nursing care of patients has moved from the home to the hospital and back again to the home. At the turn of the 21st century, it is moving yet again: to cyberspace, or to a place "created and sustained by . . . computers and communication lines . . . a virtual world . . . entered equally from anywhere . . . where nothing is forgotten and yet everything changes."[62(p1)] Telenursing practices (e.g., telephone nursing, telemetry, videoconferencing, and videomonitoring) are dramatic examples that nursing care no longer necessarily occurs in any "certain physical . . . space."[63] The "arena of direct care"[63] no longer necessarily involves nurses in physical proximity with patients nor any physical ministrations at all. Nursing increasingly happens on screen, instead of "behind the screens."[28,32]

Accordingly, although presence has always been conceived as a "multichannel"[60] intervention involving physical, psychological, and even spiritual encounters, telenursing practices eliminate the proximate body as the primary channel of communication. In the burgeoning field of telephone nursing, for example, nurses and patients rely on a "monosensory device"[64] to communicate with each other. Telephone-mediated encounters "vastly reduce the richness of the presence" of nurse to patient, as each party is only partially present to each other as a voice and thus without the full range of "sensory presence" occurring in face-to-face encounters.[64(p24)] Telephone nurses are compelled to "infer from reduced data"[64] the conditions and intentions of their patients. Moreover, as telephones "incline"[64] users toward interactions involving the communication of information, nurses must work around the telephone to convey the fullness of attentive care. To offset the reductions and inclinations of the telephone, nurses have developed protocols, standardized guidelines, and algorithms for nursing appraisal, intervention, and research over the telephone.[65,66] Yet in order to preserve their psychological and personal presence there, they also have been concerned that telephone nursing not be conceived or practiced solely in terms of protocols.[67]

Although they seem far removed from each other, both media designers and nurses share a common interest in presence: in how to create it, how to use it effectively, and how it works to generate its effects.[68] "At the heart of . . . all"[68] efforts to enhance media is the creation of the illusion that technologically mediated experiences, such as telehealth encounters and virtual reality, are not mediated at all; that is, to create the perception of presence. As Bricken noted, "psychology is the physics of virtual reality."[69(p7)] The design intentions behind distance technologies are to overcome the effects of distance and electronic mediation; that is, to simulate lifelike and full-bodied encounters in proximate space that close the distance between people and allow users to feel as if they were—as telephone company advertisements promise—reaching out to touch someone.

Both media designers and nurses want to create comfortable environments for interaction that feel immediate, intimate, and "real." But while media designers want to create the kind of "telepresence" that transports users to another place (or the feeling that "you are there"), or other people and objects to the user's place (or the feeling that "it is here"), nurses have a primary interest in creating the sense of shared space (or the feeling that "we are together").[68] Telepresence, or the "illusion of (technological) nonmediation," is successful when persons "fail to perceive or acknowledge the existence of a medium in (their) communication environment and respond as (they) would if the medium were not there."[68(p10)]

Nurses have an interest in determining how teletechnologies can be used to maximize health benefits and to enhance the felt presence of the nurse, but they also have an interest in understanding how these technologies can undermine the presence of the nurse. Telehealth practices not only call for nurses to reconceptualize presence, place, and bodies in nursing, but also to explore how these practices threaten to displace nursing. Indeed, although telenursing promises great advances for nurses, it also threatens a new kind of "spatial vulnerability" for nursing, as it is a practice already vulnerable by virtue of the in-between and "gendered space" nurses occupy in the healthcare arena.[63] Inhabiting this space—as "interface"[48]—has contributed to the cultural invisibility of nurses, if only because what is in between is hidden from view and because nurses' work, like much of what is culturally deemed woman's work, "disappears into the doneness."[70] Having a place (e.g., in society, in health care) depends on being seen,[63] but what can be seen "is determined by where we are placed."[71(p23)] Telenursing has the potential to reinforce in virtual space the ambiguity of the nurse's location in actual space. In telephone nursing, the nurse is literally invisible.

Another telecase in point is the use of the nurse as "presenter" of the patient in telemedicine (V. West, unpublished paper, 1999). Here the nurse holds instruments in place (e.g., a stethoscope or otoscope) so that a physician in a distant location can appraise a particular part of the patient's body, as it is visually or acoustically transmitted electronically. Although certainly novel and dramatic, and a way to deliver medical services to persons who might not otherwise have access to them, telediagnosis with the nurse as presenter simply reprises a longstanding function of the nurse to hold patients and/or instruments in place for physicians.[28] The nurses here are in their traditional role as the physician's hand, and they are in their traditional place, in between patient and physician. Their hands are also the connecting link between the stethoscope and otoscope placed on or in the patient's body and the telecommunications devices used to transmit images of and sounds from the patient's body to the physician. Indeed, in this form of telemedicine, the nurse's body is itself nothing more than a device—a prosthesis for the physician and a component of the Internet, linking devices and people to each other. The question for nurses is: What sort of presence is this?

Toward an Informatics of the Body and an Embodied Informatics in Nursing

In summary, among the most dramatic features of Western health care at the turn of the 21st century is the increasing turn to and triumph of "phantasmic images"[72] and virtual environments that challenge our notions of what and where human beings are. Clinical practice now comprises an array of spectacular encounters that allow clinicians and patients to traverse geographical and interior body spaces once largely denied them. The patient is no longer necessarily the corporeal person in the bed or on the examining table, but rather the hypertexted, hyperreal representation on screen in the form of a rhythm strip; black-and-white or colorized image; or numeric, graphic, digital, schematic, or other visual display. The clinician, in turn, is no longer necessarily the flesh-and-blood person next to the bed or examining table, but rather a voice on the telephone, an e-mail correspondent, an online presence, or the tele-image of a face or hand holding a medical instrument.

So effectively and authoritatively have medical images "erased the need for living, breathing, talking patient-bodies"[73(p143)] for diagnosis and care that it now appears normal and even preferable not to have any patients present at all.[74] Physicians can discuss their absent patients in imaging conferences where the images themselves take center stage.[73] Nurses look forward to a time when digital images of patient wounds will become routine components of nursing practice and computerized patient records, and when patients will be moved to greater participation in their own care because they are able to "view their ulcers" on screen.[75] In lieu of living patients per se, clinicians now treat "bad strips."[76] Patients, in turn, look to images of the interior of their bodies to legitimatize their illnesses, to prove they are sick[77] and to reassure themselves that they are well. They seek both information[78] and "solace"[79] in cyberspace.

But these virtual environments are creating new views of human beings at odds with the humanist views of them that nurses and physicians cherish and to which they still cling. They make it more challenging for clinicians to conceive of the individuality of patients and the individualization of care. For nurses especially, they trouble the distinction between human being/body and information network, and between body work and information work. Yet they offer nurses an opportunity to move toward an informatics of the body and a more embodied informatics in nursing; that is, toward an orientation to nursing education, practice, and research that celebrates the body work of nursing and reunites it with the information work of nursing. Nurses operating in this new body/information paradigm will recognize the revolutions in medical imaging, reproductive technology, and genetics as information revolutions and therefore as components of a new expanded nursing informatics. All technologies entail the generation, use, and production of information, and can therefore be conceived as information technologies and within information science frameworks. These nurses will be able to conceive of the body work of washing, toileting, and turning patients as information encounters, and ultrasonography, genetic counseling, and the entry of data into the computerized medical record as embodied encounters. Even in cyberspace, and notwithstanding the posthuman view of the fleshy body as unnecessary, the fleshy body is inescapable. There is no foray into cyberspace that does not begin with actual and particular bodies in a material world (e.g., tapping keys, moving mouses, and following hyperlinks). These nurses will be able to address the paradox of visibility for nursing and other traditionally invisible groups entailed by the increasing turn to technologically mediated vision. They will map the new geography of nursing entailed in the turn to virtual nursing environments, linking not only information to embodiment, but also representation to reality, and events and practices as seemingly disparate as karyotypes, ultrasound pictures, cardiac rhythm strips, and telephone nursing to each other.

Just as it is no longer possible to draw any certain lines between medium and message, virtuality and actuality, human and not-human, it may no longer be useful for nurses to see genetic counseling, reading rhythm strips, and telephone nursing as unrelated practices. In the era of the posthuman body, nurses must not only "think genetically,"[80] but also corporeally and informationally to see genetics, for example, as part of a larger turn to transforming life into information. Although we have for a long time understood that "all life . . . operates on information,"[81(pxi)] only recently have we begun to think of life as information, and information as life. Nurses must see body and information work as constituting each other, and the body as a source of knowledge and power for nursing. Because nurses occupy a distinctive place in the health care arena, they have a distinctive contribution to make to theorizing the body in the virtual environments of care now emerging.

In 1859, Nightingale[82] sought to differentiate what "nursing is" from "what it is not." Considering where we humans are (or are not) at the turn of the 21st century, she could not have foreseen how complicated it would become to draw such lines. For a practice discipline, such as nursing, which has sought to define its boundaries paradoxically as between boundaries, the posthuman conflation of bodies and information poses the greatest challenge yet to its secure place, presence, and identity in health care.

REFERENCES

[1]Stein J., ed. *The Random House Dictionary of the English Language*. New York: Random House; 1967.

[2]Hayles NK. The materiality of informatics. *Configurations J Lit Sci Technol*. 1993;1:147–170.

[3]Balsamo A. *Technologies of the Gendered Body: Reading Cyborg Women*. Durham, NC: Duke University Press; 1997.

[4]Hayles NK. *How We Became Posthuman: Virtual Bodies in Cybernetics, Literature, and Informatics*. Chicago: University of Chicago Press; 1999.

[5]Featherstone M, Burrows R. *Cyberspace/Cyberbodies/Cyberpunk: Cultures of Technological Embodiment*. London: Sage; 1995.

[6]Martin E. *Flexible Bodies: The Role of Immunity in American Culture from the Days of Polio to the Age of AIDS*. Boston: Beacon Press; 1994.

[7]Sharp LA. Organ transplantation as a transformative experience: Anthropological insights into the restructuring of the self. *Med Anthropol Q*. 1995;9:357–389.

[8]Oldenziel R. Review of Bernice L. Hausman's Changing Sex: Transsexualism, Technology, and the Idea of Gender. *Technol Cult*. 1998;39:179–181.

[9]Williams SJ. Modern medicine and the "uncertain body": From corporeality to hyperreality? *Soc Sci Med*. 1997;45:1041–1049.

[10]Stone AR. Will the real body please stand up? Boundary stories about virtual cultures. In: Benedikt M, ed. *Cyberspace: First Steps*. Cambridge, MA: MIT Press; 1991:81–118.

[11]Visible Human Project (2000). Available at http://www.nlm.nih.gov/research/visible/visible_human.html. Accessed November 2001.

[12]Human Genome Project (2000). Available at http://www.nhgri.nih.gov/HGP. Accessed November 2001.

[13]Marchessault J. The secret of life: Informatics and the popular discourse of the life code. *N Formations*. 1996;19:120–149.

[14]Saco D. *Cyberspace and Democracy: Spaces and Bodies in the Age of the Internet*. Minneapolis, MN: University of Minnesota; 1998. Dissertation.

[15]Thacker E. . . ./visible_human.html/digital anatomy and the hyper-texted body (1998). Available at http://www.ctheory.net . Accessed November 2001.

[16]Waldby C. *The Visible Human Project: Informatic Bodies and Posthuman Medicine*. London: Routledge; 2000.

[17]Doyle R. *On Beyond Living: Rhetorical Transformations of the Life Sciences*. Stanford, CA: Stanford University Press; 1997.

[18]Grady PA. The genetics revolution: The role of the National Institute of Nursing Research. In: Lashley FR, eds. *The Genetics Revolution: Implications for Nursing*. Washington, DC: American Academy of Nursing; 1997:27–31.

[19]Ridley M. Genome: *The Autobiography of a Species in 23 Chapters*. New York: Perennial; 2000.

[20]Blueprint of the body (2000). Available at http://www.cnn.com/SPECIALS/2000/genome. Accessed November 2001.

[21]Keller EF. The body of a new machine: Situating the organism between telegraphs and computers. In: Keller EF, ed. *Refiguring Life: Metaphors of Twentieth-Century Biology*. New York: Columbia University Press; 1995:79–118.

[22]Biocca F. The cyborg's dilemma: Progressive embodiment in virtual environments. J Comput Mediated Commun. 1997;3(2):1–30. Available at http://www.ascusc.org/jcmc/vol3/issue2/biocca2.html. Accessed November 2001.

[23]Waldrop MM. On-line archives let biologists interrogate the genome. *Science*. 1995;269:1356–1358.

[24]Nelkin D, Lindee MS. *The DNA Mystique: The Gene as a Cultural Icon*. New York: W.H. Freeman; 1995.

[25]Helmreich S. Replicating reproduction in artificial life: Or, the essence of life in the age of virtual electronic reproduction. In: Franklin S, Ragone H, eds. *Reproducing Reproduction: Kinship, Power, and Technological Innovation*. Philadelphia: University of Pennsylvania Press; 1998:207–234.

[26]Kay LE. Cybernetics, information, life: The emergence of scriptural representations of heredity. *Configurations J Lit Sci Technol*. 1997;5:23–91.

[27]Williams SJ, Bendelow G. *The Lived Body: Sociological Themes, Embodied Issues*. London: Routledge; 1998.

[28]Sandelowski M. *Devices and Desires: Gender, Technology, and American Nursing*. Chapel Hill, NC: University of North Carolina Press; 2000.

[29]Short P. Picturing the body in nursing. In: Lawler J, eds. *The Body in Nursing*. Melbourne, Australia: Churchill Livingstone; 1997:7–9.

[30]Wiltshire J. Medical science, nursing, and the future. *Nurs Inq*. 1998;5:187–193.

[31]Wilde MH. Why embodiment now? *Adv Nurs Sci*. 1999;22(2):25–38.

[32]Lawler J. *Behind the Screens: Nursing, Somology, and the Problem of the Body*. Melbourne, Australia: Churchill Livingstone; 1991.

[33]Van Manen M. Modalities of body experience in illness and health. *Qual Health Res*. 1998;8:7–24.

[34]Csordas TJ. *Embodiment and Experience: The Existential Ground of Culture and Self*. Cambridge, UK: Cambridge University Press; 1994.

[35]Fox RC, Aiken LH, Messikomer CM. The culture of caring: AIDS and the nursing profession. *Milbank Q*. 1990;68(suppl 2):226–256.

[36]Wolf ZR. *Nurses' Work: The Sacred and the Profane.* Philadelphia: University of Pennsylvania Press; 1988.

[37]Hughes EC. *Men and Their Work.* Glencoe, IL: Free Press; 1958.

[38]Dunlop MJ. Is a science of caring possible? *J Adv Nurs.* 1986;11:661–670.

[39]Davis C. Poetry about patients: Hearing the nurse's voice. *J Med Humanities.* 1997;18:111–125.

[40]Crenner CW. *Professional Measurement: Quantifying Health and Disease in American Medical Practice, 1880–1920.* Cambridge, MA: Harvard University; 1993. Dissertation.

[41]Heath D. Bodies, antibodies, and modest interventions. In: Downey GL, Dumit J, eds. *Cyborgs and Citadels: Anthropological Interventions in Emerging Sciences and Technologies.* Santa Fe, NM: School of American Research Press; 1997:66–82.

[42]Lesser M, Keane V. Nursing and bodily care. *Am J Nurs.* 1955;55:804–806.

[43]Savage J. Gestures of resistance: The nurse's body in contested space. *Nurs Inq.* 1997;4:237–245.

[44]Balsamo A. Forms of technological embodiment: Reading the body in contemporary culture. In: Featherstone M, Burrows R, eds. *Cyberspace/Cyberbodies/Cyberpunk: Cultures of Technological Embodiment.* London: Sage; 1995:215–237.

[45]Wilson RR. Cyber(body)parts: prosthetic consciousness. In: Featherstone M, Burrows R, eds. *Cyberspace/Cyberbodies/Cyberpunk: Cultures of Technological Embodiment.* London: Sage; 1995:239–259.

[46]Littlewood J. Care and ambiguity: towards a concept of nursing. In: Holden P, Littlewood J, eds. *Anthropology and Nursing.* London: Routledge; 1991:170–189.

[47]Engelhardt HT. Physicians, patients, health care institutions—and the people in between: Nurses. In: Bishop AH, Scudder JR, eds. *Caring, Curing, Coping: Nurse–Physician–Patient Relationships.* Tuscaloosa, AL: University of Alabama Press; 1983:62–79.

[48]Parker J. The body as text and the body as living flesh: Metaphors of the body and nursing in postmodernity. In: Lawler J, eds. *The Body in Nursing.* Melbourne, Australia: Churchill Livingstone; 1997:11–29.

[49]Ihde D. Image technologies and traditional culture. In: Feenberg A, Hannay A, eds. *Technology and the Politics of Knowledge.* Bloomington, IN: Indiana University Press; 1995:147–158.

[50]Barnard A, Sandelowski M. Technology and humane nursing care: (Ir)reconcilable or invented difference? *J Adv Nurs.* 2001;34:367–375.

[51]Friedman RH, Stollerman JE, Mahoney DM, Rozenblyum L. The virtual visit: Using telecommunications technology to take care of patients. *J Am Med Inf Assoc.* 1997;4:413–425.

[52]Gadow S. Touch and technology: Two paradigms of patient care. *J Religion Health.* 1984;23:63–69.

[53]Treichler PA, Cartwright L, Paley C. Introduction: Paradoxes of visibility. In: Treichler PA, Cartwright L, Penley C, eds. *The Visible Woman: Imaging Technologies, Gender, and Science.* New York: New York University Press; 1998:1–17.

[54]Lauria R. Virtual reality: An empirical–metaphysical testbed. *J Comput Mediated Commun.* 1997;3(2):1–29. Available at http://www.ascusc.org/jcmc/vol3/issue2/lauria.html. Accessed November 2001.

[55]Allen D. The nursing–medical boundary: A negotiated order? *Soc Health Illness.* 1997;19:498–520.

[56]Gardner DL. Presence. In: Bulechek GM, McCloskey JC, eds. *Nursing Interventions: Essential Nursing Treatments.* 2nd ed. Philadelphia: W.B. Saunders; 1992:191–200.

[57]Osterman P, Schwartz-Barcott D. Presence: Four ways of being there. *Nurs Forum.* 1996;31:23–30.

[58]Lawler J. Knowing the body and embodiment: Methodologies, discourses and nursing. In: Lawler J, eds. *The Body in Nursing.* Melbourne, Australia: Churchill Livingstone; 1997:31–51.

[59]Liaschenko J. Knowing the patient. In: Thorne SE, Hayes VE, eds. *Nursing Praxis: Knowledge and Action.* Thousand Oaks, CA: Sage; 1997:23–38.

[60]Bottorff JL, Morse JM. Identifying types of attending: Patterns of nurses' work. *Image J Nurs Sch.* 1994;26:53–60.

[61]Wyschogrod E. Empathy and sympathy as tactile encounter. *J Med Philos.* 1981;6:25–43.

[62]Benedikt M. Introduction. In: Benedikt M, ed. *Cyberspace: First Steps.* Cambridge, MA: MIT Press; 1991:1–24.

[63]Liaschenko J. Ethics and the geography of the nurse–patient relationship: Spatial vulnerabilities and gendered space. *Sch Inq Nurs Pract.* 1997;11:45–59.

[64]Ihde D. *Technics and Praxis: A Philosophy of Technology.* Dordrecht, Holland: D. Reidel; 1979.

[65]American Academy of Ambulatory Care Nursing. *Telephone Nursing Practice Administration and Practice Standards.* Pitman, NJ: Anthony J. Jannetti; 1997.

[66]Haas SA, Androwich IA. Telephone consultation. In: Bulechek GM, McCloskey JC, eds. *Nursing Interventions: Effective Nursing Treatments.* 3rd ed. Philadelphia: W. B. Saunders; 1999:670–684.

[67]Greenberg ME. The domain of telenursing: issues and prospects. *Nurs Econ.* 2000;18:220–222.

[68]Lombard M, Ditton T. At the heart of it all: The concept of presence. *J Comput Mediated Commun.* 1997;3(2):1–45. Available at http://www.ascusc.org/jcmc/vol3/issue2/lombard.html. Accessed November 2001.

[69]Bricken W. *Virtual Reality: Directions of Growth.* Seattle, WA: University of Washington Human Interface Technology Laboratory; 1990. Available at http://www.hitl.washington.edu/publications. Accessed November 2001.

[70]Star SL. Epilogue: Work and practice in social studies of science, medicine, and technology. *Sci Technol Hum Values.* 1995;20:501–507.

[71]Liaschenko J. The moral geography of home care. *Adv Nurs Sci.* 1994;17(2):16–26.

[72]Stafford BM. *Artful Science: Enlightenment Entertainment and the Eclipse of Visual Education.* Cambridge, MA: MIT Press; 1994.

[73]Simon CM. Images and image: Technology and the social politics of revealing disorder in a North American hospital. *Med Anthropol Q.* 1999;13:141–162.

[74]Kaplan B. Objectification and negotiation in interpreting clinical images: Implications for computer-based patient records. *Artif Intell Med.* 1995;7:439–454.

[75]Fischetti LF, Paguio EC, Alt-White AC. Digitized images of wounds: A nursing practice innovation. *Nurs Clin North Am.* 2000;35:541–550.

[76]Cartwright E. The logic of heartbeats: Electronic fetal monitoring and biomedically constructed birth. In: Davis-Floyd R, Dumit J, eds. *Cyborg Babies: From Techno-Sex to Techno-Tots.* New York: Routledge; 1998:240–254.

[77]Rhodes LA, McPhillips-Tangum CA, Markham C, Klenk R. The power of the visible: the meaning of diagnostic tests in chronic back pain. *Soc Sci Med.* 1999;48:1189–1203.

[78]Lewis D, Pesut DJ. Emergence of consumer health care informatics. *Nurs Outlook.* 2001;49:7.

[79]Klemm P, Hurst M, Dearholt SL, Trone SR. Cyber solace: Gender differences on Internet cancer support groups. *Comput Nurs.* 1999;17:65–72.

[80]Lashley FR. Genetics in nursing education. *Nurs Clin North Am.* 2000;35:795–805.

[81]Levinson P. *The Soft Edge: A Natural History and Future of the Information Revolution.* London: Routledge; 1997.

[82]Nightingale F. *Notes on Nursing: What It Is and What It Is Not.* New York: Dover; 1859/1969.

CHAPTER 10

Machine Technologies and Caring in Nursing

Rozzano C. Locsin

Because of the prominence of medical and machine technology, patient care is frequently based on procedures that prolong patients' lives, but do not fully meet their need for care. Many encounters with patients seem to involve complex equipment and technologies, which nurses monitor and document. Patient satisfaction is often determined by how well a nurse facilitates a patient's recovery, which is often associated with the competent management of machinery. As all health professionals are well aware, dependence on mechanical technology is often an indispensable ingredient of health care. However, health care consists of much more than equipment and medical techniques.

Current concerns about nursing care as dependent upon expert utilization of machine technology was vividly described to me by a student who discussed a colleague's apprehension about the quality of nursing practice in an intensive care unit. Her colleague, a professional nurse, claimed that nursing routines in the unit had become so overwhelmingly machine-oriented that she could no longer care for her patients. Most activities were centered on ventilators and cardiac monitors or documentation requirements that she believed prevented her from caring. Talking to patients and families, in her view, was often considered superfluous, and seldom viewed as a nursing priority. Such caring activities, she observed, are often considered as actions that require nursing time but with no immediate identifiable outcome. Being with a patient is considered time spent which does not influence patients' health and is therefore expendable.

Various definitions of technology exist, but one that fits nursing well is Heidegger's (1977) who described technology as a means to an end, an instrument, as well as a human activity. Cardiac monitors are technological instruments and interpretation technology of the monitor data is a human activity. Information acquired through cardiac monitoring is used as a basis for the human activities of medical and nursing care technology to maintain a patient's well-being.

Using Bush's (Sandelowski, 1983) definition of technology as people, equipment, and procedures in established patterns of interactions for the purpose of accomplishing human goals, Sandelowski (1993) describes "technology dependency" as reliance on equipment and techniques to manage the health care of patients. The effect of technology in nursing practice is also discussed by Cooper (1993) who describes critical care units as places where the challenge of machine technology in nursing is greatest. In these settings, machines provide life support to patients and are

Source: Permission from Blackwell Sciences and Sigma Theta Tau International. *Image—the Journal of Nursing Scholarship,* *27*(3), 201–203, 1995.

vital to patient care management. However, what patients often see are nurses who seem to focus more attention on the data gathered from equipment than on their human needs. That is, competence in machine technologies assumes more prominence that listening to the patient.

Machine technology can bring a patient closer to nurses because it enhances their knowledge of the person being cared for. However, such technology may also widen the gap between a nurse and patient because of an unconscious disregard of the patient as a person. While machine technology becomes a familiar work world for nurses, it may contribute to the alienation of patients for whom such a world is unfamiliar (Cooper, 1993).

The pressure for professional nurses to achieve greater technological proficiency has fostered a rethinking of the technology-caring dichotomy. Caring has gained prominence as a central expression of nursing. The current emphasis on technologic competency for quality nursing practice and the dependence on machine technology have achieved a distinction that is significant to the practice of nursing. To fully care in this increasingly sophisticated world, nurses seem to recognize that technologic proficiency is a desirable attribute—not a substitute for caring but an enhancement of caring.

Caring in nursing is described in a variety of ways (Leininger, 1988; Watson, 1985). Discussions of the issues (Jacono, 1993; Olson, 1993; Phillips, 1993; Swanson, 1993), attributes (Roach, 1987), and ingredients (Mayeroff, 1971) illustrate the current significance of the concept of caring. Leininger's (1988) claim that caring is the unifying feature of nursing is supported by Lynaugh and Fagin (1988) who state that caring is the common link that brings nurses together. Watson (1990) emphasizes that caring is the moral ideal of nursing. Roach (1992) considers caring to be the human mode of being.

Some of the dimensions of caring in nursing include caring as the tradition of nursing (Olson, 1993) and caring as a process of interaction (Phillips, 1993). Mangold (1991) defined caring as assisting other's growth in a cognitive and emotional sense toward self-actualization. Noddings (1984) suggested that caring occurs when one is completely receptive to another: The interactive nature of caring requires mutual commitment from the one giving care and the one being cared for. Phillips (1993) described caring in nursing as requiring the one giving care to respond to the needs of another. Boykin and Schoenhofer (1993) describe caring as being intentionally and authentically present for an other.

The competent use of machine technology as integral to caring has been advanced by several including Cooper (1993), Jones and Alexander (1993), Ray (1987), and Sandelowski (1993). For some, competence with machines and equipment in technologically demanding environments is the ultimate expression of nursing as caring and technologic incompetence is tantamount to not caring. Neighbors and Eldred (1993) emphasize that nurses must be able to address the complexity of nursing, and develop technologic skills to keep pace with the rapid development of new technologies in health care.

A MODEL OF TECHNOLOGIC COMPETENCE AND CARING FOR NURSING

Nurse scholars and practitioners are constantly searching for useful ways to understand and improve the practice of nursing. Boykin and Schoenhofer's (1993) framework of nursing as caring grounds my model machine and caring competence in nursing. The nursing-as-caring perspective makes the following assumptions: "Persons are caring by virtue of their being human; persons are caring moment to moment; persons are whole or complete in the moment; personhood is the process of living grounded in caring; and personhood is enhanced through participating in nurturing relationships with caring others" (p. 3). All nursing takes place within nursing situations. These situations are the shared lived experiences between nurses and patients. Within the intimacy of a nursing situation, the calls for nursing are expressed, heard, and addressed, as the patient too, seeks to be known and affirmed as a caring person. In a nursing situation, the nurse enters the world of the other with the intention of knowing him or her as a caring person. Nursing responses are specific forms of caring created within a unique situation. In the caring process, each person grows in competency including technologic competency to express himself or herself as a caring person.

Cooper (1993) states that machines and equipment are designed to be invulnerable, objective, and predictable. These features stand in contrast to the human characteristics of vulnerability, subjectivity, and unpredictability. Professional nurses are challenged to be technologically competent while simultaneously recognizing human vulnerability in responding authentically and intentionally to calls for nursing. Authenticity and intentionality are demonstrated when a nurse appropriately accepts the patient's care as requiring high levels of technical expertise. In doing so, the nurse focuses his or her activities toward knowing the person fully as a caring human being who is in the process of living his or her hopes, dreams, and aspirations. Burfitt and colleagues (1993) describe caring for critically ill patients as a mutual process in which intentions from the nurse and patient are joined to form a shared experience. This mutual process can allow each to envision healing as an outcome that might otherwise be unrecognized. Jones and Alexander (1993) state that, by proclaiming the adoption of a definition of technology that incorporates caring, the growth and evolution of nursing scholarship will be advanced.

Machine technologies and caring are the core structures, while the perspective of nursing-as-caring grounds the model for nursing. As simply technology, competence in machine technologies is exemplified by nursing assistants who are ordered to use these to determine physiological aspects of patients. A professional nurse who is technologically competent but is not a caring person knowledgeable about the patient is the ultimate example of a care giver who is not truly caring. Understanding technology as a human way to know a patient more fully as a person is the expression of the harmonious relationship between machine technology and caring in nursing.

Technologic competence requires intentionality along with compassion, confidence, commitment, and conscience (Roach, 1987). This is achieved by donning different lenses in grounding nursing practice. In this model for nursing, the lens employed is the perspective of Nursing as Caring (Boykin & Schoenhofer, 1993). It is used to conceive of machine technological competence and caring as coexisting harmoniously in nursing.

The model in Figure 10.1 shows three circles, one for each of the concepts: machine technologies and caring, technological competence, and nursing as caring. The inner circle is divided into two halves; in one half is shown the concept of machine technologies and in the other, the concept of caring. The middle circle showing the concept of technological competence is undivided. The outermost circle is divided into two; the left side showing the concept of nursing as caring, and the right side empty. The use of the circle is best explained by Boykin and Schoenhofer (1993) as illustrating the commitment of people toward knowing self and others as living

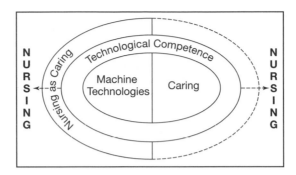

Figure 10.1 Model of Machine Technologies and Caring in Nursing. Copyright 1995, Rozzano C. Locsin.

caring and growing in caring. The inner circle shows that the core concepts of machine technology and caring exist inseparably but relate distinctly as independent entities. This independence is represented by the straight line that divides the circle into two distinct halves, while simultaneously demonstrating interconnectedness within the circle. Although the two core concepts are proximal and connected, they do not express the fullness of nursing. The competent exhibition of machine technology and caring is perceived as nursing practice if grounded on a perspective of nursing, otherwise it is simply the practice of machine proficiency.

The arrow directed to the left traversing the concepts of caring, machine technologies, technological competence, and the perspective of nursing as caring, exemplify the focus and direction of technologically competent nursing practice. It is the exhibition of proficiency in machine technology and caring. This practice occurs when machine technology is expressed competently while being grounded in the perspective of nursing as caring. Similarly, nursing practice that is exhibited without the framework of nursing as caring is plainly proficiency in machine technologies. However, there exists the potential for adeptness in machine technologies as nursing practice, even without its grounding in the perspective of nursing as caring. This occurs when machine proficiency is performed within other frameworks of nursing. This potential is exhibited as the broken lines which intersect the concepts of machine technologies, caring, and technological competence. Proficiency in machine technologies demonstrated without grounding in a nursing perspective is simply technological competence. When this occurs, the perception of people as human beings who are complete in the moment and therefore do not need to be fixed (Boykin and Schoenhofer, 1993) is nonexistent, focusing nursing practice as merely technological competence. This is the dilemma of machine technology demonstrated as technologic competence without the benefit of a perspective of nursing.

As people seriously involved in giving care know, there are various ways of expressing caring. Professional nurses will continue to find meaning in their technological caring competencies, expressed intentionally and authentically, to know another as a whole person. Through the harmonious coexistence of machine technology and caring technology the practice of nursing is transformed into an experience of caring. Professionals and patients alike can only be grateful for the vast advances in medical and machine technology, however, their inclusion must not compromise nurses' caring. As nursing professionals become more and more technically adept, they will find new and improved ways to build strong, healing connections with patients.

REFERENCES

Boykin, A., & Schoenhofer, S. (1993). *Nursing as caring: A model for transforming practice*. New York: National League for Nursing.

Burfitt, S., Greiner, D., Miers, L., Kinney, M., & Branyon, M. (1993). Professional nurse caring as perceived by critically ill patients: A phenomenologic study. *American Journal of Critical Care, 2*(6), 489–499.

Carper, B. (1977). Fundamental patterns of knowing in nursing. *Advances in Nursing Science, 1*, 13–24.

Cooper, M. (1993). The intersection of technology and care in the ICU. *Advances in Nursing Science, 15*(3), 23–32.

Heidegger, M. (1977). *The question concerning technology and other essays*. New York: Harper and Row.

Jacono, B. (1993). Caring is loving. *Journal of Advanced Nursing, 18*, 192–194.

Jones, C., & Alexander, J. (1993). The technology of caring: A synthesis of technology and caring for nursing administration. *Nursing Administration Quarterly, 17*(2), 11–20.

Leininger, M. (Ed.). (1984). *Care: The essence of nursing and health*. Thorofare, NJ: Slack.

Leininger, M. (1988). Leininger's theory of nursing: Cultural care diversity and universality. *Nursing Science Quarterly, 1*, 152–160.

Lynaugh, J., & Fagin, C. (1988). Nursing outcomes of age. *Image: Journal of Nursing Scholarship, 20*, 184–190.

Mangold, A. (1991). Senior nursing students and professional nurses' perceptions of effective caring behaviors: A comparative study. *Journal of Nursing Education, 30*, 134–139.

Mayeroff, M. (1971). *On caring*. New York: Harper and Row.

Neighbors, M., & Eldred, E. (1993). Technology and nursing education. *Nursing and Health Care, 14*(2), 96–99.

Noddings, N. (1984). *Caring: A feminine approach to ethics and moral education*. Berkeley, CA: University of California Press.

Olson, T. (1993). Laying claim to caring: Nursing and the language of training, 1915–1937. *Nursing Outlook, 41*(2), 68–72.

Phillips, P. (1993). A deconstruction of caring. *Journal of Advanced Nursing, 18*, 1554–1558.

Porter, S. (1992). The poverty of professionalization: A critical analysis of strategies for the occupational advancement of nursing. *Journal of Advanced Nursing, 17*, 723–728.

Ray, M. (1987). Technological caring: A new model in critical care. *Dimensions in Critical Care, 6*(3), 166–73.

Roach, S. (1987). *The human act of caring*. Ottawa, Canada: Canadian Hospital Association.

Sandelowski, M. (1993). Toward a theory of technology dependency. *Outlook, 41*(1), 36–42.

Swanson, K. (1993). Nursing as informed caring for the well-being of others. *Image: Journal of Nursing Scholarship, 25*, 352–357.

Watson, J. (1985). *Nursing: The philosophy and science of caring*. Boulder, CO: Colorado Associated University Press.

SECTION 2

APPLICATION OF THE SCHOLARSHIP OF NURSING IDEAS

Patrice K. Nicholas

Several philosophical and theoretical views have relevance for the development of nursing ideas. In particular, the views on ways of knowing in nursing have advanced the application of nursing knowledge in the practice settings. In Chapter 11, Carper examines the four fundamental patterns of knowing in nursing: (1) empirics, the science of nursing; (2) esthetics, the art of nursing; (3) personal knowledge, a unique personal aspect of nursing; and (4) ethics, moral knowledge in nursing. Carper addresses the importance of these ways of knowing in supporting the rationale for the discipline of nursing and the development of nursing as a practice discipline.

In Chapter 12, White reviews and critiques the four fundamental patterns of knowing in nursing and extends her analysis to include sociopolitical knowing, which is aimcd at understanding the sociopolitical context of the nurse and patient and the sociopolitical context of nursing as a practice profession.

In Chapter 13, Meisenhelder develops a vivid portrayal of the power of spirituality in the ways of knowing and in the realm of personal knowledge in nursing—one of Carper's original elements in the ways of knowing. Meisenhelder's chapter addresses the empirics of personal knowing applied to spirituality and offers specific nursing interventions to consider in clinical practice.

In Chapter 14, Barrett addresses the importance of defining nursing, science, research, and nursing-theory-guided practice. With an optimistic view on the development of the science of nursing, Barrett discusses the importance of articulating the unique contributions of the discipline of nursing and the interrelationships of nursing science, research, and practice.

In Chapter 15, Chin explores the philosophic theory of nursing art. She suggests that this theory was developed to "deepen understanding of that aspect of nursing that moves practice beyond purely technical or interpersonal skills into a realm that is a healing art form" (p. 173). Further, Chin suggests that nursing art evolves in four ways: refining synchronous narrative skills; refining synchronous movement skills; rehearsal and connoisseurship; and reflective practice in nursing. Each of these skills is essential to developing the theory, art, and practice base of nursing.

In Chapter 16, Kelly examines nursing practice within a rational, relational, and reflective perspective with application of the views of Carper, Chin, and White. Kelly applies a reflective framework as well as feminist theory and views on cultural competence to the clinical problem of domestic abuse experienced by women of different cultures.

In Chapter 17, Corless and Nicholas examine the ethics of care at the end of life. The concept of a healthy death is explored within an ethical framework that includes nursing's views of the patient-centered environment. Complex ethical issues, such as euthanasia, withholding support, and technology at the end of life are addressed. Palliative care and patient-centered care are discussed for their relevance in nursing's role at the end of life. Pizzo's chapter on grief and bereavement (Chapter 18) provides further discussion of end-of-life issues and places them within a historical perspective.

In Chapter 19, Terres examines family coping and how parents of children with disabilities adapt. She examines factors involved in parents' coping, family adaptation, and social support within a framework for family and community networks.

Sylvester and Rosenbloom-Brunto examine health issues of older adults with the application of the Neuman Systems Model. In Chapter 20, Sylvester explores adverse drug reactions in the elderly and the role of nursing in preventing adverse drug reactions. In Chapter 21, Rosenbloom-Brunto reviews the literature on delirium in the hospitalized older adult and the application of Neuman's Model in the development of a delirium risk stratification tool.

Johnson's chapter (Chapter 22) explores one of the earliest nursing perspectives—the work of Hildegard Peplau and her views on the interpersonal relationship between nurse and patient. Johnson examines the central focus of nursing within Peplau's framework and applies this knowledge in clinical nursing practice. In Chapter 23, Nicholas and colleagues examine the concepts of quality of life and cancer rehabilitation with an application to instrument development. The use of theories—both within and outside of nursing—are important in the development of appropriate instruments for use in clinical nursing practice.

This section concludes with two classic chapters by Schlotfeldt and Newman that address nursing's future. In Chapter 24, Schlotfeldt examines the structure of nursing knowledge as a priority for creating the future of nursing. In Chapter 25, Newman addresses the ways in which we create barriers to nursing praxis and the need to connect emerging theories.

CHAPTER 11

Fundamental Patterns of Knowing in Nursing

Barbara A. Carper

It is the general conception of any field of inquiry that ultimately determines the kind of knowledge the field aims to develop as well as the manner in which that knowledge is to be organized, tested, and applied. The body of knowledge that serves as the rationale for nursing practice has patterns, forms, and structure that serve as horizons of expectations and exemplify characteristic ways of thinking about phenomena. Understanding these patterns is essential for the teaching and learning of nursing. Such an understanding does not extend the range of knowledge, but rather involves critical attention to the question of what it means to know and what kinds of knowledge are held to be of most value in the discipline of nursing.

IDENTIFYING PATTERNS OF KNOWING

Four fundamental patterns of knowing have been identified from an analysis of the conceptual and syntactical structure of nursing knowledge.[1] The four patterns are distinguished according to logical type of meaning and designated as: (1) empirics, the science of nursing; (2) esthetics, the art of nursing; (3) the component of a personal knowledge in nursing; and (4) ethics, the component of moral knowledge in nursing.

EMPIRICS: THE SCIENCE OF NURSING

The term nursing science was rarely used in the literature until the late 1950s. However, since that time there has been an increasing emphasis, one might even say a sense of urgency, regarding the development of a body of empirical knowledge specific to nursing. There seems to be general agreement that there is a critical need for knowledge about the empirical world, knowledge that is systematically organized into general laws and theories for the purpose of describing, explaining, and predicting phenomena of special concern to the discipline of nursing. Most theory development and research efforts are primarily engaged in seeking and generating explanations which are systematic and controllable by factual evidence and which can be used in the organization and classification of knowledge.

Source: Carper, B. A. (1978). Fundamental patterns of knowing in nursing. *Advances in Nursing Science, 1*(1), 13–23. Reprinted with permission from Lippincott, Williams & Wilkins.

The pattern of knowing which is generally designated as "nursing science" does not presently exhibit the same degree of highly integrated abstract and systematic explanations characteristic of the more mature sciences, although nursing literature reflects this as an ideal form. Clearly there are a number of coexisting, and in a few instances competing, conceptual structures—none of which has achieved the status of what Kuhn calls a scientific paradigm. That is, no single conceptual structure is as yet generally accepted as an example of actual scientific practice "which include[s] law, theory, application, and instrumentation together . . . [and] . . . provide[s] models from which spring particular coherent traditions of scientific research." [2(p10)] It could be argued that some of these conceptual structures seem to have greater potential than others for providing explanations that systematically account for observed phenomena and may ultimately permit more accurate predictions and control of them. However, this is a matter to be determined by research designed to test the validity of such explanatory concepts in the context of relevant empirical reality.

New Perspectives

What seems to be of paramount importance, at least at this stage in the development of nursing science, is that these pre-paradigm conceptual structures and theoretical models present new perspectives for considering the familiar phenomena of health and illness in relation to the human life process; as such they can and should be legitimately counted as discoveries in the discipline. The representation of health as more than the absence of disease is a crucial change; it permits health to be thought of as a dynamic state of process which changes over a given period of time and varies according to circumstances rather than a static either/or entity. The conceptual change in turn makes it possible to raise questions that previously would have been literally unintelligible.

The discovery that one can usefully conceptualize health as something that normally ranges along a continuum has led to attempts to observe, describe, and classify variations in health, or levels of wellness, as expressions of a human being's relationship to the internal and external environments. Related research has sought to identify behavioral responses, both physiological and psychological, that may serve as cues by which one can infer the range of normal variations of health. It has also attempted to identify and categorize significant etiological factors which serve to promote or inhibit changes in health status.

Current Stages

The science of nursing at present exhibits aspects of both the "natural history stage of inquiry" and the "stage of deductively formulated theory." The task of the natural history stage is primarily the description and classification of phenomena which are, generally speaking, ascertainable by direct observation and inspection.[3] But current nursing literature clearly reflects a shift from this description and classification form to increasingly theoretical analysis which is directed toward seeking or inventing explanations to account for observed and classified empirical facts. This shift is reflected in the change from a largely observational vocabulary to a new, more theoretical vocabulary whose terms have a distinct meaning and definition only in the context of the corresponding explanatory theory.

Explanations in the several open-system conceptual models tend to take the form commonly labeled functional or teleological.[4] For example, the system models explain a person's level of wellness at any particular point in time as a function of current and accumulated effects of inter-actions with his or her internal and external environments. The concept of adaptation is central to this type of explanation. Adaptation is seen as crucial in the process of responding to environ-mental demands (usually classified as stressors), and enables an individual to maintain or reestab-lish the steady state which is designated as the goal of the system. The developmental models often exhibit a more genetic type of explanation in that certain events, the developmental tasks, are believed to be causally relevant or necessary conditions for the normal development of an individual.

Thus the first fundamental pattern of knowing in nursing is empirical, factual, descriptive, and ultimately aimed at developing abstract and theoretical explanations. It is exemplary, dis-cursively formulated, and publicly verifiable.

ESTHETIC: THE ART OF NURSING

Few, if indeed any, familiar with the professional literature would deny that primary em-phasis is placed on the development of the science of nursing. One is almost led to believe that the only valid and reliable knowledge is that which is empirical, factual, objectively descriptive, and generalizable. There seems to be a self-conscious reluctance to extend the term of knowl-edge to include those aspects of knowing in nursing that are not the result of empirical investi-gation. There is, nonetheless, what might be described as a tacit admission that nursing is, at least in part, an art. Not much effort is made to elaborate or to make explicit this esthetic pattern of knowing in nursing—other than to vaguely associate the "art" with the general category of man-ual and/or technical skills involved in nursing practice.

Perhaps this reluctance to acknowledge the esthetic component as a fundamental pattern of knowing in nursing originates from the vigorous efforts made in the not-so-distant past to exor-cise the image of the apprentice-type educational system. Within the apprentice system, the art of nursing was closely associated with an imitative learning style and the acquisition of knowl-edge by accumulation of unrationalized experiences. Another likely source of reluctance is that the definition of the term art has been excessively and inappropriately restricted.

Weitz suggests that art is too complex and variable to be reduced to a single definition.[5] To conceive the task of esthetic theory as definition, he says, is logically doomed to failure in that what is called art has no common properties—only recognizable similarities. This fluid and open approach to the understanding and application of the concept of art and esthetic meaning makes possible a wider consideration of conditions, situations and experiences in nursing that may properly be called esthetic, including the creative process of discovery in the empirical pattern of knowing.

Esthetics Versus Scientific Meaning

Despite this open texture of the concept of art, esthetic meanings can be distinguished from those in science in several important aspects. The recognition "that art is expressive rather than merely formal or descriptive," according to Rader, "is about as well established as any fact in the whole field of esthetics."[6(pxvi)] An esthetic experience involves the creation and/or appreciation of a singular, particular, subjective expression of imagined possibilities or equivalent realities which "resists projection into the discursive form of language."[7] Knowledge gained by empirical description is discursively formulated and publicly verifiable. The knowledge gained by subjective acquaintance, the direct feeling of experience, defines discursive formulation. Although an esthetic expression requires abstraction, it remains specific and unique rather than exemplary and leads us to acknowledge that "knowledge—genuine knowledge, understanding—is considerably wider than our discourse."[7(p23)]

For Wiedenbach, the art of nursing is made visible through the action taken to provide whatever the patient requires to restore or extend his ability to cope with the demands of his situation."[8] But the action taken, to have an esthetic quality, requires the active transformation of the immediate object—the patient's behavior—into a direct, nonmediated perception of what need is actually being expressed by the behavior. This perception of the need expressed is not only responsible for the action taken by the nurse but reflected in it.

The esthetic process described by Wiedenbach resembles what Dewey refers to as the difference between recognition and perception.[9] According to Dewey, recognition serves the purpose of identification and is satisfied when a name tag or label is attached according to some stereotype or previously formed scheme of classification. Perception, however, goes beyond recognition in that it includes an active gathering together of details and scattered particulars into an experienced whole for the purpose of seeing what is there. It is perception rather than mere recognition that results in a unity of ends and means which gives the action taken an esthetic quality.

Orem speaks of the art of nursing as being "expressed by the individual nurse through her creativity and style in designing and providing nursing that is effective and satisfying."[10(p155)] The art of nursing is creative in that it requires development of the ability to "envision valid modes of helping in relation to 'results' which are appropriate."[10(p69)] This again evokes Dewey's sense of a perceived unity between an action taken and its result—a perception of the means of the end as an organic whole.[9] The experience of helping must be perceived and designed as an integral component of its desired result rather than conceived separately as an independent action imposed on an independent subject. Perhaps this is what is meant by the concept of nursing, the whole patient or total patient care. If so, what are the qualities that enable the creation of a design for nursing care that eliminate or would minimize the fragmentation of means and ends?

Esthetic Pattern of Knowing

Empathy—that is, the capacity for participating in or vicariously experiencing another's feelings—is an important mode in the esthetic pattern of knowing. One gains knowledge of another person's singular, particular, felt experience through empathic acquaintance.[11,12] Empathy is controlled or moderated by psychic distance or detachment in order to apprehend and abstract what we are attending to, and in this sense it is objective. The more skilled the nurse becomes in perceiving and empathizing with the lives of others, the more knowledge or understanding will be gained of alternate modes of perceiving reality. The nurse will thereby have available a larger repertoire of choices in designing and providing nursing care that is effective and satisfying. At the same time, increased awareness of the variety of subjective experiences will heighten the complexity and difficulty of the decision making involved. *empathy = ↑ care/ options and ↑ complexity*

The design of nursing care must be accompanied by what Langer refers to as sense of form, the sense of "structure, articulation, a whole resulting from the relation of mutually dependent factors, or more precisely, the way the whole is put together."[7(p16)] The design, if it is to be esthetic, must be controlled by the perception of the balance, rhythm, proportion and unity of what is done in relation to the dynamic integration and articulation of the whole. "The doing may be energetic, and the undergoing may be acute and intense," Dewey says, but "unless they are related to each other to form a whole," what is done becomes merely a matter of mechanical routine or of caprise.[9]

The esthetic pattern of knowing in nursing involves the perception of abstracted particulars as distinguished from the recognition of abstracted universals. It is the knowing of a unique particular rather than an exemplary class.

THE COMPONENT OF PERSONAL KNOWLEDGE

Personal knowledge as a fundamental pattern of knowing in nursing is the most problematic, the most difficult to master and to teach. At the same time, it is perhaps the pattern most essential to understanding the meaning of health in terms of individual well-being. Nursing considered as an interpersonal process involves interactions, relationships, and transactions between the nurse and the patient-client. Mitchell points out that "there is growing evidence that the quality of interpersonal contacts has an influence on a person's becoming ill, coping with illness and becoming well."[13(p950)] Certainly the phrase "therapeutic use of self," which has become increasingly prominent in the literature, implies that the way in which nurses view their own selves and the client is of primary concern in any therapeutic relationship.

Personal knowledge is concerned with the knowing, encountering, and actualizing of the concrete, individual self. One does not know *about* the self; one strives simply to *know* the self. This knowing is a standing in relation to another human being and confronting that human being as a person. This "I-Thou" encounter is unmediated by conceptual categories or particulars abstracted from complex organic wholes.[14] The relation is one of reciprocity, a state of being that cannot be described or even experienced—it can only be actualized. Such personal knowing extends not only to other selves but also to relations with one's own self.

It requires what Buber refers to as the sacrifice of form, that is, categories or classifications for a knowing of infinite possibilities, as well as the risk of total commitment.

> Even as a melody is not composed of tones, nor a verse of words, nor a statue of lines—one must pull and tear to turn a unity into a multiplicity—so it is with the human being to whom I say You. . . . I have to do this again and again; but immediately he is no longer You.[14(p59)]

Maslow refers to this sacrifice of form as embodying a more efficient perception of reality in that reality is not generalized nor predetermined by a complex of concepts, expectations, beliefs, and stereotypes.[15] This results in a greater willingness to accept ambiguity, vagueness, and discrepancy of oneself and others. The risk of commitment involved in personal knowledge is what Polanyi calls the "passionate participation in the act of knowing."[16(p17)]

The nurse in the therapeutic use of self rejects approaching the patient-client as an object and strives instead to actualize an authentic personal relationship between two persons. The individual is considered as an integrated, open system incorporating movement toward growth and fulfillment of human potential. An authentic personal relation requires the acceptance of others in their freedom to create themselves and the recognition that each person is not a fixed entity, but constantly engaged in the process of becoming. How then should the nurse reconcile this with the social and/or professional responsibility to control and manipulate the environmental variables and even the behavior of the person who is a patient in order to maintain or restore a steady state? If a human being is assumed to be free to choose and chooses behavior outside of accepted norms, how will this affect the action taken in the therapeutic use of self by the nurse? What choices must the nurse make in order to know another self in an authentic relation apart from the category of patient, even when categorizing for the purpose of treatment is essential to the process of nursing?

Assumptions regarding human nature, McKay observes, "range from the existentialist to the cybernetic, from the idea of an information processing machine to one of a many splendored being."[17(p399)] Many of these assumptions incorporate in one form or another the notion that there is, for all individuals, a characteristic state which they, by virtue of membership in the species, must strive to assume or achieve. Empirical descriptions and classifications reflect the assumption that being human allows for prediction of basic biological, psychological, and social behaviors that will be encountered in any given individual.

Certainly empirical knowledge is essential to the purposes of nursing. But nursing also requires that we be alert to the fact that models of human nature and their abstract and generalized categories refer to and describe behaviors and traits that groups have in common. However, none of these categories can ever encompass or express the uniqueness of the individual encountered as a person, as a "self." These and many other similar considerations are involved in the realm of personal knowledge, which can be broadly characterized as subjective, concrete, and existential. It is concerned with the kind of knowing that promotes wholeness and integrity in the personal encounter, the achievement of engagement rather than detachment; and it denies the manipulative, impersonal orientation.

ETHICS: THE MORAL COMPONENT

Teachers and individual practitioners are becoming increasingly sensitive to the difficult personal choices that must be made within the complex context of modern health care. These choices raise fundamental questions about morally right and wrong action in connection with the care and treatment of illness and the promotion of health. Moral dilemmas arise in situations of ambiguity and uncertainty, when the consequences of one's actions are difficult to predict and traditional principles and ethical codes offer no help or seem to result in contradiction. The moral code which guides the ethical conduct of nurses is based on the primary principle of obligation embodied in the concepts of service to people and respect for human life. The discipline of nursing is held to be a valuable and essential social service responsible for conserving life, alleviating suffering, and promoting health. But appeal to the ethical "rule book" fails to provide answers in terms of difficult individual moral choices which must be made in the teaching and practice of nursing.

The fundamental pattern of knowing identified here as the ethical component of nursing is focused on matters of obligation or what ought to be done. Knowledge of morality goes beyond simply knowing the norms or ethical codes of the discipline. It includes all voluntary actions that are deliberate and subject to the judgment of right and wrong—including judgments of moral value in relation to motives, intentions, and traits of character. Nursing is deliberate action, or a series of actions, planned and implemented to accomplish defined goals. Both goals and actions involve choices made, in part, on the basis of normative judgments, both particular and general. On occasion, the principles and norms by which such choices are made may be in conflict.

According to Berthold, "goals are, of course, value judgments not amenable to scientific inquiry and validation."[18(p196)] Dickoff, James, and Wiedenbach also call attention to the need to be aware that the specification of goals serves as "a norm or standard by which to evaluate activity . . . [and] . . . entails taking them as values—that is, signifies conceiving these goal contents as situations worthy to be brought about."[19(p422)]

For example, a common goal of nursing care in relation to the maintenance or restoration of health is to assist patients to achieve a state in which they are independent. Much of the current practice reflects an attitude of value attached to the goal of independence, and indicates nursing actions to assist patients in assuming full responsibility for themselves at the earliest possible moment or to enable them to retain responsibility to the last possible moment. However, valuing independence and attempting to maintain it may be at the expense of the patient's learning how to live with physical or social dependence when necessary—for example, in instances when prognosis indicates that independence cannot be regained.

Differences in normative judgments may have more to do with disagreements as to what constitutes a "healthy" state of being than lack of empirical evidence or ambiguity in the application of the term. Slote suggests that the persistence of disputes, or lack of uniformity in the application of cluster terms, such as health, is due to "the difficulty of decisively resolving certain sorts of value questions about what is and is not important." This leads him to conclude "that value judgment is far more involved in the making of what are commonly thought to be factual statements than has been imagined."[20(p220)]

The ethical pattern of knowing in nursing requires an understanding of different philosophical positions regarding what is good, what ought to be desired, what is right; of different ethical frameworks devised for dealing with the complexities of moral judgments; and of various orientations to the notion of obligation. Moral choices to be made must then be considered in terms of specific actions to be taken in specific, concrete situations. The examination of the standards, codes, and values by which we decide what is morally right should result in a greater awareness of what is involved in making moral choices and being responsible for the choices made. The knowledge of ethical codes will not provide answers to the moral questions involved in nursing, nor will it eliminate the necessity for having to make moral choices. But it can be hoped that:

> The more sensitive teachers and practitioners are to the demands of the process of justification, the more explicit they are about the norms that govern their actions, the more personally engaged they are in assessing surrounding circumstances and potential consequences, the more "ethical" they will be; and we cannot ask much more.[21(p221)]

USING PATTERNS OF KNOWING

A philosophical discussion of patterns of knowing may appear to some as a somewhat idle, if not arbitrary and artificial, understanding having little or no connection with the practical concerns and difficulties encountered in the day-to-day doing and teaching of nursing. But it represents a personal conviction that there is a need to examine the kinds of knowing that provide the discipline with its particular perspectives and significance. Understanding four fundamental patterns of knowing makes possible an increased awareness of the complexity and diversity of nursing knowledge.

Each pattern may be conceived as necessary for achieving mastery in the discipline, but none of them alone should be considered sufficient. Nor are they mutually exclusive. The teaching and learning of one pattern does not require the rejection or neglect of any of the others. Caring for another requires the achievements of nursing science, that is, the knowledge of empirical facts systematically organized into theoretical explanations regarding the phenomena of health and illness. But creative imagination also plays its part in the syntax of discovery in science, as well as in developing the ability to imagine the consequences of alternate moral choices.

Personal knowledge is essential for ethical choices in that moral action presupposes personal maturity and freedom. If the goals of nursing are to be more than conformance to unexamined norms, if the "ought" is not to be determined simply on the basis of what is possible, then the obligation to care for another human being involves becoming a certain kind of person—and not merely doing certain kinds of things. If the design of nursing care is to be more than habitual or mechanical, the capacity to perceive and interpret the subjective experiences of others and to imaginatively project the effects of nursing actions on the lives becomes a necessary skill.

Nursing thus depends on the scientific knowledge of human behavior in health and in illness, the esthetic perception of significant human experiences, a personal understanding of the unique individuality of the self, and the capacity to make choices within concrete situations involving particular moral judgments. Each of these separate but interrelated and interdependent fundamental patterns of knowing should be taught and understood according to its distinctive logic, the restricted circumstances in which it is valid, the kinds of data it subsumes, and the methods by which each particular kind of truth is distinguished and warranted.

The major significances to the discipline of nursing in distinguishing patterns of knowing are summarized as: (1) the conclusions of the discipline conceived as subject matter cannot be taught or learned without reference to the structure of the discipline—the representative concepts and methods of inquiry that determine the kind of knowledge gained and limit its meaning, scope, and validity; (2) each of the fundamental patterns of knowing represents a necessary but incomplete approach to the problems and questions in the discipline; and (3) all knowledge is subject to change and revision. Every solution of an existing problem raises new and unsolved questions. These new and as yet unsolved problems require, at times, new methods of inquiry and different conceptual structures that change the shape and patterns of knowing. With each change in the shape of knowledge, teaching and learning require looking for different points of contact and connection among ideas and things. This clarifies the effect of each new thing known on other things known and the discovery of new patterns by which each connection modifies the whole.

REFERENCES

1. Carper, B. A. "Fundamental patterns of knowing in nursing." PhD dissertation, Teachers College, Columbia University, 1975.
2. Kuhn, T. *The structure of scientific revolutions.* Chicago: University of Chicago Press, 1962.
3. Northrop, F. S. C. *The logic of the sciences and the humanities.* New York: The World Publishing Co., 1958.
4. Nagel, E. *The structure of science.* New York: Harcourt, Brace and World, Inc., 1961.
5. Weitz, M. "The role of theory in aesthetics." In Rader, M., ed. *A modern book of esthetics* 3rd ed. New York: Holt, Rinehart and Winston, 1960.
6. Rader, M. "Introduction: The meaning of art." In Rader, M., ed. *A modern book of esthetics* 3rd ed. New York: Holt, Rinehart and Winston, 1960.
7. Langer, S. K. *Problems of art.* New York: Charles Scribner and Sons, 1957.

8. Wiedenbach, F. *Clinical nursing: A helping art.* New York: Springer Publishing Co., Inc., 1964.

9. Dewey, J. *Art as experience.* New York: Capricorn Books, 1958.

10. Orem, D. E. *Nursing: Concepts of practice.* New York: McGraw-Hill Book Co., 1971.

11. Lee, V. "Empathy." In Rader, M., ed. *A modern book of esthetics* 3rd ed. New York: Holt, Rinehart and Winston, 1960.

12. Lippo, T. "Empathy, inner imitation and sense-feeling." In Rader, M., ed. *A modern book of esthetics* 3rd ed. New York: Holt, Rinehart and Winston, 1960.

13. Mitchell, P. H. *Concepts basic to nursing.* New York: McGraw-Hill Book Co., 1973.

14. Buber, M. *I and thou.* Translated by Walter Kaufman. New York: Charles Scribner and Sons, 1970.

15. Maslow, A. H. "Self-actualizing people: A study of psychological health." In Moustakas, C. E., ed. *The self.* New York: Harper and Row, 1964.

16. Polanyi, M. *Personal knowledge.* New York: Harper and Row, 1964.

17. McKay, R. "Theories, models and systems for nursing." *Nursing Research* 18:5, September–October, 1969

18. Berthold, J. S. "Symposium on theory development in nursing: Prologue." *Nursing Research* 17:3, May–June 1964.

19. Dickoff, J., James, P. and Wiedenbach, E. "Theory in a practice discipline: Part I." *Nursing Research* 17, September–October, 1968.

20. Slote, M. A. "The theory of important criteria." *Journal of Philosophy* 63, April 14, 1966.

21. Greene, M. *Teacher as stronger.* Belmont, CA: Wadsworth Publishing Co., Inc., 1975.

Each area - empirics, esthetics, personal knowledge, & ethics must be present & interacting to approach & solve problems in nursing. All of these are crucial aspects which must be known & understood in able to teach and/or learn in nursing. All of this knowledge is in flux and not static.

CHAPTER 12

Patterns of Knowing: Review, Critique, and Update

Jill White

In 1978 Barbara Carper[1] published "Fundamental Patterns of Knowing in Nursing" in the first edition of *Advances in Nursing Science*. Based on her doctoral work, the article described her typology of patterns of knowing in nursing. These patterns she named empirics, esthetics, ethics, and personal knowing.

Carper's patterns of knowing have been much cited and commented on, albeit somewhat uncritically, in the writing of nurses over the ensuing years. As with much of nursing's written heritage, there is little connection between the number of citations and the extent of critical development that has taken place. An important exception to this, however, is the work of Jacobs-Kramer and Chinn[2] a decade after Carper's article first appeared. Jacobs-Kramer and Chinn extended Carper's framework by producing a model that elucidated their understanding of the creation and development, the expression and transmission, and the assessment of each of Carper's patterns of knowing. Their intention was for such an elucidation to facilitate the integration of these patterns of knowing in nursing into clinical practice.

The lack of recent dialogue about the patterns themselves or about the model may reflect the decreased interest in the use of models generally in nursing, part of a move from reductionist thinking. The continued citation of both Carper and Jacobs-Kramer and Chinn, however, suggests their work is still being used in teaching.

The "patterns" of Carper[1] and "model" of Jacobs-Kramer and Chinn[2] do provide convenient conceptual organizers for introducing students to different ways of knowing in nursing. The patterns and model can be used to facilitate exploration of nursing practice and to enhance understanding of the rich history of modern nursing writing. They enable the contributions of nurses from the past to be analyzed in terms of the dominant social, political, and philosophical contexts of their time and enable nurses to trace with understanding the cumulative and disparate knowledge development that contributes to the discipline of nursing.

Given that the patterns and the model are still being used in education, it is appropriate that they be reviewed and critiqued within the context of nursing knowledge development in the mid-1990s. This article offers such a review, critique, and update.

In her seminal article "Fundamental Patterns of Knowing in Nursing," Carper[1] identified the following patterns:

Source: White, J. (1995). Patterns of knowing: Review, critique, and update. *Advances in Nursing Science,* 17(4): 73–86. Reprinted with permission from Lippincott, Williams & Wilkins.

139

☐ empirics, or the science of nursing;
☐ ethics, or the moral component;
☐ the component of personal knowledge; and
☐ esthetics, or the art of nursing.

In this article the author explores each of these patterns in turn, looking first at what Carper had to say, then at the extension of this pattern within the Jacobs-Kramer and Chinn model, and finally at questions that arise with references to the current literature and each particular pattern. Table 12.1 summarizes the essential elements of Jacobs-Kramer and Chinn's model of nursing knowledge.

EMPIRICS: THE SCIENCE OF NURSING

Carper described empirics as

knowledge that is systematically organized into general laws and theories for the purpose of describing, explaining, and predicting phenomena of special concern to the discipline of nursing. . . . The first fundamental pattern of knowing in nursing is empirical, factual, descriptive, and ultimately aimed at developing abstract theoretical explanations. It is exemplary, discursively formulated, and publicly verifiable.[1(pp14–15)]

The key element here is that the "ultimate aim" of this knowing is "theory" development. Inherent in theory development is the ontological position that nature has a single or dominant reality commonly experienced and about which one can draw generalizable abstract explanations. This clearly encompasses the traditional view of scientific knowledge with its stance of objectivity and context-free replicability. This view was the dominant one in the nursing research and writ-

Table 12.1 Summary of Essential Elements: Model of Nursing Knowledge

Dimension	Empirics	Ethics	Personal	Esthetics
Creative	Describing Explaining Predicting	Valuing Clarifying Advocating	Encountering Focusing Realizing	Engaging Interpreting Envisioning
Expressive	Facts Theories Models	Codes Standards Normative-ethical theories	Self: Authentic and disclosed	Art-act
	Descriptions to impart understanding	Descriptions of ethical decision-making		
Assessment: Critical question	What does this represent?	Is this right?	Do I know what I do?	What does this mean?
	How is this representative?	Is this just?	Do I do what I know?	
Process-context	Replication	Dialogue	Response and reflection	Criticism
Credibility index	Validity	Justness	Congruity	Consensual meaning

ing at the time of Carper's doctoral work. However, it is debatable at this time whether this pattern encompasses all research-based knowing, which Jacobs-Kramer and Chinn expressed as "facts, theories, models and descriptions that impart understanding."[2(p132)]

The realist ontological position, whose assumptions allow generalization, may also be seen as including grounded theory and ethnographic research, which generate generalizable abstractions. However, the relativist position of the interpretive paradigm as represented by phenomenology, for example, also seeks to provide "descriptions that impart understanding" but would not be consistent with Carper's definition of having an ultimate aim of developing abstract theoretical explanations that could be "systematically organized into general laws and theories."[1(p14)]

It is therefore suggested that the definition of the empirical pattern of knowing needs to be modified to accommodate the relativist ontological positions of knowledge development using methodologies such as phenomenology. If not modified, nursing needs to acknowledge the limitations of this definitions in encompassing empirical knowing that seeks not to generalize, but rather through interpretation or description to put before the reader context-embedded stories whose purpose is to enrich understanding.

The inclusion of the word "understanding" by Jacobs-Kramer and Chinn[2] within the aim of the empirical pattern of knowing may be confusing; "understanding" is more commonly associated with the aim of research within the interpretive paradigm. The ontological position of the interpretive paradigm embraces the notion of multiple realities that cannot be generalized and puts this paradigm outside Carper's definition of this pattern of knowing. As discussed later, interpretive and critical research is encompassed more appropriately elsewhere.

Jacobs-Kramer and Chinn's model suggests that the pattern of empirics is expressed through "facts, theories, models and descriptions."[2(p132)] This expressive dimension may be extended to include the common mode of expression and transmission via books for academic theoretical instruction and professional journals for stimulation of professional debate.

Jacobs-Kramer and Chinn's[2] assessment dimension asks the critical questions, "What does this represent?" and "How is it representative?" The process of assessment is by replication, and the index of credibility they suggest is validity—that the knowledge can be demonstrated to be what it is thought to be. The assessment dimension is dealt with in their article in a brief paragraph that makes it somewhat difficult to fully grasp the intent of the critical questions; a critical question, one would assume, inquires about the relationships between the variables under study and the generalizability of the relationships.

In the case of grounded theory, a critical question would be the relationship to the core concepts of the other concepts and the nature of these relationships. The process of judging the trustworthiness of the results would require both sufficient detail to enable replication and application and the seeking out and offering up to professional debate of the findings. As Kuhn said, "There is no standard higher than assent of the relevant community."[3(p94)] The remaining process for ascertaining credibility is the "fit" of the new knowledge with the extant knowledge in the area at the time.

It is within this assessment dimension that the case for empirics, not including work using the interpretive or critical paradigm, gains credence. Here, clearly, the standards of credibility are not related to validity, replication, or relationships between variables or categories. If the empirical pattern were to be expanded to accommodate knowledge created through interpretive or critical work, an entirely new assessment would be required with different critical questions, processes, and credibility indices.[4] Possible modifications to the pattern of empirics within the model of nursing knowledge are proposed in Table 12.2.

ETHICS: THE MORAL COMPONENT

"The fundamental pattern of knowing identified here as the ethical component of nursing is focused on matters of obligation or what ought to be done."[1(p20)] In exploring this pattern Carper acknowledged the important place of knowledge of norms and ethical codes: "The examination of the standards, codes, and values by which we decide what is morally right should result in a greater awareness of what is involved in making moral choices and being responsible for the choices made."[1(p21)]

However, Carper goes on to caution that the complexity of the ethical issues in modern health care practice means that "moral choices to be made must be considered in terms of specific actions to be taken in specific concrete situations."[1(p21)] In extending this caution, Carper represents one of the earliest nursing writers to speak of the situational and relational importance of moral decision making, which has become fundamental to the ethic of care now so prevalent in the nursing literature.

There has been a plethora of publications in the area of moral knowing. Principal among these are the works of Benner,[5,6] Benner and Wrubel,[7] Bishop and Scudder,[8,9] Cooper,[10,11] and Watson.[12,13] Not directly within nursing but highly relevant are the works of Gilligan,[14,15] Noddings,[16] Pellegrino,[17,18] and Zaner.[19,20]

Much of this work has its origins in Gilligan's[14] critique of Kohlberg's[21] hierarchy of moral decision making. Gilligan challenged Kohlberg's contention that believing in "the primacy and universality of individual rights" was the highest form of moral development and that this represented a morally superior position to Kohlberg's penultimate stage, which embodies a "very strong sense of being responsible to the world."[14(p444)] Gilligan suggested that the focus on in-

Table 12.2 Empirics: Essential Elements

Dimension	Original Model[2]	Modifications
Creative	Describing Explaining Predicting	Describing Explaining Predicting
Expressive	Facts Theories Models Descriptions to impart understanding	Facts Theories and models described in books and professional journals Descriptions that indicate relationships
Assessment: Critical question	What does this represent? How is it representative?	What relationships were found? Under what conditions do these relationships hold?
Process-context	Replication	Replication and application Professional debate Fit with extant knowledge
Credibility index	Validity Reliability	Validity Reliability

dividual justice is a predominantly male orientation, whereas women more commonly adopt the contextual, relational, care orientation that focuses on social and moral good.

Moss[22] provided an excellent exploration of the impact of Gilligan's work over the past 15 years, particularly in relation to nursing. Together with Moss, Bishop and Scudder,[9] Benner,[6] and Watson[12,13] suggested that the moral ideal of doing what is good (that is, adopting a caring orientation), rather than that which is just, will most fruitfully be revealed through the exploration of practice rather than simply through reference to "rule-books." This, they suggested, will happen through processes of reflection, discussion, and storytelling of life and nursing practice.[6,9] Bishop and Scudder made a particularly salient point for nurses within this discussion by questioning the notion that moral decision making is about "solving" dilemmas at all: "One way in which the moral sense differs from traditional nursing ethics is that it directs us to moral dilemmas which cannot be solved but must be lived with and, when possible, ameliorated."[9(p124)]

Zaner, with reference to physicians but equally applicable to nursing, suggested "Moral life is essentially communal at its root, and it is mutuality (in all its complex forms), not autonomy, that is foundational. Nowhere is this more plainly evident than in the contexts of clinical situations dealing with ill persons."[20(p292)] Zaner went on to say that "autonomy and rights" inhibit moral decision making within health care, which requires, foundationally, cooperation and collaboration.

Cooperation is also emphasized in the work of Gadow[23] on existential advocacy. She reinforced the importance of collaboratively making "the effort to help persons become clear about what they want to do, by helping them discern their values in the situation and on the basis of that self examination, to reach decisions which express their reaffirmed, perhaps recreated, complex of values."[23(p44)] Gadow put this effort forward as a moral ideal, not duty, norm, or prescription. It is a moral enterprise through situated engagement.

Jacobs-Kramer and Chinn[2] focused on justice in their assessment dimension of this pattern. An expansion of the assessment dimension is required to accommodate an ethic of care as well as an ethic of justice. Thus, potential modifications to the ethical pattern of knowing are listed in Table 12.3.

The discussion about ethics shows how intimately linked the patterns of moral and personal knowing are. Moral knowing requires fundamentally an authentic interpersonal involvement for its development.

PERSONAL KNOWING

The pattern of personal knowing is concerned with "the knowing, encountering and actualizing of the concrete individual self. One does not know about self; one strives simply to know the self. This knowing is a standing in relation to another human being and confronting that human being as a person."[1(p18)] The pattern of personal knowing develops when the nurse approaches the patient not as an object or category of illness, but strives instead "to actualize an authentic personal relationship between two persons."[1(p19)] This pattern requires the nurse to allow the person who is the patient-client to "matter." It involves engagement as opposed to detachment.

Mayeroff, whom Carper[1] cited as a source for her notion of personal knowing, saw a special feature of caring for a person as being "able to understand [the person] and his world as if I were inside it."[24(p42)] For Mayeroff, relationship is about reciprocity, about helping the other "grow" and through this, growing oneself. However, Mayeroff's words harbor subtle paternal-

Table 12.3 Ethics: Essential Elements

Dimension	Original Model[2]	Modifications
Creative	Valuing Clarifying Advocating	Valuing the moral idea of caring Critically appraising values Existential advocacy[23] Sensitizing to other value positions Fostering articulation of everyday notions of good[6]
Expressive	Codes, standards Normative theories Descriptions of decision making	Codes, standards Normative theories Observation Storytelling to explore embedded notions of good
Assessment: Critical question	Is it right? Is it just?	Is it good? Is it just? Is it right? Does it embody caring?
Process-context	Dialogue	Dialogue Critical reflection Collaborative values elaboration
Credibility index	Justness	Justness Goodness Caring Congruence with personal values of patients

ism: "I want it to grow in its own right . . . and I feel the other's growth as bound up with my own sense of well-being."[24(p8)] Such a position mitigates against genuine reciprocity.

Mayeroff's reciprocity was elaborated on and refined in the works of Watson[12] in describing her concept of "transcendental moment," by Taylor[25] in her exposition of the "ordinariness" of nursing, in Morse's[26] work on nurse–patient relationships, and in Moch[27] in her exploration of "personal knowing," and probably most well known within nursing is Benner's[5] seminal work *From Novice to Expert.* Benner's notion of involvement and engagement was further developed collaboratively with Tanner[28] on intuition and with Wrubel[7] on the primacy of caring.

The idea of "being-with," of presence, of letting the person matter and being open to help that person make meaning out of his or her experience, is an essential feature of nursing practice. Without this knowing of self that allows an openness to the knowing of another person, nursing is only technical assistance, not involved care. In Carper's words, "It is concerned with the kind of knowing that promotes wholeness and integrity in the personal encounter, the achievement of engagement rather than detachment, and it denies the manipulative, impersonal orientation."[1(p 20)]

In the model of nursing knowledge described by Jacobs-Kramer and Chinn,[2] the pattern of personal knowing is seen as being created by "experiencing the self-encountering and focusing on self while realizing the realities and potentialities."[2(p135)] It also involves "experiencing, encountering and focusing."[2(p135)] These are not easy concepts to grasp. Carper herself said of this pattern that it "is the most problematic, the most difficult to master and to teach. At the same time, it is perhaps the pattern most essential to understanding the meaning of health in terms of individual well-being."[1](p18)

The creation of personal knowing may be enhanced through the use of art, poetry, literature, and storytelling in an endeavor to more truly "understand [the person] and his world as if I were inside it."[24](p42) An example of this is poetry about childbirth that helps the midwife "see" inside the patient's world; poems such as Sharon Doubiago's "South American Mi Hija" (in Chester[29]) show the intensity that can allow the soul to grow, whereas stories such as Anais Nin's "Birth" (in Chester[29]) illuminate the potential for the soul to shrivel if a woman is not supported by the right kind of caring. Poems such as "Sunshine Across Living Centre" in Krysl and Watson[30] help nurses "see" the humanity of nurse and patient in interaction. The expressive dimension is the self as authentic (privately known) and disclosed (revealed to others): "Personal knowledge is expressed as ourselves, through the self."[2](p135)

The assessment of this pattern comes through the "focus on the self as privately known and expressed to others. Assessment of self is a process carried out by the self through a rich inner life."[2](p135) The critical questions involve exploration for congruence between knowing what we do and doing what we know, between the authentic and disclosed self. The process through which this assessment is made is the reflection and response of others to us, which we reflect on in turn. Agan put it succinctly by suggesting that "credibility of this type of knowing is determined through *individual reflection that is informed by the responses of others.*"[31](p70) The credibility index is therefore congruence with the authentic and disclosed self.

Although the volume of literature in this area has provided much clarification and extension of the notion of personal knowing, the "essential elements" identified by Jacobs-Kramer and Chinn[2] are still pertinent. An elaboration could include, within the creative dimension, some examples of the means by which "encountering, focusing and realizing" might be facilitated (e.g., poetry, art, literature, and storytelling) and within the process-context dimension, reflection informed by the response of others (see Table 12.4).

ESTHETICS: THE ART OF NURSING

Carper suggested that the delay in explicating the esthetic pattern of knowing is associated with nursing's attempt to see itself as scientific and to "exorcise the image of the apprentice-type ed-

Table 12.4 Empirics: Personal Knowing

Dimension	Original Model[2]	Modifications
Creative	Encountering Focusing Realizing	Encountering, focusing, and realizing through practice and through art, literature, poetry, and storytelling
Expressive	Self: Authentic and disclosed	Self: Authentic and disclosed
Assessment: Critical question	Do I know what I do? Do I do what I know?	Do I know what I do? Do I do what I know?
Process-context	Response and reflection	Reflection informed by the response of others and our reflection on our response to the life-world of other
Credibility index	Congruity	Congruity

ucation system."[1(p16)] This delay has certainly been overcome, and there has been intense interest in this pattern recently. The pattern had its beginnings in the works of many early nursing writers. Wiedenbach[32] suggested that esthetic practice is making "visible through action" the nurse's perception of what the patient needs. Orem[33] spoke of the "creativity and style in design" of the provision of care. Orem also mentioned as necessary in artful practice the ability to "envision" models of helping with regard to the appropriate outcomes. Benner[5] was foremost in the development of the notion of perceiving the whole of a situation, without reference to rational processes, in her work on expert nursing practice. The concept of "intuitive" knowing developed by Benner and Tanner,[28] Rew,[34] and Agan[31] (and mentioned earlier as part of personal knowing) is an important component of perceiving and envisioning.

The design of the art-act combines all patterns of knowing in its esthetic form—it is all of and more than the other patterns: "The design, if it is to be esthetic, must be controlled by the perception of balance, rhythm, proportion and unity of what is done in relation to the dynamic integration and articulation of the whole."[1(p18)]

Carper named "empathy" as an important mode in the esthetic pattern of knowing; however, there is currently debate in the nursing literature over the appropriateness of this concept for nursing. Morse, Bottorff, Anderson, O'Brien, and Solberg suggested that "empathy was uncritically adopted from psychology and is actually a poor fit for the clinical reality of nursing practice."[35(p273)] They recommended exploration of other communication strategies that have been devalued, such as sympathy, pity, consolation, compassion, and commiseration. To these Taylor[25] might add affiliation, fun, and friendship.

Whatever the definitional outcome, the basic requirement of effective and authentic interpersonal engagement remains. This is highlighted in the recent Australian work of Taylor[25] and in the innovative work of Lumby[36] in her development of a critical feminist methodology for exploring nursing.

According to Jacobs-Kramer and Chinn,

> Esthetic knowledge finds expression in the art-act of nursing. Like personal knowledge, the expression of esthetic knowledge is not in language. We can unfold our art and retrospectively recollect and write about its features, and we can record it using electronic media, but the knowledge form itself is not what we write or record. The knowledge form *is* the art-act.[2(p137)]

They then proceeded to raise an important issue, albeit indirectly, that experience is an important component of esthetic knowing:

> As practice contexts are encountered, processes within the creative dimension of esthetics are initiated. Through the process of engagement, interpreting, and envisioning, "past" knowledge is enfolded into esthetics, and clients are uniquely cared for. As caring processes continue, new knowledge merges.[2(pp137–138)]

In putting forward experience as a necessary condition to esthetic practice, it may be necessary to include this context-specific experience as part of the creative and generative dimension, suggested by Jacobs-Kramer and Chinn as including "engaging, interpreting and envisioning." The addition of experience, particularly context-specific experience, suggests that these acts are cumulative, aligning with Benner's[5] position that expertise is context specific and not a transferable skill.

In exploring the assessment dimension within Carper's model of knowledge, Jacobs-Kramer and Chinn followed her inclusion of notions of esthetic appreciation from other art forms. They suggested that the critical question is, "What does this mean?"

Criticism requires empathy and an intent to fully appreciate what the actors meant to convey. As the art-act is criticized, credibility is discerned by reaching for consensus—a full and rich understanding of the art-act that brings together the perspectives of a community of co-askers who construct and confer meanings.[2(p137)]

Table 12.5 presents the essential elements for the esthetic pattern.

The major point of Jacobs-Kramer and Chinn's model development appears to be the unfolding of a story that suggests that each pattern may be seen by "examination of the art-act that integrates all knowledge patterns as expressed in practice . . . [as it] provides a comprehensive, context-sensitive means for enfolding multiple knowledge patterns."[2(p138)] This, they suggested, leads nursing away from "a quest for structural truth and towards a search for dynamic meaning."[2(p138)]

The model and its exposition of essential elements provide critical questions that may structure our process of inquiry, processes by which the inquiry might take place, and credibility indices to which claims of rigor may be addressed. If it is to be useful in the process of our practice-based inquiry, the model must adequately account for all patterns of knowing and their appropriate processes of inquiry.

SOCIOPOLITICAL KNOWING: CONTEXT OF NURSING

The patterns and inquiry processes in Jacobs-Kramer and Chinn's[2] model appear adequate to the description of the nurse–patient relationship and the persons of the nurse and the patient. What appears to be missing is the context—the sociopolitical environment of the persons and their interaction. This represents a fifth pattern of knowing essential to an understanding of all the others.

The other patterns address the "who," the "how," and the "what" of nursing practice. The pattern of sociopolitical knowing addresses the "wherein." It lifts the gaze of the nurse from the introspective nurse–patient relationship and situates it within the broader context in which nursing and health care take place. It causes the nurse to question the taken-for-granted assumptions about practice, the profession, and health policies.

Sociopolitical knowing may be conceptualized as including understandings on two levels: (1) the sociopolitical context of the persons (nurse and patient), and (2) the sociopolitical con-

Table 12.5 Esthetics: Essential Elements

Dimension	Original Model[2]	Modifications
Creative	Engaging Interpreting Envisioning	Cumulative experience by engaging, interpreting, and envisioning and including the "artful enfoldment" of all other patterns
Expressive	Art-act	Art-act
Assessment: Critical question	What does this mean?	What does this mean?
Process-context	Criticism	Exhibition and criticism Recognition as authentic to other nurses
Credibility index	Consensual meaning	Consensual meaning

text of nursing as a practice profession, including both society's understanding of nursing and nursing's understanding of society and its politics.

The sociopolitical context of the persons of the nurse–patient relationship fundamentally concerns cultural identity, for it is in culture that "self" is intrinsically located. This cultural location influences each person's understanding of health and disease causation, language, identity, and connection to the land. Such understanding goes well beyond Carper's[1] or Mayeroff's[24] notion of personal knowing. It is related to deeply embedded historical issues of connection to and dislocation from land and heritage.

Chopoorian suggested that "nursing ideas lack an archaeology of the social, political, and economic worlds that influence both client states and nursing roles."[37(p41)] She claimed that unequal class structure, power relationships, and political and economic power produce sexism, racism, ageism, and classism, which in turn affect health and result in illness. Chopoorian continued, "Nursing practitioners continually confront the human responses to the underlying social dynamics of poverty, unemployment, undernutrition, isolation and alienation precipitated through the structures of society."[37(pp40–41)]

Violence, drug dependence, and diabetes are examples of responses to what are inherently political rather than simply personal problems, and nurses' efforts to deal with them require nurses to articulate what they see resulting from societies' structures. Stevens suggested that nurses must provide a "critique of domination within fundamental social, political and economic structures and the analysis of how domination affects the health of persons and communities."[38(p58)] This effect includes the position and visibility of nursing in policy planning and decision making about health issues.

To have a voice in these decisions, nurses must both be articulate about what they know and do and be recognized by others as having something to contribute to debate. Nurses must have an understanding of the gatekeeping mechanisms within the political arena and their function. It is a paradox that when people are involved with nurses and nursing as patients or as concerned friends, the contribution of nurses is prized. Why then is it so quickly forgotten when these same people are influencing healthcare decisions? Diers and Fagin[39] suggested that the reason is visible in the metaphors the public associates with nursing, which include nurturance, dependence, and intimacy. These images are often reminders of personal pain and vulnerability, the natural reaction to which is suppression. To resurface an understanding of nursing is to resurface the context and all that is associated with it. Nurses must find a way of helping people remember, when they are well and politically able, what they knew of nursing when in crisis. Nurses must find the intersections between the health-related interests of the public and nursing and must become involved and active participants in these interests.

A sociopolitical understanding in which to frame all other patterns of knowing is an essential part of nursing's future in an increasingly economically driven world. Nurses must explore and expose alternative constructions of health and health care, find means of enabling all concerned to have a voice in this care provision, and develop processes of shared goverance for the future. Table 12.6 illustrates how the sociopolitical dimension might be added to the model of knowing.

As Chinn said of nursing in the next century, "it is time to construct critical analyses of our present that are informed by the ethical and political ideals that we seek. It is time to begin to envision what our future nursing might be like and to create knowledge and skills that we need to begin to make it happen."[40(p56)] Understanding the context of nursing practice is fundamental to

Table 12.6 Sociopolitical Knowing: Essential Elements

Dimension	Characteristics
Creative	Exposing and exploring alternate constructions of reality
Expressive	Transformation
	Critique
Assessment: Critical question	Whose voice is heard?
	Whose voice is silenced?
Process-context	Critique and hearing all voices
Credibility index	Shared governance, enlightenment
	Movement toward equality

this endeavor. Appreciation and exploration of all the patterns of knowing in nursing and their interactions can contribute to the future articulation and development of nursing practice and nurses' place in determining the future of nursing practice and of health care.

REFERENCES

1. Carper B. Fundamental patterns of knowing in nursing. *ANS.* 1978;1(1):13–23. Reprinted with permission from Aspen Publishers, Inc. © Copyright 1978.
2. Jacobs-Kramer M., Chinn P. Perspectives on knowing: A model of nursing knowledge. *Schol Inq Nurs Pract.* 1988;2(2):129–139. Used by permission of Springer Publishing Company, Inc., New York.
3. Kuhn T. *The Structure of Scientific Revolutions.* Chicago, IL: University of Chicago Press; 1970.
4. Sandelowski M. Rigor or rigor mortis: The problem of rigor in qualitative research revisited. *ANS.* 1993;16(2):1–8.
5. Benner P. *From Novice to Expert: Excellence and Power in Clinical Nursing Practice.* Menlo Park, CA: Addison-Wesley; 1984.
6. Benner P. The role of experience, narrative, and community in skilled ethical comportment. *ANS.* 1991;14(2):1–21.
7. Benner P., Wrubel J. *The Primacy of Caring: Stress and Coping in Health and Illness.* Menlo Park, CA: Addison-Wesley; 1989.
8. Bishop A., Scudder J., eds. *Caring, Curing, Coping.* University, AL: University of Alabama Press; 1985.
9. Bishop A., Scudder J. *The Practical, Moral and Personal Sense of Nursing.* Albany, NY: State University of New York Press; 1990.
10. Cooper M. Reconceptualizing nursing ethics. *Schol Inq Nurs Pract.* 1990;4(3):209–218.
11. Cooper M. Principle-oriented ethics and the ethic of care: Creative tension. *ANS.* 1991;14(2):22–31.
12. Watson J. *Nursing: Human Science and Human Care.* Norwalk, CT: Appleton-Century-Crofts; 1985.
13. Watson J. The moral failure of the patriarchy. *Nurs Outlook.* 1990;28(2):62–66.
14. Gilligan C. In a different voice: Women's conception of self and morality. *Harvard Educ Rev.* 1979;47:481–517.
15. Gilligan C. *In a Different Voice.* Cambridge, MA: Harvard University Press; 1982.
16. Noddings N. *Caring—A Feminine Approach to Ethics and Moral Education.* Berkley, CA: University of California Press; 1984.
17. Pellegrino E. Being ill and being healed. In: Kestenbaum V., ed. *The Humanity of the Ill.* Knoxville, TN: University of Tennessee Press; 1982.

18. Pellegrino E. The caring ethic. In: Bishop A, Scudder J, eds. *Caring, Curing, Coping.* University, AL: University of Alabama Press; 1985.

19. Zaner R. How the hell did I get here? In: Bishop A., Scudder J., eds. *Caring, Curing, Coping.* University, AL: University of Alabama Press; 1985.

20. Zaner R. *Ethics and the Clinical Encounter.* Englewood Cliffs, NJ: Prentice Hall; 1988.

21. Kohlberg L. *The Philosophy of Moral Development.* San Francisco, CA: Harper & Row; 1981.

22. Moss C. Has Gilligan's "Different Voice" made a difference? In: *Nursing Research: Scholarship for Practice.* Geelong, Victoria, Australia: Deakin Institute of Nursing Research, Deakin University; 1992.

23. Gadow S. Existential advocacy: Philosophical foundation of nursing. In: Spicker S., Gadow S., eds. *Nursing: Images and Ideals: Opening Dialogue with the Humanities.* New York, NY: Springer; 1980.

24. Mayeroff M. *On Caring.* New York, NY: Harper & Row; 1971.

25. Taylor B. Enhancement of the nursing encounter through a shared humanity. In: *Nursing Research: Scholarship for Practice.* Geelong, Victoria, Australia: Deakin Institute of Nursing Research, Deakin University; 1992.

26. Morse J. Negotiating commitment and involvement in the nurse–patient relationship. *J Adv Nurs.* 1991;16:455–468.

27. Moch S. Personal knowing: Evolving research and practice. *Schol Inq Nurs Pract.* 1990;4(2):155–165.

28. Benner P., Tanner C. Clinical judgment: How expert nurses use intuition. *Am J Nurs.* 1987;87:23–31.

29. Chester L., ed. *Cradle and All.* Boston, MA: Faber & Faber; 1989.

30. Krysl M., Watson J. Existential moments of caring: Facets of nursing and social support. *ANS.* 1988;10(2):12–17.

31. Agan R. D. Intuitive knowing as a dimension of nursing. *ANS.* 1987;10(1):64–70.

32. Wiedenbach E. *Clinical Nursing: A Helping Out.* New York, NY: Springer-Verlag; 1985.

33. Orem D. *Nursing: Concepts of Practice.* New York, NY: McGraw-Hill; 1971.

34. Rew L. Intuition and decision-making. *Image J Nurs Schol.* 1988;20(3):150–154.

35. Morse J., Bottorff J., Anderson G., O'Brien B., Solberg S. Beyond empathy: expanding expressions of caring. *Adv Nurs.* 1992;17:809–821.

36. Lumby J. *A Woman's Experience of Illness: The Emergence of a Feminist Method for Nursing.* Geelong, Victoria, Australia: Deakin University; 1993.

37. Chopoorian T. Reconceptualizing the environment. In: Moccia P, ed. *New Approaches in Theory Development.* New York, NY: National League for Nursing; 1986.

38. Stevens P. A critical social reconstruction of environment in nursing: implications for methodology. *ANS.* 1989;11(4):56–68.

39. Diers D., Fagin C. Nursing as a metaphor. *N Engl J Med.* 1981;309(2):116–117.

40. Chinn P. Looking into the crystal ball: positioning ourselves for the year 2000. *Nurs Outlook.* 1991;39(6):251–256.

CHAPTER 13

An Example of Personal Knowledge: Spirituality

Janice Bell Meisenhelder

Carper (1978) identifies personal knowledge as the "knowing, encountering and actualizing" (p. 18) of the individual self. It is the knowledge of one's own self as distinct from others. Thus, it encompasses the depths of self-awareness combined with an appreciation for that knowledge in the other. White (1995) elaborates on this definition to describe the engagement and reciprocity dimension of the nurse–patient relationship. Central to integrating personal knowledge into nursing practice is the idea of presence, being with the person in a therapeutic manner, an openness to the other "that promotes wholeness and integrity in the personal encounter" (Carper, 1978, p. 80).

Carper uses the concept of therapeutic use of self as an example of personal knowledge. One must know one's own therapeutic capacities and the needs of the other in order to use oneself in a therapeutic manner to achieve the engagement and reciprocity sought in such an encounter. One must also have met one's own needs in order to be able to focus on the other and have the capacity to give to the other.

Comfort is another example of a type of personal knowledge. This 13th-century concept conveys "consolation in time of trouble or worry, solace; a feeling of relief or encouragement, contented well-being; a satisfying or enjoyable experience" (Merriam-Webster, 2003). One knows comfort by experiencing it and identifying the relieving or pleasurable feelings associated with that particular experience. Hence, it constitutes personal experiential knowledge. We learn that which comforts us and then extend such comfort to others in word, touch, presence, knowledge, food, or environment. The ability to give comfort is based on our personal knowledge of comfort.

Another prime example of personal knowledge in nursing is spirituality. The following discussion describes spirituality, applying this concept to the elements of personal knowledge delineated by Carper (1978) and White (1995).

SPIRITUALITY: DEFINITION

Spirituality is such a broad, encompassing, and abstract term that nursing scholars continue to debate its definition (Emblem, 1992; Dyson, Cobb, & Forman, 1997; McSherry & Draper, 1998). Reed defines *spirituality* as "the propensity to make meaning through a sense of relatedness to dimensions that transcend the self in such a way that empowers and does not devalue the individual" (Reed, 1992, p. 350). Spirituality is that which gives meaning and purpose to one's life, as well as providing a transcendental experience (McCormick, Holder, Wetsel, & Cawthon,

2001). It is both the reason for living and the means for escaping the constrictions of life into a broader spectrum or experience. It is more than simply what makes life worthwhile. Spirituality leads to a sense of connectedness to or oneness with something greater than oneself, such as nature, the universe, or a Higher Being. This connectedness brings the transcendence beyond one's own time and space to a larger dimension, however the individual chooses to describe or experiences it.

Spirituality is embedded in culture, shaped by choices and experiences, and determined by one's worldview or personal philosophy. Values and beliefs lay a foundation for spiritual expression, while an innate need to connect beyond the physical and emotional spurs spiritual exploration, leading to increased understanding of one's spiritual self. Spiritual pathways include, but are not limited to, religious expressions: Beliefs regarding spiritual dimensions that are shared by a group. One's spirituality may be strongly congruent with the principles and practices of a particular religion or largely divert from orthodox theology while springing from a particular doctrine or worldview. Such doctrine may be as specific as a particular religious denomination or as open as an agnostic worldview. In all circumstances, spirituality is a highly unique and individual component of self.

Spirituality encompasses both beliefs and practices. Beliefs define what is meaningful in life, the purpose of one's existence. The experience of transcendence or connectedness is often sought through spiritual practices, such as listening to music, meditating, being surrounded by nature, speaking to a higher power, and engaging in various forms of prayer. One may experience transcendence through such deliberate practices, encounter it unexpectedly, or embrace it through connectedness with others, as in a worship experience.

SPIRITUALITY IN NURSING PRACTICE

Encountering illness often triggers spiritual hunger and exploration. The need to find meaning in the midst of suffering may well be universal in human existence. Examples of such a search lie in the primitive explanations of disease as Divine punishment and continue to emerge in research on coping with HIV infection (Barroso, 1999; Kendall, 1994; Martin, Rissmiller, & Beal, 1995; Moser, Sowell, & Phillips, 2001; Regan-Kubinski & Sharts-Hopko, 1995; Tsevat et al., 1999). Thus, spirituality is not only a foundational part of self-knowledge, but also an intrinsic part of nursing practice. So much of suffering at the end of life is spiritual suffering—the grasp for comprehending the purpose and meaning of one's life, the desperate attempt to feel connected to something larger than oneself (Peri, 1995). Alleviating such psychic pain can only be addressed with spiritual measures.

Addressing a person's spiritual needs requires personal self-knowledge of spirituality. This dimension can only be shared by nurses who have a foundational degree of spirituality—knowledge of one's own meaning in life and methods of transcendence. Without this self-knowledge, the nurse is void of any reference with which to understand the other's anguish or make an attempt to alleviate it. Because personal knowledge is "the pattern most essential to understanding the meaning of health in terms of the individual well-being" (White, 1995, p. 80), spirituality is one of the prime examples of personal knowledge in nursing. A nurse needs foundational self-knowledge of spirituality in order to have any basis for assessing or intervening on the behalf of another. Table 13.1 applies the essential elements of personal knowledge to the concept of spirituality with examples of nursing interventions.

Table 13.1 Empirics of Personal Knowing Applied to Spirituality

Dimension	Carper's Model	Spirituality	Interventions
Creative	Encountering Focusing Realizing	Encountering a connectedness with a larger force or existence, such as God, Nature or the Universe. Focusing on that which is outside of oneself that brings meaning. Realizing the meaning and purpose in life for oneself.	Encouraging spiritual practices that have led to transcendence in the past for the other. Exploring the other's self-knowledge of spiritual practices and experiences. Focusing on the values underlying the person's meaning to life. Integrating meaningful experiences and connectedness to significant others into the healthcare arena.
Expressive	Self: Authentic and disclosed	One's own meaning of life. One's own connectedness with a larger experience. Sharing such meaning and connectedness with others.	Using one's own spiritual framework as a means for understanding that of the other. Such expression may be implicit or explicit.
Assessment: Critical question	Do I know what I do? Do I do what I know?	How do I find inner peace and harmony? How congruent are my spiritual practices with my spiritual self?	Am I using my own spiritual instinct to assess for spiritual suffering in the other?
Process-context	Response and reflection	Reflection on one's own spiritual growth, own comfort with other's spirituality, and response from others on one's own spirituality.	Reflection on the spiritual needs of the other. Reflection on the response of the other to one's spiritual interventions.
Credibility index	Congruity	One's personal spirituality is consistent with that disclosed to others.	Interventions are consistent with one's spiritual understanding.

Desired outcomes of spirituality are a sense of peace, purpose, and communion. Identification of one's own spirituality is often a result of realizing what thoughts, practices, beliefs, or experiences have led to the perception of peace or inner harmony. A sense of purpose stems from the meaning of life. A sense of communion results from connectedness to a larger whole. Thus, evaluation of spiritual interventions can be based on the presence of peace, purpose, and communion in the other. Recognizing these three elements in the other provides evidence of the effectiveness of one's spiritual nursing interventions.

SPIRITUALITY AND WAYS OF KNOWING

Because each of the four patterns of knowing are interrelated and interdependent (Carper, 1978, p. 22), personal knowledge of spirituality interfaces with empirical, esthetic, and ethical knowledge. Empirical knowledge lends support to the importance of the spiritual dimension in nursing care. Hundreds of research studies have documented the relationship of spirituality to improved mental health (Koenig, McCullough, & Larson, 2001). Several extensive meta-analyses independently have concluded that there is overwhelming evidence for the preventive impact of spirituality on morbidity and mortality (Levin, 1996; Levin, Larson, & Puchalski, 1997; Matthews, McCullough, Larson, Koenig, Swyers, & Milano, 1998; Strawbridge, Cohen, & Shema, 2000).

Another cohort of research lends evidence to the frequency and effectiveness of spiritual coping with disease, trauma, or misfortune (Barusch, 1999; Chang, Noonan, & Tennsteadt, 1998; Krause, 1998, Matthews et al., 1998; Pargament, Smith, Koenig, & Perez, 1998; Pargament et al., 1999; Richards & Folkman, 1997; Woods, Antoni, Ironson, & Kling, 1999a, 1999b). Thus, empirical knowledge provides validity for the importance of this personal element in providing nursing care.

The expression of the personal knowledge of spirituality is its aesthetic quality. Spiritual expressions may be simply a quiet, still presence or a tender touch. They can incorporate counseling, disclosure, referral, or prayer. The wide and almost infinite combinations of spiritual expression are an artistic manifestation of personal knowledge that is dependent on both knowledge of one's self and the other. It is the aesthetic combination of touch, feel, movement, and verbalizing in synchrony with the needs of the other and spiritual capacity of the nurse who determines the interventions at any given moment in time.

The decisions on how, what, when, and how much spiritual expression, focus, and intervention to incorporate in any interaction lies heavily on the ethics of respecting the other and valuing that person's distinct needs and expressions. Ethical knowledge is the critical pillar in discriminating between therapeutic intervention and possible destructive intrusion. The nurse's well-developed personal knowledge of spirituality provides a secure basis from which the nurse may determine the degree of engagement based solely on the other's needs and desired nursing outcomes. This decision is an ethical one, requiring the nurse also to have knowledge of one's own boundaries and the point of departure from therapeutic professional practice into seeking control of another. Clinicians are cautioned against precisely such misuse (Koenig, 2000).

The personal knowledge of spirituality is validated by the empirical findings of the importance of spirituality to multiple dimensions of health. Spiritual interventions are created through the nurse's aesthetic knowledge and filtered and directed by the nurse's ethical knowledge. While context and manifestations of spirituality are determined by aesthetics and ethics, the content of spiritual interventions lies fundamentally in the personal knowledge of each nurse.

REFERENCES

Barroso, J. (1999). Long-term nonprogressors with HIV disease. *Nursing Research, 48*, 242–249.

Barusch, A. S. (1999). Religion, adversity and age: Religious experiences of low-income elderly women. *Journal of Sociology & Social Welfare, 26*, 125–142.

Carper, B. A. (1978). Fundamental patterns of knowing. *Advances in Nursing Science, 1*, 13–23.

Chang, B. H., Noonan, A. E., & Tennstedt, S. L. (1998). The role of religion/spirituality in coping with caregiving for disabled elders. *Gerontologist, 38*, 463–470.

Dyson, J., Cobb, M., & Forman, D. (1997). The meaning of spirituality: A literature review. *Journal of Advanced Nursing, 26*, 1183–1188.

Emblem, J. D. (1992). Religion and spirituality defined according to current use in nursing literature. *Journal of Professional Nursing, 8*(1), 41–47.

Kendall, J. (1994). Wellness spirituality in homosexual men with HIV infection. *Journal of the Association of Nurses in AIDS Care, 5*(4), 28–34.

Koenig, H. G. (2000). Religion, spirituality, and medicine: Application to clinical practice. *JAMA, 284*(13), 1708.

Koenig, H. G., McCullough, M. E., & Larson, D. B. (2001). *Handbook for Religion and Health.* New York: Oxford University Press.

Krause, N. (1998). Neighborhood deterioration, religious coping, and changes in health during late life. *Gerontologist, 38,* 653–664.

Levin, J. S. (1996). How religion influences morbidity and health: Reflections on natural history, salutogenesis and host resistance. *Social Science & Medicine, 43*(5), 849–864.

Levin, J. S., Larson, D. B., and Puchalski, C. M. (1997). Religion and spirituality in medicine: Research and education. *JAMA, 278*(9), 792–793.

Martin, M. A., Rissmiller, P., Beal, J. A. (1995). Health-illness beliefs and practices of Haitians with HIV disease living in Boston. *Journal of the Association of Nurses in AIDS Care, 6*(6), 45–53.

Matthews, D. A., McCullough, M. E., Larson, D. B., Koenig, H. G., Swyers, J. P., & Milano, M. G. (1998). Religious commitment and health status: A review of the research and implications for family medicine. *Archives in Family Medicine, 7*(2), 118–124.

McCormick, D. P., Holder, B., Wetsel, M. A., & Cawthon, T. W. (2001). Spirituality and HIV disease: An integrated perspective. *Journal of the Association of Nurses in AIDS Care, 21*(3), 58–65.

McSherry, W., & Draper, P. (1998). The debates emerging from the literature surrounding the concept of spirituality as applied to nursing. *Journal of Advanced Nursing, 27,* 683–691.

Merriam-Webster Dictionary. (2003). Accessed June 1, 2005 from http://www.m-w.com/cgi-bin/dictionary.

Moser, K. M., Sowell, R. L., Phillips, K. D. (2001). Issues of women dually diagnosed with HIV infection and substance use problems in the Carolinas. *Issues in Mental Health Nursing, 22,* 23–49.

Pargament, K. I., Cole, B., Vandecreek, L., Belavich, T., Brant, C., & Perez, L. (1999). The vigil: Religion and the search for control in the hospital waiting room. *Journal of Health Psychology, 4,* 327–341.

Pargament, K. I., Smith, B. W., Koenig, H. G., & Perez, L. (1998). Patterns of positive and negative religious coping with major life stressors. *Journal for the Scientific Study of Religion, 37,* 710–724.

Peri, T. A. (1995). Promoting spirituality in persons with acquired immunodeficiency syndrome: A nursing intervention. *Holistic Nursing Practice, 10*(1), 68–76.

Reed, P. G. (1992). An emerging paradigm for the investigation of spirituality in nursing. *Research in Nursing and Health, 15,* 349–357.

Regan-Kubinski, M. J., & Sharts-Hopko, N. (1995). Illness cognition of HIV-infected mothers. *Issues in Mental Health Nursing, 16,* 327–344.

Richards, T. A., & Folkman, S. (1997). Spiritual aspects of loss at the time of a partner's death from AIDS. *Death Studies, 21*(6), 527–552.

Strawbridge, W. J., Cohen, R. D., & Shema, S. J. (2000). Comparative strength of association between religious attendance and survival. *International Journal of Psychiatry Medicine, 30,* 299–308.

Tsevat, J., Sherman, S. N., McElwee J. A., Mandell, K. L., Simbart, L. A., Sonnenberg, F. A., Fowler, F. (1999). The will to live among HIV-infected patients. *Annals of Internal Medicine, 13*(3), 194–198.

White, J. (1995). Patterns of knowing: Review, critique, and update. *Advances in Nursing Science, 17,* 73–86.

Woods, T. E., Antoni, M. H., Ironson, G. H., & Kling, D. W. (1999a). Religiosity is associated with affective status in symptomatic HIV-infected African-American women. *Journal of Health Psychology, 4*(3), 317–326.

Woods, T. E., Antoni, M. H., Ironson, G. H., & Kling, D. W. (1999b). Religiosity is associated with affective status in symptomatic HIV-infected gay men. *Journal of Psychosomatic Research, 46,* 165–167.

CHAPTER 14

What Is Nursing Science?

Elizabeth Ann Manhart Barrett

The enigma of defining nursing science is preceded by defining nursing, science, research, and nursing theory–guided practice. The context for exploring the meaning of nursing science is provided through examination of the totality and simultaneity paradigms. Differing views of nursing as a discipline are discussed. The position is taken that nursing is a basic science with various nursing schools of thought that constitute the substantive knowledge of the discipline. Finally, a definition of nursing science is presented that is broad enough to encompass all disciplinary knowledge. Despite current challenges, an optimistic vision is emerging. The nurse theorists and other nurse scholars who are furthering the development of this work are considered to be the cultural creatives of nursing and contributors to a larger movement toward wholeness in science and in society.

DEFINITION OF NURSING

What is nursing science? Although the term is quite familiar to many nurses, its definition remains an enigma. Trying to capture the meaning accurately is perhaps almost as difficult as trying to define love, because it is interpreted in many ways. At various times as I was pulling my thoughts together to answer what at first seemed like such a simple question, I began to think this was an impossible mission.

Trying to define nursing is an age-old dilemma. Traditionally, *nursing* has been defined as a verb, meaning *to do*. Fawcett (2000a) defines the metaparadigm concept of nursing as "the actions taken by nurses on behalf of or in conjunction with the person, and the goals or outcomes of nursing actions" (p. 5). King (1990) says nursing is "a process of action, reaction, and interaction" (p. 2). Orem (1997) views nursing as "a triad of interrelated action systems" (p. 28) that compose nursing agency (Fawcett, 2000a).

Rogers (1992), on the other hand, defines *nursing* as a noun meaning *to know*. She proposes that nursing is a basic science whose phenomenon of concern is unitary human beings in mutual process with their environments. She says, "The practice of nursing is not nursing. Rather, it is the use of nursing knowledge for human betterment" (Rogers, 1994, p. 34). Parse (1997) says "nursing is a discipline, the practice of which is a performing art" (p. 73). Most commonly, *nurs-*

Source: Nursing Science Quarterly, 15(1), 51–60 (2002). Reprinted by permission of Sage Press, Inc.

ing is defined as both a noun and a verb. Orem also notes that in addition, *nursing* can be defined as a participle, as in *I am nursing* (Fawcett, 2000a).

I view nursing as a scientific art, which may seem like an oxymoron. However, I believe that the art cannot exist without the science. I define nursing as a basic science and the practice of nursing as the scientific art of using knowledge of unitary human beings who are in mutual process with their environments for the well-being of people. Personal definitions of nursing are quite varied, as they reflect our unique professional identities, as well as our philosophies of nursing and our paradigmatic propensities. This seems evident in the way nursing has been defined by the various nurse theorists as well as by other nurses. At this point, I need to make explicit what has been implicit, and that is that I speak through the bias of my own perspective.

DEFINITION OF SCIENCE

If these are some ways to look at defining nursing, what then is science? King (1997a) says *science is to know*. Parse (1997) defines *science* as "the theoretical explanation of the subject of inquiry and the methodological process of attaining knowledge in a discipline; thus, science is both product and process" (p. 74) and is arrived at through "creative conceptualization and formal inquiry" (p. 75). Others view science as product only, and propose that "science is a coherent body of knowledge composed of research findings and tested theories for a specific discipline" (Burns & Grove, 2000, p. 10). Science, as scientific knowledge, represents best efforts toward discovering truth. It is open-ended, evolving, and subject to revision and occasionally unfolds in dramatic shifts in thought.

Research is how we create science. *Research*, according to Parse (1997), is "the formal process of seeking knowledge and understanding through use of rigorous methodologies" (p. 74). Taking a narrower view, the National Institutes of Health proposes that "research means a systematic investigation designed to develop or contribute to generalizable knowledge" (Daniel Vasgird, personal communication, November 21, 2000).

WHAT IS NURSING SCIENCE? PRELUDE

After this brief look at *What is nursing?* and *What is science?* we return to the question, *What is nursing science?* Although the term *nursing science* is used liberally throughout the literature, there are few definitions. Likewise, there are also few definitions of *nursing research*. It was amazing to discover this in computer searches and in a variety of books on nursing research and nursing theory. In other words, the majority of these authors do not differentiate nursing science from science produced by nurses, or nursing research from research conducted by nurses. This is the crux of the matter.

For most sources that do offer definitions, they may not be universally acceptable, nor can they be if they represent a particular philosophy, rather than the various philosophies that guide multiple schools of thought within the discipline. Failure to define key terms and failure to specify philosophical underpinnings are grave errors in building a unique body of disciplinary knowledge, which by definition reflects more than one paradigm (Parse, 1997). In addition, definitions need to be congruent with the philosophical underpinnings. To illustrate this point, in Fitzpatrick's (2000) *Encyclopedia of Nursing Research,* nursing science is not listed in the index, nor is nursing research. What is listed is *nursing care research*, and it is defined as "research directed to understanding the nursing care of individuals and groups and the biological, physiological, social, behavioral, and environmental mechanisms influencing health and disease that are relevant to nursing care" (p. 507). This reflects a particular worldview and does not reflect the discipline as a whole.

CONTEXT OF NURSING SCIENCE

Munhall (1997) makes the important point that definitions require examination within their context and reflect assumptions as well as philosophical, political, and practical dimensions. Indeed, it is context that explains why different authors define and use the same nursing terms differently and why many terms cannot be defined universally.

In attempting to rise above the bias of personal perceptions, it is indeed a formidable task to answer the question, What is nursing science? Nevertheless, this collegial journey is justified because, as Watson (1999) says so clearly, without a language, we are invisible. Nursing will remain invisible as a distinct discipline and be viewed as a subset of medical science or social science until we have clearly defined and embraced our unique identity. Yet, in many nursing circles, this conversation is dismissed as valueless.

Before nursing science can be defined, the point about context must be addressed. Fortunately, there are several ways to contextualize nursing science, including paradigmatic schemas developed by Fawcett in 1993, and Newman, Sime, and Corcoran-Perry in 1991. In 1984, Parse (as cited in Parse, 2000) designed the original, and most widely used, paradigmatic organization of nursing knowledge based on a conceptual differentiation of the totality and simultaneity paradigms (see Table 14.1). Each of these two paradigms is a worldview that expresses a philosophical perspective about the nursing discipline's unique phenomenon of concern; all nursing knowledge is connected with this phenomenon in some way (Parse, 1997). Nursing's phenomenon of concern focuses on the human as a whole being, the environment, and health. Some authors add other concepts, such as nursing and caring.

In general, there is agreement on nursing's phenomenon of concern, expressed by Parse (1997, 2000) as the human-universe-health process. However, the definitions of these terms differ according to paradigms, thereby serving to clarify rather than confuse, since the philosophical context is now explicated. The contrast between worldviews is often explained by the two paradigmatic views of the human as a whole person, although this is only one example of difference. The totality paradigm views the whole human as a biopsychosocioculturalspiritual being who can be understood by studying the parts, yet is more than the sum of the parts. The person is separate from the changing environment, but interacts continuously with it. Health exists on a wellness–illness continuum. Most authors include King (1990), Orem (1995), Roy (1997), Betty Neuman (1996), Peplau (1952), and Leininger (1995) as totality paradigm theorists.

In the simultaneity paradigm *whole* means unitary, and the unitary human has characteristics that are different from the parts and cannot be understood by a knowledge of the parts. Moreover, the human cannot be separated from the entirety of the universe, as both change continuously in innovative, unpredictable ways, and together create health, a value defined by people for themselves (Parse, 1997, 1998, 2000; Rogers, 1994). The simultaneity theorists include Rogers (1992), Parse (1998), Margaret Newman (1990), and some, including myself, would say Watson (1999).

Although the two paradigms of nursing are different, neither is superior, and it is important to remember that a discipline requires more than one worldview of the phenomenon of concern

Table 14.1 Comparison of Nursing Paradigms

| | Simultaneity | | |
	Human Becoming	**Science of Unitary Human Beings**	**All Totality Theories**
Human being	Open being cocreating meaning in multidimensional mutual process with the universe recognized by patterns of relating	Energy field in mutual process with environmental field	Biopsychosociospiritual organism interacting with environment
	Freely chooses in situation	Participates knowingly in change	Interacts by coping with or managing the environment
Health	Cocreated process of becoming as experienced and described by the person, family, and community	A value	Physical, psychological, social, and spiritual well-being as defined by norms
Central phenomenon of nursing	Unitary human's becoming	Unitary human beings	Self-care, adaptation, goal attainment, or caring
Goal of the discipline of nursing	Quality of life	Well-being and optimal health	Promotion of health and prevention of disease
Mode of inquiry	Qualitative: Parse's research method; human becoming hermeneutic method	Quantitative and qualitative methods	Extant quantitative and qualitative methods
Mode of practice	True presence in all-at-once illuminating meaning through explicating, synchronizing rhythms through dwelling with, mobilizing transcendence through moving beyond	Patterns manifestation appraisal; pattern profile—perceptions, expressions, experiences; deliberative mutual patterning	Nursing process with nursing diagnoses

Source: From *The Human Becoming School of Thought* (p. 11) by R. R. Parse, 1998, Thousand Oaks, CA: Sage.

(Parse, 1997). These differences give rise to different methods of inquiry and practice and provide sufficient scope to encompass all disciplinary activities.

SCHOOLS OF THOUGHT

Parse (1997) has advanced the conceptualization of schools of thought and proposes that each paradigm is composed of philosophically congruent schools of thought based on similar beliefs about the essential phenomenon of concern of nursing. She states, "Each school of thought is a knowledge tradition that includes a specific ontology (belief system) and congruent methodologies (approaches to research and practice)" (p. 74). In other words, schools of thought comprise the substantive knowledge of the discipline (Parse, 1997). Figure 14.1, developed by Parse, illustrates Orem's (1995) school of thought as one example from the totality paradigm and Parse's (1998) school of thought as one example from the simultaneity paradigm.

The ontology consists of the assumptions, postulates, and principles of the framework or theory. The epistemology flows from the ontology and gives rise to both research methods and practice methods that are congruent with the framework or theory.

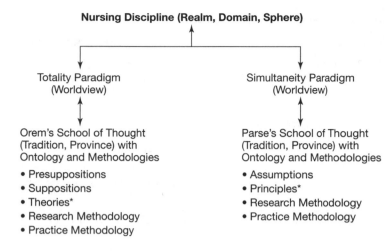

Nursing Discipline (Realm, Domain, Sphere)

Totality Paradigm (Worldview)	Simultaneity Paradigm (Worldview)

Orem's School of Thought (Tradition, Province) with Ontology and Methodologies

* Presuppositions
* Suppositions
* Theories*
* Research Methodology
* Practice Methodology

Parse's School of Thought (Tradition, Province) with Ontology and Methodologies

* Assumptions
* Principles*
* Research Methodology
* Practice Methodology

*Referred to in the literature as the theory

Source: Reprinted by permission of the Honor Society of Nursing, Sigma Theta Tau International (www.nursingsociety). From "The language of nursing knowledge: Saying what we mean," by R. R. Parse, in I. M. King and J. Fawcett (Eds.), *The language of nursing theory and metatheory* (p. 76), 1997, Indianapolis, IN: Sigma Theta Tau International Center Nursing Press.

Figure 14.1 Nursing Discipline (Realm, Domain, Sphere).

Nursing frameworks and theories have birthed numerous research instruments to measure constructs operationally defined to provide consistency with the particular framework or theory. Such instrumentation is essential to advance nursing knowledge in some frameworks and theories, notably in the totality paradigm. Rogerian science may be the only framework or theory in the simultaneity paradigm that endorses quantitative as well as qualitative methods. At least 32 instruments have been developed specifically to measure constructs reflecting 8 (King, 1990; Neuman, 1996; Orem, 1995; Pender, 1996; Peplau, 1952; Rogers, 1994; Roy, 1997; Watson, 1999) nursing science frameworks and theories (Young, Taylor, & Renpenning, 2001).

Unique Research and Practice Methodologies

Of even greater significance is the development of unique research methodologies. Table 14.2 shows Fawcett's (2000b) listing of those methods. They are all qualitative in nature. Fawcett insists that

> we must extricate ourselves from the research methods of other disciplines, such as the phenomenological methods that have their root in psychology, the grounded theory method that comes from sociology, and the randomized, controlled trials methodology that originated in agriculture and now is frequently used by pharmacologists and physicians. (p. 5)

Fawcett does, however, endorse reformulation of a method within the parameters of a nursing framework or theory. For example, Leininger (1995) reformulated ethnography, a method from

Table 14.2 Nursing Discipline–Specific Research Methodologies

Conceptual Model or Theory	Research Methodology
Rogers' Science of Unitary Human Beings	Bultemeier's Photo-Disclosure Method
	Butcher's Unitary Field Portrait Research Method
	Cowling's Unitary Pattern Appreciation Case Method
	Carboni's Rogerian Process of Inquiry
Leininger's Theory of Culture Care Diversity and Universality	Ethnonursing Research Method
Newman's Theory of Health as Expanding Consciousness	Research as Praxis Method
Parse's Theory of Human Becoming	Parse's Method of Basic Research
	Cody's Human Becoming Hermeneutic Method of Basic Research
	Parse's Preproject-Process-Postproject Descriptive Qualitative Method of Applied Research

Source: From "The state of nursing science: Where is the nursing in the science," by J. Fawcett, 2006, *Theoria: Journal of Nursing Theory, 9*(3), p. 4. Reprinted with permission.

anthropology, within the view of her nursing theory, and thereby created the ethnonursing method (Fawcett, 2000b).

In 1998, I (Barrett) proposed that unique research methods are one direct route to moving nursing toward further disciplinary definition. These methods "facilitate creation of knowledge for colleagues who practice nursing in the new way" (Barrett, 1998, p. 95). Those who use them are on the cutting edge, experiencing the passion of blazing a new trail as they sing the diversity chant of pioneers on the nursing road less traveled (Barrett, 1998).

Nursing practice methodologies are another aspect of a school of thought and are essential for making the leap from the theoretical to the practical, and clearly demonstrating the practical nature of nursing theories. Fawcett (2000b) noted that Johnson (1992), King (1990), Levine (1996), Margaret Newman (1990), Orem (1995), Rogers (1994), and Parse (1998), or scholars working with those frameworks and theories, have developed practice methodologies consistent with their work that can also form the basis for research methodologies. In other words, Fawcett (2000b), and earlier Newman (1990), proposed that information obtained during the practice of nursing can be regarded as research data.

NURSING THEORY–GUIDED PRACTICE

The American Academy of Nursing's Expert Panel on Nursing Theory–Guided Practice developed the following definition:

> Nursing theory–guided practice is a human health service to society based on the discipline-specific knowledge articulated in the nursing frameworks and theories. The discipline-specific knowledge reflects the philosophical perspectives embedded in the ontological, epistemological, and methodological processes that frame nursing's ethical approach to the human-universe-health process. (Parse et al., 2000, p. 177)

Nursing frameworks and theories provide two avenues to nursing practice by way of nursing theory–guided practice. The totality paradigm allows for adoption of evidence-based practice, defined differently in nursing than in medicine, particularly when it is nursing theory–

guided. In medicine, the gold standard for evidence-based practice is outcomes of randomized controlled trials. Evidence-based nursing, linked with the current buzzword in medicine, refers to research usage, but Ingersoll (2000) proposes a definition of evidence-based nursing that, unlike medicine's definition, does include the theory. Her definition states, "Evidence-based nursing practice is the conscientious, explicit and judicious use of theory-derived, research-based information in making decisions about care delivery to individuals or groups of patients and in consideration of individual needs and preferences" (p. 152).

Nursing theory–guided evidence-based nursing differs from evidence-based nursing in that the practice is guided by the discipline-specific knowledge reflected in the schools of thought within the totality paradigm. King (2000) has provided an example using her conceptual system. Her "theory of goal attainment within which a transaction process model was derived results in the following: Goals set lead to transactions which lead to goal attainment (outcomes) which is evidence-based practice" (p. 8).

Within the simultaneity paradigm, practice is simply nursing theory–guided or nursing science–guided. Evidence-based nursing is not compatible because it is philosophically incongruent. Its problem-oriented focus on diagnosis, interventions, and outcomes reflects the natural science approach rather than the human science approach of the simultaneity paradigm.

NURSING AS A DISCIPLINE

If nursing is a discipline, what then is a discipline? Parse (1997) describes a discipline as "a branch of knowledge ordered through the theories and methods evolving from more than one worldview of the phenomenon of concern" (p. 74). Her schema of worldviews in nursing, presented in Table 14.1, clarifies why the same words have different definitions and rather than serving to confuse, the different definitions serve to clarify when viewed within their appropriate place as the disciplinary domain.

To make matters more confusing, nursing is often called a practice discipline, or as Donaldson and Crowley described it in 1978, a professional discipline. Twenty-five years ago, many of us were still debating whether or not nursing was a profession, and we began to see these attributes on a continuum. Rather than asking if nursing was a profession, we started asking, "How professionalized is nursing?" But nursing has moved on and now the debate centers on the extent to which we are a discipline. Those who specify nursing as a professional discipline emphasize that nursing has a "social mandate to develop, disseminate, and use knowledge. In contrast, academic disciplines, such as physics, physiology, sociology, psychology, and philosophy are mandated only to develop and disseminate knowledge" (Fawcett, 2000a, p. 692). The knowledge of academic disciplines can be practiced in a corresponding profession.

According to Newman et al. (1991), a discipline is

distinguished by a domain of inquiry that represents a shared belief among its members regarding its reason for being. . . . A professional discipline is defined by social relevance and value orientations. The focus is derived from a belief and value system about the profession's social commitment, the nature of its service, and an area of responsibility for knowledge development. (p. 1)

Fawcett's (2000a) description of the discipline, as she presented it in Figure 14.2, presents nursing science and the nursing profession as the two major dimensions. Nursing research is the

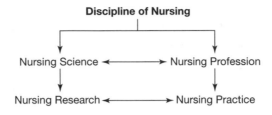

Source: From *Analysis and evaluation of contemporary nursing knowledge: Nursing models and theories* (p. 692), by J. Fawcett, 2000, Philadelphia: F. A. Davis. Reprinted with permission.

Figure 14.2 The Discipline of Nursing.

means for developing the knowledge of nursing science, and the product of the research is all the knowledge that has been developed and disseminated. The nursing profession, in a reciprocal relationship to nursing science, is actualized in nursing practice, with the major activities being used and evaluation of the knowledge previously developed and disseminated (Fawcett, 2000a).

Fawcett (2000a) summarizes the thinking of several nurse scholars when she says that "the responsibility and goal of the professional discipline of nursing is to conduct discipline-specific research using discipline-specific methodologies and to engage in discipline-specific practice" (p. 693). She echoes Parse (1999), who notes that nothing less will establish nursing as an autonomous profession and define the unique gift that we contribute to the healthcare system. Leininger (1995) also argues that professional decisions and actions by nurses require substantive disciplinary knowledge.

WHAT NURSING SCIENCE IS NOT

Before proposing a working definition of nursing science, it seems important to ask, "What is it, then, that nursing science is not?" Rogers (1992), Parse (2000), and Fawcett (2000a) are all clear that research by nurses that generates or tests theories from other disciplines is not nursing research. Furthermore, findings of such research build the knowledge base of the other disciplines. Since most nursing research falls into this category, the premise is that we are using precious resources to build a knowledge base with strong roots in other disciplines. This is not to say this research should not be done. Scholars are free to pursue whatever route to knowledge that they choose. Yet, can we call it nursing knowledge if its origins are in other disciplines? One cannot help but wonder what progress could be made in developing the nursing discipline if all nursing research, by definition, was guided by the extant nursing frameworks and theories.

This is not to say that the knowledge of other disciplines is not valuable and is not used by nurses. Of course it is. It is simply knowledge required of a learned person. Likewise, nursing knowledge can be used by others. Knowledge, per se, does not belong to anyone. It is not a commodity to be bought and sold, even though in the not too distant past, access to medical knowledge, for example, was much more difficult to obtain. We simply need to be clear on what is nursing knowledge and what is not. However, there is a difference between access to information and the use of the discipline-specific knowledge to provide a professional service that constitutes the practice of a particular discipline. Furthermore, knowledge that is not nursing knowledge simply does not reflect the uniqueness of what nurses and nursing are about. In contrast, it is nursing knowledge from both paradigms that allows us to build our discipline so that nursing services reflect nursing's distinctive schools of thought.

PUBLIC'S VIEW OF NURSING

Perhaps one reason the public is often unclear in defining what is unique about nursing is related to the fact that they may not have experienced the *real thing*. In other words, they may not have experienced being honored and cared for knowledgeably as humans who are whole and who are living life in an ever-changing and all-encompassing environment. Equally as important, they may not have experienced that their nurse caregivers are themselves humans who are aware of their wholeness and of living their life in an ever-changing and all-encompassing environment. The mutuality of the experience is what distinguishes this from the usual experience of clients who receive less than this standard of care. Instead, for the most part, the public views *nursing* as a verb that means doing, and nurses as those who carry out tasks of a certain nature. What nurses do is based on what nurses know. It is time to ask, "What is the foundational knowledge that drives the modus operandi of nursing practice?" Nursing theory–guided practice allows the discipline to escape from its low profile and create waves that demonstrate to the public why nursing services are essential to health and well-being.

WHAT IS NURSING SCIENCE? REVISITED

Finally, we return to the question, *What is nursing science?* The definition, I propose, must be broad enough to encompass all disciplinary knowledge and cannot focus on only one paradigm. Nor can the primary focus be on the activities of our science, such as theory development and research; rather, the essential focus is on knowledge. The most definitive perspective that was located appeared in the Scholarly Dialogue column of *Nursing Science Quarterly* in 1997 when nurse scholars (Daly et al., 1997) from Australia, Canada, Finland, Great Britain, Italy, Japan, Sweden, and the United States answered the question, *What is nursing science?* Only a few of their answers can be presented here. Daly (as cited in Daly et al., 1997), from Australia, said, "Nursing science is an identifiable, discrete body of knowledge comprising paradigms, frameworks, and theories" (p. 10). Mitchell (as cited in Daly et al., 1997), representing Canada, said, "Nursing science represents clusters of precisely selected beliefs and values that are crafted into distinct theoretical structures" (p. 10). Cody (as cited in Daly et al., 1997), from the United States, had this to say about the discipline and nursing science:

> The discipline encompasses all that nursing is and all that nurses do, overlaps with other disciplines and is more than the theory and research base. The discipline of nursing requires knowledge and methods other than nursing science, but nursing science is the essence of nursing as a scholarly discipline; without it there would be no nursing, only care. (p. 12)

The nursing theory movement is a global endeavor. It is important to recognize that nurse theorists in other parts of the world are developing their formulations of nursing science. The Roper-Logan-Tierney (Roper, Logan, & Tierney, 2000) model, originating in Scotland, dates back to the 1970s and Gustafsson and Porn's (as cited in Gustafsson, 2000) sympathy-acceptance-understanding-competence model, originating in Sweden, emerged in the 1990s.

The structure of the definition of nursing theory–guided practice as defined by the American Academy of Nursing's Expert Panel (Parse et al., 2000) was used as a guide to formulate the following definition as a work in progress:

> Nursing science, a basic science, is the substantive discipline-specific knowledge that focuses on the human-universe-health process articulated in the nursing frameworks and theories. The discipline-specific knowledge resides within schools of thought that reflect differing philosophical perspectives that give rise to ontological, epistemological, and methodological processes for the development and use of knowledge concerning nursing's unique phenomenon of concern.

The critical dimensions of this definition guide nursing's ongoing search for substantive disciplinary knowledge.

The Significance of Nursing Science

It is not enough to ask, *What is nursing science?* An equally important question is *What is the significance of nursing science?* Cody (as cited in Daly et al., 1997) warned that nursing's difficulty in articulating our uniqueness in the healthcare area has put the survival of nursing as a distinct discipline at risk. In a similar vein, Nagle (1999) says our future is "a matter of extinction or distinction" (p. 71). She notes that in view of fiscal constraints, the increasingly technological work environment, healthcare restructuring, the introduction of generic workers, and a dependent mode of practice, the viability of nursing seems less likely. She points out that practice defined by tasks that do not necessitate discipline-specific knowledge will not differentiate nurses' work. She wonders if we can answer the question, "What distinguishes the practice of nurses from that of a provider by any other name?" (Nagle, 1999, p. 76). The answer to that question can be found in nursing's schools of thought. Yet, it is absolutely imperative that we articulate our uniqueness to the public and other healthcare personnel, as well as articulating differences in nursing practice expected from the different paradigms.

Perhaps the strongest voice warning nurses of the consequences of what she sees as the impending demise is Fawcett (2000b), who recently asked, when considering the state of nursing science, *Where is the nursing in the science?* She analyzed 116 articles published in 1999 by *Nursing Research, Research in Nursing and Health,* and the *Western Journal of Nursing Research.* Only 4% were grounded in an existing conceptual model of nursing. Only 24% were testing an existing nursing theory. No studies were designed to generate a new nursing theory based on a nursing conceptual model. Interestingly, 39% were grounded in theories and conceptual models from other disciplines. The remaining 33% were not based on any theory or conceptual model. Over two thirds had nothing to do with nursing science as defined by nursing's schools of thought.

Truly, one begins to wonder if the adjective *nursing* in nursing science and nursing research, as it is used in mainstream nursing, is a euphemism disguising what our scholarship is really all about. Perhaps the terminology of nursing science has simply become jargon. For some, the coupling of the words *nursing* and *science* would seem a contradiction in terms. Others pay lip service to nursing science, and that is as far as it goes. Others use the words, but define them in ways that do not relate to nursing frameworks and theories, or simply do not define them distinctively from science in its general sense.

The Courage of Nurse Scholars

Orem (1995) urged nurse scholars to "have the courage to take a position about why people need nursing and about what nursing can and should be" (p. 414). This is surely necessary if we are to realize the vision of King (1997b), who has "a dream that nurses will be at the center of health-care delivery in the 21st century" (p. 16). Nursing frameworks and theories provide the power that gives the vision substantive form. Fawcett (2000a), summarizing the words of Orlando (1987) and Allison and Renpenning (1999), says,

> The development, dissemination, utilization, and and clinical evaluation of explicit nursing discipline-specific conceptual-theoretical-empirical systems will end the journey on the dependent path . . . and will facilitate . . . the journey along the independent path of professional nursing (Orlando, 1987, p. 412). . . . [This is] the only way that nursing can move from a "silent service" recognized primarily by its absence (Allison & Renpenning, 1999, p. 26) to a very public service, the need for which is widely recognized. (Fawcett, 2000a, p. 697)

Cody (as cited in Daly et al., 1997) believes that "in these frameworks lies the hope of clarifying nursing's unique contribution to health care in an important way and thus further enhancing nursing as a scholarly discipline" (p. 13). Moreover, this exemplifies the freedom and autonomy of distinctive nursing territory that Watson (1999) describes in her portrayal of nursing-qua-nursing as opposed to nursing-qua-medicine and provides a language that makes nursing visible to the public and other professionals (Orem, 1997; Watson, 1999). So, as I see it, nursing frameworks and theories as the basis of the definition of nursing science are essential ingredients in the survival of the discipline. They are perhaps the sine qua non of nursing.

Present Challenges

Indeed, the challenges to all registered nurses are daunting. Yet, nurse educators, in particular, have great power to turn the tide away from an atheoretical focus on skills (Fawcett, 2000b) or technical competencies based on knowledge derived from other disciplines (Nagle, 1999). A large volume of literature explaining how various nursing conceptual models and theories can be applied in nursing situations is available (Fawcett, 2000a). Unless the tide turns, students cannot learn enough to identify and study phenomena central to nursing's concern or to build practices that allow for delivery of discipline-specific care (Fawcett, 2000b). Cody (as cited in Daly et al., 1997) laments the continued identification of nursing with medicine and warns that "vast numbers of nurses continue to emerge from entry-level programs with only an applied-science knowledge base for nursing" (p. 13). The increased emphasis on theory and research in the mainstream of nursing education, unfortunately, often does not concern nursing discipline-specific theory or discipline-specific research. Until this situation changes, the future of our discipline is at risk.

It is of absolute importance that we foster scholars and identify students and nurses with the potential to become scholars. What appears to be nursing's lack of substantive scholarship has created a brain drain. The bright ones are going elsewhere, because nursing is often perceived as an occupation with minimum educational requirements for licensure. Of employed registered nurses, 58% have less than a bachelor of science in nursing, and only 0.6% hold earned doctorates (American Association of Colleges of Nursing, as cited in Phillips, 2000). Anderson (2000) asks, "Why would a young person choose nursing?" She answers:

> Nursing does not reward education either with salary or role differentials; nursing does not have a clearly articulated career path aligned with education; nursing is dominated by people without a college education, and nursing departments are administered by persons who have less education than their fellow administrators. Finally, and importantly, nurses are not valued within the institutions in which they practice except when they are, as they are now, in short supply. So, who is it we *can* recruit? (p. 257)

It is predicted that by 2020 there will be a dire shortage of nurses (O'Neill, 2000). According to O'Neill, unless nursing is viewed as a substantive scientific discipline, today's bright Generation Xers, who could solve the long-standing issues that Anderson (2000) discussed, will not be attracted to nursing.

Anderson (2000) suggests, as others have before her, that the only long-range solution is to require a postbaccalaureate degree for entry into practice. Although this is a worthy proposal, the futility of the 1985 proposal requiring a baccalaureate for entry into practice has not faded from memory. In the meantime, it is crucial that nurse scholars from the various frameworks and theories collaborate to develop a description of nursing portraying the substantive nature of the nursing discipline. Videos, films, novels, compact disks, and other media, such as lay publications, can be used to present a realistic portrayal of nursing scholarship, a counterpoint to anti-educationism and anti-intellectualism so often associated with the profession.

FUTURE OPTIMISM

Although many have lamented the demise of nursing, and Wieck (2000) even considered a future where there may be no nurses at all, I remain optimistic. This optimism flows from the incredible changes in nursing science that have transpired in the last 50 years along with the movement of nursing education into institutions of higher learning. In 1964, Rogers proclaimed that "nursing is a learned profession" (p. 31) and that "scholarship is the hallmark of higher education" (p. 63). In 1952, Peplau published *Interpersonal Relations in Nursing*, the first book describing a nursing theory, and nursing science has been evolving ever since. Rogers (1970) laid out the blueprint for a science of nursing in *An Introduction to the Theoretical Basis of Nursing*. In the past 25 years, major milestones have been achieved through the creative work of the nurse theorists and other nurse scholars who are participating in the ongoing scholarship of nursing science. We enter the 21st century with a strong global effort to actualize nursing's potential for delivering discipline-specific care to all people. This progress has been so noticeable that perhaps it has created a countermovement. For those who discard nursing science as insignificant, I reply that nursing science is a force to be reckoned with and it is here to stay. Devaluing nursing science is devaluing nursing. Yet, we must honor those in nursing with different views, lest we fall into the trap so often experienced by nurses, the trap of destroying ourselves from within. We can respect and appreciate differences, rather than being threatened by them. Beginning with

Nightingale's lamp, it has always been better to light one candle than to curse the darkness. Perhaps pre-science nursing has entered the dark phase of obsolescence; perhaps nursing science is a light shining into the darkness, transforming nursing's identity.

I am encouraged, rather than discouraged, that more than one-fourth of the articles published in 1999 in three major nursing research journals were nursing theory–guided. I am encouraged that since 1988, *Nursing Science Quarterly* has provided an avenue in which all articles link to nursing frameworks and theories. I am encouraged by other nursing theory journals such as the Swedish publication, *Theoria: Journal of Nursing Theory,* and *Visions: The Journal of Rogerian Nursing Science.* I am encouraged by the project of Roy and colleagues that identified, critically analyzed, and synthesized the contributions of 163 published studies, dissertations, and theses that were completed between 1970 and 1995 and based on Roy's adaptation model (Roy, 1997). Roy's (1999) book that presented this work, *The Roy Adaptation Model–Based Research: 25 Years of Contributions to Nursing Science,* won a very prestigious science award, the Alpha Sigma Nu national Jesuit Book Award. This is the first time the award has been given to the discipline of nursing (Callista Roy, personal communication, November 6, 2000). I am encouraged by the many other nursing theory–guided books too numerous to name.

I am encouraged by the movement in other disciplines toward a science of wholeness. Nursing's paradigms view wholeness as a basic axiom of the human-universe-health process, our disciplinary phenomenon of concern. At the turn of the century, there was a paradigm shift from classical physics to modern physics. In nursing, Rogers (1970) took a quantum leap from the medical model and created a similar paradigm shift from a particulate view to a unitary worldview of people and their environments.

CULTURAL CREATIVES OF NURSING

Ray and Anderson (2000), a sociologist-psychologist team who conducted 13 years of research on more than 100,000 Americans, described the emergence over the last generation of the *cultural creatives.* Beginning to grow more rapidly in the 1960s to now 50 million adults in this country, this group of people have shifted their values and their worldviews, and they may be shifting the culture itself. The cultural creatives have a more holistic orientation toward health and care deeply about ecology; about social justice, peace, and relationships; and about spirituality, self-actualization, and self-expression. They are both socially concerned and inner-directed. They are activists, volunteers, and participants in worthy causes. They often use the perspective of whole systems, see the *big picture*, and believe the world is too complex for linear, analytic thinking. Ray and Anderson propose that the cultural creatives have been relatively invisible, but that they will have an enormous impact on society once they realize their numbers. They say that the creative minority can carry us away from a fall and toward a renaissance. This is exactly how I see the persons in the nursing theory movement.

In nursing, the nurse theorists were the original cultural creatives. Starting with Nightingale, they have changed the nursing world, leaving their distinctive marks on the discipline. This minority of nurse theorists, many who could not be mentioned in this article, and those who learn, use, and expand their work, are creating a shift that will radically change the face of nursing in the 21st century. Particularly if they unite as a group with each other in support of the various worldviews, frameworks, and theories that constitute the *big picture* of nursing science, their power will be exponential. Like Robert Frost (1967) describing the traveler who comes to a fork in the road, it will make all the difference which way the men and women of nursing turn. Those who embrace nursing frameworks and theories are bringing more nurses along with them on the road less traveled. This path is antithetical to traditional definitions of nursing, nursing care, and the nursing knowledge base. The implications of the nursing theory movement are heresies of the first order. For example, will the diffusion of these nursing knowledge innovations become nursing's legacy to revolutionary healthcare reform?

Yes, those in the nursing theory movement are a minority on the road less traveled. Although the possibility cannot be ruled out that history will reveal that they are lone voices crying in the wilderness, I believe that will not be the case because this group is part of a larger movement in science, in society, in the universe. Nurse scholars who work within the new way of thinking about nursing are the cultural creatives of the discipline. You will be hearing more from them in the future. As the saying goes, *You haven't seen anything yet.* Those who walk down that road less traveled would do well to remember Margaret Mead's (as cited in Barrett, 1990) prophetic insight: "Never doubt that a small group of thoughtful, committed citizens can change the world; indeed it's the only thing that ever has" (p. xxi).

REFERENCES

Allison, S. E. & Renpenning, K. (1999). *Nursing administration in the 21st century.* Thousand Oaks, CA: Sage.

Anderson, C. A. (2000). The time is now. *Nursing Outlook, 48,* 257–258.

Barrett, E. A. M. (1990). Preface. In E. A. M. Barrett (Ed.), *Visions of Rogers' science-based nursing* (pp. xxxi–xxiii). New York: National League for Nursing.

Barrett, E. A. M. (1998). Unique nursing research methods: The diversity chant of pioneers. *Nursing Science Quarterly, 11,* 94–96.

Burns, N., & Grove, S. K. (2000). *The practice of nursing research: Conduct, critique & utilization* (4th ed.). Philadelphia: Saunders.

Daly, J., Mitchell, G. J., Toikkanen, T., Millar, B., Zanotti, R., Takahashi, T., et al. (1997). What is nursing science? An international dialogue. *Nursing Science Quarterly, 10,* 10–13.

Donaldson, S. K., & Crowley, D. M. (1978). The discipline of nursing. *Nursing Outlook, 26,* 113–120.

Fawcett, J. (1993). From a plethora of paradigms to parsimony in world views. *Nursing Science Quarterly, 6,* 56–58.

Fawcett, J. (2000a). *Analysis and evaluation of contemporary nursing knowledge: Nursing models and theories.* Philadelphia: F. A. Davis.

Fawcett, J. (2000b). The state of nursing science: Where is the nursing in the science? *Theoria: Journal of Nursing Theory, 9*(3), 3–10.

Fitzpatrick, J. J. (Ed.). (2000). *Encyclopedia of nursing research.* New York: Springer.

Frost, R. (1967). The road not taken. In R. Frost (Ed.), *Complete poems of Robert Frost* (p. 131). New York: Holt, Rinehart & Winston.

Gustafsson, B. (2000). The SAUC model for confirming nursing. *Theoria: Journal of Nursing Theory, 9*(1), 6–21.

Ingersoll, G. L. (2000). Evidence-based nursing: What it is and what it isn't. *Nursing Outlook, 48,* 151–152.

Johnson, D. E. (1992). The origins of the behavioral system model. In F. N. Nightingale (Ed.), *Notes on nursing: What it is, and what it is not* (Commemorative ed., pp. 23–27). Philadelphia: J. B. Lippincott.

King, I. M. (1990). *A theory for nursing: Systems, concepts, process.* Albany, NY: Delmar. (Original work published in 1981).

King, I. M. (1997a). Knowledge development for nursing: A process. In I. M. King & J. Fawcett (Eds.), *The language of nursing theory and metatheory* (pp. 19–25). Indianapolis, IN: Center Nursing Press.

King, I. M. (1997b). Reflections on the past and a vision of the future. *Nursing Science Quarterly, 10,* 15–17.

King, I. M. (2000). Evidence-based nursing practice. *Theoria: Journal of Nursing Theory, 9,* 71–78.

Leininger, M. (1995). Culture care theory, research, and practice. *Nursing Science Quarterly, 9,* 38–41.

Levine, M. E. (1996). The conservation principles: A retrospective. *Nursing Science Quarterly, 9,* 18–41.

Munhall, P. L. (1997). Deja vu, parroting, buy-ins, and an opening. In I. M. King & J. Fawcett (Eds.), *The language of nursing theory and metatheory* (pp. 79–87). Indianapolis, IN: Center for Nursing Press.

Nagle, L. M. (1999). A matter of extinction or distinction. *Western Journal of Nursing Research, 21,* 71–82.

Neuman, B. M. (1996). *The Neuman systems model* (3rd ed.). Norwalk, CT: Appleton & Lange.

Newman, M. A. (1990). Newman's theory of health as praxis. *Nursing Science Quarterly, 3,* 37–41.

Newman, M. A., Sime, A. M., & Corcoran-Perry, S. A. (1991). The focus of the discipline of nursing. *Advances in Nursing Science, 14*(1), 1–6.

O'Neill, E. (2000, November). *Workplace Issues in Nursing.* Paper presented at the annual conference of the American Academy of Nursing, San Diego, CA.

Orem, D. E. (1995). *Nursing: Concepts of practice* (5th ed.). St. Louis, MO: Mosby.

Orem, D. E. (1997). Views of human beings specific to nursing. *Nursing Science Quarterly, 10,* 26–31.

Orlando, I. J. (1987). Nursing in the 21st century: Alternate paths. *Journal of Advanced Nursing, 12,* 405–412.

Parse, R. R. (1997). The language of nursing knowledge: Saying what we mean. In I. M. King & J. Fawcett (Eds.), *The language of nursing theory and metatheory* (pp. 73–77). Indianapolis, IN: Center Nursing Press.

Parse, R. R. (1998). *The human becoming school of thought: A perspective for nurses and other health professionals.* Thousand Oaks, CA: Sage.

Parse, R. R. (1999). The discipline and the profession. *Nursing Science Quarterly, 12,* 275.

Parse, R. R. (2000). Paradigms: A reprise. *Nursing Science Quarterly, 13,* 275–276.

Parse, R. R., Barrett, E., Bourgeois, M., Dee, V., Egan, E., Germain, C., et al. (2000). Nursing theory–guided practice: A definition. *Nursing Science Quarterly, 13,* 177.

Pender, N. J. (1996). *Health promotion in nursing practice* (3rd ed.) Stamford, CT: Appleton & Lange.

Peplau, H. (1952). *Interpersonal relations in nursing.* New York: Putnam.

Phillips, J. R. (2000). Rogerian nursing science and research: A healing process for nursing. *Nursing Science Quarterly, 13,* 196–203.

Ray, P. H., & Anderson, S. R. (2000). *The cultural creatives: How 50 million people are changing the world.* New York: Harmony Books.

Rogers, M. E. (1964). *Reveille in nursing.* Philadelphia: F. A. Davis.

Rogers, M. E. (1970). *An introduction to the theoretical basis for nursing.* Philadelphia: F. A. Davis.

Rogers, M. E. (1992). Nursing science and the space age. *Nursing Science Quarterly, 5,* 27–34.

Rogers, M. E. (1994). The science of unitary human beings. *Nursing Science Quarterly, 7,* 33–35.

Roper, N., Logan, W., & Tierney, A. J. (2000). *The Roper-Logan-Tierney model of nursing.* New York: Churchill Livingstone.

Roy, C. (1997). Future of the Roy model: Challenge to redefine adaptation. *Nursing Science Quarterly, 10,* 42–48.

Roy, C. (1999). *The Roy adaptation model-based research: 25 years of contributions to nursing science.* Indianapolis, IN: Center Nursing Press.

Watson, J. (1999). *Postmodern nursing and beyond.* New York: Churchill Livingstone.

Wieck, K. L. (2000). A vision for nursing: The future revisited. *Nursing Outlook, 48,* 7–8.

Young, A., Taylor, S. G., & Renpenning, K. (2001). *Connections: Nursing theory, research, and practice.* St. Louis, MO: Mosby.

CHAPTER 15

Toward a Theory of Nursing Art

Peggy L. Chinn

The purpose of this chapter is to present a philosophic theory of nursing art. The theory was developed to deepen understanding of that aspect of nursing that moves practice beyond purely technical or interpersonal skills into a realm that is a healing art form. The healing art form of nursing involves integrating all aspects of nursing into a coherent whole, and the theory describes, and explains philosophically, how this happens.

It is important to understand that I am not projecting empirical theory. Rather I am presenting a philosophic theory that offers a conceptual definition of the art of nursing—explanations as to how nursing art evolves as a distinct aspect of nursing practice and explanations of artistic validity in nursing. Unlike empirical theory, what I propose is not intended to be subjected to empirical testing, but rather to be considered from a logical, philosophic, and aesthetic perspective. In philosophy, aesthetics is the study of that which is artistically valid. Notions such as beauty, for example, enter into logical explorations, but cannot be subjected to empirical investigation. Likewise, in developing this theory, I considered the notion of a unitary, coherent whole within a complex action and interaction—the art and act of nursing. This idea is analogous to the idea of beauty in traditional aesthetics.

The following section explains the background from which this theory has been developed. The subsequent sections present assumptions on which the theory is based—a conceptual definition of nursing art as a pattern of knowing in nursing and as a distinct way of being in nursing and theoretical explanations as to how nursing art evolves as a distinct aspect of what nursing is.

DEVELOPMENTAL BACKGROUND

Ideas that have come together to form this theory are grounded in an investigation conducted in Denver, Colorado, from 1990 through 1996 (Chinn, 1994; Chinn & Kramer, 1999; Chinn, Maeve, & Bostick, 1997). In the course of this investigation, I worked with nurses in five different units of two hospitals. I also worked with two colleagues, M. Katherine Maeve and Cynthia Bostick, who were doctoral students during the course of the study. Katherine pursued work in the area of nursing narrative and storytelling (Maeve, 1994). Cynthia, who is also a profes-

Source: The nursing profession, tomorrow and beyond, Chaska, N.L. (Ed), (2001), pp. 287–297. Reprinted by permission of Sage Press, Inc.

sional dancer, pursued her doctoral dissertation on movement and its relationship with creativity in practice (Bostick, 1997).

I observed 12 nurses in their practice for three to four 2-hour sessions. We each reflected on the observation period and journaled. About 2 to 3 days later, we discussed our experience and reflections on their practice. Because a main purpose of my inquiry was to create a method for developing aesthetic knowledge in nursing, I used a discussion approach that integrated hermeneutic interpretation and aesthetic criticism (Chinn, 1994). In other words, I shared insights concerning (a) meanings that I perceived in their practice, (b) symbolic messages conveyed in what they did and how they did it, and (c) reflective details about aesthetic qualities such as rhythm, synchrony of movements and interactions, and overall coherence of their practice in relation to the whole scenario in which they acted. For example, in one observation, I noticed that the nurse, upon entering a patient's room, moved around the space, briefly touching various things. The space that she touched became the space within which she maintained her practice for the duration of her stay in the room. In some instances she moved within a broad space that included others in the room; in other instances she moved within a relatively confined space that included only bed and patient. When we met for our discussion, I reflected on the symbolic meanings of "setting the stage" for her practice encounter in this time and space.

Groups of nurses who volunteered to participate in the inquiry met weekly to discuss ideas concerning the art of nursing and to share stories of practices. Charlene Eldridge volunteered to take black and white photographs of selected nurses as they practiced; these were spontaneous photographs that were not rehearsed in any way. We met in groups to discuss what the photographs revealed about the art of nursing.

STEPS FOR PERSONAL GROUNDING

Because staying focused on the art of nursing as aesthetics—and not as an empirical phenomenon—was so difficult. I took steps to keep myself grounded in art experiences and in healing as an art form. I completed a 1,000-hour massage therapy program at the Colorado School of Healing Arts in Denver. This program explicitly taught massage as a healing art, integrating motive, intention, action, and spirit into the skill of therapeutic massage. Although there were similarities in philosophy between what we learned in massage therapy and what I believed about nursing, never in my nursing education had I experienced the same kind of explicit acknowledgment of, and intentional focus on, nursing as a healing art. Needless to say, this discovery inspired for me a very different vision of what nursing can become and how it can be taught.

The study of music deepened my understanding of what it means to learn an art form and what it means to teach an art form effectively. I have had the good fortune of working with master teachers and continue to study and practice, playing a traditional folk harp. This experience provides grounding in aesthetics and brings to awareness some distinctions between empirical methods and aesthetic methods.

Exploratory Course Offering

At the University of Connecticut in the Spring of 1998, I proposed and taught a one-time exploratory course titled "An Introduction to the Art of Nursing" for freshmen and sophomore students. (See http://www.nursing.uconn.edu/ to find a link to the syllabus for this course.) I remain in touch via e-mail with these students to explore further ideas and insights that have emerged in developing a theory of nursing art. The course's content and processes were designed from the findings of my Denver study. After the first three weeks of focusing on the art form of nursing, the course integrated allopathic and holistic skills, practicing in class with a focused eye toward developing the skill as a nursing caring/healing art form. Skills included those that can be used by any lay person, such as taking vital signs, wound care, foot care and massage, use of hot and cold, and so forth. Each week we discussed an excerpt from Nightingale's "Notes on Nursing" (1969) pertinent to the topic of the week, focusing on the significance of what we were learning for developing nursing as a caring and healing art form. For example, the week that we worked with music and movement as a therapeutic modality, I read Nightingale's note on the healing properties of music and the type of music that is beneficial to the sick (Nightingale, 1969, p. 67). This reading prompted rich discussion of how nurses facilitate healing by mindful, intentional use of music and movement. The 1998 course was based on a premise that directly challenges preconceived ideas that students need to master technical skills before beginning to integrate elements of interpersonal dynamics into their practice. Instead I felt that introducing students to nursing as an art form first, using basic technical skills as the "carrier" of the art form, can have a number of advantages. With that sequence, students will acquire skills more easily, they will view the worth of what they do as nurses differently, and they will perceive themselves to be actively engaging in a caring and healing process. From everything that I have observed to date, this indeed is the case.

ASSUMPTIONS

Assumptions on which my theory of nursing art is based come from my beliefs about nursing and about the nature of art. First, nursing is a healing art. This concept is growing in significance as nurses turn increasingly to holistic healing modalities that enhance their participation in healing processes. Even though holistic modalities can greatly expand nursing's potential, I also believe that everything that traditionally has been a part of nursing practice can be viewed as a medium for the healing process.

Art requires two kinds of knowledge (Chinn & Kramer, 1999; Eisner, 1985). The first is knowledge of human experiences toward which our art form is directed—suffering, pain, birth, life transitions, stress, illness, and so forth. Art also requires knowledge of the art form itself, which is the focus of my own work and substance of this theory.

Art is present in all activity that involves forming elements into a whole. Most instances of art are not subjected to critical reflection nonvalued as art. However, when we bring elements together to form a whole, we experience art.

Art expands perceptual abilities beyond what is, to what might be. Art moves us to another plane, another potential, another possibility. When someone reads a novel or views a painting or sees a performance, he or she is moved into the realm of experience represented by the art form. This "move" is an inner, emotional, mental, spirit-self move that is in a realm of perception that arises from aesthetics.

All art requires skill in technical aspects of the art. My experience in learning to play the harp certainly brought this into focus. However, I also learned during the first two weeks of lessons that, because of what my teacher imagined a simple song could sound like and her ability to convey that possibility to me, I could produce a beautiful, artistically valid song. The technical skill for the simple song was not difficult and so, as I mastered the relatively easy technical skill, I also could focus on artistic qualities that my teacher guided me to integrate as I played. At first, I could only play one song, but it sounded heavenly!

Art requires imagination and intuition to bring elements into a creative whole. When I play the harp, I do need skill to pluck the right strings, in a particular order and with rhythm to produce a recognizable tune. This technical skill needs to be developed "in my fingers" for each new tune I play, and technical challenges gradually progress as I gain expertise and skill. What makes a tune a beautiful song is the imagination of feeling that I want to bring into the sound and the intuitive following of various musical possibilities that emerge in the song. This creative imagination, when nurtured from the moment of beginning to learn the skill, multiplies the meaning of the skill into a place of the imagination so that the emerging and developing skill becomes a carrier for the art. Because of this dynamic, even as the skill is developing, artistic quality comes through, making learning a thing of joy and beauty.

Art seeks unique expressions. One of my first songs—the Quaker hymn "Simple Gifts"—speaks to deep satisfaction that comes from giving and taking, of living in company of friends and finding joy and delight in simple gifts we offer one another. This common human experience is conveyed both in words and in the music itself, which has a soothing tone, with movements of notes and rhythm that also suggest a deep longing for the kind of nurturing connections that are possible in community. Each time I play the song, it acquires unique expressions that emerge in the moment.

Finally, art is a bodymind experience and it elicits bodymind responses. This is the aspect of art that makes it difficult to understand as a component of nursing. We are accustomed to understanding nursing as a mind experience only. To move to the bodymind concept is a considerable challenge.

Conceptual Meanings of Nursing Art

Joy Johnson (1994) conducted a philosophic analysis of nursing literature that used the term "art of nursing." Johnson found five distinct meanings associated with idea of the art of nursing. I will discuss each of these briefly in terms of the assumption that nursing art requires knowledge of the experience toward which our art is directed, and knowledge of the art form itself.

Johnson (1994) found that the art of nursing meant the grasping of meaning in a situation. Grasping meaning is associated primarily with knowledge of the experience toward which our art form is directed. Nurses must know the nature of the experiences of illness, life transitions, grief, tension, stress, and so forth. Nurses must be able to sense the nature of a particular experience in any situation. It is within the contexts of these experiences that nursing art is practiced, and it is toward these experiences that nursing art is directed. But this reality does not address the art form itself.

Another meaning that Johnson found is the ability to establish a meaningful connection. This ability repeatedly appeared in my discussions with practicing nurses in the Denver study. Those nurses clearly identified meaningful connection as the reason for practicing artfully. The art, those practicing nurses said over and over, is what makes connection possible. Consistent with Jeanne LeVasseur's ongoing work (LeVasseur, 1999), this aspect of nursing art suggests something about outcome, or the object of nursing art. However, the connection that is established as nursing art is practiced still does not address the art form itself.

Johnson also found that the art of nursing has been associated with the ability to perform nursing activities skillfully. This aspect of nursing art also appeared frequently in my discussions with nurses in the Denver study. Those nurses often said: "it is not what you do, but how you do it." Still, they were at a loss to speak to the form, to describe exactly what they meant by "how you do it."

Johnson (1994) further identified meanings associated with the ability to determine rationally a course of action and the ability to conduct practice morally. These two abilities are part of what enters into the picture when all elements of nursing practice come together to form a whole, but as distinct entities of practice these abilities do not address the art form.

CONCEPTUAL DEFINITION OF THE FORM OF NURSING ART

The definition of nursing art that emerged from the Denver study remains the conceptual foundation for this theory of nursing art and focuses on the art form itself. (Chinn & Kramer, 1999):

> The nurse's synchronous arrangement of narrative and movement into a form that transforms experiences into a realm that would not otherwise be possible. The arrangement is spontaneous, in-the-moment, and intuitive. The ability to make the moves that are transformative grounded in a deep understanding of nursing, including relevant theory, facts, technical skill, personal knowing, and ethical understanding, and this ability requires rehearsal in deliberative application of these understandings. (p. 90)

This definition first identifies elements that nurses use to form a whole: narrative and movement. Using these elements in a synchronous fashion, the nurse transforms experiences into a realm that would not otherwise be possible. Although it is possible to focus on the nurse's movement or narrative, what emerges is a whole that is greater than the sum of the parts and includes the total picture of the situation, including others with whom the nurse interacts.

Arrangement of narrative and movement is spontaneous, in-the-moment, and intuitive. This component of our definition emerged from nurses in the art study, using improvisational theater as an analogy for what they experience as the art of nursing. However, consistent with improvisational arts, in order to interact spontaneously and intuitively in the situation, nursing art requires rehearsal. In the art study, nurses spoke of their years of practice as "rehearsal time," but also began to imagine what it might have been like if they had been able to work in a studio with expert teachers, coaches, and directors to help them refine their artistic potential early in their practice.

The ability to form art in nursing practice is also grounded in deep understanding of nursing, including theory, technical skill, personal knowing, and ethical understanding. The studio can provide some practice that integrates this understanding, but clinical experience is truly the ground from which this integration arises.

In Barbara Carper's initial presentation of nursing's patterns of knowing, she spoke to the tension between elements of an art form and that which emerges as the whole (Carper, 1978). Carper said: "The design, if it is to be esthetic, must be controlled by perception of the balance, rhythm, proportion and unity of what is done in relation to the dynamic integration and articulation of the whole" (p. 18).

ONTOLOGY OF NURSING ART

Art is a distinct aspect of nursing practice. Nursing art arises from aesthetic knowing. Empirical, personal, and ethical knowing cannot give rise to nursing art. For example, an empirical theory of pain and comfort informs what a nurse does and contributes to making judgments in alleviating pain, but such a theory does not, and cannot, provide insight as to *how* to carry out the nursing actions and interactions involved in alleviating pain. *How* the nurse *is* in this context comes from the nurse's aesthetic sensibilities and senses.

In our work with Carper's patterns of knowing, Maeona Kramer and I distinguished between knowledge, which is the epistemological dimension that focuses on what we know and how we come to know it, and the ontological dimension, which is what it means to be a nurse, to experience the practice of nursing (Chinn & Kramer, 1999). We conceptualized the core of nursing as practice as the ontological perspective of what nursing is.

Nursing is that which arises from each of the four fundamental patterns of knowing in nursing. Each pattern of knowing has a nondiscursive form of expression, which is what we can discern in nursing practice and what forms the ontological elements that form nursing practice, as depicted in Figure 15.1.

Scientific competence arises from empiricism. Moral and ethical comportment arises from ethics. Therapeutic use of self arises from personal knowing and transformative art and acts arise from aesthetics. When we witness nursing practice, we perceive the whole of what is happening and cannot perceive the elements of practice in isolation from the whole. At the same time, we can discern what we would characterize as scientific competence and differentiate it from moral and ethical comportment. As an example, consider what it takes to recognize a person. You know the sound of a person's voice, appearance of that person's face, and size and configuration of that person's body. You can distinguish each of these elements that make it possible to recognize the person, but all are required for a full and accurate perception of who the person is.

For purposes of developing a theory of the art of nursing, I am proposing a shift in focus for basic elements of nursing practice. From the perspective of nursing art, aesthetics is viewed as an integrating pattern, whereby the art form itself provides foundation for transformative art and acts, which in turn integrate moral and ethical comportment, scientific competence, and therapeutic use of self, as illustrated in Figure 15.2. That is, it is the art that brings all elements together to form a whole of nursing practice.

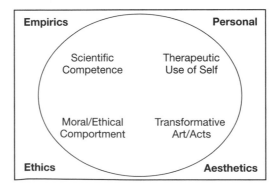

Source: Excerpted from Chinn, P. L., & Kramer, M. K. (1999). *Theory & nursing: Integrated knowledge development* (5th ed.) St. Louis: Mosby

Figure 15.1 Ontology of Nursing Practice.

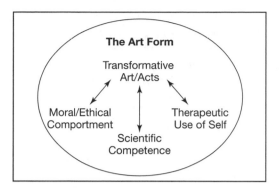

Figure 15.2 Art as an Integrating Pattern.

How Nursing Art Evolves

Nursing art evolves in four ways—the four "R's":

- ☐ refining synchronous narrative skills,
- ☐ refining synchronous movement skills,
- ☐ rehearsal and connoisseurship, and
- ☐ reflective practice in nursing, with a critic or connoisseur.

Each of these processes requires more than learning skills. They require developing a mindful way of bringing caring and healing intention into being, into experience.

Refining Synchronous Narrative Skills

Narrative skills involve both what is said or not said, as well as how it is said. In developing narrative skills, the major focus is on how a person speaks, sounds, and develops timing and rhythm to convey caring and healing intention. Voice tone is an important aspect of artistic narrative skill. In the "Introduction to the Art of Nursing" class, we used various exercises to explore possible voice tones and considered which tones conveyed caring and healing intention. The students then used different voices in narrative exchanges, giving and receiving feedback as to what voice tone and expression conveyed.

Effective storytelling is a skill that, until now, most nurses have taken for granted. In the Denver art study, we began to recognize the central role that storytelling played in the day-to-day practice of nursing. Nurses talked about stories they told their patients, stories they told one another at end of the day, and how they used storytelling to try to understand and improve their practice. Many nurses wrote down their stories for the group, which provided opportunities for recasting stories and rehearsing alternative story lines (Maeve, 1994). Recasting stories became a form of rehearsal, whereby nurses challenged one another to envision different possibilities for the story and to rehearse narratives that would move struggles of the story toward a different end. With each telling of a story, reflective insights deepened and possibilities for future encounters broadened. For example, one of the nurses told of being asked by a dying woman: "Will I know when I am dead?" The actual response to this question had been very unsatisfactory. In response to her account of what happened, many different story lines emerged with different ways of responding, different rhythms, timing, and synchrony in how various scenarios could unfold. This process deepened everyone's perception of what might be possible in a similar situation.

Artistic Validity of Narrative

Developing narrative skills requires an understanding of what constitutes artistic validity: What are the artistic qualities of narrative? Overall, artistic quality depends on the formation of a valid whole. From a narrative perspective, this means that the nurse's voice tone, expression, and substance of the narrative interaction are synchronous with intentions brought to the interaction. Within a nursing context, intention is consistent with caring and healing. Artistic quality depends on a "right relationship," which is also reflected in the idea of synchrony. A right relationship between what is expressed and how it is expressed must be evident, involving synchrony with movement of the self and the other and the nurses' timing and rhythm in bringing the experience together to form a valid whole that conveys caring and healing intention.

Refining Synchronous Movement Skills

Narrative skills have been given some attention in nursing, but movement has been reduced to a brief introduction to body mechanics. Movement skills involve much more than body mechanics, and indeed, when viewed from an artistic perspective, body mechanics take on new and significant meanings. Movement skills involve personal style in both large and fine motor movement, refined balance, finesse, timing, and synchrony. Skills include knowing how to deliberately form movements to convey a motive, intention, or feeling. Touch, which we often consider as a separate entity, from an artistic perspective is one phase in an entire movement sequence. It is the movement that brings touch to actuality that conveys meaning of the touch. We actually gained this insight by studying black and white photographs of nurses in the art study. The photographs prompted many different stories around what might have been happening when the pictures were taken. When a photograph showed a nurse touching a patient, the story could not emerge by focusing on the touch itself. The story and meanings symbolized in the situation came from imagining what moves had preceded and what moves followed the moment of touch.

Artistic Validity of Movement

Artistic qualities of movement, like those of narrative, focus on forming a valid whole, characterized by balance and finesse in both large and fine motor movements. Movement exhibits synchrony in timing and rhythm. Each nurse exhibits a personal style of movement that is refined over time but, like personality itself, has an enduring quality that conveys unique ways in which this particular nurse moves. In order to be artistically valid, movement in a nursing art context conveys caring and healing intentions. Movement of the nurse must be synchronous with both the narrative and with movement of others in the situation.

REHEARSAL AND CONNOISSEURSHIP

The next element that explains how nursing art evolves is rehearsal and connoisseurship. Rehearsal can be done without a connoisseur (e.g., teacher, coach, director, or critic), but presence of a connoisseur enhances awareness of what the art form is expressing and how well it is conveying the intended message.

Rehearsal brings movement and narrative together. Exercises that we used in the art course to refine narrative and movement skills focused largely on one or the other, but when we began rehearsal, one could not happen without the other. For example, at first we rehearsed what to say when first approaching a new patient, with particular attention on voice tone and words that convey caring and healing intention for interactions and relationships. Then we focused on how to move into a new situation, examining various body moves and stances that convey different intentions. These separate exercises constituted refining narrative and refining movement skills. When we began to work with particular nursing modalities, narrative and movement came together. We rehearsed entire sequences that included (a) the first approach, (b) introduction, (c) questions to become acquainted, (d) explanations as to what will happen in this encounter (e.g., taking a blood pressure reading), (e) movement of the body and hands to accomplish the task in a way that conveyed caring and healing intention, (f) explanations as to what happened or what was observed, and (g) words and movements to bring the encounter to a close.

Rehearsal Purpose

Each rehearsal included students who were "acting" the scenario and one or more student observers who were specifically noticing artistic qualities in the rehearsal (the connoisseurs). This kind of rehearsal nurtures reflective capacities that refine artistic capabilities. It gives the nurse artist an opportunity to notice differences between good timing and rhythm from poor timing and rhythm, for example. The observer or connoisseur provides feedback to students who are enacting the scenario, encouraging them to reach new dimensions—feeling what it is like to achieve coordinated movement, for example, when that has seemed particularly difficult. Learning to become a connoisseur and learning and rehearsing an art form at the same time are essential for reflective practice. Connoisseurship makes it possible to see the art form beneath what appears on the surface, to notice artistic qualities, and to reach toward the intended artistic expression.

Rehearsal reveals creative potential because the connoisseur encourages the artist to take risks. The connoisseur is able not only to "mirror" what actually has happened, but also to show, demonstrate, and inspire something else that might happen in the scenario—some new possibility for developing the art form. Even if the connoisseur is a student colleague, the connoisseur is an expert teacher, the best of coaches, the most inspiring of directors. The connoisseur provides a "mirror" for the artist's technical skill and artistic qualities. The best connoisseur gives accurate feedback as to how performance is executed. If it is not done well, the focus is on how to do it better. My harp teacher, for example, never says, "That sounds terrible." Instead, she says, "Try playing it like this (and she demonstrates) and listen to the difference. Now try it again."

Connoisseur Role

The connoisseur interprets perceived motive, intention, and feeling. My harp teacher says in an excited voice, for example, "That made me feel like I was running and now I am breathless." Now changing her voice to a slow pace, lower pitch, and lilting rhythm, she says, "This is a lullaby—slow it down and make me feel like going to sleep!" Then, when I play the piece like a lullaby (and not like a march), she says, "Oh, how sweet that sounds! I can just imagine holding this little baby until it sleeps."

The connoisseur presents imaginary situations and helps the student imagine new situations and project new creative possibilities. In "Introduction to the Art of Nursing Class" for example, we imagined situations that were different from those we had rehearsed, changing story lines and playing out scenarios with new story lines that called forth new creative skills and possibilities.

Most important, the connoisseur interprets artistic validity, giving the artist a way to see the art from another perspective. Doing so involves

- explaining symbolic elements that hold promise for transforming experience,
- connecting specific elements of artistic quality with perceived meanings and intentions that are conveyed, and
- connecting what art inspires as new possibilities for the future.

Reflective Practice with a Connoisseur

Finally, what emerges—from refining narrative and movement and from rehearsal with a connoisseur—comes into play as reflective practice. Reflective practice is the ultimate rehearsal studio and makes possible refinement of practice itself. Reflective practice brings what is rehearsed into practice and brings skills of connoisseurship to bear on nursing practice for the nurse and for others. Practice presents infinite complexities that usually are not present in rehearsal and provides infinite possibilities for reflection. Practice reveals ethical, empirical, and personal insights that emerge in artistic practice and provides a ground from which to envision new possibilities for the nurse artist.

CONCLUDING STATEMENT

In this chapter, I presented a theory of nursing art that includes assumptions, conceptual meanings of nursing art, a definition of the form of nursing art, and explanations as to how nursing art evolves. This theory can inform the teaching and practice of nursing art and can lead to scholarly aesthetic inquiry in the form of artistic criticism that arises from connoisseurship.

The question remains: Why nurture the art of nursing? My response to this critical question lies within our definition of nursing art, which states that "nursing art transforms experience from what is, to what might be possible." This transformation is the heart of our caring and healing practice—the ability to participate in experiences in such a way as to inspire new possibilities and to facilitate a healing path.

REFERENCES

Bostick, C. (1997). *Dance movement and its effects on rhythmic flow and nursing practice.* Unpublished PhD dissertation, University of Colorado, Denver.

Carper, B. A. (1978, October). Fundamental patterns of knowing in nursing. *Advances in Nursing Science, 1*(1), 13–23.

Chinn, P. L. (1994). Developing a method for aesthetic knowing in nursing. In P. L. Chinn & J. Watson (Eds.), *Art & aesthetics in nursing* (pp. 19–40). New York: National League for Nursing Press.

Chinn, P. L. & Kramer, M. K. (1999). *Theory & nursing: Integrated knowledge development* (5th ed.). St. Louis: Mosby.

Chinn, P. L., Maeve, M. K., & Bostick, C. (1997). Aesthetic inquiry and the art of nursing. *Scholarly Inquiry for Nursing Practice, 11*(2), 83–96.

Eisner, E. (1985). *Learning and teaching the ways of knowing: Part II.* Chicago: University of Chicago Press.

Johnson, J. L. (1994). A dialectical examination of nursing art. *Advances in Nursing Science, 17*(1), 1–14.

LeVasseur, J. J. (1999). Toward an understanding of art in nursing. *Advances in Nursing Science, 21*(4), 48–63.

Maeve, M. K. (1994). Coming to moral consciousness through the art of nursing narratives. In P. L. Chin & J. Watson (Eds.), *Art & aesthetics in nursing* (pp. 67–89). New York: National League for Nursing.

Nightingale, Florence (1969). *Notes on nursing: What it is and what it is not.* New York: Dover. (Original work published 1860).

CHAPTER 16

Wading Through Muddy Waters: The Intersection of Feminist Theory, Cultural Competence, and Ethics in the Care of Battered Women

Ursula Kelly

INTRODUCTION

Nursing is viewed as both an art and a science, incorporating a variety of ways of knowing. Nursing practice is rational, relational, and reflective. Expert nursing practice involves the integration of a variety of ways of knowing and being and their utilization in relationship with another human being. Nursing practice involves the application of nursing knowledge at the individual level, enabling human transformation within the experience of the health continuum.

Several patterns of knowing were first articulated by Carper (1978), modified by Jacobs-Kramer and Chinn (1988), and added to by White (1995). Carper (1978) identified four patterns of knowing: (1) empirics, the science of nursing; (2) ethics, the moral component; (3) personal knowledge; and (4) esthetics, the art of nursing. Jacobs-Kramer and Chinn's (1988) modifications were designed to redirect nursing away from "a quest for structural truth and towards a search for dynamic meaning" (p. 138). White (1995) added the dimension of sociopolitical knowing to place the nurse–patient relationship in context; that is, the sociopolitical environment within which the persons and their interactions take place.

This chapter will consider the clinical problem of domestic abuse experienced by women of different cultures to demonstrate the development and application of knowledge in nursing practice. Both a feminist perspective and ethical knowledge will be brought to bear on the discussion. Differences in cultural experiences of domestic abuse, as well as cultural disparities between patients and nurses, pose ethical dilemmas for nurses. The ethical judgments that nurses make relative to domestic abuse direct nursing practice. The essential question is, "Who decides what is domestic abuse and what is not?" The answer to this question across cultures requires a systematic application of relevant knowledge in order to reach an ethical judgment or position, which in turn directs nursing practice.

DOMESTIC ABUSE, ETHICS, AND NURSING

Domestic abuse is a significant health problem for women around the globe. In Latin America and the Caribbean, 30 to 50% of adult women with partners experience psychological abuse and

10 to 35% experience physical abuse (Buvinic, Morrison, & Shifter, 1999). Estimates of the prevalence of domestic violence in the United States range from 960,000 to more than 2 million incidents per year (Bachman & Saltzman, 1996; U.S. Department of Justice, 1998). Domestic abuse is recognized as the number one public health problem facing women and is associated with a multitude of specific health problems (McCauley et al., 1995). Healthcare providers are mandated to screen for and intervene in cases of domestic violence (AMA, 1992; ANA, 1991; JCAHCO, 1995).

The population of the United States is becoming more ethnically diverse. According to projections, ethnic minorities will make up 50% of the U.S. population by the year 2050 (U.S. Bureau of the Census, 1991). Nurses and other healthcare providers are being called upon to recognize and be responsive to the different values and needs of this diverse population. Practicing with cultural competence is considered a standard of care in nursing.

The intersection of domestic abuse and culture provides many challenges for nursing practice. Nurses struggle to understand the values, beliefs, and choices of battered women. The struggle to understand is even greater across cultures. For the purposes of this chapter, domestic abuse is restricted to mean intimate partner violence against women by men. The ethical questions are "Who decides what is domestic abuse and what is not?" and "Are there universal standards of behavior that can be applied to adults?" The answers to these questions are simpler with regards to cases of child abuse, where there are assumptions of lack of power, lack of freedom, and vulnerability. In contrast, women are generally assumed to have power, freedom, and choice, adding to the barriers to understanding the reality of battered women's lives, in any culture.

The problem of domestic abuse will be considered first from a traditional ethical perspective. Feminist theory and feminist ethics, as well as the concepts of cultural competence and multiculturalism, will be brought to bear on the ethical questions just raised. The competing demands of feminism and cultural competence will be discussed, and emerging concepts will be presented that reconcile the ethical and philosophical conflicts inherent in providing nursing care to battered women across cultures.

ETHICS AND DOMESTIC ABUSE: THE HISTORICAL VIEW

Only recently has domestic abuse emerged as a publicly recognized problem. Historically, the nature of relationships between intimates was considered a private and personal matter, inappropriate for public discourse and shameful if made public. From an ethical perspective, historically women were viewed as lacking rationality and, therefore, were not viewed as moral beings worthy of moral consideration (Rachels, 1999). This is exemplified in the writings of Aristotle as long ago as 350 B.C. and subsequently by Kant. More recently, Kohlberg (1984) asserted that women's moral development was inferior to that of men. Because of the combined effect of the privacy afforded domestic abuse and traditional ethical views of women, domestic abuse remained, until recently, outside the realm of ethical consideration and judgment and outside the scope of nursing practice.

ETHICS AND DOMESTIC ABUSE: THE 21ST CENTURY

On the surface, by the standards of the 21st century, the question of the ethics of domestic abuse would seem so obvious as to be inane. Basic ethical principles of justice and autonomy find abuse of an individual by another unethical, particularly in the context of an intimate relationship. All individuals, women and men, are seen as rational free agents worthy of equal consideration. This perspective leads to a conception of the "generalized other" in self–other relations (Benhabib, 1992, p. 280). The generalized other lacks individuality and individual circumstance and is related to us by norms of formal equality and reciprocity.

The overriding ethical principle applied here is that every individual is a rational being entitled to the same duties and rights we would want to ascribe to ourselves. In this context, domestic abuse is seen as wrong and as an issue not only worthy of public discourse, but as a public health problem to be addressed by society. The rights of women are now seen as universal human rights. The 1993 United Nations Conference on Human Rights declared "women's rights are an inalienable, integral, and indivisible part of universal human rights," and, further, that these rights are not subordinate to the state or cultural considerations (Marshall, Thomasma, & Bergsma, 1994, p. 325).

Despite the simplicity of the ethical argument, nurses' judgments about domestic abuse across cultures are complicated by personal feelings, as well as cultural considerations, which may be misguided. Of course, many nurses see the simplicity of the case and view domestic abuse in any scenario as unethical or wrong. Others may see domestic abuse as wrong by our cultural standards (for us), but not by another culture's standards (for them). Another judgment is that domestic abuse is universally wrong, but that women from some other cultures do not know that, and they would not agree, so it is futile to address it. Finally, in considering other cultures, some nurses conclude that domestic abuse in those cultures is normal and expected and is therefore acceptable.

The question of the morality of domestic abuse is easily answered using traditional ethical principles. However, the questions of the universality of rights and who decides what constitutes domestic abuse take on added complexity with the inclusion of both feminist and multicultural perspectives (see Table 16.1).

Feminist Theory

Feminism is not a monolithic entity. There are a variety of different types of feminism; most share a few common tenets, but diverge with regard to philosophical stances, goals, and ontological assumptions. Despite wide variations in feminist perspectives, common definitions and principles of feminism have been articulated in the literature. Feminism is primarily concerned with the oppression and emancipation of women. Sampselle (1990) identified three basic tenets that have emerged in feminist philosophy: (1) affirmation of gender equity; (2) the value of an individual to society based on the capacity to contribute, rather than sex or gender characteristics; and (3) women's right to sovereignty over their bodies. Epistemological issues in feminist theory include the assertions that (1) women can be knowers (Belenky et al., 1986), and their

Table 16.1 Comparison of Ethical Approaches

Ethical Approach	Traditional	Feminist	Cultural	Interactive Universalism
Philosophical approach	Rational	Relational/contextual	Relational/contextual	Rational and relational
Other in relation to self	Generalized	Concrete	Concrete	Generalized and concrete

knowledge is legitimate (Stanley & Wise, 1990); (2) knowledge is relational and contextual (Campbell & Bunting, 1991); and (3) practice must have gender-sensitive reflexivity (Ginzberg, 1995). Both cultural and radical feminisms recognize and value differences between the sexes, whereas liberal feminism historically has stressed rationality and equality between the sexes, minimizing differences.

The application of feminist theory leads to the same judgment on domestic abuse as traditional ethical reasoning, that it is unethical. However, feminist moral reasoning involves different assumptions. The feminist reasoning process is contextual and relational, as opposed to rational. The "concrete other" replaces the generalized other of traditional ethics. The concrete other is viewed as a rational individual with a concrete history, identity, and personality (Benhabib, 1992). Relationships are governed by the norms of equity and complementary reciprocity. Sherwin (1992) applied feminist philosophy to ethics and described feminist ethics as inclusive of both justice and caring. An ethics of care alone would lead to "feminine" ethics, which is inadequate in its lack of commitment to considerations of justice.

Cultural Competence

Cultural competence is used both as a concept and as a model within nursing. Cross et al.'s (1989) definition of cultural competence reflects the common traits of many authors' definitions, "a set of congruent behaviors, attitudes, and policies that come together in a system, agency, or among professionals and enable [them] to work effectively in cross-cultural situations" (p. 13). Orlandi et al. (1992) stressed cultural competence as entailing personal awareness and willingness to work with the values and individuals from the community. Campinha-Bote's (1999) model of cultural competence in health care includes specific cultural awareness, knowledge, skills, encounters, and desire.

The nursing model of cultural competence takes the emic view that individuals within the culture are knowers. At its extreme, cultural competence takes a position of cultural relativism, and consequently, ethical relativism. Cultural relativists claim that (1) different cultures have different moral codes, (2) there is no universal truth in ethics, (3) the moral code within a society determines what is right within that society, and (4) it is arrogant for one culture to judge another's conduct (Rachels, 1999).

Like feminism, the model of cultural competence is relational and contextual, views the other as concrete, and recognizes the importance of differences among individuals. However, culture has primacy over gender in this model. Multiculturalism does not allow for universals, including universal human rights. Thus, the intersection of feminist nursing and culturally competent nursing has inherent conflicting principles and assumptions.

FEMINISM AND CULTURAL COMPETENCE

Several feminist scholars have addressed this apparent conflict in principles. At the most basic level is the recognition that there are commonalities among women, regardless of culture. Feminists also have deconstructed the concept of culture as homogenous and equitable within itself. Okin (1999) claimed that most cultures seek the subordination of women by men as a primary aim. Differences within cultures are often ignored in favor of those between cultures. For example, North Americans tend to view Hispanic cultures as approving of domestic abuse, citing the cultural norm of *machismo* and the prevalence of abuse, ignoring differences within any one Hispanic culture in how domestic abuse is viewed and addressed. Frye's (1983) feminist analysis of oppressive systems can be applied to cultures as well. She asked the following questions of such a system: (1) Who constructs and maintains it? (2) Whose interests are served? (3) Who benefits? and (4) Who suffers?

Meleis et al. (1995), utilizing a feminist perspective, defined culturally competent care as "care that takes into account issues related to diversity, marginalization, and vulnerability due to culture, race, gender, and sexual orientation" (p. 4). Cultural knowledge taken out of context of situated constraints and universal humanistic values is marginalizing (Meleis & Im, 1999). The concept of marginalization reconciles the concerns of feminism and culture and offers a new way of knowing.

The questions of this chapter, "Who decides what is domestic abuse and what is not?" and "Are there universal standards of behavior that can be applied to adults?" can now be seen in a new light and partially answered. Two problems persist, however. Domestic abuse is not a dichotomous entity. It includes a range of behaviors, including emotional, psychological, physical, and sexual abuse. Individuals, as well as groups, define abuse differently, some include nonphysical abuse and some do not. Where is the line to be drawn between universal rights and cultural practices? A behavior that one person or culture may see as merely a sign of an unhealthy relationship, for example, insulting one's partner, may be seen as abusive to another individual or culture. The second problem involves language. Specifically, meaning and subtlety easily can be misunderstood across languages. For example, *abuse*, which is defined in many ways in one culture, may be given very different meanings in another.

In responding to the question of "Who decides?" each group is subject to criticism. Feminists are criticized by cultural rights groups as imposing cultural imperialism. Cultural rights groups adhering to cultural norms are accused of ethical relativism. Battered women themselves often are dismissed as either culturally indoctrinated or as suffering from battered women's syndrome or denial.

APPLICATION TO ADVANCED NURSING PRACTICE

Nurses face a number of responsibilities and mandates in providing care to battered women across cultures. Nurses are charged with moral, ethical, and professional responsibilities to provide culturally competent care that conveys respect to the individual and advocacy that meets standards of care, including identifying and intervening in cases of domestic abuse. An understanding of marginalization and an emerging model of knowledge development (Meleis & Im, 1999) offer direction in meeting these potentially conflicting responsibilities.

In applying ethics, the approach of interactive universalism provides for an inclusion of the concerns of feminism and culture (Benhabib, 1992). Interactive universalism includes consideration of both the generalized and the concrete other. One can both recognize universals, including universal human rights, and attend to the specifics of a case, applying the principles of justice and care. Interactive universalism is an analytical-utopian view that provides an integrated view of humans, both women and men, deconstructing the dichotomies created by the language of feminism and culture.

Interactive universalism as an ethical approach parallels the application of situation-specific knowledge in nursing. Extant knowledge is brought to bear upon a specific situation and incorporated into what can be known in an individual nurse–patient interaction and clinical context, as well as a cultural context.

The application of ethical knowledge to the clinical problem of domestic abuse across cultures clarifies the role of cultural differences. Cultural differences often are perceived as barriers to clinical care and nursing knowledge. Through applied ethics, it is argued that domestic abuse does not have to be accepted simply because of perceived differences in cultures. These differences no longer pose barriers to nursing practice. Recognition of the universals of human rights, human experiences, and humanness allows for movement forward in the process of transformation, for both the nurse and the patient.

This application of ethical, feminist, and cultural knowledge to the clinical problem of intimate partner abuse is a small first step toward the development of a gender-sensitive theory of women's health. Im and Meleis (2001), in "An international imperative for gender-sensitive theories in women's health," asserted that the development of gender-sensitive theories would enable nurses to "transcend androcentric and ethnocentric views on women's health, decrease gender inequity in health care, enhance women's well-being, and ultimately contribute to knowledge development in nursing" (p. 309). They identified six major components of such theories: (1) gender as a central factor in women's health, (2) women's own voices and experiences, (3) diversities and complexities of women's experiences, (4) theorists' perspectives, (5) sociopolitical contexts, and (6) guidelines for action (Im & Meleis, 2001). With these components as a backdrop, using a relational narrative in practice can facilitate the emergence of newly constructed meanings for both the nurse and the patient, and as such, enable human transformation.

Clinical Exemplar

Iliana is a 36-year-old Colombian woman. She is Spanish-speaking only and has a fourth grade education. She presents to a nurse practitioner for prenatal care in her first trimester. The setting is an urban neighborhood health center that serves an ethnically diverse population. As part of her initial visit, the nurse practitioner screens her for intimate partner abuse, according to the health center's protocol. Rather than answering with a simple "Yes" or "No," Iliana replies that her partner has "un caracter fuerte," a phrase that literally translated means "a strong character." This could have been the end of the discussion, with mandatory screening completed and no sign of abuse.

The nurse practitioner speaks Spanish, but not fluently. Recognizing the potential for misunderstanding, even without language barriers, the nurse practitioner asks Iliana what she means by "un caracter fuerte." She learns that Iliana's partner is controlling, demanding, moody, and quick-tempered, though Iliana justifies his behavior as the result of stress at work. Over the course of the next several visits, the nurse practitioner asks Iliana more about her life, her process of immigration, and her current experiences.

Iliana has suffered a lifetime of abuse. She started working at age 9. She came to the United States in order to provide financially for her three children in Colombia. She immigrated illegally and unknowingly served as a mule for a drug dealer. She was arrested at the airport in Miami, and after much difficulty, was allowed to leave on probation. She lives in constant fear of deportation. She met the abuser on the day she arrived alone in a new city. He took her in, and she felt indebted to him. She became pregnant within a few months of meeting him, and they got married. He started beating her the week after they got married, made her sleep on the bare floor, and dragged her around the apartment by her hair. Iliana is desperate and afraid, but feels she has no options, because he is supporting her and she is indebted to him. More than anything, she needs to provide for her children in Colombia and will withstand whatever is necessary to ensure their well-being, including staying with the abuser. This represents another possible end-point in the discussion between Iliana and her nurse practitioner about the abuse. Iliana is acknowledging the abuse, but views it as inevitable, and is unwilling to leave the abuser.

The nurse practitioner, practicing within an understanding of the complexities of Iliana's situation, takes the conversation further, seeking a richer understanding for both Iliana and herself about Iliana's experiences and opportunities. They develop a mutually trusting relationship with open communication. The nurse practitioner offers hope, a vision that Iliana's life can be different and free from abuse. She frames the abusive behavior as unacceptable, regardless of the abuser's financial support, Iliana's upbringing, her feelings of gratitude, or her belief in God's will. She tells her that no human being deserves to be treated this way.

The nurse practitioner gains a more developed understanding of the incredible tangible and intangible barriers Iliana faces in escaping the abuse and the abuser. She assists Iliana in identifying her strengths and self-worth as a survivor and provider for her children. She provides Iliana with information about available battered women's services, including a Spanish-speaking support group, as well as childcare, employment, and legal services. Immediately following the birth of her fourth child, nearly one year after the abuse began, Iliana escapes to a battered women's shelter and obtains a protective order. She is successful in obtaining child support from the abuser and begins the long process of healing from the abuse, both physically and psychologically.

CONCLUSION

This chapter used the clinical problem of intimate partner abuse to discuss the application of existing theories and the need for the development of gender-specific theories to guide nursing care of women. Despite the conclusions reached in this discussion, the reality is that domestic abuse of women is still considered by many nurses and patients to be a taboo issue, one that is rife with the potential for misunderstanding, particularly across cultures. Nurses practicing within a monolithic theoretical or cultural perspective will fail to address women's health needs effectively. Current feminist theory, ethics, and a model of cultural competence bring important perspectives to the clinical care of women, particularly women who are being abused. Together they incorporate the components of a gender-specific theory that can contribute to nursing knowledge and guide nursing practice to enhance women's well-being.

REFERENCES

AMA Council on Scientific Affairs. (1992). Violence against women: Relevance for medical practitioners. *JAMA, 267,* 3184–3189.

ANA. (1991). *Position statement on physical violence against women.* Washington, D.C.: Author.

Bachman, R., & Saltzman, L. E. (1996). *Violence against women: Estimates from the redesigned survey* (NJC No. 154348). Washington, D.C.: U.S. Department of Justice.

Belenky, M. F., Clinchy, B. M., Goldberger, N. R., & Tarule, J. M. (1986). *Women's ways of knowing: The development of self, voice, and mind.* New York, NY: Basic Books.

Benhabib, S. (1992). The generalized and the concrete other. In E. Frazer, J. Hornsby, & S. Lovibond (Eds.), *Ethics: A feminist reader.* Cambridge: Blackwell.

Buvinic, M., Morrison, A., & Shifter, M. (1999). Violence in the Americas: A Framework for action. In A. R. Morrison & M. L. Biehl (Eds.), *Too close to home: Domestic violence in the Americas* (pp. 3–34). Washington, D.C.: Inter-American Development Bank.

Campbell, J. C., & Bunting, S. (1991). Voices and paradigms: Perspectives on critical and feminist theory in nursing. *Advances in Nursing Science, 13*(3), 1–15.

Campinha-Bote, J. (1999). A model and instrument for addressing cultural competence in healthcare. *Journal of Nursing Education, 38*(5), 203–207.

Carper, B. (1978). Fundamental patterns of knowing in nursing. *Advances in Nursing Science, 1*(1), 13–23.

Cross, T. L., Barzon, B. J., Dennis, K. W., & Isaacs, M. R. (1989). *Towards a culturally competent system of care.* Washington, D.C.: CASSP Technical Assistance Center.

Frye, M. (1983). *The Politics of Reality: Essays in Feminist Theory.* Freedom, California: Crossing Press.

Ginzberg, R. (1995). Feminism, science, and nursing. In A. Omery, C. E. Kasper, & G. G. Page (Eds.), *In search of nursing science*, (pp. 93–105). Thousand Oaks, CA: Sage Publications.

Im, E., & Melcis, A. (2001). An international imperative for gender-sensitive theories in women's health. *Journal of Nursing Scholarship, 33*(4), 309–314.

Jacobs-Kramer, M., & Chinn, P. (1988). Perspectives on knowing: A model of nursing knowledge. *Scholarly Inquiry for Nursing Practice, 2*(2), 129–139.

JCAHCO. (1995). *Accreditation mannual for hospitals.* Oakbridge Terrace, IL: Author.

Kohlberg, L. (1984). *The psychology of moral development: The nature and validity of moral stages* (Vol. II). San Francisco: Harper & Row.

Marshall, P., Thomasma, D., & Bergsma, J. (1994). Intercultural reasoning: The challenge for international bioethics. *Cambridge Quarterly of Healthcare Ethics, 3*, 321–328.

McCauley, J., Kern, D. E., Kolodner, K., Dill, L., Schroeder, A. F., DeChant, H. K., Ryden, J., Bass, E. B., & Derogatis, L. R. (1995). The "battering syndrome": Prevalence and clinical chararacteristics of domestic violence in primary care internal medicine practices. *Annals of Internal Medicine, 123*(10), 737–746.

Meleis, A. I., & Im, E. O. (1999). Transcending marginalization in knowledge development. *Nursing Inquiry, 6*, 94–102.

Meleis, A. I., Isenberg, M., Koerner, J. E., Lacey, B., & Stern, P. (1995). *Diversity, marginalization, and culturally competent health care issues in knowledge development.* Washington, D.C.: American Academy of Nursing.

Okin, S. M. (1999). Is multiculturalism bad for women? In J. Cohen, M. Howard, & M. C. Nussbaum (Eds.), *Is multiculturalism bad for women?* (pp. 9–24). Princeton, NJ: Princeton University Press.

Orlandi, M., Weston, R., & Epstein, L. (1992). *Cultural competence for evaluators* (DHHS Pub. No. (ADM)92-1884). Rockville, MD: Office for Substance Abuse Prevention.

Rachels, J. (1999). *The elements of moral philosophy* (3rd ed.). Boston: McGraw-Hill.

Sampselle, C. M. (1990). The influence of feminist philosophy on nursing practice. *Image: Journal of Nursing Scholarship, 22*(4), 243–247.

Sherwin, S. (1992). Ethics, "Feminine" ethics, and feminist ethics. In S. Sherwin (Ed.), *No longer patient: Feminist ethics in health care* (pp. 35–57). Philadelphia: Temple University.

Stanley, L., & Wise, S. (1990). Method, methodology, and epistemology in feminist research processes. In L. Stanley (Ed.), *Feminist praxis* (pp. 20–60). London: Routledge.

U.S. Bureau of the Census. (1991). *Statistical abstract of the United States: 1991.* Washington, D.C.: Author.

U.S. Department of Justice. (1998). *Violence by intimates: Analysis of data on crimes by current or former spouses, boyfriends, and girlfriends.* Washington, D.C.: Author.

White, J. (1995). Patterns of knowing: Review, critique, and update. *Advances in Nursing Science, 17*(4), 73–86.

CHAPTER 17

Healthy Death: The Ethics of Care at the End of Life

Inge B. Corless
Patrice K. Nicholas

The phrase *healthy death* would seem to be an oxymoron; that is, how can a death be healthy? In this chapter, we will examine how a patient-centered environment can facilitate healthy dying and death. Our focus will be to examine some of the ethical issues that may impede healthy dying.

BACKGROUND

Interest in ethical issues concerning the care of patients was renewed in the 20th century by the examination during the second Nuremberg Trial, the Doctors' Trial, of the behavior of Nazi healthcare providers during World War II. Nazi physicians and health officials were charged with experimenting on human subjects, primarily prisoners in concentration camps. The trial concluded on August 19, 1947; seven of the defendants were sentenced to death, five to life imprisonment, four to prison terms ranging from 10 to 25 years, and seven others were acquitted (Shuster, 1997). Brigadier General Telford Taylor, Chief of Counsel for War Crimes, set the stage for the conduct of the trial by noting in his opening statement that physicians were held to a higher standard of conduct than were other individuals: "He opined that the fatal experiments on human subjects were especially evil since they were performed by physicians who pledged by the Hippocratic oath to do no harm" (Kagarise & Sheldon, 2000, p. 39).

Following the Nuremberg Trials, the Nuremberg Code on the Ethics of Human Research was created. Its importance is reflected in the following appraisal: "The Nuremberg Code is the most important document in the history of the ethics of medical research" (Shuster, 1997, p. 1436). Although geared toward physicians who conduct primary research, many of the 10 principles have been incorporated into patient care. The 10 principles are:

> . . . voluntary consent; an expected beneficial outcome; prior experimentation on animals; avoidance of unnecessary pain and horror; avoidance of risk or disablement; risk taking not to exceed expected advantages; protection against the possibility, however slight, of injury, disablement, or death; scientifically and technically qualified experimenters; the subject's freedom to retract consent; and the experimenter's obligation to stop the experiment. (Kagarise & Sheldon, p. 40)

Shuster (1997) argues that the Nuremberg Code reflects the importation of patient rights into a code for research (p. 1438). We assert that the formulation of patient rights has been abetted, likewise, by the development of codes for the practice of research.

Although these principles have evolved to become the standard for the conduct of research, additional specifications of the rights of patients have been developed. The Declaration of Lisbon on the Rights of the Patient was adopted by the 34th World Medical Assembly in September/October 1981 (Bulletin of the Pan American Health Organization, 1990). Two of the principal rights of this declaration are particularly relevant to this chapter. These are: "The patient has the right to accept or refuse treatment after receiving adequate information" and "The patient has the right to die in dignity" (Bulletin of the PAHO, pp. 621–622). Although the right to die in dignity is not mentioned specifically, *A Patient's Bill of Rights*, approved by the American Hospital Association House of Delegates on February 6, 1973, contains other principles germane to the discussion in this chapter, including the right to considerate and respectful care; to complete and current information about diagnosis, treatment, and prognosis; information necessary to give informed consent; and the right to refuse treatment and be informed of the consequences of this action (Bulletin of the PAHO, 1990).

In 1979, the Belmont Report, which elaborated ethical principles to be used when conducting research on human subjects, noted three ethical principles that have become the basis for discussion of clinical decision making (National Commission for the Protection of Human Subjects, 1979). The three ethical principles discussed in the Belmont Report are respect for persons, beneficence, and justice. Respect for persons is elaborated further in subsequent documents to include autonomy and the protection of persons with impaired or diminished capacity (Tolle, 1991, 1993). The International Guidelines for Ethical Review of Epidemiological Studies applies these principles to informed consent, maximizing benefit, minimizing harm, confidentiality, and conflict of interest (Tolle, 1991).

The basic bioethical principles employed in most ethical discussions are the so-called Georgetown principles. These principles include beneficence, autonomy, and justice as well as nonmaleficence and fidelity (Otte & Allen, 1987). In brief, these principles can be defined as follows:

- ☐ **Beneficence:** Promoting the good of others or contributing to another's welfare.
- ☐ **Nonmaleficence:** The obligation to avoid harming or injuring others.
- ☐ **Autonomy:** The right to self-determination, noninterference, and liberty with the obligation to respect the autonomy, liberty, and rights of others.
- ☐ **Justice:** The principle of fairness by which each person is given his or her fair share.
- ☐ **Fidelity:** The moral obligation to keep promises, meet commitments, and fulfill contracts.

These principles are the foundation for what is termed *principle-based ethics and decision making*.

Another approach is the ethics of care. Caring "refers to care for, emotional commitment to, and willingness to act on behalf of persons with whom one has a significant relationship" (Beauchamp & Childress, 1994, p. 85). The focus in an ethics of care is on relationships and on maximizing the good of all concerned: "Having a certain emotional attitude and expressing the appropriate emotion in acting are morally relevant factors, just as having the appropriate motive is morally relevant" (Beauchamp & Childress, 1994, p. 89). This is a major change from an emphasis on cognition alone: "The person who acts from rule-governed obligations without appropriately aligned feelings such as worry when a friend suffers seems to have a moral deficiency" (Beauchamp & Childress, 1994, p. 89).

Thus, taking into consideration the needs and feelings of others is central to the ethics of care, as is a situation-specific analysis. It is interesting that Churchill and Siman (1986) assert that "Principles are also situation-specific, in the sense that they are appropriate in some settings, but not in others. For example, patient autonomy is an important ideal in the care of chronically ill patients, but it has a greatly diminished role in emergency care" (p. 463). Problems arise when emergency care is provided to a chronically ill person whose previously specified wishes are not utilized in rendering care. In such cases, the patient's autonomy is violated, as well as his or her person. Ethics of care is directed to specific situations, whereas principle-based ethics is concerned with equity. In a real-life situation, these approaches need to be utilized judiciously so that an optimum outcome can be achieved. In the next section, we will consider some of the issues and the ethical dimensions that have made approaches to caregiving less than clear-cut.

Caregiving Issues

The emphasis on truth-telling in medical practice has undergone a major revision. As Churchill (1979) notes, "The issue of whether a physician should tell patients the truth about the nature of their illness is a very old one" (p. 218). He continues, "It is widely argued, and probably widely practiced, that the obligation of a physician to tell the truth is suspended when the truth might become an agent of harm" (p. 218). While the emphasis in previous decades was on telling a responsible member of the family "the bad news," this dilemma has been resolved in recent years in favor of telling the patient directly, often with family members present. Physicians were concerned with taking away "hope," and many discussions and articles by terminally ill healthcare providers weighed in on one side of the argument or the other. Currently, the issue is not so much one of truth-telling about a diagnosis, but more one of truth-telling about treatment options and prognosis. It is here that there may be less than full disclosure. This lack of candor reflects, at worst, the healthcare provider's discomfort in conveying bad news; at best, the provider's optimism about the outcome of therapy. Truth-telling is basic to all of the other issues to be discussed in this chapter. It is also basic to a patient-centered environment.

Issues surrounding withholding or withdrawing treatment have received increased attention for a number of different reasons. With the advent of high-technology critical care units, providers can intervene to achieve short-term goals, and given the wishes of families that "everything be done," physicians utilize the tools at hand to solve one immediate crisis after another. The "everything be done" mentality has led to questions of when further treatment is futile. Questions about quality of life have been accelerated by the sight of individuals in a persistent vegetative state, without consciousness, who are maintained on life support machinery. The issue here is the withdrawal of technological support.

The question of withholding support has been accelerated by the hospice and palliative care movements where the emphasis has been on supporting the patient and family to achieve comfort at the end of life. Not imposing burdensome technologies in ways that would prolong dying has been a major consideration. At the same time, a demographic phenomenon is occurring, namely, the aging of the population. Given competing access to resources that are becoming increasingly scarce, how should these resources be used? In effect, how many people and which ones get into the lifeboat when there is a sinking ship?

Another issue is the impact of managed care, with its emphasis on the prudent use of financial resources. It is in this arena that questions of futility occur. Given that most end-of-life expenditures occur in the last month of life, managed care plan officials might consider promoting physician-assisted suicide as a cost-saving measure. According to Emmanuel and Battin (1998), however, "The most reasonable estimate is a savings of $627 million, less than 0.07 percent of total health expenditures" (p. 171). Emmanuel and Battin effectively counter the argument of shortening life predicated on futility based on financial considerations.

Other considerations, primarily the imposition of burdensome technologies on a patient whose quality of life will not improve, are relevant to the question of withdrawing/withholding support. This array of factors is complicated further by family members and others who may have various psychological and financial reasons for wanting life prolonged or shortened. Given this mix of stakeholders, what is an ethical framework for decision making?

Pellegrino (2000) suggests that "There are four practical ethical questions that must be answered in any clinical decision to withhold or withdraw life-sustaining treatment: (1) Who decides? (2) By what criteria? (3) How are conflicts among decision makers resolved? (4) How is conflict prevented?" (p. 1065). The "who decides" is now clearly agreed upon to be the patient, if that individual has decision-making capacity. Questions about the capacity of an individual to make decisions often arise when those decisions are in conflict with the wishes of relevant others. At such times, the capacity of the individual to make crucial decisions may be called into question:

> Decision-making capacity depends on the ability to communicate, to comprehend the nature and gravity of the decision, to make a reasoned judgment based on one's own values, to persist in that judgment, and to do so in a manner consistent with previously expressed values and beliefs. (Pellegrino, 2000, p. 1066)

Clearly, a patient-centered environment will strive to foster healthcare decisions that are made in accord with the patient's wishes.

Are there any limitations to the primacy given to the patient or surrogate's decision making? Pellegrino (2000) outlines such circumstances. He notes that the moral authority of the patient and surrogate are:

> limited under the following conditions: (1) when the patient's decision produces identifiable, serious, probable harm to identifiable others; (2) when the physician is asked to violate his or her personal and professional ethical integrity; (3) when the patient deliberately attempts to injure himself or herself; or (4) when the treatment requested is clinically futile or contraindicated. (p. 1066)

These limitations to moral authority are areas where there is often intense discussion among healthcare providers.

Although bioethicists see no distinction between the withdrawal and the withholding of clinical treatment, withdrawal of in situ interventions is often a greater ethical challenge for clinicians. Rhymes, McCullough, Luchi, Teasdale, and Wilson (2000) argue that even very low burden interventions may be withdrawn from chronically ill patients. The question of whether such withdrawal constitutes assisted suicide has been raised. Rhymes et al. clarify this issue in the following way. They distinguish between a new and an existing condition:

Thus when a physician extubates a patient with respiratory failure who then dies of that failure, or—deactivates a pacemaker in a patient who may then die of cardiac arrest, the physician is not introducing a new pathology as a cause of death. Rather in both cases, an existing disease pathology is allowed to complete its natural history. (pp. 1062–1063)

A parallel question is whether foregoing life support is suicide. To answer this question, it is important to investigate the nature of the life support. For some, the answer revolves around whether the life support is ordinary or extraordinary. Brock (1984) suggests that simply determining whether a treatment is ordinary or extraordinary is fraught with the problems of definition. Instead, some assessment of benefits and burdens of treatment is more to the point, particularly for the patient. He notes that "competent patients are morally entitled to refuse any life-sustaining treatment that they judge to be sufficiently burdensome, so as to make life no longer worth living with that treatment" (p. 347). The intent, therefore, is to eliminate a burdensome treatment so as not to impair quality of life. The intent is not to eliminate life itself.

Although not usually considered in this fashion, the issue of double effect applies to this situation. The Doctrine of Double Effect is often raised when morphine sulfate is given in sufficient doses to subdue pain, because it has the secondary effect of slowing respirations and, in some eyes, hastening death. Unless a massive dose of morphine is given that is disproportionate to the need for pain relief, such is not the case. But if it were, is the intent death or the relief of pain? Most ethicists agree that death as a means of relieving pain is not morally acceptable (Brock, 1984). And some would argue that the double effect is itself a spurious concept, arguing that in giving large doses where the effect is pain relief followed by death, intent is immaterial. Clinicians would argue strongly to the contrary.

Another issue is the withholding of basic life support (i.e., nutrition and hydration). Looking at the issue from a slightly different perspective, the question becomes one of the force-feeding of individuals who may not want such ministrations. And perhaps that is the right perspective. No one is suggesting that intake be withheld from individuals who want food and drink and find meals pleasurable. The question of intake becomes problematic when the patient is actively refusing such intake or when the patient is not conscious. McCann, Hall, and Groth-Juncker (1994) studied the effects of limiting food and drink to that requested by their terminally ill cancer patients and found that "Providing food and fluids only as needed to relieve the patient's discomfort can be an effective means of fulfilling a patient's wishes while alleviating discomfort" (p. 1266).

Fulfilling a patient's wishes is at the heart of a patient-centered environment. The question may arise as to what those wishes are. When the patient is unable to speak for him or herself, family members may disagree as to the appropriate mode of action. To increase the probability that the patient's wishes will be respected, healthcare institutions are required to ask the patient whether he or she has or would like to complete an advance directive. One such form is the Physician Orders for Life-Sustaining Treatment (POLST) (Tolle, Tiden, Nelson & Dunn, 1998). The POLST form is grouped into A and B sections. Section A is concerned with resuscitation and has boxes to check resuscitate or do not resuscitate. Section B contains progressive amounts of intervention, from comfort measures only (including measures to relieve pain and suffering) to comfort measures plus limited intervention (oxygen, suction, manual treatment of airway obstruction, and wound care). Advanced interventions include the interventions just listed plus monitors, cardiac rhythms, medications, and intravenous fluids. Finally, Full Treatment includes everything mentioned previously plus cardiopulmonary resuscitation, intubation, and defibrillation (Tolle, 1998, p. 4). This form was designed for long-term care facilities where residents were invited to consider the sort of care they wanted to receive. Such forms are not necessary when the patient is aware of his or her life-shortening condition and is preparing to enjoy whatever life remains while preparing for death.

The ethical issues discussed in this chapter have primacy in acute care institutions and in those long-term care facilities where a form such as the one just described is not in routine use. When individuals become hospice patients, they know their remaining life is limited. Part of the intake procedure is an acknowledgment of this fact and that the hospice will not engage in so-called heroics. In hospice, aggressiveness is limited to comfort care and not the preservation of life at all costs in individuals with a terminal illness. Given this emphasis on low-tech care, it would seem that the costs of care might be lower for the individual who dies in the care of a hospice program.

Although Medicare payments for all patients for the last year of life averaged just over $26,000 per decedent, spending for the last year of life of Medicare recipients in hospices accounted for 25% of total expenditures (Hogan, Lynn, Gabel, Lunney, O'Mara, & Wilkinson, 2000). It is interesting that total payments for those who had some hospice in the last year of life were greater than for those without hospice care. This finding is accounted for by the fact that some of the nonhospice patients had unanticipated deaths that occurred prior to the use of much medical care. A "descriptive analysis showed total costs for hospice users are no different from other decedents, but that Medicare's share of costs is higher" (p. 48). Nonetheless, although institutional death added very little additional cost for hospice patients, it added significantly to the costs of care for nonhospice patients. Home death is less expensive for both hospice and nonhospice patients.

Palliative care, although concerned with costs, is predicated on loftier notions of quality of care and appropriateness of care. The emphasis in palliative care is also on comfort, but it is comfort in tandem with care oriented toward cure or the limitation of the deleterious effects of the disease process or its treatment. Thus palliative care may be delivered earlier in the disease trajectory than is typical for hospice care.

The importance of palliative care in tertiary-care facilities is underscored by a study by Somogyi-Zalud, Zhong, Hamel, and Lynn (2002) that examined the use of life-sustaining treatments in hospitalized patients 80 years and older. Of the 1266 patients in the study, 72 died during the study enrollment. Seventy percent of these individuals, whose median age was 86, reported a fair or poor quality of life. Although "70% wanted their care focused on comfort rather than prolonging life, and 80% had a do-not-resuscitate order—the majority (63%) of the patients received one or more life-sustaining treatments before they died" (p. 930). Procedures applied to these individuals included ventilator care (43%), cardiopulmonary resuscitation (18%), surgery (17%), cardiac catheterization (15%), blood transfusion (14%), and hemodialysis (6%). Although it might be argued that these procedures were utilized for the 30% of the patients who had not indicated they wanted comfort care, such a scenario is not likely to pertain to all in that group. What then accounts for such an outcome?

Did the family demand that everything be done for their loved one, with healthcare providers reluctantly complying? Or was there a little-discussed medical practice occurring; namely, the use of older and/or dying persons to practice various procedures with full knowledge that they were not likely to be of benefit to the dying person? The ethical argument here is that the practice is for the greater good of society, that doctors will know how to perform procedures when they may in fact have a positive impact. The greater good of the use of dying persons as "educational material" overrides the needs of the person so used. Obviously, this is diametrically opposed to the concept of patient-centered care.

PATIENT-CENTERED CARE

Patient-centered care and the patient-centered environment have evolved as critical elements in end-of-life care. Hospice proponents advocated for this change after decades of the sterile environment of hospital rooms being the setting for death. As important as the physical environment is, and it is important, it is the centrality of the patient that is the key to care that is transformative for all concerned.

Patient-centered care and the patient-centered environment in end-of-life care are the hallmark of hospice care. In fact, hospice patients often are encouraged to bring in not only treasured mementos to their hospice room if they are in a facility, but also pieces of furniture to make their hospice room more homelike. The environment is emphasized in order to create a serene atmosphere that is supportive of the patient.

As important as the environment is, hospice care also is being provided in environments that many may consider the least desirable. Hospice care is being provided in Angola, a Louisiana prison noted for the toughness of its inhabitants. Nonetheless, prisoner volunteers are providing hospice care to their fellow inmates. The innovativeness of this program was recognized by an honorary mention for a Circle of Life Award presented by the American Hospital Association.

The environment is not only physical, but there is also a psychosocial environment that can enrich the lives of patients, families, and caregivers. We will consider the psychosocial environment in this final part of the chapter. The following example shows how a patient-centered approach can enhance end-of-life care.

Mrs. A was a patient in an acute care facility. Her physician had asked the hospice program director to engage in a consultation to investigate what else might be provided to this patient, well-loved by her family and the mother of two teenage girls. One morning at 7:00 A.M., when the hospice program director was visiting Mrs. A., she was greeted with "Where's my drink?" Somewhat taken aback, the hospice program director responded "Where's your drink?" "Yes, something with a little something in it!" With that clarification, the hospice program director queried Mrs. A on her favorite beverages. Gin and wine were two of the potables mentioned. The hospice program director commented "It sounds like you would like to have a party." "Yes that's what I would like" responded Mrs. A. With Mrs. A's sister sitting beside her at the bedside, the hospice program director ventured "What about Friday night? That's a good night for a party." All agreed that the party would be held the next evening. While at first the hospice program director volunteered to bring the beverages, it seemed more prudent to have family members be the beverage bearers.

The next evening the family assembled at the patient's bedside. She was attired in a new bed jacket, with hair groomed and makeup to suit the festive occasion. She had a gift to present to the friends whose anniversary it was. A three-tiered hospital cart was festooned with food. The young people in the family had brought guitars and other musical instruments. There was music and laughter. Unfortunately, the program director had neglected to inform the evening nursing supervisor who inquired about the noise. When confronted, the hospice program director explained the situation to the nursing supervisor, who was supportive of the party. That was Friday evening. The party was a going-away party. Mrs. A died the following Tuesday.

The application of principle-based ethics and/or care-based ethics requires judgment and an assessment of the situation. To state that one approach to ethical questions is more applicable in one situation is not to denigrate the value of another approach to ethics. Had the program director used a principle-based response to the above situation, she might have said "You'll have to be sure to have a drink when you leave the hospital." Instead, the hospice program director used a care-based approach with the following result.

Months after Mrs. A died, the family told the hospice program director that when they thought of the hospital, they thought of the party. What a nice way to think of a hospital when a loved one dies there. This is the essence of a patient-centered environment.

REFERENCES

Beauchamp, T. L., & Childress, J. F. (1994). *Principles of biomedical ethics* (4th ed.). New York: Oxford University Press.

Brock, D. W. (1984). Death and dying. In *Principles of Biomedical Ethics* (4th ed.). New York: Oxford University Press, 329–356.

Bulletin of the Pan American Health Organization. (1990). Special issue on bioethics. *Bulletin of the Pan American Health Organization 24*(1).

Churchill, L. R. (1979). Interpretations of dying: Ethical implications for patient care. *Ethics in Science & Medicine 6*:211–222.

Churchill, L. R., & Siman, J. J. (1986). Principles and the search for moral certainty. *Social Science Medicine 23*(5):461–468.

Emmanuel, E. J., & Battin, M. P. (1998). What are the potential cost savings from legalizing physician-assisted suicide? *The New England Journal of Medicine 339*(3):167–172.

Hogan, C., Lynn, J., Gabel, J., Lunney, J., O'Mara, A., & Wilkinson, A. (2000). Medicare beneficiaries costs and the costs of care in the last year of life. Final Report. Washington, D.C.: Medicare Payments Advisory Commission. Available at http://www.rand.org/health/researchareas/endoflifecare.html.

Kagarise, M. J., & Sheldon, G. F. (2000). Translational ethics: A perspective for the new millennium. *Archives of Surgery 135*(1):39–45.

McCann, R. M., Hall, W. J., & Groth-Juncker, A. (1994). Comfort care for terminally ill patients: The appropriate use of nutrition and hydration. *JAMA 272*(16):1263–1266.

National Commission for the Protection of Human Subjects of Biomedical and Behavioral Research. (1979). The Belmont Report—Ethical principles and guidelines for the protection of human subjects of research. *OPRR Reports.* U.S. Government Printing Office: 1988.

Otte, D. M., & Allen, K. S. (1987). Ethical principles in the nursing care of the terminally ill adult. *Oncology Nursing Forum 14*(5):87–91.

Pellegrino, E. D. (2000). Decisions to withdraw life-sustaining treatment: A moral algorithm. *JAMA 283*(8):1065–1067.

Rhymes, J. A., McCullough, L. B., Luchi, R. J., & Wilson, N. (2000). Withdrawing very low-burden interventions in chronically ill patients. *JAMA 283*(8):1061–1063.

Shuster, E. (1997). Fifty years later: The significance of the Nuremberg Code. *The New England Journal of Medicine 337*(20):1436–1440.

Somogyi-Zalud, E., Zhong, Z., Hamel, B. M., Lynn, J. (2002). The use of life-sustaining treatments in hospitalized persons aged 80 and older. *Journal of the American Geriatrics Society 50*(5):930–934.

Tolle, S. W., Tilden, V. P., Nelson, C. A., & Dunn, P. M. (1998). A prospective study of the efficacy of the physician order form for life-sustaining treatment. *Journal of the American Geriatrics Society 46*(9): 1170–1171.

Tolle, S. W. (1991). *International guidelines for ethical review of epidemiological studies.* Geneva: CIOMS.

Tolle, S. W. (1993). *International guidelines for biomedical research involving human subjects.* Geneva: CIOMS.

CHAPTER 18

Grief and Bereavement: Guidance for Primary Care Providers

Angela S. Pizzo

More than 2 million people die in the United States each year (O'Connor, 2002). Hundreds of women miscarry every year, and nearly 50 percent of marriages end in divorce (O'Connor, 2002). Loss and the resulting grief are almost inevitable. If grief and bereavement are prevalent in American society, the mystery lies in the great amount of discomfort felt by those caring for a person who is mourning. Expressions of sympathy are oftentimes stated in a meaningless tone and offers of help are seldom followed up on (Parkes, 2001).

The scope of primary care practice includes caring for bereaved persons. The *Diagnostic Statistical Manual* (DSM) of the American Psychiatric Association includes "bereavement" among a group of "other conditions that may be the focus of clinical attention," allowing clinicians to consider grief as a primary diagnosis (Parkes, 2001, p. 6). Grieving patients may present with physical or psychiatric complaints. However, the course of bereavement usually fails to follow a traceable trajectory; therefore, the patient and healthcare provider may be left with feelings of uncertainty (Casarett, Kutner, & Abrahm, 2001). In addition, clinicians may not possess the skills needed to identify the various types of grief or to determine when grief becomes a complication or a risk factor for the overall health of the patient. The nature of a loss can profoundly affect the pattern of grief; unexpected losses may be particularly traumatic and overwhelming, whereas a loss that is anticipated may allow the patient more time to prepare (Hamburg, 1998). Moreover, mourning varies based on the emotional style of the individual, ranging from stoicism to hysteria, which also presents as a challenge to providers (Hamburg, 1998). Culture and tradition also must be considered in order to better understand the patient's grief pattern.

BACKGROUND

Grief has been defined within numerous contexts and by a variety of authorities. The process of grief and bereavement is highly individualized; there is no right or wrong way to grieve. The course and duration of grief are variable and depend on the factors influencing the grief response. The health consequences of bereavement have been studied to determine the effects of grief and loss on the human body and spirit. Some authors argue that the features of the loss play an important role in the griever's outcome and identify different types of grief based on these features.

Definitions of Grief and Bereavement

The American Academy of Family Physicians (AAFP, 2002) states that "grief is a normal, healthy response to loss" and that "healing from a loss involves coming to terms with the loss" (p. 1). Critical to this definition is the understanding of loss. One of the greatest losses is the loss of life. Although the death of a loved one generally results in severe grief, other losses have the ability of generating strong grief responses, such as the loss of one's health. Rando (1984), an expert in the study of bereavement, argues that loss is a natural part of human existence. Losses can be physical or tangible, such as losing a possession or the death of a relative, or psychosocial or symbolic, such as a divorce or a job demotion (Rando, 1984, 2003).

Rando (1984) further challenges that grief is "the process of psychological, social, and somatic reactions to the perception of loss" (p. 15). This definition implies that grief is based on the unique, individualistic perception of the loss and that the loss does not require validation by others for the person to experience grief. The majority of discussions regarding grief concur that grief is a natural, expected reaction and that the absence of it actually implies an abnormality. Grief is intense mental suffering or distress that may manifest itself as a variety of symptoms (Peretz, 1990). Although the term *bereavement* often is interchanged with grief in the layperson's vernacular, bereavement refers to the state of feeling, thought, and activity that is a consequence of the loss (Peretz, 1990). An individual who has experienced a loss is said to be bereaved, that is, deprived of someone or something important. Bereavement is the condition that causes the grief response (Pine, 1986); it is "the state of having suffered a loss" (Rando, 1984, p. 16). Bereavement may last 6 months to a year or longer, depending on the circumstances of the loss and the individual (Peretz, 1990). Although surges of strong grief may occur with reminders or anniversary dates of the incident, bereavement lasting for years is considered to be complicated, and the person may be at risk for adverse health outcomes.

Reactions to Grief

Although individuals grieve in different ways, common symptoms of grief have been identified. The following are some of the typical physiological manifestations of grief: anorexia and gastrointestinal disturbances, weight loss, insomnia, crying, palpitations, physical exhaustion, emptiness or heaviness, a feeling of a lump in the throat, nervousness and tension, decreased libido or hypersexuality, lack of energy and psychomotor retardation, restlessness and searching for things to do, and shortness of breath (AAFP, 2002). Most clients will state that they find themselves oscillating between opposing feelings: avoidance of reminders of the loss may alternate with the deliberate cultivation of memories (Solsberry, 1984).

Rando (1984) outlines three main reactions to grief that are common and completely healthy. The avoidance phase involves the desire to avoid the acknowledgment of the loss. There is a normal desire to escape the overwhelming situation. The person is usually dazed, confused, and unable to fully comprehend the loss. Patients will generally describe a feeling of numbness. When the shock begins to wear off, denial may evolve as a coping mechanism, which may serve as "emotional anesthesia" to therapeutically numb the pain (Rando, 1984, p. 29). The griever then moves into the confrontation phase in which the shock is diminished and the grief is intense; extreme emotions such as anger, sadness, guilt, and panic are typical reactions (Rando, 1984).

Depression and despair with an overall lack of concern for self may also be present. The reestablishment phase involves the gradual decline of grief and the beginning of emotional and social reentry back into everyday life occurs (Rando, 1984). Grievers do not forget the loss, but they learn to adapt to the deficit in their life.

Parkes (2001) comments specifically on the anger and guilt that are common during bereavement. From his studies, Parkes (2001) found that many widows seem to regard the pain of grieving as an unfair punishment. They are angry with the person they have lost and view death as something that is done to a person. They seek someone to blame for the loss and the resulting pain; therefore, the deceased, healthcare providers, or God may be blamed. In addition, self-blame is prevalent when there may be regret for a lack of accomplishments or unmet expectations (Parkes, 2001). Losing an identity is also a disappointment and cause of anger and blame. Instead of a wife, the person now realizes she is a widow. Thinking of another as a widow or bereaved person may also instigate particular stereotypes, resulting in different traits being ascribed to the person (Solsberry, 1984). The grieving process will eventually paint her a new identity of a partnerless half, but also as a woman who is independent and hopefully content with herself.

Factors Influencing Grief Reactions

Although the aforementioned grief reactions are typical of the majority of bereaved persons, responses do reflect individual differences. Grief may be a very intense experience or a mild one, depending on a variety of factors. Healthcare providers should not only understand an individual's grief reactions, but also be mindful of the factors influencing these responses. The factor most often cited as weighing heavily on the grief process is the nature or meaning of the loss to the bereaved (Rando, 1984). The nature of the attachment plays a critical role in bereavement; the intensity of the grief is usually correlated with the intensity of the relationship with the lost person or object. In the case of death, the grief reaction typically increases in severity proportionate to the intensity of the love in the relationship between the bereaved and the deceased (Worden, 1982). The grief reaction will generally be more difficult if the deceased was a central component of the griever's daily physical or emotional functioning.

If death is the defining loss, the mode of death becomes a factor that influences bereavement. Unexpected deaths seem to generate more emotional disturbance given the unexpected nature of the loss (Parkes, 2001). Individuals tend to be more numb, more tearful, and possess more guilt; they are at risk for depression years after the grieving period; initial reactions of numbness and disbelief persist longer; and social withdrawal is more prevalent than in grief concerning anticipated deaths (Parkes, 2001). Preoccupied memories of the loss, especially if the death was painful or witnessed, may meet the criteria for posttraumatic stress disorder (PTSD) and prevent happy recollections of the deceased. These intrusive memories may in turn interfere with the normal grieving process. Suicides most often fall under the category of unexpected deaths and usually cause bereaved persons to blame themselves for not preventing the death. Furthermore, Parkes (2001) addresses "disenfranchised grief," which results from losses that cannot be openly acknowledged, socially validated, or publicly mourned, such as death from AIDS, death of an extramarital attachment, abortion, loss of a pet, or a psychological loss such as from Alzheimer's disease (p. 134).

Another psychological factor that influences the grief reaction is an individual's coping behaviors and aspects of his or her personality. Prayer is a healthy coping mechanism, whereas drugs and alcohol are detrimental to the grief process (Rando, 1984). Self-esteem, values, beliefs, attitudes, desires, needs, emotions, and strengths are all elements of personality that play a part in determining the difficulty of grief. Increasing age and gender have been linked to grief reactions and to emotional coping mechanisms (Chen et al., 1999; Costello & Kendrick, 2000). Additional factors include an individual's level of maturity and intelligence; past experiences with loss; social, cultural, ethnic, and religious background; the presence of secondary losses, such as loss of income, loss of housing, or change in other relationships; and presence of concurrent stresses or crises (Rando, 1984). When strain increases above adaptable thresholds to severe levels, efficiency decreases rapidly, and a person is simply unable to cope with the situation.

Health Consequences of Grief and Bereavement

It has been hypothesized that grief and bereavement have adverse health consequences. In their early work, Klerman and Clayton (1984) recognized that bereavement predisposes people to physical and mental illness, may precipitate illness and death, aggravates existing illnesses, and causes an increased use of health services. Sick populations have been found to have higher rates of bereavement in the year before the illness is diagnosed (Klerman & Clayton, 1984). This finding suggests a correlation between bereavement and the subsequent development of an illness. In addition to the aforementioned physical complaints, an exacerbation in risky behaviors such as smoking, drinking, and drug use has also been noted (Klerman & Clayton, 1984).

Although grief is not considered an illness, the DSM acknowledges bereavement as a diagnosis that is normal for 3 months (Klerman & Clayton, 1984). Yet, this time frame seems shorter than the usual period of time that is required to regain psychological equilibrium. Nevertheless, epidemiologic evidence exists to suggest that some individuals are at an increased risk for mortality after bereavement. The origin of the phrase "broken heart" dates back to biblical times, with the image of severe grief actually causing damage to the heart (Parkes, 2001).

The classic work of Elisabeth Kübler-Ross addresses the stages of grief. In 1969, Kübler-Ross published her book, *On Death and Dying*, which focused on the lessons doctors, nurses, clergy, and families can learn from dying patients. Her five stages of coping with imminent death are well known in the healthcare field and among the general public. Stage one, denial and isolation, explains the shock that functions as a buffer to the reality of the grief; denial is a healthy way of dealing with an uncomfortable and painful situation and allows patients to collect themselves (Kübler-Ross, 1969). Denial is usually a temporary defense that over time is replaced by partial acceptance. The second stage, anger, develops as denial dissipates; feelings of rage, envy, and resentment are common (Kübler-Ross, 1969). Bargaining, the third stage, involves pleas made to an authoritative figure to return or reverse the loss so that grieving can be avoided (Kübler-Ross, 1969). Many bargains are likely to be silently made with God or vocalized to a healthcare provider in a desperate attempt to postpone the inevitable. The fourth stage, depression, sets in when the great sense of loss is realized and the patient begins to endure the pain and suffering (Kübler-Ross, 1969). Acceptance, the final stage, entails the transition into confronting the situation at face value and learning to live with the loss or the threat of loss (Kübler-Ross, 1969). Kübler-Ross cautions, however, that this stage should not be mistaken for a happy time. Furthermore, many experts argue that it is normal for true acceptance to never be achieved after a significant loss.

Types of Grief

Several categories of grief have been established. Categories of grief include anticipatory, acute, chronic, delayed or absent, and at-risk or complicated. Even though these categories may be helpful in putting a patient's grief in context, these types often overlap because loss often involves complex life situations.

Anticipatory

Anticipatory grief is "the phenomenon involving mourning, coping, interaction, planning, and psychosocial reorganization that is initiated in response to the awareness of the impending loss and the recognition of associated losses in the past, present, and future" (Rando, 1986, p. 24). Anticipatory grief is more than a warning sign of a situation to come. Although most grieving is triggered at the onset of a loss, with anticipatory grief the grieving process actually begins with the anticipation of the loss so that the grieving occurs both before and after the actual loss. No fixed volume of grief exists, thus it is incorrect to assume that the grief that is experienced during the anticipatory phase will decrease the grief experienced once the loss occurs (Rando, 1986). In most instances, anticipatory grief allows for the absorbing of the reality of the loss over time; the finishing of unfinished business, including expressing feelings and resolving conflict; and the making of plans for the future (Rando, 1984). Preparations may be therapeutic, and individuals begin to learn how to live with the prospect of the loss. Although the threat of loss may provoke separation anxiety, the person has the opportunity to begin to accept the loss before it occurs.

Acute

Acute grief refers to the initial stages of grief in an acute situation. This type of grief is characterized by initial grief reactions that are normal, such as denial, sobbing or intense crying spells, anxiety, numbness, derealization, and somatic symptoms (Casarett et al., 2001). Clinicians may be uncomfortable around patients who are acutely grieving, because the emotions are intense and may be distressing and dramatic. An important service that should be offered to acutely bereaved patients is presence (Casarett et al., 2001). Sitting with the client and being a witness to the expression of grief is valuable support that should not be underestimated by the healthcare provider.

Chronic

"A chronic grief reaction is one which is prolonged, is excessive in duration, and never comes to a satisfactory conclusion" (Worden, 1982). With chronic grief, grief reactions are continuously exhibited that are more appropriate in the early stages of loss. Yearning for the lost person or object and preoccupied thoughts and memories may persist for years after the bereavement (Parkes, 2001). Uncontrollable crying is frequent, as is extreme social withdrawal, placing these individuals at risk for clinical depression and suicide (Parkes, 2001). These individuals have not gone on to lead effective, satisfying lives. The process of mourning has no resolution, and these patients find little meaning in their lives (Rando, 1984). They continue to avoid situations that remind them of the loss, the grief, and the associated pain. Chronic grief is fairly easy to diagnose, because grievers are usually aware that they are not getting through the period of mourning. The chronically bereaved will generally state, "I'm not getting back to living" or "I need help to be myself again" (Worden, 1982, p. 59). This type of reaction requires the identification of unresolved tasks, the determination of the reasons for the unresolved tasks, and the implementation of interventions focused on resolving these issues.

Delayed or Absent

When reactions to bereavement are delayed, the individual may not possess any emotional reaction at the time of the loss. Delayed grief reactions are sometimes referred to as inhibited, suppressed, or postponed grief (Worden, 1982). If there are no pressing responsibilities forcing the person to deal with the loss, grief reactions may be delayed for years (Rando, 1984). A subsequent loss can later trigger a full grief reaction to the prior loss that was never dealt with. During the delayed period, the patient may have somatic complaints of insomnia, panic attacks, irrational anger, and social withdrawal. Occasions have been documented where grieving patients have developed a hypochondriacal condition in which they develop symptoms resembling the symptoms suffered by the dead person during the last illness (Parkes, 2001).

Absent grief is the lack of a grief reaction altogether. Grief is either consciously denied or the bereaved person is in shock (Rando, 1984). Such grievers may appear to be coping effectively, yet they are often tense and short-tempered (Solsberry, 1984). Although absent grief is relatively uncommon, it is considered to be pathologic if it continues for weeks or months. Denial to this extreme is detrimentally postponing awareness of what must eventually be faced; it is not beneficial, like the initial denial that positively enables the patient to reduce fear by pacing the decision-making process (Solsberry, 1984). Individuals with delayed or absent grief may be at risk for the development of depression due to the component of denial (Parkes, 2001).

Complicated and At-Risk

According to Rando (1994), complicated grieving is the phenomenon of compromise, distortion, or failure to accomplish one or more of the six 'R' processes of mourning. She describes these six processes as healthy accommodations of any loss: recognize the loss, react to the separation by experiencing the pain, recollect and reexperience the deceased or object by realistically remembering, relinquish old attachments and the old assumptive world, readjust to move adaptively into the new world without forgetting the old, and reinvest (Rando, 1994). With complicated grief, these goals are not achieved, and the person may deny, repress, or avoid the loss and the full realization of its implications. The bereaved may hold onto the loss and avoid relinquishing old ideas and concepts.

Rando (1994) also outlines seven syndromes of complicated grief: absent mourning, delayed mourning, inhibited mourning, distorted mourning (i.e., severe anger or guilt), conflicted mourning, unanticipated mourning, and chronic mourning where there is a problem with closure.

Rosell (1990) offers more specific symptoms. Although delay or absence of grieving is one of the most alarming warning signs, overactivity without a sense of the loss, acquisition of symptoms belonging to the last illness of the deceased, and a loss of social interaction patterns also are red flags for complicated grief (Rosell, 1990).

Complicated grief places individuals at risk for mental or physical illness (Rando, 1994). However, the at-risk grief process may be difficult to identify, because the experience of grief varies greatly among individuals (Casarett et al., 2001). Awareness of the risk factors that place individuals at risk is most likely more helpful in defining the profile of complicated grief. Age and gender have been researched to determine whether there are poorer outcomes in specific groups. Several studies have demonstrated that younger widows, those under age 65, frequently consult healthcare providers for assistance with emotional problems during the first 6 months after bereavement (Parkes, 2001). Sedative consumption remains the same before and after bereavement in older people, but increases sevenfold in people younger than 65 during the first 6 months of bereavement (Parkes, 2001). Furthermore, 10 to 17 percent of elderly widows are estimated to experience levels of depression equivalent to those found in psychiatric clinics at some point during the first year of bereavement (Parkes, 2001). These findings may be attributed to the possibility that psychiatric problems in elderly grievers are due to the multiplicity of losses which occur more frequently in old age, such as the death of a spouse, loss of income in retirement, and the loss of friends.

Regarding gender differences, females are more likely to experience psychological problems than males after bereavement; males are more likely to die of a myocardial infarction after a loss (Parkes, 2001). Researchers believe this conclusion may be linked to the repressed grief some males harbor, which could place added stress on the heart. Men may feel it is necessary to contain their own grief in order to care for their family.

Effects on Family

Many significant losses occur within the context of a family unit, disrupting the natural homeostasis to which the family members are accustomed (Worden, 1982). Families differ in their ability to express and tolerate feelings and emotions; if the expression of specific feelings is not accepted in the family, the grief process can be altered for individual members, as well as the entire family system. A family that is emotionally integrated will be better able to help each other cope with a loss without much involvement of outside services (Worden, 1982). A less integrated family, however, may exhibit abnormal grief reactions. Unresolved grief may serve as a risk factor for family pathology and may contribute to pathological relationships across generations (Worden, 1982). In addition, children grieve differently than adult family members. A child's bereavement is often intermittent, shutting out others and evading any communication about grief (Parkes, 2001). Young boys typically express grief aggressively, whereas girls have a tendency to become compulsive caregivers (Parkes, 2001).

A common oversight of clinicians counseling grieving individuals is the basic medical needs of the bereaved family (Hyman, 1990). The grieving family may ignore serious medical problems, both acute and chronic ones. Follow-up appointments for conditions such as hypertension and diabetes should be scheduled in a timely manner without interrupting the grief process but with mindfulness of inappropriate postponement of essential care (Hyman, 1990). Bereaved families also lack adequate rest. Support systems should be identified to assist with household tasks such as grocery shopping, cooking, and cleaning in order to prevent physical exhaustion. If mild sedatives or sleep agents are prescribed, their use should be monitored and reassessed on a regular basis.

Cultural Perspectives

Although there is great variation as to how grief is expressed, anthropological studies have failed to reveal any society in which people do not show some sign of grief (Parkes, 2001). Culture provides "norms for labeling the consequences of loss, priorities for ranking loss among other stressful life events, expectations about social support and coping styles, and sanctioned idioms for articulating personal and family distress" (Kleinman, Kaplan, & Weiss, 1984, p. 204). Cultural heritage is a key component of the context in which humans live and is reflected in human responses, including grief (Cowles, 1996).

Although the development of physical complaints following bereavement is common in the general population, it is thought that somatization is more common among ethnic minorities, especially those members who belong to the working class and who possess lower levels of education (Kleinman et al., 1984). Sex-role conditioning in Western cultures has also been documented as heavily influencing bereavement. American males are conditioned to be in control and avoid expressing their feelings; crying is poorly tolerated (Rando, 1984). American females are conditioned not to display anger and to relinquish power and control; decision making stereotypically is labeled as a male's job in Western cultures (Rando, 1984). Puerto Rican women are expected to express their grief dramatically through seizure-like attacks and uncontrollable emotions (Kleinman et al., 1984). Similarly, Southeast Asian American groups participate in public displays of sobbing and wailing; however, in private settings, these grievers are expected to be contained and stoical, demonstrating endurance in the face of adversity (Kleinman et al., 1984). In Greek and Portuguese cultures, individuals have been known to enact grief over a death for the rest of their lives, demonstrating loyalty to the memory of the dead (Kleinman et al., 1984). In contrast, grief in American culture is expected to be transient and resolved quickly, with successful outcomes measured in terms of developing new relationships and participating in rewarding activities.

Migration and acculturation may prove to be problematic for members of American minority groups who possess few traditional resources for carrying out culturally expected bereavement practices (Kleinman et al., 1984). Immigrants may be uncomfortable with American rituals, beliefs, and values. Because it is difficult to predict in advance whether members of a given ethnic group will maintain traditional values or replace them with those of the dominant culture, healthcare providers must determine which practices are relevant to individuals in a particular episode of bereavement (Kleinman et al., 1984). Few studies have been conducted regarding the needs of individuals from various cultures. A 1996 study by Cowles concluded that although the experience of grief is unique to each individual, "differences exist between cultural groups in the traditions, rituals, and the expressions of grief" (p. 293). "We all feel the same," stated a participant of the study who was of African heritage, yet cultural differences warrant special attention (Cowles, 1996, p. 293).

BEREAVEMENT CARE

Healthcare providers are generally unaware of their role in the bereavement process. Yet, evidence exists that the public would like grief issues to be addressed by their clinicians. The establishment of hospice programs and numerous support groups to assist the bereaved is proof that patients want grief issues to receive more attention (Campbell & Thill, 2000; Green, 1984; Parkes, 2001). A wide range of reasons seems to prevent providers from adequately responding to grieving patients, from time constraints and personal discomfort to lack of formal training and reimbursement issues. Nevertheless, education is required to decrease these barriers and to reaffirm that the general practitioner truly has a valuable role in the grief process.

All primary care providers should first develop a philosophy of involvement with bereaved patients, addressing any personal limitations. Care should be personalized, responding to individual needs; however, the clinician must maintain a sense of self without distancing him or herself too much from the patient (Humphrey, 1986; Parkes, 2001; Silverman, 2000), thus healthcare providers must be comfortable with their own feelings of grief and loss. Clinicians need to learn to rely on their own support systems during difficult grief situations with patients, utilizing the support of their colleagues, clergy, mental health professionals, and family and friends, while remembering to maintain patient confidentiality.

General Principles of Bereavement Care

The general principles of bereavement care can be employed by any healthcare provider. The goals of these basic principles are to validate the patient's feelings of grief, answer questions, show compassion, assess for complicated grief, identify support systems, and offer other types of grief help, which are discussed in the following sections (Parkes, 2001). An effective provider is one who is an active listener; the bereaved patient needs time to talk and vent their emotions. Providers should listen in a nonjudgmental manner and with acceptance; listening is healing (O'Connor, 2002). The griever should be allowed to cry or express strong emotions such as anger. Encouraging the griever to identify, accept, and express all feelings of grief is an important initial intervention. Recollection of the loss or deceased should be encouraged as the patient learns to recognize, actualize, and accept the loss (Rando, 1984). If the patient is resisting the grief process, the presence of defense mechanisms should be explored as well as the reasons behind such coping. Reflection of what the provider is observing or hearing is a useful way of having the patient think about his or her reactions (Rando, 1984).

The loss does not need to be explained in religious or philosophical terms. Identification of religious and spiritual beliefs does, however, help the clinician to localize relevant sources of support. Furthermore, the provider should not unrealistically make the situation positive. Validating and normalizing the patient's grief are critical in making patients realize that what they are feeling is normal and typical. The therapeutic value of the gift of presence cannot be underestimated; being present for the bereaved and accepting the feelings of grief are an important role of the primary care provider (Rando, 1984). Warm silence allows time and space for quiet communication. Excess conventional expressions of sympathy should be avoided; there is no one proper thing to say, but trite phrases may widen the gap between the bereaved and nonbereaved.

Providing help with simple decisions is also within the realm of primary care. Clinicians should remember that although they will be unable to take away the pain grief causes, they will be able to facilitate the grief process for their patients while assessing for any complications. Follow-up phone calls have proven to be effective in reaching out to bereaved patients in a concrete way, because many patients will not call their provider if they need help. The importance of telephone support from nursing staff in support of bereaved families has been established in the oncology literature (Kaunonen, Aalto, Tarkka, & Paunonen, 2000; Kaunonen, Tarkka, Laippala, & Paunonen-Ilmonen, 2000).

Types of Help

The first source of help for most bereaved patients is family members and friends; nevertheless, family and friends may fail to provide adequate support beyond the acute grief period (Parkes, 2001). Because perception of one's family as unsupportive may be a predictor of poor outcome after bereavement, patients should be offered services such as counseling and support groups.

Bereavement Counseling

Bereavement counseling is generally provided by psychiatrists, psychologists, and social workers if utilized on a regular basis (Parkes, 2001). Counseling can range from individual to family therapy and from home to office consultation. Hospice workers are a good example of informal counseling services that can occur in the privacy of the home. Hospice nurses and volunteers help family members to plan ahead for the loss and anticipate grief, including preparing for what life will be like without the loved one. With such preparation, individuals are better able to cope with bereavement when the loss occurs (Parkes, 2001).

Bereavement counseling that is offered through psychiatric, psychologic, or social services is generally very structured. The goals of such therapy include the following: increase the reality of the loss, help the bereaved deal with both expressed and latent affect, assist the bereaved to overcome any impediments to readjustment after the loss, and encourage healthy and emotional withdrawal from the deceased or lost object in order to feel comfortable reinvesting emotion in other relationships or activities (Worden, 1982). Most experts believe that grief counseling should be offered to all individuals, and strongly encouraged for individuals with complicated grief responses (Parkes, 2001; Worden, 1982). A counselor who possesses the attitudes of empathy, genuineness, and nonjudgmental acceptance will enable the client to talk, to stop fearing and condemning his or her feelings, and to eventually accept the loss and experience the grief (Cutcliffe, 1998). These attitudes must be conveyed by responses in order to have any healing benefits. Patterns of defense being used to avoid the pain of the loss are identified. Such defense mechanisms may include protection against intimacy, protection against feelings, and suicidal thoughts as a fantasy of relief from the pain (Cutcliffe, 1998).

Mutual-Help Groups

Mutual-support, or self-help, groups are associations of people who have experienced a major bereavement and who unite for the purpose of mutual aid (Osterweis, 1984). Because these individuals have been through grief, they understand similar situations of grief and, therefore, are qualified to help others. These groups provide their members with person-to-person exchange based on identification and reciprocity, access to specialized information, the opportunity to share coping techniques based on realistic expectations for optimal functioning, and an increased sense of personal worth (Osterweis, 1984; Silverman, 2000). In addition, self-help partnerships serve as an opportunity to help others by providing role models as well as an arena for advocacy and social change.

Support Groups

Support groups are structured groups in which the format of the discussion focuses on specific topics of importance to bereaved people (Parkes, 2001). Support groups can help prevent isolation and provide acceptance of grief through social support. Group members develop a sense of connection because they feel the same way, which can be a source of comfort (Rando, 1984). The environment of these groups can be formal, as in a seminar, or informal, such as a roundtable discussion. Professionals experienced in bereavement and grief counseling generally lead such groups. Like mutual-help groups, grieving individuals typically utilize support groups later in the bereavement process.

Family Support

Various programs are aimed at the entire family unit. Interventions from home-based family meetings to weekend camps for parents and children have been employed. Although little research has been conducted on family grief therapy, researchers hypothesize that interventions targeted at the family increase the warmth in the relationships between family members and help prevent depression (Parkes, 2001). After the death of a family member, role assignments are typically made subtly, and individuals may feel pressured into assuming their new role and assigned duties; the scapegoating role is sometimes imposed on one of the younger and more vulnerable family members (Worden, 1982). In addition, alliances between family members may form based on individual grieving processes. Roles and alliances should be addressed in family support programs in order to assist in restoring the equilibrium in the family unit.

Clergy

In the past, clergy would visit bereaved individuals in their homes, whether or not they had a previously established relationship with the griever. Many religious figures have since abandoned the tradition of visiting bereaved parishioners they do not know; however, individuals who know their priest are more likely to seek out this type of support (Parkes, 2001). If spiritual beliefs are assessed by the primary care provider, finding support from the person's religion can be encouraged. Clergy visits are most beneficial when visitors have decreased in numbers after the loss, when the bereaved is often faced with the harsh reality of the grief. Clergy help by listening and can provide spiritual advice if warranted (Parkes, 2001).

Pharmacological Support

Psychopharmacological treatment is not the preferred treatment for grief (Weisman, 1998). Antidepressants, such as selective serotonin reuptake inhibitors, are beneficial if the griever develops depression. However, medication for the normal grief process should be limited so that the agents do not interfere with grief responses. When prescribed, medications may be used to promote sleep and relieve anxiety. Benzodiazepines can be used for insomnia and anxiety; however, a short course of therapy is recommended with this class of drugs due to the possibility of the development of tolerance, physical dependence, and rebound anxiety (Lehne, 2001). A small dose of tranquility may be helpful as long as the drug stops short of sedation and does not interfere with the right to mourn (Weisman, 1998).

Online Resources

For patients who have access to the Internet, online resources may be effective intervention tools for providing information and support. GriefNet (2005, www.griefnet.org) is described as "an Internet community of persons dealing with grief, death, and major loss." The Web site features 47 e-mail support groups and is directed by Cendra Lynn, Ph.D., a clinical grief psychologist, death educator, and traumatologist. GROWW, Grief Recovery ONLINE (2005) for ALL Bereaved, is another online resource, offering message boards, chat rooms, and information on news and gatherings. This online mutual self-help organization allows grieving peers to be paired in order for bereaved persons to see "a mirror image of someone describing exactly" the same feelings (GROWW, 2005). This validation of feelings helps individuals with acute grief reactions move through the grief process and later help newly bereaved individuals. HospiceNet (2005) also supplies extensive bereavement information for patients and families facing a life-threatening illness. Links on this site include a guide to grief, spiritual readings, frequently asked questions, and hospice stories, as well as connections to available services. Anticipatory guidance handouts are available in English and Spanish at Familydoctor.org (American Academy of Family Physicians, 2005), which is sponsored by the American Academy of Family Physicians.

Conclusion

Grief and bereavement are unavoidable processes that most individuals will experience in their lifetime. The irony is the overall lack of awareness that exists in caring for bereaved persons in the scope of primary care. A critical component of primary care is tending to the health needs of the whole person, including body, mind, and spirit. Grief affects all aspects of a patient's wellness, disrupting the equilibrium that normally allows for everyday functioning. Bereaved individuals need to know that what is happening to them is completely normal; their feelings require validation. Clinicians must learn to be attentive to individual needs in addition to assessing grief responses for any signs of complications. An effective provider is one who is an active listener, one who listens to the patient in a nonjudgmental manner and with acceptance. The provider is present to facilitate identification, acceptance, and expression of all feelings of grief. The importance of talking about loss was even recognized by Shakespeare in his famous work *Macbeth*: "Give sorrow words; the grief that does not speak whispers the o'erfraught heart and bids it break" (Shakespeare, 1908, p. 125).

Healthcare providers who familiarize themselves with the grieving process will ultimately be better caregivers. Self-reflection about personal attitudes toward bereavement, including personal experiences, can help illuminate and dissipate any existing fears about caring for bereaved persons. The primary healthcare provider needs to make the care and comfort of grieving patients a priority in order to be a true healer. Although "at such dark times . . . the hurt seems incurable, the wound grievous, and there is no healing" (Aronson, 1986, p. 89), the primary provider equipped with the aforementioned skills can shine some hope on a bleak and painful situation.

References

American Academy of Family Physicians (2002, May). Grieving: Facing illness, death and other losses. Retrieved February 20, 2005, from http://familydoctor.org/handouts/079.html.

Aronson, S. M. (1986). A physician's acquaintance with grief. In T. A. Rando (Ed.), *Loss and anticipatory grief* (pp. 89–93). Lexington, MA: D. C. Health and Company.

Campbell, M. L., & Thill, M. (2000). Bereavement follow-up to families after death in the intensive care unit. *Critical Care Medicine, 28*(4), 1252–1253.

Casarett, D., Kutner, J. S., & Abrahm, J. (2001). Life after death: A practical approach to grief and bereavement. *Annals of Internal Medicine, 134,* 208–215.

Costello, J. & Kendrick, K. (2000). Grief and older people: The making or breaking of emotional bonds following partner loss in later life. *Journal of Advanced Nursing, 32*(6), 1374–1382.

Cowles, K. V. (1996). Cultural perspectives of grief: An expanded concept analysis. *Journal of Advanced Nursing, 23,* 287–294.

Cutcliffe, J. R. (1998). Hope, counselling, and complicated bereavement reactions. *Journal of Advanced Nursing, 28,* 754–761.

GriefNet, Inc. (2005). Welcome to GriefNet.org. Retrieved February 20, 2005, from http://www.griefnet.org.

Green, M. (1984). Roles of health professionals and institutions. In M. Osterweis, F. Solomon, & M. Green (Eds.), *Bereavement: Reactions, consequences, and care* (pp. 215–235). Washington, D.C.: National Academy Press.

GROWW, Inc. (2005). GROWW: Grief recovery ONLINE for ALL bereaved. Retrieved February 20, 2005, from http://www.groww.org.

Hamburg, P. (1998). Breaking bad news. In T. A. Stern, J. B. Herman, & P. L. Slavin (Eds.), *The MGH guide to psychiatry in primary care* (pp. 159–165). New York: McGraw-Hill.

HospiceNet. (2005). HospiceNet. Retrieved February 20, 2005, from http://www.hospicenet.org.

Humphrey, M. A. (1986). Effects of anticipatory grief for the patient, family member, and caregiver. In T. A. Rando (Ed.), *Loss and anticipatory grief* (pp. 63–79). Lexington, MA: D. C. Health and Company.

Hyman, G. A. (1990). Medical needs of the bereaved family. In A. H. Kutscher, S. Bess, S. G. Klagsbrun, M. E. Siegel, D. J. Cherico, L. G. Kutscher, D. Peretz, & F. E. Selder (Eds.), *For the bereaved: The road to recovery* (pp. 190–192). Philadelphia: The Charles Press.

Kaunonen, M., Aalto, P., Tarkka, M.-T., & Paunonen, M. (2000). Oncology ward nurses' perspectives of family grief and a supportive telephone call after the death of a significant other. *Cancer Nursing, 23,* 314–324.

Kaunonen, M., Tarkka, M.-T., Laippala, P., & Paunonen-Ilmonen, M. (2000). The impact of supportive telephone call intervention on grief after the death of a family member. *Cancer Nursing, 23,* 483–491.

Kleinman, A., Kaplan, B., & Weiss, R. (1984). Sociocultural influences. In M. Osterweis, F. Solomon, & M. Green (Eds.), *Bereavement: Reactions, consequences, and care* (pp. 199–212). Washington, D.C.: National Academy Press.

Klerman, G. L., & Clayton, P. (1984). Epidemiologic perspectives on the health consequences of bereavement. In M. Osterweis, F. Solomon, & M. Green (Eds.), *Bereavement: Reactions, consequences, and care* (pp. 15–44). Washington, D.C.: National Academy Press.

Kübler-Ross, E. (1969). *On death and dying.* New York: Touchstone.

Lehne, R. A. (2001). *Pharmacology for nursing care* (4th ed.). Philadelphia: WB Saunders.

O'Connor, K. (2002). Good grief—dealing with ordinary people experiencing the extraordinary. *AORN, 76,* 498–499.

Osterweis, M. (1984). Bereavement intervention programs. In M. Osterweis, F. Solomon, & M. Green (Eds.), *Bereavement: Reactions, consequences, and care* (pp. 239–278). Washington, D.C.: National Academy Press.

Parkes, C. M. (2001). *Bereavement: Studies of grief in adult life* (3rd ed.). Philadelphia: Taylor & Francis.

Peretz, D. (1990). Understanding your mourning: A psychiatrist's view. In A. H. Kutscher, S. Bess, S. G. Klagsbrun, M. E. Siegel, D. J. Cherico, L. G. Kutscher, D. Peretz, & F. E. Selder (Eds.), *For the bereaved: The road to recovery* (pp. 24–37). Philadelphia: The Charles Press.

Pine, V. R. (1986). An agenda for adaptive anticipation of bereavement. In T. A. Rando (Ed.), *Loss and anticipatory grief* (pp. 39–54). Lexington, MA: D. C. Health and Company.

Rando, T. A. (1984). *Grief, dying, and death: Clinical investigations for caregivers.* Champaign, IL: Research Press.

Rando, T. A. (1986). A comprehensive analysis of anticipatory grief: Perspectives, processes, promises, and problems. In T. A. Rando (Ed.), *Loss and anticipatory grief* (pp. 3–37). Lexington, MA: D. C. Health and Company.

Rando, T. A. (1994). Complications in mourning traumatic death. In I. B. Corless, B. B. Germino, & M. Pittman (Eds.), *Dying, death, and bereavement: Theoretical perspectives and other ways of knowing* (pp. 253–271). Boston: Jones and Bartlett.

Rosell, A. (1990). Lindemann's studies on reactions to grief. In A. H. Kutscher, S. Bess, S. G. Klagsbrun, M. E. Siegel, D. J. Cherico, L. G. Kutscher, D. Peretz, & F. E. Selder (Eds.), *For the bereaved: The road to recovery* (pp. 73–76). Philadelphia: The Charles Press.

Shakespeare, W. (1908). *Tragedy of Macbeth* (E.C. Black, Ed.). Boston: Ginn and Company. (Original work published circa 1606).

Silverman, G. K., Jacobs, S. C., Kasl, S. V., Shear, M. K., Maciejewski, P. K., Noaghiul, F. S., & Prigerson, H. G. (2000). Quality of life impairments associated with diagnostic criteria for traumatic grief. *Psychological Medicine, 30,* 857–862.

Solsberry, V. (1984). Adults' reactions to bereavement. In M. Osterweis & M. Green (Eds.), *Bereavement: Reactions, consequences, and care* (pp. 47–68). Washington, D.C.: National Academy Press.

Weisman, A. (1998). The patient with acute grief. In T. A. Stern, J. B. Herman, & P. L. Slavin (Eds.), *MGH guide to psychiatry in primary care* (pp. 177–180). New York: McGraw-Hill.

Worden, J. W. (1982). *Grief counseling and grief therapy: A handbook for the mental health practitioner.* New York: Springer Publishing.

CHAPTER 19

Family Coping and Adaptation In Planning Support Services for Parents of Children with Chronic Disabilities

Nancy M. Terres

An essential part of planning the home care of children with severe chronic illnesses and disabilities is consideration of parent support needs. Home care of these children can be difficult, absorbing considerable amounts of time, energy, and resources. The assumption that parents will need and use support services forms the foundation of early hospital discharge planning for children with complex care needs and is the rationale for the existence of support groups and other family-centered services. Yet, some families do not accept support services or limit those services that they will accept. People may not use a particular support service for a number of different reasons. Rather than speculate on parent motivations, an examination of the literature and theory on family coping and personal styles of managing crisis can guide the clinician in understanding how to approach families about support services and identifying the best time to do so.

This chapter will describe how a family may experience a child's disability, identify the characteristics of parent coping, and describe family types and styles of functioning that may encourage or discourage support service use. Using the Resiliency and Adaptation Model, this chapter will also describe the role of support services in family adaptation to chronic childhood disability and offer guidelines for how and when to encourage service use.

CHRONIC ILLNESS AND DISABILITY AS A FAMILY CRISIS

Overall, the chronic illness or disability of a child creates a crisis in the family that is strikingly similar to classic grief responses. Although some studies focus on the grief response to the birth of a child with disabilities as a process with a beginning and an end (Cohen, 1962; Epperson, 1977; Goodman, 1967; Kennedy, 1970; Solnit & Stark, 1961), others see the grief as lifelong, moving in and out of various stages in response to significant occasions, such as birthdays, the first day of school, or changes in the child's health or functional status (Lee, Strauss, Wittman, Jackson, & Carstens, 2001; Olshansky, 1962; Scornaienchi, 2003; Wikler, Wasow, & Hatfield, 1981).

Fortier and Wanlass (1984) believe that specific interventions are of most use to families if introduced at a time in the crisis continuum when the family is most likely to be receptive. Although the idea seems conceptually sound, clinicians are well aware that people do not always react in such clearly defined ways. Families in a denial stage of grief can and do accept services, even if they believe that the services are not necessary, and families are able to meet their child's needs long before any sense of closure is achieved. Seeking support is a feature of each of the stages of grief, but the kinds of support services offered and the way in which parents use them may vary widely depending on where parents are in the grieving process. Parents absorbed in early grief states may not welcome services from outside the family, but prefer to absorb the impact of the child's illness and needs before determining what services they most need.

Besides dealing with grief, after the child's hospital discharge there is a stage of adjustment lasting approximately 6 months. During this time, parent feelings range from relief about the child's being home to frustration with home care nurses and the receding of support received during the child's hospitalization. In the time immediately after hospital discharge, parents strive to achieve a sense of normalcy for the child and family (Feinberg, 1985; Johnson, 2000; Morse, Wilson, & Penrod, 2000). Ultimately, the child becomes integrated into the daily life of the family, as the family realizes what they can manage and what exceeds their resources. Families may not begin to seek specific support services until the later stages of adjustment, which Feinberg estimates to be about a year into the family's adjustment process. Families whose children are hospitalized for a prolonged period of time may need help with the child's home care, but may not be willing to give the care over to a stranger, such as a home care nurse, or aide right away. They might not be willing or feel the need at that time to leave the child for any period of time for something like respite care.

FACTORS INVOLVED IN PARENT COPING

The Role of Appraisal in Coping

Coping begins when an individual perceives stress. Stress is a transactional process between the environment and the availability of resources and is influenced by individual patterns of appraisal (Lazarus & Folkman, 1984; McCubbin & McCubbin, 1988; Trute & Hiebert-Murphy, 2002). *Appraisal* concerns the way in which parents regard the child's illness or disability in terms of its seriousness and its impact on family functioning. Some parents might view a serious head injury as a temporary problem that will heal quickly, and the child will return to full function before leaving the hospital. Other parents might see a heart murmur as potentially heralding a full cardiac arrest and lifelong debility. The parents' appraisal is likely to be influenced by their culture, their usual coping style, by the amount information about the child's condition conveyed to them, the way in which the information is presented or processed, and their stage of grieving (Danielson, Hamel-Bissel, & Winstead-Fry, 1993; Fadiman, 1997; Fortier & Wanlass, 1984; Kellegrew, 2000; King, 2001; Klein, 1993; Lazarus & Folkman, 1984). Parents may not understand or appraise their situation as requiring support services.

Levels of Meaning

Another way to conceptualize appraisal is in terms of the *levels of meaning* that the child's illness or disability has for families (Patterson & Garwick, 1994; Patterson, Holm, & Gurney, 2004). *Level one* involves situational meanings, or how the child's condition coincides with other family stresses or the pile-up of demands. A shared definition of the stressor is a part of this level. If families disagree on their definition of the situation, arranging supportive care can be more complex. An example is a mother who sees the child's situation as long term and involving the use of many resources, while the father views the situation as not as serious as described and believes that support resources are unnecessary.

Along those same lines, Tunali and Powers (1992) suggest that factors involved in coping may actually be the *result* of coping, but note that the processes (i.e., the psychological strategies) remain unexplained. The processes may have a role in how families regard their unmet needs. One coping process that could affect the conceptualization of unmet needs is *redefinition*. With redefinition, the family reconsiders what constitutes the fulfillment of a need and develops alternative means to achieving it (Saylor, 1990). If they can no longer find time for leisure activities, for example, leisure time may be redefined as unimportant or greatly reduced in importance. Similarly, families might decide that they are the only ones who can or should meet the needs of the child with chronic illness and disability, and that outside support services are not needed or are not in the child's best interests (Curran & Bongiorno, 1986; Shannon, 2004).

Level two is characterized by how the family views itself. This stage includes the functioning of each of the family members, their definition of external and internal boundaries, each person's role assignment, and the rules and norms for interactional behavior. Families at this level may regard outside support services as intrusive to the family's functioning or as not within the purview of nonfamily members. Other families might view support services as the only means by which parents can fulfill their obligations to other family members.

At *level three*, family members' orientation is turned to the world outside the family. This stage influences how families interpret reality, their core assumptions about their environment, and their purpose in life (Logan, Radcliffe, & Smith-Whitley, 2002; Patterson & Garwick,1994). A general sense of optimism, a sense of control, and strong family cohesion and hardiness correlate with positive outcomes for the child and the family (McKernon, Holmbeck, Colder, Hommeyer, Shapera, & Westhoven, 2001; Svavarsdottir, McCubbin, & Kane, 2000). Families at this stage might reconsider the role of support resources in promoting family cohesion and hardiness.

If parents persist in their preference not to use support services, rather than letting the matter drop, the issue should be raised again at another opportune time, because reluctance to use resources could affect the child's outcome and parent coping (Patterson, 2002). Coping involves a mobilization of effort, whereby interventions, resources, or behaviors are called forth to manage the stress. Managing stress includes developing strategies to reduce, minimize, master, or tolerate the impact of the child's illness on the family (Dunn, Burbine, Bowers, & Tantleff-Dunn, 2001; Folkman, Lazarus, Gruen, & DeLongis, 1986). Caregiver burden is associated with the use of fewer coping strategies (Patterson, Holm, & Gurney, 2004; Ray & Ritchie, 1993) and is increased when there are unmet support needs (Thyen, Sperner, Morfield, Meyer, & Ravens-Sieberer, 2003). Factors that protect individuals from the negative psychological consequences of stress include feelings of self-confidence and an easy-going disposition as well as tenaciousness, a disinclination to use avoidance coping, and the availability of family support (Dunn et al., 2001; Holahan & Moos, 1986; Katz & Kessel, 2002; Shannon, 2004). Families whose coping styles include a positive belief system and the use of noncritical family networks are more likely to adapt and experience less psychological distress (Frey, Greenberg, & Fewell, 1989; Green, 2001; Ray & Ritchie, 1993; Trulsson, & Klingberg, 2003).

Steps to Coping

Patterson (1995) describes specific steps that parents can take to manage their stress around the care of the child with chronic illness and disability. The steps involve marshalling internal resources into positive action, so that the need for control of the stress results in reducing the demands on the family; learning more about the child's care to gain some sense of mastery over the situation; and maintaining and allocating resources for the family. To manage their personal tensions, parents might engage in activities such as exercise or going to the movies. Changing the way they think about their situation, such as viewing the child's condition as an opportunity to develop new skills, is another step. Many of Patterson's examples require support resources that can contribute to the care of the child, freeing the parents to attend to the needs of the family as a whole or to engage in stress-relieving activities.

That families new to the care of a child with chronic illness and disability would be particularly stressed is not surprising. Besides dealing with grief, these parents must learn a new caregiver role and how to gather the appropriate support resources. Stress and vulnerability can deplete coping resources over time, probably accounting for why parents caring for ventilator-assisted children for longer than two years fared worse than parents with less home-care experience (Parra, 2003; Quint, Chesterman, Crain, Winkleby, & Boyce, 1990). Informal support resources also may dwindle over the years, after high initial levels of support (Morrow, Carpenter, & Hoagland, 1984; Terres, Thyen, & Perrin, 1995; Wegener & Aday, 1989). To maintain and develop coping resources, families need to draw on informal and formal support networks, including financial, emotional, and practical support throughout phases of the child's life (Bregman, 1980; Williams et al., 2002).

Parent Personality Factors and Coping

Even when parents can identify a potential social support system, they may not be able to effectively use the system in order to cope with their stress (Terres et al., 1995). The ability to use support resources and otherwise cope with the stress of the child's care seems to be related to parent personality factors. Parental neuroticism and family conflict, for example, are negatively related to coping, whereas positive relationships were seen with the quality of the marital relationship, locus of control, family cohesion, family expressiveness, the amount of parental social support, and the ability of the family to advocate for themselves and the child (Lewis & Vitulano, 2003; Shannon, 2004; Sloper, Knussen, Turner, & Cunningham, 1991).

Patterns of coping characterized as *practical coping* and *wishful thinking* are correlated with outcome. Practical coping involves using strategies that directly affect the parents' ability to manage the child's care, such as seeking home-care services, school programs, and financial resources. Wishful thinking is more passive in that it involves hoping that things will get better or that needs will somehow be met. Mothers who employ practical coping perceive a significantly greater satisfaction with life than mothers who use wishful thinking (Penley, Tomaka, & Wiebe, 2002; Sloper et al., 1991; Sloper & Turner, 1992). Mothers who show good adaptation also show high extroversion, low neuroticism scores, and fewer unmet needs for help with child-related problems, whereas fathers' positive adaptation was associated with low use of wishful thinking as a coping strategy (Sloper & Turner, 1992).

Emotion-focused and *problem-focused* coping are two types of coping strategies. Emotion-focused, or palliative, coping is directed at the somatic, or feeling, level. Problem-focused, or adaptive, coping is directed at altering the situation causing the stress (Folkman et al., 1986; Hauser-Cram, Warfield, Shonkoff, & Krauss, 2001; Zakowski, Hall, Klein, & Baum, 2001). Emotion-focused coping strategies are positively associated with maternal distress, whereas problem-focused coping was associated with decreased stress (McCrae & Costa, 1986; Park, Armeli, & Tennen, 2004). A lower level of perceived stress is associated with the use of more adaptive than palliative coping methods (Frey, Greenberg, & Fewell, 1989; Lindqvist, Carlsson,

& Sjoden, 2000; Macrodimitris & Endler, 2001; Miller, Gordon, Daniels, & Diller, 1992; Thompson, Gustafson, Hamlet, & Spock, 1992). The use of formal support services is more of a problem-focused strategy. Families seeking more emotion-focused coping might seek other sources of support, such as friends or support groups, rather than a concrete service not as directly related to providing emotional support.

Beliefs about control appeared in other studies about parental coping strategies. A relationship was seen between coping and whether a parent had an external or internal locus of control (Carver, Scheier, & Weintraub, 1989; Johnson, 2004; Parkes, 1984; Petrosky & Birkimer, 1991). Individuals with an external locus of control believe that situations that happen to them and what is required to remedy them exist completely outside themselves, and instead rest with fate, chance, external circumstances, or with other people. Individuals with an internal locus of control believe that solutions originate from within, that change can be affected through the use of one's own efforts and abilities (Rotter, 1966). People with internal locus of control find social support to be an effective coping resource, whereas people with external locus of control do not (Dean & Ensel, 1982; Lefcourt, Martin & Salen, 1984; Park et al., 2004; Sandler & Lakey, 1982).

External locus of control could be associated with a wishful thinking coping style, whereas an internal locus of control would more likely result in practical coping. Social support requires the mobilization of personal resources to tap into support networks and to use the support networks to alter or modify stress. The use of resources tends to be an active process. People with external locus of control are inclined to react more passively to the stress, because, fundamentally, they do not believe that what they can do themselves will substantially alter their situation. Parents with external locus of control might, theoretically, be expected to use formal support services less often and less effectively or require more assistance in accessing and maintaining supports than parents with internal locus of control.

The influence of gender socialization and belief systems may also influence coping. While both mothers and fathers demonstrated a predominance of problem-solving coping strategies, mothers were much more likely to seek support and use positive reappraisal, whereas fathers focused on self-controlling approaches (Heaman, 1995; Pelchat, Lefebvre, & Perreault, 2003; Trute, 1995).

FAMILY ADAPTATION

Whereas coping implies process, adaptation implies outcome. Outcomes may be adaptive or maladaptive, depending on how the child and the family system as a whole are affected. Positive adaptation is facilitated by personal strengths of family members, strengths of the family as a unit, and community support, and may be influenced by *family type* (McCubbin & McCubbin, 1988; Saloviita, Italinna, & Leinonen, 2003).

The classification of family type has created particular controversy, as researchers seek to define the characteristics of various kinds of families and to predict the effect of various interacting variables on the trajectory of the development of these family types (Cluff & Hicks, 1994; Cluff, Hicks, & Madsen, 1994; Olson, 1994). Understanding the interaction of variables within family types can point toward a potential direction for intervening to relieve family stress in ways most tailored to the particular family type.

McCubbin and McCubbin (1987), building on the family stress theory of Reuben Hill (1949) and Wesley Burr (1973), developed a regenerative model of family stress. The Double

ABCX Model of Adjustment and Adaptation (McCubbin & Patterson, 1983) and the Typology Model of Family Adjustment and Adaptation, also called the T-Double BCX Model of Family Adjustment and Adaptation (McCubbin & McCubbin, 1987), focus on various family resistance, appraisal, and coping strategies in the face of stress. The Resiliency Model of Family Stress, Adjustment, and Adaptation (the Resiliency and Adaptation model) emphasizes the processes involved in family adaptation to stress (McCubbin, Thompson, & McCubbin, 1996).

Family Types

The Resiliency and Adaptation model includes four family types: (1) unpatterned, (2) intentional, (3) structuralized, and (4) rhythmic (McCubbin & McCubbin, 1988). *Unpatterned families* put minimal emphasis on structure and routines and conduct their lives with little evidence of either. In another framework, such as the Circumplex model, they might be called *chaotic* families (Olson, Russell, & Sprenkle, 1983). *Intentional families* place value on family structure and routines, but there is little evidence of either in actual family functioning. Conversely, *structuralized families* conduct their daily lives with routines that promote family time together, but they are reluctant to embrace the structure as an ideal. *Rhythmic families* value routines and support activities that foster a sense of shared purpose, togetherness, and predictability. When compared with other family types, rhythmic families demonstrate more evidence of family bonding and flexibility, as well as evidence of more positive adaptation, as indicated by family, marital, child development, and community satisfaction, and a greater overall sense of family well-being.

Even with the apparent ability of rhythmic families to adapt more positively, there is no reason to believe that rhythmic families would be more likely to use support services than the other family types. Unpatterned families might use support services when a case manager is available to help them organize themselves around the requisite arrangements. Family types that value structure, especially structure that promotes family time together, may be more likely to use services that would facilitate that goal. Support services can free parents from the burden of the child's care to attend to other family members and activities, provided they are perceived in that manner. Support services such as respite care may also be perceived as taking the parents or the child away from the family, thereby conflicting with family values and goals.

Family Characteristics Contributing to Adaptation

Certain characteristics within families help them to recover or regenerate from stressors. *Regenerative* family types (McCubbin, Thompson, Pirner, & McCubbin, 1988) are characterized by their level of family *hardiness* and family *coherence*. Hardiness refers to the family's internal strengths and durability and includes a sense of meaningfulness in life, involvement in activities, and a commitment to learn and explore new experiences. Family coherence, as a coping strategy, involves "family emphasis on acceptance, loyalty, pride, faith, trust, respect, caring, and shared values in the management of tension and strain" (McCubbin & McCubbin, 1988, p. 250). Family expression and lack of family conflict, elements of coherence, are associated with outcomes in parents' physical and mental health, life satisfaction, and family environment (Sloper et al., 1991; Svavarsdottir et al., 2000).

Caregivers with a strong sense of coherence are more likely than others to cope in situation-specific appropriate ways (McCubbin & Patterson, 1981; Olson, McCubbin, Bowen, Larson,

Muxem, & Wilson, 1989). A sense of coherence is related to management of the meaning of the situation, the selection of reasonable coping strategies, and the avoidance of potentially maladaptive or unhealthy behaviors (Gallagher, Wagenfeld, Baro, & Haepers, 1994). Familes who have moderate levels of both cohesion and adaptability will function more adequately over the life cycle and be better able to adapt to normative and situational stressors (Olson et al., 1983).

How coherence and hardiness appear in families is described by the four types of families in the Regenerative Model of family systems. The first of these types is *vulnerable* families, who are low in family coherence and family hardiness. Vulnerable families are less in control of what happens to them, are more passive and complacent in their functioning, and are less able to mobilize toward activity and learning new things.

The second family type is the *secure* family. These families score high in hardiness, but low in coherence. Secure families cope with stresses by becoming upset, showing less caring and understanding and more blaming. However, these families also demonstrate a sense of purpose. They can plan ahead, they are more active and in control, they value their efforts, and they feel that life is meaningful.

Durable families are high in coherence, but low in hardiness. Although these families demonstrate a lower sense of purpose and meaningfulness in life and a lack of being appreciated, they have a high regard for their coping abilities. They are less reactive, more caring, and maintain more emotional stability.

Regenerative families are high in both hardiness and cohesiveness. These families maintain emotional calm and stability and cope by accepting stressful life events and working together to solve problems. They plan ahead and feel in control. They are caring, loyal, and tolerant of hardships. As with rhythmic families, regenerative families demonstrate more adaptive family functioning and greater levels of satisfaction than other family types.

Stages of Adaptation

The Resiliency Model of Family Stress and Adaptation has two phases: the *adjustment* phase and the *adaptation* phase. Each phase contains similar elements that influence adjustment to the stressor. In the adjustment phase, the stressor (the onset of the illness or realization of the disability) occurs, and the magnitude of the impact on the family is influenced by family vulnerability related to any concurrent family strains, family transitional stages, and the pile up of demands (Wiegner & Donders, 2000). For example, the child's diagnosis might occur a month before the birth of another child in the family. Or perhaps a grandparent has recently had a stroke and the child's parents are the closest relatives. Maybe the family has recently moved to the area from another state or one parent or the other has just found new employment. Because each one of these events presents its own demands and stresses, they would all add to the burden the family experiences around the child's illness or disability.

The demands on the family do not, necessarily, have to constitute individual negative stressors. New employment, for instance, may be a welcome relief from a previous undesirable employment situation. Nevertheless, each transition creates demands on the family system that compete for the family's resources and have the potential for intensifying the family's stress response and ability to cope with any one demand or stressor. Families dealing with a number of concurrent stresses or demands may find the arrangement of support services to be part of the pile up of demands rather than a means of coping (Patterson & Garwick, 1994).

Family vulnerability interacts with the previously described family types and established patterns of family functioning. Family types and their patterns of functioning interact with family resistance resources. Family resistance resources represent a family's abilities to address and manage the stress while maintaining adaptive family functioning. Good communication skills, a sense of family cohesiveness, and an ability to make use of support systems are examples of resources that help families resist the impact of the stressor.

Family resistance resources influence and are influenced by the family's appraisal of the stressor (serious, temporary, life-threatening, manageable, overwhelming, etc.). The family's appraisal of the situation influences their problem-solving and coping strategies. Families will not employ coping strategies to deal with severe disability if they do not appraise the situation to be serious. They will select coping resources based on the perceived need, secondary to their appraisal of the situation (Mellin, Neumark-Sztainer, & Patterson, 2004). The family's ability to cope with the stressor ultimately leads to the family's positive or negative adjustment to the stressor.

The adaptation phase of the Resiliency Model of Family Stress and Adaptation represents the dynamic processes involved in adapting to the care of the child with chronic illness and disability over time. Children grow and pass through various stages of development. Families also go through various developmental stages, from couples without children to couples with grown children who haved moved away from the family home. Each change creates its own demands on the family (Carter & McGoldrick, 1980). Some families might be dealing with the transition from being a couple without children to first-time parenthood when their child's illness or disability occurs or is discovered. Other couples might have planned their lives with the last child leaving the family home when that child is severely injured and returned to the home in a completely dependent capacity. An accumulation of family life changes can affect the system's ability to cope and affect a positive outcome. For example, an accumulation of family life changes was associated with a decline in pulmonary function in children with cystic fibrosis (Patterson & McCubbin, 1983; Patterson, McCubbin, & Warwick, 1990).

During the course of the life of a child with chronic illness and disability, various additional crises are common. Children may be rehospitalized, their symptoms may worsen, or families may receive bad news about the child's prognosis. With each change or crisis, the family reappraises the crisis situation and its relationship to their appraisal of the original stressor. They bring new skills and new patterns of functioning to the process and may develop and refine their problem-solving and coping skills to meet the needs that arise from the crisis. The role of social support in influencing parent patterns of functioning, problem solving, and coping is a prominent feature of the adaptation phase.

SOCIAL SUPPORT AND FAMILY ADAPTATION

The influence of social support on a family's ability to adapt to caring for a child with chronic illness and disability surfaces continually in the research literature. Models of coping and social support emphasize the essential nature of one for the other (Beresford, 1994; Dunst, Trivette, & Cross, 1986; Quittner, Glueckauf, & Jackson, 1990; Robinson, Jackson, & Townsley, 2001; Schilling, Gilchrist, & Schinke, 1984; Sherman & Cocozza, 1984; Taanila, Syrjala, Kokkonen, & Jarvelin, 2002). Support, individual strengths, and family strengths play interactive and mutually supportive roles in the life of resilient families (McCubbin & McCubbin, 1987, 1988; McCubbin, Thompson, Thompson, McCubbin, & Kaston, 1993).

The family's reaction to stress has been described as an active process of managing available resources to facilitate adaptation (Flynt & Wood, 1989; Patterson, 2002). *Available resources* refers to the family's social network and services that are designed to assist and support the family in the care of the child. The availability of support affects the family's appraisal of events and determines which strategies the family can use (Fong, 1991; Mullins, Aniol, Boyd, Page, & Cheney, 2002; Patterson, 2002; Redfield & Stone, 1979).

Types of Social Support

Cobb (1976) describes three types of social support and two types of stress support. Social support includes: (1) *emotional support,* to shore up the individual during difficult times; (2) *esteem support,* which contributes to the way in which individuals feel about themselves; and (3) *network support,* which involves belonging to an interconnection of communication that involves mutual support and mutual understanding. Stress support includes: (1) *appraisal support* (i.e., information, feedback), which allows the family to assess how they are doing with life tasks in the crisis; and (2) *altruistic support,* which is information received in good will from others giving something of themselves.

Social support can protect both parents and children from the physical and emotional consequences of life's stresses (Cobb, 1976; Helitzer, Cunningham-Sabo, VanLeit, & Crowe, 2002; Mullins et al., 2002). Families satisfied with their support networks report fewer of the physical and emotional problems significantly related to time demands placed on the parents. Social support of parents influenced child adjustment in the domains of community acceptance, developmental progress, the level of child behavior problems, and the ability of parents to become involved in home and community activities. Families with more social support had children who were more accepted and integrated into the community. Limitations on children were correlated with an increase in the child's age and a decrease in social support. The level of difficulty of the child's behavior was also mediated by social support, perhaps by enhancing the parent–child relationship, the child's developmental potential, and the communication patterns between parents and children (Dunst et al., 1986; Wilder & Granlund, 2003).

The structural characteristics of support reflect the degree to which an individual is embedded in a social context and by the existence and interconnectedness of social relationships. *Social embeddedness* includes marital status, participation in community organizations, and contact with friends (Barrera, 1986). The characteristics of the social network include its size, density, multiplexity, and symmetry or reciprocity. *Density* refers to the extent to which members have a relationship with each other independent of the person seeking support. *Multiplexity* is the number of kinds of aid available. *Symmetry* or *reciprocity* is the degree to which the support relationships are balanced in giving and receiving support (Barrera, 1986; Krahn, 1993). The *reachability* of the support system is another important feature (Barrera, 1986). A strong family network that lives in a geographically distant area may have severe limitations in its ability to offer the kinds of support that best relieves the family's distress.

Social support is subject to the parents' appraisal in terms of the amount of support and its ability to relieve the parents' distress or burden of care. No particular number of support resources is likely to help families when they do not feel supported. Because the perception of social support is more important to outcome than the actual receipt of services (Garwick, Patterson, Bennett, & Blum, 1998; Heitzmann & Kaplan, 1988; Olson & Esdaile, 2000), the assessment of amount of social support is not as important as the parents' perception of that support.

Parent Perceptions of Support

Support is linked more to internal than external processes (Turner & Marino, 1994). The perceived availability of support is related to the parents' decision to seek out the support, as well as to the provision of support by individuals (Barrera, 1986; Krahn, 1993; Pelletier, Godin, Lepage, & Dussault, 1994). Externally oriented individuals report receiving more enacted support than do individuals with an internal orientation, but a stress-buffering effect of enacted support was shown for people with internal locus of control (Sandler & Lakey, 1982).

Although any threats to existing support systems can be extremely stressful, supportive friends, family, and professionals can pose their own sources of stress to families (Garwick et al., 1998; Patterson et al., 1997; Patterson, Jernell, Leonard, & Titus, 1994; Waisbren, 1980). Family members are not always perceived to be available or supportive to parents (Garwick et al., 1998; Herman & Thompson, 1995; Seligman & Darling, 1989; Thyen, Terres, Yazdgerdi, & Perrin, 1998). Individuals in the support network may be critical of the parents' care of the child or impose their own demands on the already stressed parents. That extended family members do not intuitively meet parents' needs is a source of disappointment and is interpreted by the families as a lack of understanding or lack of caring about the parents' stress (Terres et al., 1995).

A close look at the families' support networks may reveal that groups of family and friends do not so much desert the parents but become smaller and denser (Kazak & Marvin, 1984; Kazak, Reber, & Carter, 1988; Krahn, 1993). Parents' social skills are related to their ability to extend their social networks (Kirkham, Schilling, Norelius, & Schinke, 1986; McKinney & Peterson, 1987; Monroe & Steiner, 1986). Parents' skills in pulling together and using a support system is a predictive factor in how successful families are in adapting to the birth of a disabled child (Dunn et al., 2001; Trute & Hauch, 1988).

Although support services for families of children with chronic illness and disability are important to adaptation, the services must be perceived as helpful and not mandated. Unrequested, imposed assistance can result in eroded self-confidence (Affleck, Tennen, Rowe, Roscher, & Walker, 1989; Krahn, 1993). A family's utilization of services is correlated with positive outcome only when the services assist positive family functioning (Hauser, DiPlacidio, Jacobson, Willett, & Cole, 1993; Trulsson, & Klingberg, 2003). Parents of children assisted by technology are clear in expressing their need for support services (Terres et al., 1995). But the services may disrupt the family in ways that impart additional stressors. Services that are unreliable, that are not geared to the family's needs, or that disrupt the day-to-day functioning of the family impose additional burdens. Parents have identified that professionals are most supportive when they provide (a) information, (b) emotional support for the parent, (c) regular personal contact, and (d) ideas to help with the care of the child. Parents do not relate the *type* of professional to any aspect of helpfulness (Sloper & Turner, 1992).

In the broader social network analysis of important relationships, all such linkages do not involve the provision of social support (Wellman, 1981). Parents of children with disabilities generally perceive themselves to be lonely and socially isolated. Social isolation can be one of the most stressful aspects of caring for a disabled child (Bradshaw & Lawton, 1978; Quine & Pahl, 1989; Terres et al., 1995). The loneliness parents express is directly linked to a lack of social support (Dean & Ensel, 1982; Florian & Krulik, 1991). The source of parents' isolation has also been linked to a sense of stigma that parents feel is connected to disability (Green, 2003; Saylor, 1990; Woolfson, 2004). Families withdraw from socializing with friends in order to protect themselves from rejection (Schilling & Schinke, 1984). Families with severely disabled children are significantly more restricted in social activities (Kazak & Marvin, 1984). Besides the restrictions on the family's time, the economic restrictions imposed by chronic illness and disability can limit parents' participation in a wide variety of activities (Doolittle, 1998; Heyman et al., 2004; Newacheck & Kim, 2005; Terres et al., 1995).

Parents may turn away from social support because they view the use of such assistance as an indication of their incompetence or as an affront to their sense of self-reliance (Brett, 2004; Mitchell, & Sloper, 2002). Education is one way to enhance a parent's sense of competence and reduce stress and has been described by parents as an area of greatest need (Mitchell & Sloper, 2002; Pisterman et al., 1992; Sloper & Turner, 1992). This approach has much in common with family-centered programs that incorporate education and support to empower families to feel competent and in control in the face of the crises and changing needs that come with the care of children with chronic illness and disability (Dempsey & Dunst, 2004; Helitzer et al., 2002; Itzhaky & Schwartz, 2000; Kirkham et al., 1986; Lash & Wertlieb, 1993; Seligman & Darling, 1989; Turnbull & Turnbull, 1986).

Chronic parenting stress is associated with lowered perceptions of emotional support and greater symptoms of depression and anxiety. There is evidence for the efficacy of early connection with support services, rather than introducing services primarily in times of stress. Social support is often used to moderate or alleviate a stress that has already occurred. However, Quittner and colleagues (1990) contend that social support is most effective when it *mediates* rather than *moderates*, or buffers, stress. Instead of waiting until the family is stressed, social support can come between the family and the stress to decrease or lessen its effects on the family (Quittner et al., 1990; Tak & McCubbin, 2002).

Support Groups

The kinds of services parents require can be guided more by conventional wisdom than proof of the ability of the service to meet family needs in substance or structure. Support groups, for example, are assumed to be a way in which parents can meet other parents of children with chronic illness and disability and find support. However, groups are not always positive resources for people. The benefit of a group depends on environmental conditions, group conditions, participant characteristics, and intended outcomes (Ainbinder et al., 1998; Galinsky & Schopler, 1994; Law, King, Stewart, & King, 2001). The appropriate support group may not be available within a certain geographic area. Attendance at support groups often is poor (Smith, Gabard, Dale, & Drucker, 1994). Restrictions on the parents' time to attend groups, the lack of child care to free the parent to attend a group, and the lack of mobility of the child (as in the case of some children assisted by technology) which keeps parents from bringing the child to the group, all are possible reasons why groups are not well attended. Some parents reject a referral to a group because they either do not like groups in general or they view groups as taking on other people's problems when they have enough of their own (Terres et al., 1995). Formal support services, including support groups, often are used by parents in times of crisis and after other sources of support have been tried (Smith et al., 1994; Unger & Powell, 1980). In any case, there is no evidence that participation in a support group is enough or even the best way to provide support to families coping with the care of children with chronic illness and disability.

ENCOURAGING SUPPORT USE

Over time, the burden of care and the effect of personal strain on the parents of children with chronic illness and disability can exact a toll, compromising their ability to care for the child and threatening the child's achievement of an optimal level of health and development. Support services were designed to prevent parents from reaching such a critical level of stress.

When negotiating support use with families, the clinician must keep in mind that such discussions are part of a partnership the clinician forms with the parents. Parents are the final decision makers as to whether a certain support service would be helpful for them and their child. The decision to engage support services is a process for many families that may undergo many changes and adjustments over time (Brett, 2004). Some parents are more exacting in their support requirements than others. The severity of the child's illness or disability and the general burden of care posed for the parent is a powerful influence on whether parents are willing to deal with the intrusion for the relief that comes with it. Parents may feel differently about this at various times. Therefore, a parent who does not accept services at one time might welcome the opportunity to accept them at other times (Freedman & Boyer, 2000).

When parents initially refuse support services, the clinician should not wait for the family to raise the issue of support again. Because support use is so closely tied to positive outcome for families of children with chronic illness and disability, assessment of support needs and how services that are in place are meeting those needs should be part of every professional encounter. The kinds of support parents require and the timing of that support can vary depending on parent coping and family styles. The old mental health model, which presumes a certain level of motivation to exist when parents seek services themselves, is generally not appropriate for most families of children with chronic illness and disease. Parents are often too overwhelmed and absorbed with the care of the child to be able to spend the time making the multiple telephone calls that may be required to arrange support (Shannon, 2004; Terres, 1999). Parents often welcome the clinician's offer to make the phone call for them, and to do so would be more in keeping with the family and coping styles of some parents than the mental health models of the past would presume.

Conversely, some parents prefer to maintain greater control in planning and managing their own support services (Balling & McCubbin, 2001; Holm, Patterson, & Gurney, 2003). In such a situation, the clinician serves as a consultant to the parent, and as such must be well informed of the support services available, how parents can gain access to them, and what role the parent prefers the clinician to have in helping arrange the services. If a breadth of knowledge about available support is not realistic, or if the setting or clinical demands do not allow time for arranging services, the clinician must be aware of case management resources and how a parent can gain access to those services. In some states, case management is available through various states' Departments of Public Health. Similar services may also be available through Associations for Retarded Citizens and Departments of Mental Health.

When parents are not ready for certain services, for example, a support group, they can still be given telephone numbers, addresses, and online references they can use when ready. When services are time sensitive, such as when waiting lists are involved, parents unsure of the service should be encouraged to put themselves on the waiting list, with the understanding that they can request to be passed over for the service if they still do not feel ready once the service becomes available. Respite care, certain developmental services, and institutional placement are examples of such time-sensitive services.

Parents who do not have formal services in place may be receiving considerable amounts of informal support from friends, family, and community networks. Some parents find these supports to be more comfortable for their style, whereas others feel that constantly drawing on informal resources eventually imposes an unacceptable imposition on the resource. In any case, over time, because these resources can diminish, the clinician must be aware of what formal resources can step into place.

In an American culture of self-reliance and independence, families may need reassurance that asking for help is not a sign of weakness or personal incompetence. In times when families live distances apart and neighbors feel less connected to each other, we may forget that mutual support is also a part of our national history. From pioneer days through the Great Depression to more recent times of war and tragedy, citizens have relied on each other through trying times. Healthcare clinicians of all types are the modern links for parents to the kinds of support that will help optimize the health and outcomes for both the child and the parent.

REFERENCES

Affleck, G., Tennen, H., Rowe, J., Roscher, B., & Walker, L. (1989). Effects of formal support on mothers' adaptation to the hospital-to-home transition of high-risk infants: The benefits and costs of helping. *Child Development, 60,* 488–501.

Ainbinder, J. G., Blanchard, L. W., Singer, G. H. S., Sullivan, M. E., Powers, L. K., Marquis, J. G., & Santelli, B. (1998). A qualitative study of parent to parent support for parents of children with special needs. *Journal of Pediatric Psychology, 23,* 99–109.

Balling, K., & McCubbin, M. (2001). Hospitalized children with chronic illness: Parental caregiving needs and valuing parental expertise. *Journal of Pediatric Nursing, 16*(2), 110–119.

Barrera, M. (1986). Distinctions between social support concepts, measures, and models. *American Journal of Community Psychology, 14,* 413–445.

Beresford, B. A. (1994). Resources and strategies: How parents cope with the care of a disabled child. *Journal of Child Psychology and Psychiatry, 35,* 171–209.

Bradshaw, J., & Lawton, D. (1978). Tracing the causes of stress in families with handicapped children. *British Journal of Social Work, 8,* 181–192.

Bregman, A. M. (1980). Living with progressive childhood illness: Parental management of neuromuscular disease. *Social Work in Health Care, 5,* 387–408.

Brett, J. (2004). The journey to accepting support: How parents of profoundly disabled children experience support in their lives. *Paediatric Nursing, 16*(8), 14–18.

Burr, W. (1973). *Theory construction and the sociology of the family.* New York: John Wiley & Sons.

Carter, E., & McGoldrick, M. (Eds.). (1980). *The family life cycle: A framework for family therapy.* New York: Gardner.

Carver, C. S., Scheier, M. F., & Weintraub, J. K. (1989). Assessing coping strategies: A theoretically based approach. *Journal of Personality and Social Psychology, 56,* 267–283.

Cluff, R. B., & Hicks, M. W. (1994). Superstition also survives: Seeing is not always believing. *Family Process, 33,* 479–482.

Cluff, R. B., Hicks, M. W., Madsen, C. H. (1994). Beyond the Curcumplex Model: 1. A moratorium on curvilinearity. *Family Process, 33,* 455–470.

Cobb, S. (1976). Social support as a moderator of life stress. *Psychosomatic Medicine, 38,* 300–314.

Cohen, P. (1962). The impact of a handicapped child on the family. *Social Casework, 43,* 137–142.

Curran, N. Q., & Bongiorno, H. H. (1986). Parents' perspectives: Focus on need. In C. L. Salisbury & J. Intagliata (Eds.), *Respite care* (pp. 89–97). Baltimore: Paul Brooks.

Danielson, C. B., Hamel-Bissel, B., & Winstead-Fry, P. (1993). *Families, health and illness: Perspectives on coping and intervention.* St. Louis: Mosby.

Dean, A., & Ensel, W. M. (1982). Modeling social support, life events, competence, and depression in the context of age and sex. *Journal of Community Psychology, 10,* 392–408.

Dempsey, I., & Dunst, C. J. (2004). Helpgiving styles and parent empowerment in families with a young child with a disability. *Journal of Intellectual & Developmental Disability, 29*(1), 40–51.

Doolittle, D. K. (1998). Welfare reform: Loss of supplemental security income (SSI) for children with disabilities. *Journal of the Society of Pediatric Nurses, 3,* 33–44.

Dunn, M. E., Burbine, T., Bowers, C. A., & Tantleff-Dunn, S. (2001). Moderators of stress in parents of children with autism. *Community Mental Health Journal, 37*(1), 39–52.

Dunst, C. J., Trivette, C. M., & Cross, A. H. (1986). Mediating influences of social support: Personal, family, and child outcomes. *American Journal of Mental Deficiency, 90,* 403–417.

Epperson, M. (1977). Families in sudden crisis. *Social Work in Health Care, 2,* 265–273.

Fadiman, A. (1997). *The spirit catches you and you fall down.* New York: Farrar, Straus & Giroux.

Feinberg, E. A. (1985). Family stress in pediatric home care. *Caring, 4,* 38–44.

Florian, V., & Krulik, T. (1991). Loneliness and social support of mothers of chronically ill children. *Social Science and Medicine, 32,* 1291–1296.

Flynt, S. W., & Wood, T. A. (1989). Stress and coping of mothers of children with moderate mental retardation. *American Journal on Mental Retardation, 94,* 278–283.

Folkman, S., Lazarus, R. S., Gruen, R. J., & DeLongis, A. (1986). Appraisal, coping, health status, and psychological symptoms. *Journal of Personality and Social Psychology, 50,* 571–579.

Fong, P. L. (1991). Cognitive appraisals in high- and low-stress mothers of adolescents with autism. *Journal of Consulting and Clinical Psychology, 59,* 471–474.

Fortier, L. M., & Wanlass, R. L. (1984). Family crisis following the diagnosis of a handicapped child. *Family Relations, 33,* 13–24.

Freedman, R. I., & Boyer, N. C. (2000). The power to choose: Supports for families caring for individuals with developmental disabilities. *Health and Social Work, 25*(1), 59–68.

Frey, K. S., Greenberg, M. T., & Fewell, R. R. (1989). Stress and coping among parents of handicapped children: A multidimensional approach. *American Journal of Mental Retardation, 94,* 240–249.

Galinsky, M. J., & Schopler, J. H. (1994). Negative experiences in support groups. *Social Work in Health Care, 20,* 77–95.

Gallagher, T. J., Wagenfeld, M. O., Baro, F., & Haepers, K. (1994). Sense of coherence, coping, and caregiver role overload. *Social Science and Medicine, 39,* 1615–1622.

Garwick, A. W., Patterson, J. M., Bennett, F. C., & Blum, R. W. (1998). Parents' perceptions of helpful vs unhelpful types of support in managing the care of preadolescents with chronic conditions. *Archives of Pediatric and Adolescent Medicine, 152,* 665–671.

Goodman, L. (1967). Continuing treatment of parents with congenitally defective infants. *Social Work, 9,* 92–97.

Green, S. E. (2001). Grandma's hands: Parental perceptions of the importance of grandparents as secondary caregivers in families of children with disabilities. *International Journal of Aging and Human Development, 53*(1), 1–33.

Green, S. E. (2003). "What do you mean 'what's wrong with her?'": Stigma and the lives of families of children with disabilities. *Social Science & Medicine, 57*(8), 1361–1374.

Hauser, S. T., DiPlacido, J., Jacobson, A. M., Willett, J., & Cole, C. C. (1993). Family coping with an adolescent's chronic illness: An approach and three studies. *Journal of Adolescence, 16,* 305–329.

Hauser-Cram, P., Warfield, M. E., Shonkoff, J., & Krauss, M. W. (2001). Children with disabilities: A longitudinal study of child development and parent well-being. *Monographs of the Society for Research in Child Development, 66*(3), 1–114.

Heaman, D. J. (1995). Perceived stressors and coping strategies of parents who have children with developmental disabilities: A comparison of mothers with fathers. *Journal of Pediatric Nursing, 10,* 311–320.

Heitzmann, C. A., & Kaplan, R. M. (1988). Assessment of methods for measuring social support. *Health Psychology, 7,* 75–109.

Helitzer, D. L., Cunningham-Sabo, L. D., VanLeit, B., & Crowe, T. K. (2002). Perceived changes in self-image and coping strategies of mothers of children with disabilities. *Occupational Therapy Journal of Research, 22*(1), 25–33.

Herman, S. E., & Thompson, L. (1995). Families perceptions of their resources for caring for children with developmental disabilities. *Mental Retardation, 33,* 73–83.

Heyman, M. B., Harmatz, P., Acree, M., Wilson, L., Moskowitz, J. T., Ferrando, S., & Folkman, S. (2004). Economic and psychologic costs for maternal caregivers of gastrostomy-dependent children. *Journal of Pediatrics, 145*(4), 511–516.

Hill, R. (1949). *Families under stress.* New York: Harper & Row.

Holahan, C. J., & Moos, R. H. (1986). Personality, coping, and family resources in stress resistance: A longitudinal analysis. *Journal of Personality and Social Psychology, 51,* 389–395.

Holm, K. E., Patterson, J. M., & Gurney, J. G. (2003). Parental involvement and family-centered care in the diagnostic and treatment phases of childhood cancer: Results from a qualitative study. *Journal of Pediatric Oncology Nursing, 20*(5), 301–313.

Itzhaky, H., & Schwartz, C. (2000). Empowerment of parents of children with disabilities: The effect of community and personal variables. *Journal of Family Social Work, 5*(1), 21–36.

Johnson, B. S. (2000). Mother's perceptions of parenting children with disabilities. *MCN: The American Journal of Maternal/Child Nursing, 25*(3), 127–132.

Johnson, M. (2004). Approaching the salutogenesis of sense of coherence: The role of 'active' self-esteem and coping. *British Journal of Health Psychology, 9*(Pt 3), 419–432.

Katz, S., & Kessel, L. (2002). Grandparents of children with developmental disabilities: Perceptions, beliefs, and involvement in their care. *Issues in Comprehensive Pediatric Nursing, 25*(2), 113–128.

Kazak, A., & Marvin, R. (1984). Differences, difficulties and adaptation: Stress and social networks in families with a handicapped child. *Family Relations, 33,* 67–77.

Kazak, A. E., Reber, M., & Carter, A. (1988). Structural and qualitative aspects of social networks in families with young chronically ill children. *Journal of Pediatric Psychology, 13,* 171–182.

Kellegrew, D. H. (2000). Constructing daily routines: A qualitative examination of mothers with young children with disabilities. *American Journal of Occupational Therapy, 54*(3), 252–259.

Kennedy, J. (1970). Maternal reactions to the birth of a defective baby. *Social Casework, 51,* 410–416.

King, S. V. (2001). "God won't put more on you than you can bear": Faith as a coping stratefy among older African American caregiving parents of adult children with disabilities. *Journal of Religion, Disability, and Health, 4*(4), 7–24.

Kirkham, M. A., Schilling, R. F., Norelius, K., & Schinke, S. P. (1986). Developing coping styles and social support networks: An intervention outcome study with mothers of handicapped children. *Child: Care, Health and Development, 12,* 313–323.

Klein, S. D. (1993). The challenge of communicating with parents. *Journal of Developmental and Behavioral Pediatrics, 14,* 184–191.

Krahn, G. L. (1993). Conceptualizing social support in families of children with special needs. *Family Process, 32,* 235–248.

Lash, M., & Wertlieb, D. (1993). A model for family-centered service coordination for children who are disabled by traumatic injuries. *ACCH Advocate, 1,* 19–27.

Law, M., King, S., Stewart, D. & King, G. (2001). The perceived effects of parent-led support groups for parents of children with disabilities. *Physical and Occupational Therapy in Pediatrics, 21,* 29–48.

Lazarus, R. S., & Folkman, S. (1984). *Stress, appraisal, and coping.* New York: Springer.

Lee, A. L., Strauss, L., Wittman, P., Jackson, B., & Carstens, A. (2001). The effect of chronic illness on roles and emotions of caregivers. *Occupational Therapy in Health Care, 14*(1), 47–60.

Lefcourt, H. M., Martin, R. A. & Salen, W. E. (1984). Locus of control and social support: interactive moderators of stress. *Journal of Personality and Social Psychology, 47*, 378–389.

Lewis, M., & Vitulano, L. A. (2003). Biopsychosocial issues and risk factors in the family when the child has a chronic illness. *Child and Adolescent Psychiatric Clinics of North America, 12*(3), 389–399.

Lindqvist, R., Carlsson, M., & Sjoden, P. O. (2000). Coping strategies and health-related quality of life among spouses of continuous ambulatory peritoneal dialysis, haemodialysis, and transplant patients. *Journal of Advanced Nursing, 31*(6), 1398–1408.

Logan, D. R., Radcliffe, J., & Smith-Whitley, K. (2002). Parent factors and adolescent sickle cell disease: Associations with patterns of health service use. *Journal of Pediatric Psychology, 27*(5), 475–484.

Macrodimitris, S. D., & Endler, N. S. (2001). Coping, control, and adjustment in Type 2 diabetes. *Health Psychology, 20*(3), 208–216.

McCrae, R. R., & Costa, P. T. (1986). Personality, coping and coping effectiveness in an adult sample. *Journal of Personality, 54*, 385–405.

McCubbin, H. I., & McCubbin, M. A. (l987). Family stress theory and assessment: The T-Double ABCX model of family adjustment and adaptation. In H. I. McCubbin & A. Thompson (Eds.), *Family adjustment inventories for research and practice* (pp. 3–32). Madison: University of Wisconsin.

McCubbin, H. I., & McCubbin, M. A. (1988). Typologies of resilient families: Emerging roles of social class & ethnicity. *Family Relations, 37*, 247–254.

McCubbin, H. I., & Patterson, J. M. (1983) The family stress process: The Double ABCX Model of adjustment and adaptation. In H. I. McCubbin, M. Sussman, & J. Patterson (Eds.), *Advances and developments in family stress theory and research* (pp. 7–37). New York: Haworth.

McCubbin, H. I., & Patterson, J. M. (1981). *Systematic assessment of family stress, resources, and coping: Tools for research, education, and clinical intervention.* St. Paul, MN: Department of Family Social Science, Family Stress and Coping Project.

McCubbin, H. I., Thompson, A. I., & McCubbin, M. A. (1996). *Family assessment: Resiliency, coping, and adaptation. Inventories for research and practice.* Madison: University of Wisconsin.

McCubbin, H., Thompson, A., Pirner, P., & McCubbin, M. (1988). *Family types and family strengths: A life cycle and ecological perspective.* Minneapolis: Burgess.

McCubbin, H. I., Thompson, E. A., Thompson, A. I., McCubbin, M., & Kaston, A. (1993). Culture, ethnicity, and the family: Critical factors in childhood chronic illness and disabilities. *Pediatrics, 91*, 1063–1070.

McKernon, W. L., Holmbeck, G. N., Colder, C. R., Hommeyer, J. S., Shapera, W., & Westhoven, V. (2001). Longitudinal study of observed and perceived family influences on problem-focused coping behaviors of preadolescents with spina bifida. *Journal of Pediatric Psychology, 26*(1), 41–54.

McKinney, B., & Peterson, R. A. (1987). Predictors of stress in parents of developmentally disabled children. *Journal of Pediatric Psychology, 12,* 133–150.

Mellin, A. E., Neumark-Sztainer, D., & Patterson, J. M. (2004). Parenting adolescent girls with type 1 diabetes: Parents' perspectives. *Journal of Pediatric Psychology, 29*(3), 221–230.

Miller, A. C., Gordon, R. M., Daniels, R. J., & Diller, L. (1992). Stress, appraisal, and coping in mothers of disabled and nondisabled children. *Journal of Pediatric Psychology, 17*, 587–605.

Mitchell, W., & Sloper, P. (2002). Information that informs rather than alienates families with disabled children: Developing a model of good practice. *Health and Social Care in the Community, 10*(2), 74–81.

Monroe, S. M., & Steiner, S. C. (1986). Social support and psychopathology: Interrelations with pre-existing disorder, stress, and personality. *Journal of Abnormal Psychology, 95*, 29–39.

Morrow, G. R., Carpenter, P. J., & Hoagland, A. C. (1984). The role of social support in parental adjustment to pediatric cancer. *Journal of Pediatric Psychology, 9*, 317–329.

Morse, J. M., Wilson, S., & Penrod, J. (2000). Mothers and their disabled children: Refining the concept of normalization. *Health Care for Women International, 21(8),* 659–676.

Mullins, L. L., Aniol, K., Boyd, M. L., Page, M. C., & Cheney, J. M. (2002). The influence of respite care on psychological distress in parents of children with developmental disabilities: A longitudinal study. *Children's Services: Social Policy, Research, and Practice, 5*(2), 123–138.

Newacheck, P. W., & Kim, S. E. (2005). A national profile of health care utilization and expenditures for children with special health care needs. *Archives of Pediatrics & Adolescent Medicine, 159*(1), 10–17.

Olshansky, S. (1962). Chronic sorrow: A response to having a mentally defective child. *Social Casework, 43*, 190–193.

Olson, D. H. (1994). Curvilinearity survives: The world is not flat. *Family Process, 33*, 471–478.

Olson, J., & Esdaile, S. (2000). Mothering young children with disabilities in a challenging urban environment. *American Journal of Occupational Therapy, 54*(3), 307–314.

Olson, D., McCubbin, H. I., Bowen, H., Larson, A., Muxem, A., & Wilson, M. (l989). *Families and what makes them work* (2nd ed.). Newbury Park, CA: Sage.

Olson, D. H., Russell, C. S., & Sprenkle, D. H. (l983). Circumplex model VI. Theoretical update. *Family Process, 22*, 69–83.

Park, C. L., Armeli, S., & Tennen, H. (2004). Appraisal-coping goodness of fit: A daily Internet study. *Personality & Social Psychology Bulletin, 30*(5), 558–569.

Parkes, K. R. (1984). Locus of control, cognitive appraisal, and coping in stressful episodes. *Journal of Personality and Social Psychology, 46*, 655–668.

Parra, M. M. (2003). Nursing and respite care services for ventilator-assisted children. *Caring, 22*(5), 6–9.

Patterson, J. M. (1995). Promoting resilience in families experiencing stress. *Pediatric Clinics of North America, 42*, 47–63.

Patterson, J. M. (2002). Understanding family resilience. *Journal of Clinical Psychology, 58*(3), 233–246.

Patterson, J. M., & Garwick, A. W. (1994). Levels of meaning in family stress theory. *Family Process, 33*, 287–304.

Patterson, J. M., Garwick, A. W., Bennett, F. C., & Blum, R. W. (1997). Social support in families of children with chronic conditions: Supportive and nonsupportive behaviors. *Journal of Developmental and Behavioral Pediatrics, 18*, 383–391.

Patterson, J. M., Holm, K. E., & Gurney, J. G. (2004). The impact of childhood cancer on the family: A qualitative analysis of strains, resources, and coping behaviors. *Psycho-Oncology, 13*(6), 390–407.

Patterson, J. M., Jernell, J., Leonard, B. J., & Titus, J. C. (l994). Caring for medically fragile children at home: The parent–professional relationship. *Journal of Pediatric Nursing, 9*, 98–106.

Patterson, J. M., & McCubbin, H. I. (1983). The impact of family life events and changes on the health of a chronically ill child. *Family Relations, 32*, 255–264.

Patterson, J. M., McCubbin, H. I., & Warwick, W. J. (l990). The impact of family functioning on health care in children with cystic fibrosis. *Social Science in Medicine, 31*, 159–164.

Pelchat, D., Lefebvre, H., & Perreault, M. (2003). Differences and similarities between mothers' and fathers' experiences of parenting a child with a disability. *Journal of Child Health Care, 7*(4), 231–47.

Pelletier, L., Godin, G., Lepage, L., & Dussault, G. (1994). Social support received by mothers of chronically ill children. *Child: Care Health Development, 20*, 115–131.

Penley, J. A., Tomaka, J., & Wiebe, J. S. (2002). The association of coping to physical and psychological health outcomes: A meta-analytic review. *Journal of Behavioral Medicine, 25*(6), 551–603.

Petrosky, M. J., & Birkimer, J. C. (1991). The relationship among locus of control, coping styles, and psychological symptom reporting. *Journal of Clinical Psychology, 47*, 336–345.

Pisterman, S., Firestone, P., McGrath, P., Goodman, J. T., Webster, I., Mallory, R., & Goffin, B. (1992). The effects of parent training on parenting stress and sense of competence. *Canadian Journal of Behavioral Science, 24*, 41–58.

Quine, L., & Pahl, J. (1989). Stress and coping in families caring for a child with severe mental handicap: A longitudinal study. *Institute of social and applied psychology and centre for health service studies.* Cambridge: University of Kent.

Quint, R. D., Chesterman, E., Crain, L. S., Winkleby, M., & Boyce, W. T. (1990). Home care for ventilator-dependent children. *American Journal of Diseases of Children, 144*, 1238–1241.

Quittner, A., Glueckauf, R. L., & Jackson, D. N. (1990). Chronic parenting stress: Moderating versus mediating effects of social supports. *Journal of Personality and Social Psychology, 59*, 1266–1278.

Ray, L. D., & Ritchie, J. A. (1993). Caring for chronically ill children at home: Factors that influence parents' coping. *Journal of Pediatric Nursing, 8,* 217–225.

Redfield, J., & Stone, A. (1979). Individual viewpoints of stressful life events. *Journal of Consulting and Clinical Psychology, 47,* 147–154.

Robinson, C., Jackson, P., & Townsley, R. (2001). Short breaks for families caring for a disabled child with complex health needs. *Child and Family Social Work, 6*(1), 67–75.

Rotter, J. B. (1966). Generalized expectancies for internal versus external control of reinforcement. *Psychological Monographs, 81,* (1), 1–28.

Saloviita, T., Italinna, M., & Leinonen, E. (2003). Explaining the parental stress of fathers and mothers caring for a child with intellectual disability: A Double ABCX model. *Journal of Intellectual Disability Research, 47,* 300–312.

Sandler, I. N., & Lakey, B. (1982). Locus of control as a stress moderator: The role of control perceptions and social support. *American Journal of Community Psychology, 10,* 65–80.

Saylor, C. (1990). The management of stigma: Redefinition and representation. *Holistic Nursing Practice, 5,* 45–53.

Schilling, R. F., Gilchrist, L. D., & Schinke, S. P. (1984). Coping with social support in families of developmentally disabled children. *Family Relations, 33,* 47–54.

Schilling, R. F., & Schinke, S. P. (1984). Personal coping and social support for parents of handicapped children. *Children and Youth Services Review, 6,* 195–206.

Scornaienchi, J. M. (2003). Chronic sorrow: One mother's experience with two children with lissencephaly. *Journal of Pediatric Health Care, 17*(6), 290–294.

Seligman, M., & Darling, R. B. (1989). *Ordinary families, special children: A systems approach to childhood disability.* New York: Guilford Press.

Shannon, P. (2004). Barriers to family-centered services for infants and toddlers with developmental delays. *Social Work, 49*(2), 301–308.

Sherman, B. R., & Cocozza, J. J. (1984). Stress in families of the developmentally disabled: A literature review of factors affecting the decision to seek out-of-home placements. *Family Relations, 33,* 95–103.

Sloper, P., Knussen, C., Turner, S., & Cunningham, C. (1991). Factors related to stress and satisfaction with life in families of children with Down's syndrome. *Journal of Child Psychology and Psychiatry, 32,* 655–676.

Sloper, P., & Turner, S. (1992). Service needs of families of children with severe physical disability. *Child: Care, Health and Development, 18,* 259–282.

Smith, K., Gabard, D., Dale, D., & Drucker, A. (1994). Parental opinions about attending parent support groups. *Children's Health Care, 23,* 127–136.

Solnit, A., & Stark, M. (1961). Mourning the birth of a defective child. *The Psychoanalytic Study of the Child, 16,* 523–527.

Svavarsdottir, E. K., McCubbin, M. A., & Kane, J. H. (2000). Well-being of parents of young children with asthma. *Research in Nursing and Health, 23*(5), 356–358.

Taanila, A., Syrjala, L., Kokkonen, J., & Jarvelin, M. (2002). Coping of parents with physically and/or intellectually disabled children. *Child: Care, Health and Development, 28*(1), 73–86.

Tak, Y. R., & McCubbin, M. (2002). Family stress, perceived social support and coping following the diagnosis of a child's congenital heart disease. *Journal of Advanced Nursing, 39*(2), 190–198.

Terres, N. M. (1999). *The use of respite care services for parents of children with chronic illness and disability.* Dissertation Abstracts International 60 (04), 1890B. (UMI No. 9925242).

Terres, N. M., Thyen, U., & Perrin, J. M. (1995). *Factors contributing to parent satisfaction with services for the home care of technologically dependent children.* Unpublished doctoral qualifying paper. Medford, MA: Tufts University.

Thompson, R. J., Gustafson, K. E., Hamlett, K. W., & Spock, A. (1992). Stress, coping, and family functioning in the psychological adjustment of mothers of children and adolescents with cystic fibrosis. *Journal of Pediatric Psychology, 17,* 573–585.

Thyen, U., Sperner, J., Morfield, M., Meyer, C., & Ravens-Sieberer, U. (2003). Unmet health care needs and impact on families with children with disabilities in Germany. *Ambulatory Pediatrics, 3*(2), 74–81.

Thyen, U., Terres, N. M., Yazdgerdi, S. R., & Perrin, J. M. (1998). Impact of long-term care of children assisted by technology on maternal health. *Journal of Developmental and Behavioral Pediatrics, 19*, 273–282.

Trulsson, U., & Klingberg, G. (2003). Living with a child with a severe orofacial handicap: Experiences from the perspectives of parents. *European Journal of Oral Sciences, 11*(1), 19–25.

Trute, B. (1995). Gender differences in the psychological adjustment of parents of young, developmentally disabled children. *Journal of Child Psychology & Psychiatry & Allied Disciplines, 36*, 1225–1242.

Trute, B., & Hauch, C. (1988). Social network attributes of families with positive adaptation to the birth of a developmentally disabled child. *Canadian Journal of Community Mental Health, 7*, 5–16.

Trute, B., & Hiebert-Murphy, D. (2002). Family adjustment to childhood developmental disability: A measure of parent appraisal of family impacts. *Journal of Pediatric Psychology, 27*(3), 271–280.

Tunali, B., & Powers, T. G. (1992). Creating satisfaction: A psychological perspective on stress and coping in families of handicapped children. *Journal of Child Psychology and Psychiatry, 34*, 945–957.

Turnbull, A. P., & Turnbull, H. R. (1986). *Families, professionals, & and exceptionality.* Columbus, OH: Merrill.

Turner, R. J., & Marino, F. (1994). Social support and social structure: A descriptive epidemiology. *Journal of Health and Social Behavior, 35*, 193–212.

Unger, D. G., & Powell, D. R. (1980). Supporting families under stress: The role of social networks. *Family Relations, 29*, 566–574.

Waisbren, S. E. (1980). Parents' reactions after the birth of a developmentally disabled child. *American Journal of Mental Deficiency, 84*, 345–351.

Wegener, D. H., & Aday, L. A. (1989). Home care for ventilator-assisted children: predicting family stress. *Pediatric Nursing, 15*, 371–376.

Wellman, B. (1981). Applying network analysis to the study of support. In B. H. Gottlieb (Ed.), *Social networks and social support* (pp. 171–200). Beverly Hills: Sage.

Wiegner, S., & Donders, J. (2000). Predictors of parental distress after congenital disabilities. *Journal of Developmental and Behavioral Pediatrics, 21*(4), 271–277.

Wikler, L., Wasow, M., & Hatfield, E. (1981). Chronic sorrow revisited: Parent versus professional depiction of the adjustment of parents of mentally retarded children. *American Journal of Orthopsychiatry, 51*, 63–70.

Wilder, J., & Granlund, M. (2003). Behavior style and interaction between seven children with multiple disabilities and their caregivers. *Child: Care, Health and Development, 29*(6), 559–567.

Williams, P. D., Williams, A. R., Graff, J. C., Hanson, S., Stanton, A., Hafeman, C., Licbcrgen, A., Leuenberg, K., Setter, R. K., Ridder, L., Curry, H., Barnard, M., & Sanders, S. (2002). Interrelationships among variables affecting well siblings and mothers in families of children with a chronic illness or disability. *Journal of Behavioral Medicine, 125*(5), 411–424.

Woolfson, L. (2004). Family well-being and disabled children: A psychosocial model of disability-related child behavior problems. *British Journal of Health Psychology, 9*, 1–13.

Zakowski, S. G., Hall, M. H., Klein, L. C., & Baum, A. (2001). Appraised control, coping, and stress in a community sample: A test of the goodness-of-fit hypothesis. *Annals of Behavioral Medicine, 23*(3), 158–165.

CHAPTER 20

Common Adverse Drug Reactions in the Elderly: Application of the Neuman Systems Model and the Role of Nursing

Debra C. Sylvester

Adverse drug reactions (ADRs) rank fifth among the top preventable threats to the health of older people (Berenson, 2000). The most common cause of ADRs is polypharmacy, the concurrent use of multiple prescriptions or over-the-counter medications by a single patient. Polypharmacy is especially common among elderly patients. A number of studies over the past decade have revealed that the typical elderly person uses an average of two to six prescribed medications and one to four over-the-counter medications on a daily basis (Larsen & Hoot Martin, 1999). Polypharmacy is the leading risk factor for ADRs.

The more medications a patient takes, the greater the risk for ADRs. A recent literature review indicates that the potential for an ADR is 6% when patients take two medications, 50% when they take five different medications, and 100% when they take eight or more medications (Larsen & Hoot Martin, 1999). Further evidence that ADRs are a serious and common problem for the elderly is that numerous hospital admissions for people over 65 are the direct result of ADRs. The problem of polypharmacy has been recognized as a critical issue at various levels of health care. At the federal level, the problem is so extensive that the U.S. Department of Health and Human Services named it the principal medication safety issue in its Healthy People 2010 document (U.S Department of Health and Human Services, 2000).

At the provider level, nurses who care for elders are faced with the daunting task of managing the care of elderly patients on complex, risky, and sometimes unnecessary, medication regimens. At the patient level, the more complex the regimen, the more difficult it is for the patient to manage it. Side effects are more likely in such situations. Additionally, due to the increasing costs of drugs, many older persons on fixed incomes may conserve medications by reducing or skipping doses.

This chapter addresses the issues of medication administration in the elderly within the framework of Betty Neuman's Systems Model. In addition, the application of the Neuman Model is used to examine the physical and cognitive changes resulting from common medications that pose risks to the elderly, as well the role of nursing in preventing ADRs.

BACKGROUND

Several contributing factors make elderly people particularly vulnerable to ADRs. These include coexisting illness, patient expectations, and age-related considerations. Each of these factors presents a challenge for the elderly, many of whom are confronted with comorbid chronic illnesses, differing expectations of medication management, and other age-related issues such as sensory losses, particularly visual and auditory changes.

Coexisting Illness

The incidence of coexisting chronic conditions requiring multiple medications increases with age. Eighty percent of people over the age of 65 have at least one chronic condition, and 50% have more than one. Multiple medications are usually prescribed to manage these conditions. In addition, patients often have multiple providers for care, resulting in multiple prescriptions and a lack of coordination or communication between providers about regimens (Larsen & Hoot Martin, 1999).

Patient Expectations

The literature indicates that up to 75% of all visits to a provider result in a patient receiving a written prescription (Larsen & Hoot Martin, 1999). Patients of all ages may consider a visit to a physician as worthwhile only if they complete the visit with a prescription for their health problem. Because of this belief that a "successful" visit is linked with prescriptions, polypharmacy becomes a greater potential problem, especially if patients are seen by multiple providers.

Age-Related Considerations

The most complex contributor to ADRs is the effect of aging. For those who live at home, diminished physical and instrumental activities of daily living have been associated with an increased number of prescription medications (Hanlon, Schmadel, Ruby, & Weinberger, 2001). Further, age-related changes in the elderly significantly alter pharmacokinetics and pharmacodynamics. Pharmacokinetics relates to how the body absorbs a drug into the bloodstream, distributes the medication to the site of action, and excretes the drug from the body. Pharmacokinetics includes the processes of drug absorption, distribution, metabolism, and excretion.

With aging, the proportions of fat, lean tissue, and body water content are reduced. Water content, total body mass, and lean body mass all decrease, whereas the percentage of body fat increases. In addition, a decrease in muscle mass and a loss of subcutaneous tissue occurs. These changes affect the relationship between medication concentration and solubility in the body (Larsen & Hoot Martin, 1999).

The problem with fat-soluble medications is the increased fat composition of the elderly, which affects the distribution of these medications. For instance, benzodiazapines, barbiturates, phenothiazides, and phenytoin are stored in fat tissues. This process results in decreased medication concentration in the blood stream; however, the actions of the medications are prolonged by a slow release from the adipose tissue, resulting in increased duration of action and increased half-life. Fat-soluble sleeping medications, such as flurazepam, temazepam, and triazolam, often leave patients with prolonged residual drowsiness in the morning because of their long half-life. Tricyclic antidepressants such as thorazine and phenobarbital are examples of fat-soluble medications with an increased half-life (Larsen & Hoot Martin, 1999).

The distribution process for all medications includes plasma protein concentration and protein binding. Older adults have less serum albumin than younger adults. This allows more of one medication to be free to interact with other medications or causes increased levels of the medication in the blood stream. Medications particularly affected by decreased serum albumin levels are naproxen, phenytoin, tolbutamide, and warfarin (Larsen & Hoot Martin, 1999). Further, protein binding decreases by 15 to 25% in patients over age 60. Medications highly bound to plasma proteins and affected by the decreased binding include diazepam, meperidine, phenytoin, furosemide, tolbutamide, and warfarin.

Metabolism is the breakdown of a medication in the body. The liver is primarily responsible for medication metabolism. Aging decreases liver mass, alters hepatic blood flow, and reduces protein synthesis and enzymatic activity. Commonly prescribed medications most affected by age-related liver changes include meperidine, barbiturates, propranolol, and tricyclic antidepressants. The result is that elderly people metabolize medications at a slower rate (Larsen & Hoot Martin, 1999).

Excretion is how the body gets rid of a medication. Most medications are excreted through the renal system. Age-related changes in the renal system affect medication excretion. Age-related reduction in blood flow and decreased glomerular filtration rate cause a buildup of medications in the renal system. The elderly have a glomerular filtration rate of only 60 to 70% of normal (Larsen & Hoot Martin, 1999).

Medications that are commonly prescribed to the elderly and excreted through renal elimination include acetazolamide, amantadine, aminoglycosides, atenolol, cimetidine, digoxin, lithium, and vancomycin. Because these medications are excreted more slowly as people age, the medications have more potential to reach toxic levels. Medications with a narrow therapeutic range and high toxic potential, such as digoxin and gentamicin, are most affected by age-related changes to the renal system.

Pharmacodynamics is the effect a medication has on the individual and how the medication interacts with receptors at the site of action. The elderly have increased sensitivity to some medications due to changes in receptor numbers, past preceptor alterations, or decreased homeostatic mechanisms. Specifically, the elderly tend to have greater central nervous system response to benzodiazapines (e.g., diazepam, chlordiazepoxide, flurazepam, and triazolam). Some medications have exhibited decreased sensitivity in the elderly (e.g., propranolol, atenolol, and metoprolol) (Larsen & Hoot Martin, 1999).

REVIEW OF THE LITERATURE

Beers (1997) developed specific criteria for identifying inappropriate use of medications in older adults. Some classes of frequently prescribed medications pose special risks for the elderly, whether they are used alone or in combination with some other drugs. According to Routledge and colleagues (2003), NSAIDs, antihypertensives, cardiovascular drugs, anticoagulants, and benzodiazapines are responsible for 60% of ADRs.

Nonsteroidal Anti-inflammatory Drugs (NSAIDs)

NSAIDs are a problem even when taken alone. There is widespread consumption of these drugs in the United States, with 70% of people 65 years of age or older taking them at least weekly and around 50% taking them daily. The most common adverse effects of NSAIDs are gastrointestinal manifestations, such as gastric ulceration and hemorrhage, which usually occur without signs of dyspepsia, abdominal pain, or nausea. The risk of gastrointestinal bleeding due to NSAIDs, which is often life threatening, is greater in persons older than age 60. In persons over the age of 60 who have a history of gastrointestinal bleeding, the risk is even higher. Ibuprofen, diclofenac, and salicylates may be slightly less likely to cause upper gastrointestinal bleeding than other anti-inflammatories. In addition, other adverse reactions of NSAIDs include renal impairment, sodium retention, and bleeding diathesis from platelet dysfunction (Chutka, Evans, Fleming, & Mikkelson, 1995).

The effect of NSAIDs is magnified when taken with other medications. Patients concurrently receiving corticosteriods and NSAIDs were found to have a risk of peptic ulcer disease that was 15 times greater than that of nonusers of either drug. The risk of upper gastrointestinal hemorrhage increases more substantially when NSAIDs are combined with warfarin (Routledge, O'Mahony, & Woodhouse, 2003).

NSAIDs also increase the serum concentration of digoxin and attenuate the effects of beta-adrenergic blockers, ACE inhibitors, and thiazides. The nephrotoxic effects of triamterene are also potentiated by NSAIDs (Chutka, Evans, Fleming, & Mikkelson, 1995). Further, NSAIDs should be used with caution in the elderly population, due to the increased risk of gastrointestinal bleeding and ADRs with other medications. Of all the NSAIDs, indomethacin (Indocin, Indocin SR) produces the most central nervous system side effects and should be avoided in the elderly (Beers & Berkow, 2000). In patients who have not had relief with less toxic analgesics, NSAIDs should be used at the lowest effective dose for the shortest period of time. In cases of mild to moderate pain, acetaminophen has been shown to be safer yet just as effective as NSAIDs (Beers & Berkow, 2000).

Antihypertensive Drugs

Aggressive management of hypertension is one of the most important concerns in care of the elderly. The main types of antihypertensive drugs are diuretics, calcium-channel blockers, beta-adrenergic blocking agents, and beta blockers.

In the management of hypertension, diuretics are often the first choice for medication management for elderly patients because they reduce cardiovascular morbidity and mortality rates. Lower doses of thiazide diuretics may successfully control hypertension in the elderly, with less risk of hypokalemia and hyperglycemia than higher doses (Beers, 1997). Long-acting calcium-channel blockers such as amlodipine, felodipine, and sustained-release nifedipine also appear effective in reducing cardiovascular events in the elderly. Short-acting nifedipine should not be used because of increased mortality risk in the elderly. Beta-adrenergic blocking agents such as propranolol and metoprolol have a potential to produce central nervous system (CNS)-adverse reactions such as vivid dreams, depression, fatigue, and impotence and induce brochospasm in people with asthma and COPD. In addition, when used in the elderly, beta-adrenergic blocking agents can worsen symptoms of claudication for people with peripheral arterial disease. Patients with diabetes may also experience hypoglycemic episodes and hypertension with beta-adrenergic blocking agents.

Cardiovascular Drugs

Cardiovascular disease is the leading cause of death in the United States and is treated with lifestyle changes and medications. In a study by Gurwitz et al. (2003) of elderly enrolled in an HMO, cardiovascular drugs were the most frequently prescribed drug class, with 53% of patients prescribed this class of medications. Cardiovascular drugs have been implicated in a larger percentage of ADRs. Cardiovascular drugs with potentially serious ADRs in the elderly include digoxin, dipyridamole, and disopyramide.

Digoxin is prescribed for the treatment of congestive heart failure, tachyarrhythmias, atrial fibrillation, and atrial flutter. Digoxin clearance decreases an average of 50% in elderly patients with normal serum creatinine levels. Therefore, doses should not exceed 0.125 mg/day, except when used to treat atrial arrhythmias. The potential for toxicity is enhanced when drugs such as verapamil hydrochloride, amiodarone, or quinidine are used concomitantly. Caution is necessary when digoxin is used in conjunction with diuretics, because this may exacerbate renal impairment and lead to digitalis toxicity. Some elderly patients are more sensitive to the effects of digitalis than others and may exhibit evidence of digitalis toxicity even with therapeutic drug concentrations. Some researchers suggest that electrocardiography is helpful in detecting toxicity (Chutka, Evans, Fleming, & Mikkelson, 1995). In 2003, Juurlink and colleagues reported that patients admitted with digoxin toxicity were about 12 times more likely to have been treated with clarithromycin in the previous week. Thus, new prescriptions and the effect of additional medications on toxicity should be examined (Juurlink et al., 2003).

Dipyridamole frequently causes orthostatic hypotension in the elderly. Increased risk of bleeding may occur when taken with anticoagulants and NSAIDs. If possible, dypyridamole should be avoided in the elderly. Disopyramide is used to treat premature ventricular contractions and is the most potent negative inotrope. Therefore, it may induce heart failure in the elderly. Because of this, the use of disopyramide should be considered carefully.

Anticoagulants

The anticoagulant warfarin is a frequently prescribed drug in the elderly population. When taken with other drugs it can lead to severe ADRs. Medications that increase the effect of warfarin include aspirin, phenylbutazone, bactrim, metronidzole, fluconazole, cimetidine, and prilosec. Medications that decrease the effect of warfarin include amytal, nembutal, seconal, rifampin, carbamazepine, doridam used for insomnia, dilantin, Vitamin K, oral contraceptives, cholestyramine, and colestipol.

Drugs that promote bleeding when taken with warfarin include aspirin and other salicylates, dipyridamole, indocin, heparin, thrombolytic agents, methotrexate, phenylbutazone, glutcocorticoids, and tamoxifen. Beers (1997) found that ticlopidine was more toxic in the elderly population.

Psychotropic Medications

Based on work by Beers (1997), a number of psychotropic medications should be avoided in the elderly population, including amitriptyline alone or in combination products, due to strong anticholingeric and sedating effects; barbiturates other than phenobarbital, meperidine, and meprobamate, due to their addictive properties; Librium, alone or in combination with Valium, due to long half-lives and the risk of sedation and increased falls; doxepin, due to strong anti-cholinergic and sedating properties; and benzodiazapines (long acting).

A study by Berenson (2000) indicated that 40% of benzodiazapine prescriptions are written for the elderly. In a study of homebound older adults, Golden and colleagues (1999) found that benzodiazapines were the second most commonly prescribed medication and that many older adults were prescribed two different benzodiazapines, with many prescriptions exceeding the recommended dosages. The greatest concern in the study by Golden et al. was the use of benzo-diazapines and their role as a risk factor for falls and hip fractures. Additionally, the Golden study found that 7.6% of older adults were prescribed more than one type of benzodiazapine at the same time. Several studies have found that benzodiazapines contribute to mental status changes and falls that result in serious injury and incontinence. This occurs due to their long du-ration of action because of diminished drug metabolism in the elderly. Benzodiazapines should also be used with caution in the elderly; long-acting benzodiazapines should be avoided due to risk of accumulation and toxicity (Beers, 1997).

Gastrointestinal complaints are one of the most common reasons for primary care visits. H2-receptor histamine antagonists are commonly prescribed to the elderly population for a variety of gastrointestinal symptoms. Cimetidine was the first H2-receptor antagonist to be released and is a cytochrome P-450 enzyme inhibitor. It reduces the metabolism of drugs such as phenytoin, carbamazepine, theophylline, warfarin, and quinidine. As a result, the half-life of these drugs can be increased when used in conjunction with cimetidine.

Ranitidine has a similar but weaker effect. Close monitoring and dose adjustment may be necessary. The other H2 antagonists do not exhibit this enzyme inhabitation, and thus would not be expected to interact with the previously described medications. These drugs have a rather be-nign side-effect profile (Chutka, Evans, Fleming, & Mikkelson, 1995). Gastrointestinal anti-spasmodic drugs are highly anticholinergic and generally produce toxic effects in the elderly. These include Bentyl, Levsin, Probanthine, and Librax.

In 2003, Juurlink and collegues examined common drug-to-drug interactions among the el-derly that resulted in hospitalizations for drug toxicity. They found that patients with diabetes treated with sulfonylureas such as glyburide are at risk for hypoglycemia when taking sulfon-amide antibiotics such as cotrimoxazole. In patients taking angiotensin-converting enzyme (ACE) inhibitors and a potassium-sparing diuretic, this combination was found to cause poten-tially life-threatening hyperkalemia (Juurlink et al., 2003).

DISTINGUISHING ADRS FROM GERIATRIC SYNDROMES

The term *geriatric syndrome* refers to a complex of symptoms with high prevalence among older people. Geriatric syndromes result from multiple diseases and/or multiple risk factors. One rea-son providers fail to recognize ADRs in the elderly is that they may produce similar symptoms as other common geriatric syndromes. These common symptoms include urinary incontinence, falls, and cognitive changes.

Drug-Induced Urinary Incontinence

Urinary incontinence is the involuntary leakage of urine from the urethra. Transient incon-tinence is a reversible form of incontinence caused by problems outside the urinary tract. Transient incontinence caused by medication is called *drug-induced incontinence*. Alpha blockers are one class of drugs that can affect continence. Stress incontinence has been reported in women taking certain antipsychotics (e.g., thioridazine, clozapine, chlorpromazine, haloperidol). Antidepressants and antihistamines can make urinary incontinence symptoms worse and decrease flow rates in men. Diuretics are known to precipitate or worsen incontinence in all patients.

In evaluating the cause of a new onset of incontinence, it is important to determine if the person has started any new medications or stopped any medications prior to the new onset of incontinence. Nurses also have a role in determining if urinary tract infection or other serious underlying conditions and possible causes may exist. In addition, it is essential to evaluate for comorbid disease and functional ability.

Drug-Induced Falls

Falls are one of the most common, and often most serious, problems facing elderly persons. Falling is associated with considerable mortality, morbidity, reduced functioning, and premature nursing home admissions (American Geriatrics Society, 2001). In the United States, falls are the leading cause of accidental death and the seventh leading cause of death overall in persons over the age of 65 (Beers & Berkow, 2000). The use of drugs is a major risk factor for falls, and the risk of falling increases as the number of medications taken increases (Leipzeg, Cumming, & Tinetti, 1999).

The Guidelines on the Prevention of Falls in Older Persons published in the *Journal of the American Geriatrics Society* (2001) indicate that for all settings (community, long-term care, hospital, and rehabilitation), there are consistent associations between the use of psychotropic medications (neuroleptics, benzodiazapines, and antidepressants) and increased falls. Miller (2002) found that the rate of falls among nursing home residents who were current benzodiazapine users increased 44% on average, compared to patients who were not prescribed these medications, and that the risk of falls was greatest when they first began taking the medication or as doses were increased. Cooper (1996) found that the combination of a benzodiazepine and an antipsychotic medication contributed to falls in elderly patients.

Cardiac, Analgesic, and Antihypertensive Drugs

In a meta-analysis by Leipzig et al. (1999), cardiac and analgesic drugs (such as digoxin, antiarrhythmics, and diuretics) were less likely to be associated with an increased risk of falls in older adults. However, older adults taking more than one antihypertensive drug were found to have an increased risk of falls.

Over-the-Counter Medications

According to Gordon (2000), over-the-counter (OTC) medications have the potential to contribute to the risk of falls due to their effects on psychomotor function and their potential interaction with other medications. Many OTC preparations for pain, colds, and sleep contain alcohol or anticholinergic agents, both of which increase the risk of falls. The anticholinergic agent diphenhydramine is a commonly used ingredient in OTC products and has been associated with an increased risk of falls.

Miller (2002) reported that although studies have identified hundreds of medications that can contribute to falls, not all conclusions with respect to specific medications are consistent.

Because it is impossible to memorize every medication, nurses must cautiously examine what receptors the medication interacts with and the potential effect of that mechanism on the risk of falls. Studies indicate that the use of more than three or four medications is associated with an increased risk of recurrent falling (Leipzeg, Cumming, & Tinetti, 1999).

Drug-Induced Cognitive Impairments

Drug-induced changes in mental status can generally be categorized into two types: delirium and dementia. Drug-induced delirium is an acute confusional state, whereas drug-induced dementia is a more chronic change in mental status. Delirium is a syndrome characterized by disturbance in consciousness (with reduced clarity of awareness of the environment) and change in cognition, including alteration in attention, disorganized thinking, disturbed psychomotor activity, and an abnormal sleep-wake cycle. In studies of elderly hospital patients, drugs have been reported as the cause of delirium in 11 to 30% of cases; medication toxicity occurs in 2 to 12% of patients presenting with suspected dementia (Moore & O'Keefe, 1999).

Nearly every drug class can cause either drug-induced delirium or dementia in older persons. The elderly may be especially prone to developing drug-induced cognitive impairment due to age-related changes in drug pharmacokinetics and pharmacodynamics. The elderly are also at greater risk of drug-induced confusion than younger people because of decreased functional reserve of the CNS due to changes in brain perfusion, changes in neurotransmitter systems.

Due to the potential for severe CNS-adverse reactions, the Health Care Financing Administration developed new guidelines on medications with potential for adverse outcomes. These medications include pentazocine, long-acting benzodiazepines, amitriptyline, doxepin, meprobamate, disopyramide, digoxin, methyldopa, chlorpropamide (if hypoglycemia results), gastrointestinal antispasmodic drugs, and barbiturates.

Anticholinergic medications are important causes of acute and chronic confusional states. Nevertheless, polypharmacy with anticholinergic compounds is common, especially in nursing home residents. Recent studies have suggested that the total burden of anticholinergic drugs may determine development of delirium rather than any single agent. Also, anticholinergic effects have been identified in many drugs other than those classically thought of as having major anticholinergic effects (Moore & O'Keefe, 1999).

Psychoactive drugs are important causes of delirium. Narcotic agents are among the most important causes of delirium in postoperative patients. Long-acting benzodiazepines are the most common drugs to cause or exacerbate dementia. Delirium was a major complication of treatment with tricyclic antidepressants, but seems less common with newer agents. Anticonvulsants can cause delirium and dementia.

Drug-induced confusion with nonpsychoactive drugs is often idiosyncratic in nature, and the diagnosis is easily missed unless clinicians maintain a high index of suspicion. Histamine H2-receptor antagonists; cardiac medications, such as digoxin and beta-blockers; corticosteroids; NSAIDs; and antibiotics can all cause acute, and, less commonly, chronic, confusion.

Centrally acting sympathetic antihypertensive agents, sedating antipsychotic drugs, opioids, digitalis, anti-Parkinsonian drugs, antidepressants, and corticosteroids also are associated with greater risk relative to other classes of medications. Drug-induced confusion can be limited by avoiding polypharmacy and adhering to the approach of "start low and go slow." This approach is aimed at initiating lower doses to elders and increasing doses at a slower rate if medication goals are not reached. Special care is needed when prescribing for people with cognitive impairment. Early diagnosis of drug-induced confusion and withdrawal of the offending agent or agents is essential.

APPLICATION OF THE NEUMAN SYSTEMS MODEL

Betty Neuman developed the Neuman Systems Model in the 1970s as a teaching tool for nursing students. The aim of the model is to provide nurses with a structure and an analytical framework for assessment and interventions to reduce stressors and maintain or restore a client to a state of wellness. The model was based on Neuman's framework that included the theories and philosophic approaches of other experts in stress and illness. The Neuman Model is based on systems theory and the concepts of stress and reactions to stress; the person is viewed as a multidimensional whole, in constant dynamic interaction with the environment (Neuman & Fawcett, 2002).

The Neuman Model (Neuman, 1990, 1995; Neuman & Fawcett, 2002; Neuman & Young, 1972) examines the impact of stressors on health. A stressor is any force that can potentially affect a person's health. Stressors may be intrapersonal, for example, emotions and feelings; interpersonal, for example, role expectations; or extrapersonal, for example, job or financial pressures.

Neuman sees the person as a multidimensional, whole, dynamic system with interrelationships between five variables or factors: physiological, those related to structures of the body; psychological, those related to mental processes and relationships; sociocultural, those functions that relate to social and cultural expectations; developmental, those processes related to growth and development; and spiritual beliefs, the belief in a higher power influencing one's life. Attaining balance, harmony, and wellness through these five variables is the desired outcome of nursing interventions and the basis for utilizing the model.

Neuman (1995) represents the Neuman Systems Model as a series of concentric circles. Within the model, the person has a basic core structure, comprising survival mechanisms, including organ function, temperature control, genetic structure, response patterns, and ego, and what are termed *knowns* and *commonalities*. This core is protected by lines of resistance: the normal lines of defense and the flexible lines of defense. The lines of resistance surround the basic core structure and are activated by invasion of the normal line of defense by stressors. The lines of resistance aim to protect the core structure and maintain homeostasis of the system to keep the individual at baseline functioning. The normal line of defense represents the person's level of wellness or baseline functioning. When the normal line of defense is penetrated and rendered ineffective, the person will present with symptoms of instability or illness. The flexible line of defense represented in the Neuman model acts as a buffer to the person's stable or baseline level of functioning. Ideally, this line of defense prevents stressor invasions of the person, keeping the system free from stressor reactions and symptomatology. Essentially it acts to prevent stressors from impacting the health of the individual (Neuman & Fawcett, 2002).

Neuman defines nursing as actions that assist individuals, families, and groups to maintain a maximum level of wellness. The primary aim of nursing is stability of the patient–client system through nursing interventions to reduce stressors. The Neuman Model (Found on: http://www.neumann.edu/academics/undergrd/nursing/model.asp, Neuman Systems Model Home Page, 2005) categorizes interventions by nurses as primary, secondary, and tertiary. The goal of *primary prevention* is to promote client wellness by preventing stressors and reducing risk factors, thus protecting and maintaining the client's baseline functioning. The goal of *secondary prevention* is to provide appropriate treatment of symptoms to attain optimal client system stability or wellness; treatment would occur following symptoms. Maximizing the client's internal and external resources would be considered in an attempt to strengthen internal lines of resistance, thus reducing the reaction. The goal of *tertiary prevention* is to maintain wellness after treatment. Essentially, the prevention strategies in the Newman Model are necessary to retain, attain, and maintain the health and stability of the client.

DISCUSSION

Gerontology nurses can use the Neuman Systems Model as a tool in the care of the elderly patient. The Neuman Systems Model is a wellness model, and as such it views aging as a normal process rather than as an abnormal disease state. Despite the issues of loss and change in function that often accompany aging, the older person is viewed as healthy within Neuman's Model. The Neuman physiological wellness component can be conceptualized as a loss of flexibility and buffering ability in the lines of defense. These losses represent a change in the ability to fend off the effects of stressors. For the sake of this discussion, the stressor is an ADR experienced by older person.

In the elderly, the lines of defense and the lines of resistance may be weakened due to pharmacotherapy and the potential for adverse drug reactions. This problem may manifest in an elderly person with symptoms in the form of toxic effects of medications, alteration in cognitive function, increased instability, falls, and various other symptoms. The role of the nurse in gerontology practice is to examine the patient holistically, consider which medications may be causing adverse symptoms, identify nursing actions to be taken, and initiate appropriate treatment interventions. Sometimes the intervention may be eliminating the medication or substituting medications.

Nurses must be cognizant of the importance of the aging process and its potential influence on adverse drug reactions. In addition, nurses must become familiar with the effects of aging on medications and implement strategies to avoid adverse drug reactions. Also, advanced practice nurses must be educated about improving prescribing practices for the elderly population.

Recent literature suggests that as many as 28% of hospitalizations of elderly patients are related to adverse drug reactions (Conry, 2000). Approximately 95% of these ADRs are preventable. Gurwitz and colleagues (2003) examined the incidence and preventability of adverse drug reactions among elderly patients in an ambulatory clinical setting. In their study, 26% of ADRs were found to be preventable, and of these, 38% were considered life-threatening. These preventable adverse drug reactions occurred at the prescribing and monitoring stages of treatment in more than 80% of the cases. The results of these studies highlight the importance of careful prescribing and patient education. Drawing on these studies and the review of literature in this chapter, the following recommendations for preventing adverse drug reactions in the elderly can be made.

RECOMMENDATIONS FOR NURSING

The elderly are vulnerable to ADRs for a number of reasons. These include coexisting conditions and complex medication regimes, as well as changes in pharmacodynamics, pharmackinetics, and polypharmacy. Because of this vulnerability, it is necessary to have a comprehensive approach to the history and physical examination of the elderly client.

Nurses should examine medication management in elders within the framework of the "start low, go slow" approach. When prescribing for the elderly, it is often most appropriate to start most drugs at half the usual dose. Doses that may still be in the normal range for younger patients may be toxic for elderly patients. When reviewing lab results, the nurse should keep in mind that therapeutic windows narrow with age.

When it comes to prescriptions, nurses should try to "keep it simple." Ways to do this include prescribing drugs that need only be taken once daily and changing to a single combination pill instead of adding an additional pill. Conducting a comprehensive medication history with every new patient and encouraging all patients to bring in all of their medications at least quarterly (known as "brown bagging it") are critical. In particular, if different clinicians are prescribing for elders, careful review is needed. The medication review should include all OTC products (including vitamins, herbal remedies, and health foods). Nurses must be alert for duplicate medications from the same drug class. When performing home visits, nurses must ask patients to gather up all of their medications and then ask them to point out which ones they take and when. The nurse must also be alert for patients' stockpiling of medications.

Patient Education

The most important preventative measure against ADRs in older adults is patient education. Patient education can enhance the flexible lines of defense within the Neuman Systems Model. Patient education may require sufficient time to help patients become more adept at self-care and medication management, thus enhancing the flexible lines of defense. It is always helpful to provide information to patients in writing, especially when new medications are added to their regime or when medications are discontinued. Any changes in dosages and timing should be written down for the patient. Most importantly, the patient should be informed of what side effects to expect and what effects could be life-threatening. The patient and the family should know which signs and symptoms should be reported immediately and which ones can wait until the next visit.

Reviewing medication adherence during each visit with a patient is essential. The rate of noncompliance has been estimated to be between 25 and 59% in the elderly, and 50% in the elderly with chronic conditions (Berenson, 2000). The nurse should ask whether the patient is experiencing any side effects and whether he or she is taking the medications as prescribed. If side effects are present, the nurse should advise the patient on strategies to reduce their impact. Other important questions that the nurse should inquire about are whether the patient is having any difficulty remembering when to take medications. It is also important to discourage patients from doubling up on doses of certain medications if a dose is missed.

Finally, patients should be asked if they have difficulty paying for medications or if they have transportation to get their prescriptions filled. Patients should be encouraged to use only one pharmacy or mail-order company whenever possible. Most major drug chains are computerized and have medications flagged for certain reactions. When multiple pharmacies or mail-order companies are used, pharmacists may not be able to detect ADRs.

CONCLUSION

This chapter addressed the importance of nursing practice in the medication management of elders. The Neuman Systems Model provides the framework for considering the lines of defense that exist for elderly patients who are taking medications. Recommendations for nurses include the following: being knowledgeable about aging-related changes and medications; being alert to appropriate medications for the elderly and knowing which ones should be avoided; reducing polypharmacy and keeping regimes as simple as possible; conducting comprehensive medication reviews with patients; and communicating effectively verbally and in writing about medications and potential side effects.

The Neuman Systems Model is a useful tool for the nurse to use in the evaluation and treatment of the elderly with a variety of conditions. The Neuman Systems Model can be used to evaluate the stressors that may be occurring in an elder and the potential influence of pharmacotherapy. Stressors may be extrapersonal, such as a lack of financial resources to purchase medications. Stressors may also be interpersonal, such as the elderly patient's disagreements with the nurse or family members about medication treatment or adherence. Stressors may also be intrapersonal, such as an elder who may not recognize symptoms of memory loss, thus not remembering to take medications and perhaps being reluctant to share this information with others, or who is not fully aware of his or her memory loss issues.

Finally, the application of theoretical frameworks or models to the nursing care of the gerontology patient is important. In this chapter, the use of the Neuman Model provided the analysis for a systems approach for medication management in the elderly. Lines of defense—whether intrapersonal, interpersonal, or extrapersonal—are critical to consider when challenged by the possibility of ADRs in the elderly.

REFERENCES

American Geriatrics Society. (2001). Guidelines for the prevention of falls in older persons. *Journal of the American Geriatrics Society, 49*(5), 664–672.

Beers, M. (1997). Explicit criteria for determining potentially inappropriate medication use by the elderly: An update. *Archives of Internal Medicine, 157*(14), 1531–1536.

Beers, M., & Berkow, R. (2000). *The Merck manual of geriatrics* (Rev. ed.). Whitehouse Station, NJ: Merck Research Laboratories.

Berenson, L. D. (2000). Polypharmacy in the elderly. Retrieved November 10, 2003, from http://www.nsweb.nursingspectrum.com/ce/ce214.htm.

Chutka, D. S., Evans, J. M., Fleming, K. C., & Mikkelson, K. P. (1995). Drug prescribing for elderly patients. *Mayo Clinic Proceedings, 70*(7), 685–693.

Conry, M. (2000). Polypharmacy: Pandora's medicine chest? *Geriatric Times, 1*(3). Retrieved November 20, 2003 from http://www.geriatrictimes.com/g001028.html.

Fuller, G. (2000). Falls in the elderly. American Academy of Family Physicians. Retrieved November 20, 2003, from http://www.aafp.org/afp/20000401/2159.html.

Golden, A., Preston, R., Barnett, S., Llorente, M., Hamdan, K., & Silverman, M. (1999). Inappropriate medication prescribing in homebound older adults. *Journal of the American Geriatrics Society, 47*(8), 948–953.

Gordon, A., Preston, R., Barnett, S., Llorente, M., Hamdan, K., & Silverman, M. (1999). Inappropriate medication prescribing in homebound older adults. *Journal of the American Geriatrics Society, 47*(8), 948–953.

Gurwitz, J., Field, T., Harold, L., Rothschild, J., Debellis, K., Seger, A., et al. (2003). Incidence and preventability of adverse drug reactions among older persons in the ambulatory setting. *Journal of the American Medical Association, 289*(9), 1107–1116.

Hanlon, J. T., Schmadel, K. E., Ruby, C. M., & Weinberger, M. (2001). Suboptimal prescribing in older inpatients and outpatients. *Journal of the American Geriatrics Society, 49*(2), 200–209.

Juurlink, D. N., Mamdani, M., Kopp, A., Laupacis, A., & Redelmeier, D. A. (2003). Drug–drug interactions among elderly patients hospitalized for drug toxicity. *Journal of the American Medical Association, 289*(13), 1652–1658.

Larsen, P. D., & Hoot Martin, J. L. (1999). Polypharmacy and elderly patients. *The Association of Perioperative Registered Nurses, 69*(3), 619–622.

Leipzeg, R., Cumming, R., & Tinetti, M. (1999). Drugs and falls in older people: A systematic review and metaanalysis. Cardiac and analgesic drugs. *Journal of the American Geriatrics Society, 47*(1), 40–50.

Miller, C. (2002). The connection between drugs and falls in elders. *Geriatric Nursing, 23*(2), 109–110.

Moore, A., & O'Keefe, S. (1999). Drug-induced cognitive impairment in the elderly. *Drugs Aging, 15*(1), 15–28.

Neuman, B. (1990). The Neuman Systems Model: A theory for practice. In M. E. Parker (Ed.), *Nursing theories in practice*. New York: National League for Nursing.

Neuman, B. (1995). *The Neuman Systems Model* (3rd ed.). Stamford, CT: Appleton & Lange.

Neuman, B., & Fawcett, J. (2002). *The Neuman Systems Model* (4th ed., Rev.). Upper Saddle, NJ: Prentice Hall.

Neuman, B., & Young, R. J. (1972). The Betty Neuman Model: A total person approach to viewing patient problems. *Nursing Research, 21*(3), 385–394.

Routledge, P. A., O'Mahony, M. S., & Woodhouse, K. W. (2003). Adverse drug reactions in elderly patients. *British Journal of Clinical Pharmacology, 57*(2), 121–126.

U.S. Department of Health and Human Services. (2000). Health People 2010: Understanding and Improving Health. Washington, D.C.: U.S. Government Printing Office.

CHAPTER 21

Delirium in the Hospitalized Older Adult: Development of a Delirium Risk Stratification Tool

Deborah A. Rosenbloom-Brunto

Delirium is a potentially reversible disturbance in consciousness, characterized by an acute onset and fluctuating course of impaired cognitive functioning (American Psychiatric Association, 1999). It is the most frequent complication in hospitalized older adults, occurring in up to 60% (Inouye, Bogardus, et al., 1999). Delirium is associated with increased length of hospitalization, functional decline, the need for subsequent institutionalization, and increased morbidity and mortality (Inouye, Schlesinger, & Lyndon, 1999). Multiple system illnesses, comorbidities, the use of psychoactive medications, and age place the older hospitalized adult at risk for developing delirium. Although in the past delirium has been viewed as a transient disorder, evidence shows that symptoms can persist long after hospital discharge, affecting rehabilitation, cognition, and independent functioning (O'Keeffe & Lavan, 1997). Despite the availability of tools to identify delirium (Hart, Best, & Sessler, 1997; Inouye et al., 1990; Pompei, Foreman, & Cassel, 1995; Trzepacz, Baker, & Greenhouse, 1987), delirium remains unrecognized by the clinician in as many as 66 to 84% of patients experiencing this complication and is often incorrectly attributed to dementia, depression, or a normal consequence of aging (Inouye, 1994). Prevention and early detection of delirium with implementation of appropriate interventions can directly affect the older adult's hospital course and outcome.

Palmateer and McCartney (1985) and Foreman (1993) found that because nurses have insufficient knowledge about cognitive deficits, delirium is often not recognized in hospitalized patients. Eden and Foreman (1996) identified lack of knowledge on the part of nurses and physicians regarding the diagnostic and testing methods for detecting delirium and ineffective communication between staff members in relaying symptoms marking the onset of delirium as significant factors in the underrecognition of delirium. This discussion will address defining characteristics, etiology, risk factors, and management of delirium in the hospitalized older adult. It will also propose an assessment tool that can be used in the acute care setting to identify individuals at high risk for developing acute confusion. This tool may be useful to assist direct care providers in prevention, early recognition, and management of delirium as an acute complication of hospitalization in the older adult.

BACKGROUND

Defining Characteristics of Cognitive Disturbances

Delirium

Delirium is an acute disorder of attention and cognition that is characterized by a variety of clinical features. A continuum of symptoms ranging from minimal clouding of consciousness to global cognitive impairment to psychosis can develop (Meagher et al., 2000). Impairments range from quiet disorientation to agitation. In *The Diagnostic and Statistical Manual for Mental Disorders, Fourth Edition* (DSM-IV), the American Psychiatric Association (1994) describes delirium as being characterized by alterations in cognition, attention, sleep-wake patterns, and psychomotor activity. The DSM-IV criteria for delirium are outlined in Appendix A. Changes in cognition directly affect the individual's ability to acquire, process, store, and retrieve information about self, body, and the surrounding environment. Clinical manifestations may be subtle and fluctuate during the course of the day, which compounds assessment and identification. A patient may be lethargic with slow response time during one encounter and hours later be restless and agitated.

Delirium can be characterized as having three motoric subtypes: (1) hyperactive–hyperalert, (2) hypoactive–hypoalert, and (3) mixed (Meagher et al., 2000; O'Keeffe & Lavan, 1997; Sandberg et al.,1999). Hyperactive–hyperalert patients demonstrate increased psychomotor activity in the form of rapid speech, restlessness, agitation, and irritability. The more common clinical presentation of delirium is the hypoactive–hypoalert subtype, which manifests with lethargy, slowed speech, decreased alertness, and decreased psychomotor activity. Such patients are often overlooked or misdiagnosed because they are not disruptive. The diagnosis is further complicated by those patients who manifest fluctuating symptoms, changing from hyperalert to hypoalert during the course of a delirious episode, and thus are classified as having mixed symptomatology. Delirium remains unrecognized by the clinician in as many as 66 to 84% of patients due to its variability and may be incorrectly attributed to dementia, depression, or an expected consequence of aging (Inouye, Schlesinger, & Lyndon, 1999).

Dementia

Most older adults with the chronic confusion of dementia are alert and able to maintain attention until later in the progression of the disease. Dementia is characterized by an insidious onset and progressive course of impairment in short- and long-term memory; loss of judgment, impulse control, and abstract thinking abilities; and changes in personality and behavior that often are irreversible (APA, 1994). Attention span is typically intact until late in the chronic course. Comprehensive scales of cognitive function, such as the Alzheimer's Disease Assessment Scale-Cognitive subscale (ADAS-cog, where lower scores signify higher cognitive functioning), can provide objective data for an accurate diagnosis (Panisset, Stern, & Gauthier, 1996). Dementia is often not diagnosed due to the prevalent bias that cognitive changes are an expected consequence of aging (Livingston, 1994). In contrast, delirium is manifested as an abrupt onset of reduced ability to maintain and shift attention, typically with an identifiable and reversible cause.

Depression

In depression, symptoms such as apathy, changes in mood, and slowed speech may mimic the clinical picture seen in the hypoalert variant of delirium (APA, 1999). The depressed older adult may also present with symptoms suggesting dementia, such as memory loss, distractibility, disorientation, and apathy. The hallmarks that distinguish depression are dysphoric mood and loss of pleasure in usual activities (APA, 1994).

Older adults are particularly at risk for depression due to situational factors such as bereavement and changes in health status or functional capacity. Between 10 to 15% of older adults have significant depressive symptomatology (Beekman, Copeland, & Prince, 1999). The presentation of depression in older adults may be atypical. Low mood may be masked, and anxiety or memory impairment may be the principal presenting symptoms (Rosenstein, 1998). A number of scales are available to measure depressive symptoms, the most widely used being the Hamilton Depression Rating Scale (Hamilton, 1960) and the Beck Depression Inventory (Beck, 1972). These tools may not be ideal for screening older adults for depression because they include a number of somatic items that may be positive in older adults who are not depressed (Rosenstein, 1998). Specific scales for older adults such as the Geriatric Depression Scale (Yesavage et al., 1983) avoid somatic items and can help improve detection of or rule out depression as the etiology of cognitive changes in the older adult.

Functional Psychoses

This psychiatric disorder is diagnosed based on the presence of positive symptoms, such as systematic and persistent delusions, hallucinations, disorganized speech and behavior, and the presence of negative symptoms, such as flat affect and avolition, that last for at least one month (APA, 1994). An insidious onset of symptoms typically occurs in early adult life, and relapse rates after treatment are high (Andreasen, 1999). A family history of psychotic disorders is often present. The affected individual experiences social and occupational dysfunction as a result of the disturbances in thought processes and perception and impaired coping. In contrast, the false beliefs or sensory perceptions that may be present in the older adult suffering from delirium are transient and lack a recurrent pattern.

Etiology of Delirium

Risk factors can be divided into predisposing and precipitating factors (Inouye & Charpentier, 1996). Predisposing factors are present at the time of the admission and reflect the baseline vulnerability of a patient. Precipitating factors are noxious insults or hospital-related factors that contribute to the development of delirium. Patients with high vulnerability to delirium may develop delirium with any precipitating factor, even if it is minor, but those with low vulnerability are resistant to the development of delirium even with noxious insults. Investigations over the past decade have identified numerous risk factors for delirium, as shown in Appendix B (APA, 1999; Inouye et al., 1993; Inouye & Charpentier, 1996; O'Keeffe, 1996). These studies have concluded that the most powerful risks for developing delirium are present before admission and include preexisting cognitive impairment, infection, age, and self-reported alcohol abuse.

The etiologic basis of delirium in the older hospitalized adult is multifactorial comprising physiologic, psychologic, nutritional, and environmental influences. Physiologic factors have been found to be the major contributor to the development of delirium in older hospitalized adults (Inouye & Charpentier, 1996). Physiologic factors can be divided into four categories: (1) primary cerebral diseases (e.g., meningitis), (2) systemic diseases that affect the brain (e.g., electrolyte imbalance/dehydration), (3) exogenous toxic substances (e.g., medication toxicity), and (4) substance withdrawal (e.g., from medications or alcohol intake).

Medication toxicity is a leading cause of delirium in older adults (Inouye & Charpentier, 1996). Psychoactive drugs have been found to be the leading iatrogenic cause of delirium. Benzodiazepines, narcotics, and other psychoactive drugs are associated with 3 to 11 times increased risk for delirium (Inouye, Schlesinger, & Lyndon, 1999). The number and rate of increasing psychoactive medication increases the risk of delirium by 4 to 10 times. In older adults, benzodiazepines have been associated with increased confusion and oversedation (Hassan, Fontaine, & Nearman, 1998). Extreme variability exists in the pharmacokinetics of these agents according to age, ethnicity, drug metabolizing ability, and drug excretion. The half-life of narcotics can increase sixfold in acutely ill elderly patients (Francis, 1996). In 1999, the American Psychiatric Association published Practice Guidelines for the Diagnosis and Treatment of Delirium, which included a list of the most common substances that can cause delirium through intoxication or withdrawal, as shown in Appendix C.

Management of Delirium

There are several approaches in the management of delirium. These include: primary prevention, secondary prevention, creating a safe environment, restorative care, and managing behavioral disturbances.

Primary Prevention

In a 1999 study of 852 general medical patients over the age of 70, strategies for primary prevention of delirium resulted in a 40% reduction in the odds of developing delirium (Inouye et al., 1999). The protocol in this study focused on risk factor reduction via the following measures: repeated reorientation of the patient, provision of cognitively stimulating activities, nonpharmacologic sleep protocol to enhance normalization of the sleep-wake cycles, early mobilization activities and range of motion exercises, timely removal of catheters and restraints, and early correction of dehydration. These strategies can also be used to reduce the duration of identified delirium and prevent its complications.

Secondary Prevention

Treatment goals for delirium management are aimed at eliminating the sources of the delirium and ensuring that the older adult remains safe and comfortable until the delirium is resolved. General areas of patient management involve interpreting reality, maintaining normalcy, meeting basic needs, and managing behavioral disturbances. Patients with delirium are often very active and agitated, and patient safety can prevent challenges for providers. These patients are the ones who remove treatment lines most often in an effort to free themselves from an uncomfortable stimulus (Foreman, Wakefield, Culp, & Milisen, 2001).

Creating a Safe Environment

Because patients with delirium are easily disoriented, a comfortable environment and a predictable schedule can be therapeutic. Targeted interventions, including frequent reorientation and the presence of familiar objects from home, can help to support the delirious older adult (Kahn et al., 1998). Visual orientation cues, such as accurate clocks and calendars, can also be helpful. Sensory awareness should be reinforced by the patient wearing eyeglasses or hearing aides as usual. The patient should be in a room that can be observed closely by members of the healthcare team. Bright lights should be avoided during the day, and a night light or bathroom light should be used at nighttime. Stimuli, including visitors, may need to be minimized with agitated, hyperactive patients, whereas the hypoactive, withdrawn patient will need additional stimuli.

Restorative Care

Neurologic dysfunction can compromise the older adult's ability to achieve full recovery and independence following hospitalization (Dyson, 1999). During the acute care stay, the older adult who develops delirium may require assistance with some or all of the activities of daily living, including eating and drinking, urination and defecation, bathing and skin care, and range of motion or ambulation. As with all patients, a maximal level of independence and functioning should be encouraged with assistance as necessary. All procedures, activities, and any changes in the patient's routine or environment should be explained explicitly.

Managing Behavioral Disturbances

Pharmacological approaches to managing delirium and associated agitation should be used only after giving adequate attention to correction of modifiable contributing factors. It is essential to realize that delirium could be a manifestation of an acute life-threatening problem that requires immediate attention, such as hypoxia, hyperglycemia, hypoglycemia, or metabolic derangements. After such concerns have been addressed, severely agitated patients should be considered for pharmacological management of delirium in order to prevent injury to the patient or others.

Benzodiazepines, which are used most commonly in the treatment of anxiety, are not recommended for the management of delirium because of the likelihood of oversedation, exacerbation of confusion, respiratory suppression, and prolongation of the confusional state; however, they remain the drug of choice for delirium tremens and seizures (Fraser et al., 2000; Riker, Fraser, & Cox, 1994). The amnesic qualities of benzodiazepines make these agents especially useful when noxious or unpleasant procedures are required. In certain populations, including the elderly, patients with underlying dementia, and those already suffering from delirium, benzodiazepines can lead to increased confusion and agitation.

Haloperidol is the neuroleptic agent most widely used to treat delirium in the acute care setting (Fraser et al., 2000). Potential advantages of haloperidol include the fact that it does not suppress the respiratory drive and that it is largely nonsedating. The drug is usually well tolerated from both the hemodynamic and the respiratory standpoint. The incidence of paradoxical reactions with haloperidol versus lorazepam has been shown to be significantly less (Riker, Fraser, & Cox, 1994). Side effects to consider include hypotension; acute dystonia; extrapyramidal effects; and anticholinergic effects, such as dry mouth, constipation, and urinary retention. The most dangerous potential adverse effect of using high-dose haloperidol is torsades de pointes, a potentially lethal ventricular arrhythmia, which is characterized by a prolonged QT interval.

Screening Tools

Several instruments have been developed to screen patients for signs and symptoms of delirium. These instruments have been reviewed from different perspectives (Foreman, 1993; Levkoff et al., 1991; McDougall, 1990; Rapp et al., 2000). The Clinical Assessment of Confusion (CAC-A) (Versmeech, 1990), the Confusion Rating Scale (CRS) (Williams et al., 1979), and the NEECHAM Confusion Scale (Neelon, Champagne, Carlson, & Funk, 1996) were developed for use in clinical nursing practice. All were developed based on criteria identified by nurses as symptoms of acute confusion. The CAC-A, a 25-item observational scale, has shown low sensitivity (0.36) for delirium (Pompei et al., 1994, 1995). The CRS, a 4-item observational scale, has shown moderate validity and sensitivity and is recommended as an initial screening tool (Williams et al., 1979). The NEECHAM Confusion Scale is a 9-item observation-rated scale with good validity and reliability, but it does not differentiate between acute and chronic cognitive impairment.

The Confusion Assessment Method (CAM) was developed for use by trained nurses and physicians to improve the assessment of delirium in nonpsychiatric settings (Inouye et al., 1990). The CAM has four features: (1) an acute onset of mental status changes and a fluctuating course, (2) inattention, (3) disorganized thinking, and (4) a level of consciousness other than alert. Patients are determined to be delirious, or CAM positive, if they have both features 1 and 2 and either 3 or 4. The CAM is the most widely implemented and user-friendly method of objectively measuring delirium, and it has a sensitivity of 94 to 100%, a specificity between 90 and 95%, and excellent interobserver reliability (Inouye et al., 1990). The CAM has been compared to other instruments by external reviewers and has been found to have the best combination of ease, speed of use, data acquisition, reliability, and validity (Smith, Breitbart, & Meredith, 1995; Trzepacz et al., 1987). Despite the availability of a number of screening tools for delirium, inconsistent use in the acute care setting continues to be the norm (Martin & Haynes, 2000).

Application of the Neuman Systems Model

The Neuman Systems Model proposed by Betty Neuman is a dynamic, open systems approach to patient care in which nursing is concerned with the whole person (Neuman, 1982, 1990, 1995; Neuman & Fawcett, 2002). The patient is a dynamic composite of interrelationships among physical, psychological, sociocultural, developmental, and spiritual factors. Each individual is an open system in reciprocal interaction with the environment with a goal of maintaining system stability (Neuman & Fawcett, 2002). The person, with a core of basic structures, is seen as being in constant, dynamic interaction with the environment. Around the basic core structures are lines of defense and resistance that protect the individual's psyche.

The model is based on theories of stress adaptation and on Gestalt theory, and views the person as being a multidimensional whole in constant dynamic interaction with the environment (Neuman & Fawcett, 2002). The role of the nurse is seen in terms of degrees of reactions to stressors and the use of primary, secondary, and tertiary interventions to maintain the stability of the system. The Neuman Systems Model encourages the nurse to be an active participant with the client and aware of all of the variables affecting an individual's response to stressors (Neuman, 1982, 1990, 1995; Neuman & Fawcett, 2002).

Nursing

Neuman (1982) defines *nursing* as actions that assist individuals, families, and groups to maintain a maximum level of wellness. The primary goal of nursing is to assist in the retention, attainment, or maintenance of client system stability through nursing interventions to reduce stressors. Nursing is prevention as intervention (Neuman, 1995; Neuman & Fawcett, 2002; Neuman Systems Model Home Page, 2005). Nursing interventions via primary, secondary, and tertiary prevention can strengthen flexible lines of defense and resistance to stressors, and promote adaptation. Primary prevention relates to identification and reduction of possible or actual risk factors associated with environmental stressors before a reaction has occurred. Secondary prevention refers to treatment after the development of symptoms to reduce noxious effects and to attain optimal client system stability. Tertiary prevention involves maintaining optimal wellness and supporting existing strengths following treatment. Neuman pointed out that more than one prevention modality can be used at a time. This reflects the nursing profession's concern with all of the variables affecting an individual's response to stress.

Person

Neuman sees the person as being a multidimensional, whole, dynamic system with interrelationships between five primary variables (Neuman, 1982, 1990, 1995; Neuman & Fawcett, 2002). These variables are physical, psychological, sociocultural, developmental, and spiritual. The person has a basic core structure comprised of survival mechanisms, including organ function, temperature control, genetic structure, and ego development. The flexible lines of defense and lines of resistance function to protect the core. The person is seen as being in a state of constant change in reciprocal interaction with the environment.

Health

Neuman sees health as being equated with wellness. She has described health as a state in which all variables are in balance (Neuman, 1982, 1990, 1995; Neuman & Fawcett, 2002). Because the person is in constant interaction with the environment, the person's state of wellness is in dynamic equilibrium rather than a steady state.

Environment

The environment is seen to be the totality of the internal and external forces that surround a person and with which he or she interacts with at any given time. These forces include stressors that can affect the person's normal lines of defense and thereby affect the stability of the system.

Use of the Neuman Systems Model facilitates goal-directed, unified, holistic approaches to patient care. The model provides the nurse with guidelines for assessment of the whole person, utilization of the nursing process, and implementation of preventative and early interventions. Interventions can occur at a primary level to strengthen the flexible lines of defense, at a secondary level to help restore the client system to equilibrium by treating symptoms that occur after penetration of the lines of defense by a stressor, or at a tertiary level to prevent further damage and maintain stability after reconstitution has occurred.

The Neuman Systems Model is applied in this chapter to examine the older adult's dynamic state of equilibrium and the reaction or possible reaction to stressors as a result of environmental conflict. Delirium in the hospitalized adult can be conceptualized as the individual's response to stressors that threaten system stability. Therefore, nurses, as the hospitalized older adult's most consistent care providers, have an obligation to determine the needs and the concerns of the client system. Ideally, primary prevention of delirium should begin with screening hospitalized older adults for risk factors for the development of delirium upon admission. As a secondary prevention strategy, nurses should identify mental status changes. The nursing role in tertiary prevention of delirium involves interventions to provide restorative and psychosocial care after the diagnosis of delirium is present. To accomplish this goal effectively, nurses must have the knowledge and assessment skills to recognize changes in cognition that threaten the older adult's well-being.

REVIEW OF THE LITERATURE

The diagnosis of delirium is often difficult to make because of its fluctuating nature and different presentations. Nurses have been shown to be in a strategic position to observe changes at an early stage because they have frequent, consistent contact with patients (Foreman, 1990; Inouye et al., 1993; Schor et al., 1992). Francis (1992) studied recognition of delirium by physicians and nurses and found that nurses were more likely to detect it because they recognized subtle changes in mental status and used information from spouses.

Various studies have examined knowledge and awareness of nurses regarding symptoms of delirium (Foreman, 1993; Morency, Levkoff, & Dick, 1994; Palmateer & McCartney, 1985; Yeaw & Abbate, 1993). Palmateer and McCartney (1985) and Foreman (1993) found that because nurses have insufficient knowledge of cognitive deficits, many patients who develop delirium are not recognized. Morency et al. (1994) studied nurses' ability to recognize symptoms of delirium in older acute care patients. Each patient was interviewed daily by a trained assistant using the Delirium Symptom Interview (DSI) (Albert et al., 1992). The day-shift nurse was asked for her own observations and the presence and absence of DSM-III symptoms daily. The two sets of observations were compared. Thirty-eight percent of patients had delirium on admission or developed it during the hospital stay. Of all the symptoms of delirium, nurses assessed disorientation best, with a sensitivity of .81. Disturbances in sleep-wake cycle, disturbances of consciousness, and increased or decreased psychomotor activity were correctly recognized in about two-thirds of patients. The nurses observed fluctuating behavior and speech disturbances in only half of the patients. Recognition of perceptual experiences showed a sensitivity of .41. The researchers observed that the nurses were protective of patients when questioned about speech disturbances and offered explanations for the symptoms. Morency et al. (1994) concluded that nurses tend to focus on orientation and fail to recognize the behavioral aspects of delirium. Yeaw and Abbate (1993) interviewed registered nurses after a day shift in which the nurses had cared for a confused, nondemented patient. This study also concluded that nurses recognized disorientation best.

Souder and O'Sullivan (2000) compared nurses' documented observations with standardized assessment of cognitive status in 42 medically hospitalized patients. The standardized assessment showed impaired performance in 24 to 67% of all patients. Chart review showed no documentation on impaired cognitive status in any of these patients. Souder and O'Sullivan concluded that nurses limited their assessment to orientation and therefore missed many cases of cognitive problems in their patients. In addition, cognitive decline is often accepted as a normal consequence of aging, which contributes to delay or neglect in the diagnosis of delirium (Inouye, 1994). In patients with known dementia, changes in cognition and behavior are seldom seen as important (Inouye et al., 1999).

Simon, Jewell, and Brokel (1997) described a process-improvement project completed on an orthopedic unit in which systematic cognitive screening and observation of behavior led to improved detection of delirium. The authors emphasized the importance of collaboration between nurses and physicians in this process. A study by Bowler et al. (1994) showed that when doctors and nurses pooled their observations and collaborated on assessments, improvement of detection of psychiatric disorders in older medical inpatients occurred.

Lacko and colleagues (1999) studied the effect of using a standardized protocol to identify delirium in older hospitalized patients. Nurses on the intervention unit were taught about normal changes of aging, the process of delirium, and methods for recognizing this condition. A test of orientation, memory, and the CAM were used by nurses on a daily basis. On the intervention unit, 8 out of 32 patients developed delirium, and nurses detected and documented all cases correctly. Rapp et al. (2000) implemented a protocol with a combination of three instruments: the Mini-Mental Status Exam (Folstein, Folstein, & McHugh, 1975), the NEECHAM Confusion Scale, and the CAM. Nurses were trained in use of the instruments and initially reported being uncomfortable asking patients about their mental status. After some practice, nurses demonstrated improved assessment skills, increased recognition, and better communication with other professionals. Nurses were positive about the protocol, but expressed reservations about the time that screening takes.

Because most nurses are focused on disorientation in terms of cognitive assessment, most authors recommend a combination of education and the implementation of standardized systematic cognitive tests (Bostrom, 1992; Morency, 1990; Palmateer & McCartney, 1985; Souder & O'Sullivan, 2000). For successful implementation of delirium screening, nurses need instruments that are based on observation and that can be easily incorporated into routine assessments (Neelon et al., 1996; Williams et al., 1979). Screening tools need to be easy to use and interpreted to promote consistent use (Inouye et al., 1990).

DISCUSSION

Delirium is a serious problem in older hospitalized adults. Knowledge of delirium and its presentation, causes, and consequences has increased since the introduction of standardized criteria for diagnosis of delirium. Ideally, use of these standardized criteria in clinical practice should facilitate recognition of symptoms and multidisciplinary communication. Despite the availability of a number of tools to screen for delirium in the older hospitalized adult, consistent use in the acute care setting has not always been standard practice. Studies indicate that delirium continues to be overlooked or misdiagnosed, most often due to lack of understanding and awareness of this problem.

Many investigations over the past decade, using a variety of patient populations, have identified numerous risk factors for the development of delirium (APA, 1999). The most frequently implicated risk factors are shown in Appendix B (Francis & Kapoor, 1990; Inouye et al., 1990; Levkoff et al., 1992; Marcantonio et al., 1994). Knowledge of the risk factors for delirium should enable providers to focus on patients at risk. Although screening instruments have been developed to detect delirium, a tool for primary prevention is not widely available. A risk stratification tool based on these risk factors is proposed in Appendix D.

INTERPRETATION OF THE RISK STRATIFICATION TOOL

For each risk factor that is present, one point is scored. A total score is tabulated upon completion of the tool. A score of 0 to 3 is classified as low risk, 4 to 7 as moderate risk, and above 8 points as high risk. Scoring for the tool is based on the finding that with three or more risk factors, the likelihood of developing delirium is approximately 60% (Inouye & Charpentier, 1996). Based on the patient's risk stratification score, appropriate nursing and medical interventions can be implemented. The identified physiologic, psychologic, sociologic, and/or environmental elements that place the older adult at risk for delirium should be eliminated or minimized. Strategies include administering medications judiciously, preventing infection, maintaining fluid volume, and promoting electrolyte balance. In addition, all older hospitalized adults should experience a therapeutic environment that promotes safety and comfort. The difference in the approach to caring for high- versus low-risk patients will be in the frequency and number of orientation clues and environmental support.

CONCLUSION

Delirium is a common complication in many hospitalized older adults that continues to be overlooked or misdiagnosed. Prompt identification of patients at risk for delirium is important to prevent the negative outcomes associated with its development. Education regarding the expected changes of aging and the unique needs of the older adult population can help providers prevent delirium. A concise and easy-to-use risk stratification tool, such as the one described in this paper, may assist in this goal. This proposed instrument for systematic screening should be examined for its reliability, validity, and applicability for clinical nursing practice.

REFERENCES

Akins, J., & Onega, L. L. (2000). Acute confusion assessment instruments: Clinical versus research usability. *Applied Nursing Research, 13*, 37–45.

Albert, M. S., Levkoff, S. E., Reilly, C., Liptzin, B., Pilgrim, D., Cleary, P. D., Evans, D., & Rowe, J. W. (1992). The Delirium Symptom Interview: An interview for detection of delirium symptoms in hospitalized patients. *Journal of Geriatric Psychiatry and Neurology, 5*, 14–21.

American Psychiatric Association. (1994). *Diagnostic and statistical manual of mental disorders* (4th ed.). Washington, D.C.: Author.

American Psychiatric Association. (1999). Practice guidelines for the diagnosis and treatment of patients with delirium. *American Journal of Psychiatry, 156*, 1–20.

Andreasen, N. C. (1999). Symptoms, signs, and diagnosis of schizophrenia. *Lancet, 346*, 477–481.

Beck, A. T. (1972). Measuring depression: The depression inventory. In T. A. Williams, M. M. Katz, & J. A. Shield (Eds.), *Recent advances in the psychobiology of the depressive illnesses* (pp. 299–302). Washington, D.C.: U.S. Government Printing Office.

Beekman, A. T., Copeland, J. R., & Prince, M. J. (1999). Review of community prevalence of depression in later life. *British Journal of Psychiatry, 174*, 307–311.

Bostrom, A. C. (1992). Early identification of confusion in hospitalized elderly patients. *Michigan Nurse, 65*, 11–12.

Bowler, C., Boyle, A., Branford, M., Cooper, S. A., Harper, R., & Lindesay, J. (1994). Detection of psychiatric disorders in elderly medical inpatients. *Age and Aging, 23*, 307–311.

Dyson, M. (1999). Intensive care unit psychosis, the therapeutic nurse–patient relationship, and the influence of the intensive care unit setting: Analyses of interrelating factors. *Journal of Clinical Nursing, 8*, 284–290.

Eden, B. M., & Foreman, M. D. (1996). Problems associated with underrecognition of delirium in critical care: A case study. *Heart and Lung: Journal of Acute and Critical Care, 25*(5), 388–400.

Folstein, M. G., Folstein, S. E., & McHugh, P. R. (1975). Mini-Mental State: A practical guide for grading the cognitive state of patients for clinicians. *Journal of Psychiatric Research, 12*, 189–198.

Foreman, M. D. (1990). The cognitive and behavioral nature of acute confusional states. *Scholarly Inquiry for Nursing Practice: An International Journal, 5*, 3–20.

Foreman, M. D. (1993). Acute confusion in the elderly. *Annual Review of Nursing Research, 11*, 3–30.

Foreman, M. D., Wakefield, B., Culp, K., & Milisen, K. (2001). Delirium in elderly patients: An overview of the state of the science. *Journal of Gerontological Nursing, 28*(4), 12–20.

Francis, J. (1992). When do physicians and nurses recognize and document delirium? *Journal of the American Geriatric Society, 40*, 829–838.

Francis, J. (1996). Drug-induced delirium. *Central Nervous System Drugs, 5*, 103–114.

Francis, J., & Kapoor, W. N. (1990). Delirium in hospitalized elderly. *Journal of General Internal Medicine, 5*, 65–79.

Fraser, G., Prato, B. S., Riker, R., Berthiaume, D., & Wilkins, M. L. (2000). Frequency, severity, and treatment of agitation in young versus elderly patients. *Pharmacotherapy, 20*, 75–82.

Hamilton, M. (1960). Rating scale for depression. *Journal of Neurology, Neurosurgery, and Psychiatry, 23*, 56–61.

Hart, R. P., Best, A. M., & Sessler, C. N. (1997). Abbreviated cognitive test for delirium. *Journal of Psychosomatic Research, 43*, 417–423.

Inouye, S. K. (1994). The dilemma of delirium: Clinical and research controversies regarding diagnosis and evaluation of delirium in hospitalized elderly medical patients. *American Journal of Medicine, 97*, 278–288.

Inouye, S. K., & Charpentier, P. A. (1996). Precipitating factors for delirium in hospitalized elderly persons: Predictive model and interrelationship with baseline vulnerability. *JAMA, 275*, 852–857.

Inouye, S. K., van Dyck, C. H., Alessi, C. A., Balkin, S., Siegal, A. P., & Horowitz, R. I. (1990). Clarifying confusion: The confusion assessment method. *Annals of Internal Medicine, 113*, 941–949.

Inouye, S. K., Viscoli, C., Horowitz, R. I., Hurst, L. D., & Tinetti, M. E. (1993). A predictive model for delirium in hospitalized elderly medical patients based on admission characteristics. *Annals of Internal Medicine, 119*, 474–481.

Inouye, S. K., Bogardus, S. T., Charpentier, P. A., Leo-Summers, L., Acampora, D., & Holford, T. R. (1999). A multicomponent intervention to prevent delirium in hospitalized older patients. *New England Journal of Medicine, 340*, 669–676.

Inouye, S. K., Schlesinger, M. J., & Lyndon, T. J. (1999). Delirium: A symptom of how hospital care is failing older persons and a window to improve quality of hospital care. *American Journal of Medicine, 106*, 565–573.

Kahn, D., Cook, T., Carlise, C., Nelson, D., Kramer, M., & Milman, R. (1998). Identification and modification of environmental noise in an ICU setting. *Chest, 114*, 535–540.

Lacko, L., Bryan, Y., Cellasega, C., & Salerno, F. (1999). Changing clinical practice through research. *Clinical Nursing Research, 8*, 245–250.

Levkoff, S., Liptzin, B., Clearly, P., Reilly, C. H., & Evans, D. (1991). Review of research instruments and techniques used to detect delirium. *International Psychogeriatrics, 3*, 253–271.

Levkoff, S., Evans, D. A., Liptzin, B., Clearly, P., Lipsitz, L. A., & Wetie, T. T. (1992). Delirium: The occurrence and persistence of symptoms among elderly hospitalized patients. *Archives of Internal Medicine, 152*, 334–340.

Livingston, G. (1994). The scale of the problem. In A. Burns & R. Levy (Eds.), *Dementia* (1st ed., pp. 21–35). London: Chapman and Hall.

Marcantonio, E. R., Goldman, L., Mangione, C. M., Ludwig, L. E., Muraca, B., & Haslauer, C. M. (1994). A clinical prediction rule for delirium after elective noncardiac surgery. *JAMA, 271*, 134–139.

Martin, J. H., & Haynes, L. C. (2000). Depression, delirium, and dementia in the elderly patient. *AORN Journal, 72*(2), 209–217.

McDougall, G. J. (1990). A review of screening instruments for assessing cognition and mental status in older adults. *Nurse Practitioner, 15*, 18–28.

Meagher, D. J., Hanlon, D. O., Mahoney, E. O., Casey, P. R., & Trzepacz, P. T. (2000). Relationship between symptoms and motoric subtype of delirium. *Journal of Neuropsychiatry and Clinical Neuroscience, 12*, 51–56.

Morency, C. R. (1990). Mental status changes in the elderly: Recognizing and treating delirium. *Journal of Professional Nursing, 6*, 356–365.

Morency, C. R., Levkoff, S. E., & Dick, K. L. (1994). Research considerations delirium in hospitalized elders. *Journal of Gerontological Nursing, 20*, 24–30.

Neelon, V. J., Champagne, M. T., Carlson, J. R., & Funk, S. G. (1996). The NEECHAM Confusion Scale: Construction, validation, and clinical testing. *Nursing Research, 45*, 324–330.

Neuman, B. (1982). *The Neuman Systems Model: Application to nursing education and practice.* Norwalk, CT: Appleton-Century-Crofts.

Neuman, B. (1990). The Neuman Systems Model: A theory for practice. In M. E. Parker (Ed.), *Nursing theories in practice.* New York: National League for Nursing.

Neuman, B. (1995). *The Neuman Systems Model* (3rd ed.). Norwalk, CT: Appleton & Lange.

Neuman, B., & Fawcett, J. (Eds.). (2002). *The Neuman Systems Model* (4th ed.). Upper Saddle River, NJ: Prentice Hall.

Neuman Systems Model Home Page. (2005). Retrieved on February 20, 2005 at http://www.neumansystemsmodel.com.

O'Keeffe, S. (1996). Predicting delirium in elderly patients: Development and validation of a risk stratification model. *Age and Aging, 25*, 317–321.

O'Keeffe, S., & Lavan, J. (1997). The prognostic significance of delirium in older hospitalized patients. *Journal of the American Geriatric Society, 45*, 174–178.

Palmateer, L. M., & McCartney, J. R. (1985). Do nurses know when patients have cognitive deficits? *Journal of Gerontological Nursing, 11*, 6–16.

Panisett, M., Stern, Y., & Gauthier, S. (1996). *Clinical diagnosis and management of Alzheimer's disease* (pp. 129–139). London: Dunitz.

Pompei, P., Foreman, M. D., Rudberg, M. A., Inouye, S. K., Braund, V., & Cassel, C. K. (1994). Delirium in hospitalized older persons: Outcomes and predictors. *Journal of the American Geriatric Society, 42*, 809–815.

Pompei, P., Foreman, M., & Cassel, C. K. (1995). Detecting delirium among hospitalized older patients. *Archives of Internal Medicine, 155,* 301–307.

Rapp, C. G., Wakefield, B., Kundrat, M., Mentes, J., Tripp-Reimer, T., Culp, K., Mobily, P., Akins, J., & Onega, L. L. (2000). Acute confusion assessment instruments: Clinical versus research usability. *Applied Nursing Research, 13,* 37–45.

Riker, R., Fraser, G., & Cox, P. (1994). Continuous infusion of haloperidol controls agitation in critically ill patients. *Critical Care Medicine, 22*, 433–440.

Rosenstein, L. D. (1998). Differential diagnosis of the major progressive dementias and depression in middle and late adulthood: A summary of the literature of the early 1990s. *Neuropsychology Review, 8,* 109–167.

Sandberg, O., Gustafson, Y., Brannstrom, B., & Bucht, G. (1999). Clinical profile of delirium in older patients. *Journal of the American Geriatric Society, 47*, 1300–1306.

Schor, J. D., Levkoff, S. E., Lipsitz, L. A., Reilly, C. H., Cleary, P. D., Rowe, J. W., & Evans, D. A. (1992). Risk factors for delirium in hospitalized elderly. *Journal of the American Medical Association, 267*, 827–831.

Simon, L., Jewell, N., & Brokel, J. (1997). Management of acute delirium in hospitalized elderly: A process improvement project. *Geriatric Nursing, 18*, 150–154.

Smith, M. J., Breitbart, W. S., & Meredith, M. P. (1995). A critique of instruments and methods to detect, diagnose, and rate delirium. *Journal of Pain Symptom Management, 10*, 35–77.

Souder, E., & O'Sullivan, P. S. (2000). Nursing documentation versus standardized assessments of cognitive status in hospitalized medical patients. *Applied Nursing Research, 13*, 29–36.

Trzepacz, P. T., Baker, R. W., & Greenhouse, J. (1987). A symptom rating scale for delirium. *Psychiatry Resource, 23*, 89–97.

Versmeech, P. E. (1990). The Clinical Assessment of Confusion-A. *Applied Nursing Research, 3*, 128–133.

Williams, M. A., Holloway, J. R., Winn, M. C., Wolanin, M. D., Lawler, M. L., Westwick, C. R., & Chin, M. H. (1979). Nursing activities and acute confusional states in hospitalized elderly patients. *Research in Nursing and Health, 28*, 25–35.

Yesavage, J. A., Brink, T. L., Rose, T. L., Lum, O., Huang, V., Adey, M. B., & Leirer, V. O. (1983). Development and validation of a geriatric depression screening scale: A preliminary report. *Journal of Psychiatric Research, 17*, 37–49.

Yeaw, E. M., & Abbate, J. H. (1993). Identification of confusion among the elderly in an acute care setting. *Clinical Nurse Specialist, 75*, 192–197.

APPENDIX A

DSM-IV Criteria for Delirium

A. Disturbance of consciousness (i.e., reduced clarity of awareness of the environment) with reduced ability to focus, sustain, or shift attention.

B. A change in cognition (such as memory deficit, disorientation, language disturbance) or the development of a perceptual disturbance that is not better accounted for by a preexisting, established, or evolving dementia.

C. The disturbance develops over a short period of time (usually hours to days) and tends to fluctuate during the course of the day.

D. There is evidence from the history, physical examination, or laboratory findings that the disturbance is caused by one of the following:
   i. the direct physiological consequence of a general medical condition
   ii. the direct result of medication use or substance intoxication (Substance Intoxication Delirium)
   iii. the direct result of a withdrawal syndrome (Substance Withdrawal Delirium)
   iv. the direct result of one of the above etiologies (Delirium Due to Multiple Etiologies)

Source: Reprinted with permission from the Diagnostic and Statistical Manual of Mental Disorders, copyright 2000. American Psychiatric Association.

APPENDIX B

Risk Factors for Delirium

Age over 70	BUN/Creatinine ratio > 18
Transfer from a nursing home	Renal failure (Creatinine > 2.0 mg/dl)
Prior history of depression	Liver disease (Bilirubin > 2.0 mg/dl)
Prior history of dementia	History of congestive heart failure
History of stroke, epilepsy	Cardiogenic or septic shock
Alcohol abuse within a month	HIV infection
Administration of psychoactive medications	Tube feeding
Drug overdose or illicit drug use within one week	Rectal or bladder catheters
Hypo or hypernatremia	Central venous catheters
Hypo or hyperglycemia	Malnutrition
Hypo or hyperthyroidism	Use of physical restraints or posey vest
Hypothermia or fever	Visual or hearing impairment

Appendix C

Substances That Can Cause Delirium Through Intoxication or Withdrawal

Drugs of Abuse	Medications	Toxins
Alcohol	Anesthetics	Anticholinesterase
Cannabis	Analgesics	Organophosphate insecticides
Cocaine	Antiasthmatic agents	Carbon monoxide
Hallucinogens	Anticonvulsants	Carbon dioxide
Inhalents	Antihistamines	Volatile substances (e.g., fuel)
Opioids	Antihypertensives	Organic solvents
Phencyclidine	Antimicrobials	
Sedatives	Antiparkinsonian agents	
Hypnotics	Corticosteroids	
	Gastrointestinal medications (e.g., H2 blockers)	
	Muscle relaxants	
	Immunosuppressive agents	
	Psychotropic medications	

Appendix D

Delirium Risk Assessment Tool

Score 1 point for each risk factor:

Age > 70__	Renal failure__ (Creatinine > 2)
Transfer from a nursing home__	Liver disease__ (Bilirubin > 2)
History of stroke/seizure disorder__	Cardiogenic/septic shock__
Psychoactive medications (Benzodiazepines, narcotics, sedatives)__	Malnutrition__
Hypothermia/Fever__	Dehydration__
Hypo/Hypernatremia__	Use of physical restraints__

TOTAL SCORE____   **Low risk 0–3, moderate risk 4–7, high risk > 8**

Providing a Framework for the Nurse–Patient Relationship: The Nursing Theory of Hildegard Peplau

Lea A. Johnson

The work of Hildegard Peplau offers an important contribution to nursing practice in many settings. Although originally developed in the context of the psychiatric setting, the work of Peplau has relevance across the clinical spectrum because of its focus on the interpersonal relationship between the nurse and the client. Peplau's views on the evolution of the nurse–client relationship are as valid in contemporary nursing practice as when the theory was introduced in 1952.

To understand Peplau's theory of nursing, one should begin with her definition of nursing and the nursing process. Peplau viewed nursing as a "significant, therapeutic, interpersonal process" that works in cooperation with other human processes to make health possible (Peplau, 1952, p. 16). Further Peplau suggested that:

> In specific situations in which a professional health team offers health services, nurses participate in the organization of conditions that facilitate natural, ongoing tendencies in human organisms. Nursing is an educative instrument, a maturing force, that aims to promote forward movement of personality in the direction of creative, constructive, productive, personal, and community living. (p. 16)

In terms of nursing's metaparadigm, Peplau's examination of the views of person, environment, health, and nursing was unique. *Person* was described as "an organism who strives in its own way to reduce tension generated by needs" (p. 82). She defined *health* as a "word symbol that implies forward movement of personality and other ongoing human processes in the direction of creative, constructive, productive, personal, and community living" (p. 12). Rather than define society, she spoke of *environments* in terms of "forces existing outside the organism and in the context of culture from which mores, customs, and beliefs are acquired" (p. 163).

Her views on psychodynamic nursing were avant-garde. She described nursing as "being able to understand one's own behavior to help others identify difficulties, and to apply principles of human relations to the problems that arise at all levels of experience" (Peplau, 1952, p. 13). Thus, the key to nursing from Peplau's perspective was the development of the interpersonal relationship between nurse and patient. In her writings and public appearances, she often offered these views on nursing:

What is the central focus of nursing? What is the heart of nursing? Is it warmth, sympathy or tender loving care, or is it perceptive observations and intelligent interpretation, or perhaps leadership? The answer is interpersonal relations. (Peplau, 1964, p. x)

Peplau began developing her ideas on interpersonal relations and their role in the nurse–patient relationship shortly after completing her diploma-school training. In her first nursing job, she cared for a young woman with pneumonia who had just given birth to twins. The woman had wanted to come to the hospital as soon as possible; however, her husband refused to bring her until they had sexual intercourse. The woman was very distraught over this treatment by her spouse and wanted to talk, but Peplau and her fellow healthcare workers, feeling uncomfortable with the situation, ignored her emotional state and concentrated on treating her physical condition. Despite the fact that pneumonia was quite curable and the childbirth had gone well, the woman soon died. This patient's death made a lasting impression on Peplau, as she believed that the woman's psychological needs had been ignored by staff and that her fragile emotional state may have played a major role in her death. This became the starting point for Peplau's nursing theory. Never again would she neglect a patient's psychological needs out of ignorance or personal discomfort with the situation (Peplau, 1975).

PEPLAU'S VIEW OF NURSING ROLES

As she explored the importance of the nurse–patient relationship, Peplau identified six nursing roles that could emerge from this relationship (Peplau, 1952).

Stranger

At the beginning of the nurse–patient relationship, the nurse meets the patient and offers a basic level of respect. Because the nurse and the patient do not know each other, they are strangers; yet they must begin to forge the nurse–patient relationship. It is at this initial meeting that many conscious and unconscious feelings are formed that will follow and influence the nurse's ability to help the patient. In this stage, the nurse establishes a communication link with the patient and his or her family members, developing the initial groundwork for the evolution of the relationship.

Resource

In this role, the nurse answers specific questions and interprets any technical language, plans, or procedures needing clarification. Technical language may be difficult for clients to understand, thus the nurse can minimize anxiety in difficult circumstances.

Teacher

Peplau divides the role of teacher into two categories: instructional, which includes disseminating literature and providing information, and experiential, which uses the patient's base of experience to guide the learning (Peplau, 1964a). As patients share their thoughts, the nurse can assess what is needed and how best to proceed.

Leadership

The nurse's leadership role is heavily influenced by the nursing management, be it autocratic, laissez-faire, or democratic. Patients look to the nurse for leadership in managing their care; the nurse's ability to lead is dictated, in part, by the views and management style of superiors. Peplau believed that democratic management is best because it allows patients to become active participants in the design of their own nursing plans.

Surrogate

Nurses take on a surrogate role with their patients. More often than not, they remind the patient of someone in their past—a relative, a close friend, or perhaps a teacher. The patient often verbalizes these feelings to the nurse, and the nurse explores the relationship with the patient. In so doing, nurses further the establishment of trust in the nurse–patient relationship, and by being themselves they help the patient recognize the difference between the nurse and a symbolic figure. As this role progresses, the nurse–patient relationship moves forward from the initial state of dependence to independence, with the goal of adult interdependence.

Counselor

The role of counselor is often the nurse's most challenging role. In this role, the nurse helps patients process how they feel about their current health-related situation and experiences and then integrate these feelings into their lives rather than disassociate them. Not everyone can counsel or do it well. Counseling is not about giving advice. It entails reflecting, restating, observing, and being able to understand a patient's silence during a conversation. The nurse must feel confident in the role to be an effective counselor.

FOUR PHASES OF THE NURSE–PATIENT RELATIONSHIP

Peplau identified four phases in the nurse–patient relationship: orientation, identification, exploitation, and resolution. Throughout each phase of the nurse–patient relationship, the nurse may function in several of the roles previously discussed (Peplau, 1952).

Orientation

The orientation phase of the nurse–patient relationship begins with the patient exhibiting a "felt need" (Peplau, 1952, p. 22) for help from a professional. Nurses have a number of goals during this phase. First, they assess the situation, taking note of the patient's physical and psychological needs. This requires both an objective and a subjective assessment. Second, they assess the needs of the family or significant other present. They then begin to work with the patient (and family) to establish a relationship. Together they redefine and clarify the existing problem or felt need. The patient becomes an active participant in the process, asking questions and developing a basic comfort level with the nurse.

Identification

In the identification phase, the patient has grown accustomed to the nurse. This is the stage in which patients decide who can best meet their needs, and who interacts with them accordingly. The patient adopts one of three modes of interaction: either responding passively and becoming dependent on the nurse; becoming independent or autonomous from the nurse; or becoming interdependent, in which case they communicate and work together. The goal during identification is simple: Patients should become more certain of their capability to deal with the problem, thereby gaining a feeling of inner strength.

Exploitation

The patient next moves into the exploitation phase. The patient begins to make full use of the services offered. The power in the relationship shifts from the nurse to the patient as the patient begins to take some control of the situation. The patient is still a patient, but he or she is beginning to plan and focus on new goals—such as leaving the hospital. The nurse's ability to be supportive during this change is key to maintaining the therapeutic relationship. The nurse must remain nonjudgmental and provide a nonthreatening atmosphere that allows the patient to move toward independence.

Resolution

In the resolution phase, the patient's needs have been met via the collaborative nurse–patient relationship. It is time to end the therapeutic relationship and move on in life. The patient moves away from identifying with the nurse and breaks the bond. This is a collaborative effort that should result in both the patient and the nurse becoming stronger individuals.

COMPARING PEPLAU'S PHASES TO THE NURSING PROCESS

Parallels often are drawn between Peplau's four phases and today's nursing process. In fairness to Peplau, one must remember that this theory was developed more than a half century ago, at a time when nursing and society were far different than they are today.

Peplau identified the variables in nursing as needs, conflict, frustration, and anxiety, with anxiety playing a major role (Peplau, 1952). Peplau believed these variables had to be addressed in the nurse–patient relationship so that the patient could grow. This is not to say that these variables no longer exist, but in today's approach to nursing, the patient's personal variables comprise only part of the picture. Family dynamics, financial resources, community services, and the patient's home environment also are taken into account (Belcher & Fish, 2002). Add to the picture the need for health promotion and health maintenance, and one can see the growing breadth of the nurse's role in the nurse–patient relationship.

In comparing Peplau's phases with the nursing process, one can draw an immediate parallel between *orientation* and *assessment*. In today's nursing process, assessment is the phase in which data collection begins and ends; in Peplau's model it continues throughout. Peplau's model does not have the sophistication of today's nursing diagnosis; however, she believed that in orientation the "patient clarifies his first whole impression of his problem" (Peplau, 1952, p. xx).

As mutual goals begin to develop, the nurse moves on to the planning components of the nursing process. The *planning* stage is nurse directed and based on the nurse's knowledge and ability to develop a plan to help the patient. In Peplau's *identification* phase, the action is patient initiated, because patients respond to those who can meet their needs.

A clear relationship exists between Peplau's *exploitation* phase and the *implementation* phase of the nursing process. In both phases, the individualized plan of care already has been formed; thus, the goal is to move toward completion of the identified goals. Once again, this difference arises in the initiation of action. In Peplau's exploitation phase, the patient is the one seeking beneficial services, whereas in the nursing process the state of implementation is structured according to the nurse's prescribed plan. In other words, exploitation is patient directed, whereas implementation requires action on the part of the nurse and the patient and possibly other healthcare providers or even the patient's family.

The final step in the nursing process is evaluation. Although *resolution* is not the same as *evaluation*, the nurse in Peplau's model must make the evaluation that the patient's goals have been met and the relationship is ready for termination. In this way, evaluation does take place in Peplau's model (Belcher & Fish, 1980).

Overall, a major difference between Peplau's phases of interaction and the nursing process is in *defining the end*. For Peplau, the model is linear; there is a definite beginning (orientation) and an end (resolution). However, the nursing process is cyclical, with the possibility of both long- and short-term goals. Reliance on the nurse's knowledge, training, and technical skills, rather than communication strengths, gives the nursing process greater structure and makes it much easier to implement without the challenge that accompanies the therapeutic relationship Peplau described (Simpson, 1993).

A model is only valuable if it works. And Peplau's model does work. How this translates to today's current acute care setting is seen in the following case study.

CLINICAL APPLICATION

During one of my clinical experiences, I was assigned to a surgical unit where many of the patients were recovering from trauma. Although few patients on this unit had psychiatric diagnoses, the impact of chronic illness, loss, or trauma frequently led patients to suffer psychiatric symptoms—most often symptoms of depression.

Orientation

My first day on the clinical unit I was assigned six patients, one of whom was Mr. R. Mr. R kept to himself, and although he had cellulitis of the right foot, he was ambulatory. This patient physically turned away from staff whenever they entered the room. When I introduced myself, Mr. R was very polite and patiently allowed his prescribed care. However, he refused to converse and carefully avoided eye contact. He seemed very sad.

Each time I entered the room, I tried to establish rapport, if not by spoken word, then through action, but it was not easy. Despite the fact that most patients were discharged within a few days, Mr. R remained on the floor week after week. According to his chart, the foot would soon be amputated if the situation did not improve. Although the medical and nursing staff attended to Mr. R's physical needs, the nursing staff's workload was such that no one had any extra time to spend with him.

For three weeks, I tried to communicate with this patient without much success. Mr. R continued his cold shoulder with staff, and his condition remained the same. I finally gave up trying to establish rapport and resigned myself to the fact that this was one patient I simply couldn't reach. As my patient list changed from week to week, I continued to check in on Mr. R, the interaction consisting of a one-sided "Hi, Mr. R" or a friendly wave as I wheeled another patient down the hall. Mr. R sat alone in his room all day, every day, facing the window or watching television. One afternoon while on break, I stepped into the empty visitor lounge to collect my thoughts. Braced up against the window in a corner of the room was Mr. R. He had hobbled out of his room to explore. He immediately turned toward me and asked me to sit down and talk. I was stunned.

Identification

During the next half hour, Mr. R began to open up and share his feelings. He spoke of his fear of amputation and how he believed his life was a mess. His wife of 30 years had died of cancer two years ago, about that same time he was diagnosed with cancer of the cervical lymph nodes. The cancer was operable; however, the surgery left a long scar that he believed disfigured him. He carefully watched my face as he spoke of his disfigurement, looking to see if I, as a woman, would find his scar repulsive. I carefully registered no reaction. Mr. R then spoke in greater detail of his past life. He said he'd been a poor parent and too strict with his children. The end result was that none of his five children now wanted anything to do with him. So he was alone. After his wife died, he had given up on God and his church community. At this point in the conversation, it became more and more difficult for him to continue.

Exploitation

Our conversation was broken by numerous silences, yet guided by the use of reflection, observation, and restating. Mr. R brightened a bit as he spoke of his life prior to hospitalization, how he had become a skilled woodworker and now made children's toys. He wanted to return to work. He said his wood was his life. He questioned whether it would be possible to paint some of his children's toys while hospitalized. He began exploring the idea of having some of his unpainted toys delivered to the hospital so his work could continue. I restated his interest in exploring the idea, a notion he expanded and made into a goal.

When I returned to see Mr. R the following day, he was no longer in his room. Instead he had "set up shop" in the visitors lounge and was surrounded by his paints. When I entered the lounge, he was smiling from ear to ear. His previously flat affect became cheerful and animated as he spoke with pride of his past accomplishments. He announced his idea of painting "figures for the children of each nurse on the floor." He also wanted and was ready to talk more about his foot and how he might manage if he lost it. Although I already knew the story from his chart, he told me about his injury. He said he had feared amputation, but no longer. He thought he could handle it.

Mr. R's painting quickly absorbed most of his time; however, with the activity Mr. R came to the realization that he could regain his independence to some extent, even while hospitalized. Each day I was on the floor he waved me in to see his latest "creation." Slowly, a set of Disney characters began to take shape, first the Seven Dwarfs, followed by Snow White. Then several more sets. As the days passed, Mr. R appeared stronger both physically and psychologically. He stopped turning away from staff. He became talkative and took more of an interest in getting up and taking control of his situation. Within a week and a half of his renewed interest in his work, Mr. R was discharged, his cellulitis resolved.

Resolution

On our last visit, I knew even before entering his room that he was being discharged because out at the nurses' station a complete set of Mr. R's wooden figures was on display. During our last encounter, Mr. R told me of his future plans of building and selling rocking horses. He had gone so far as to order the wood. Sensing it was time to terminate the relationship, we shook hands and wished each other well. Mr. R then reached into his bag and produced a small block of wood he wanted me to have. It was not Snow White or one of the Seven Dwarfs, but a carving of one of Santa's elves, a brightly dressed toymaker sporting a genuine look of surprise.

Certainly not every nurse–patient relationship has these well-defined phases, but this author believes that most nurses can look back on their patients and relate Peplau's theory to those instances in which they developed a therapeutic nurse–patient relationship. The validity and reliability of these phases also has been established by Forchuk and Brown (1989).

APPLYING THEORY IN EVERYDAY NURSING PRACTICE

Although Peplau's theory can work well, it is not without its limitations. Some detractors might say that the theory belongs more in a psychiatric setting than in an acute care setting. Accustomed to such criticism, Peplau often countered that 77% of all hospital beds are in some way psychiatrically related hospitalizations (Peplau, 1964c, p. 3). (As like Mr. R, many patients experience symptoms of depression.) Research has confirmed the high incidence of mental disorders in patients seen by primary care providers (Miranda, Hohmann, Attkisson, & Larson, 1994).

From a research perspective, Peplau's model provides the ability to test hypotheses based on interpersonal processes. For more than 50 years, her model has formed the basis for research studies providing objective, valid findings (Howke et al., 2002). However, Peplau's model contains several inherent weaknesses that should be addressed (Simpson, 1993).

Communication Skills

Peplau's model requires the nurse to have well-developed communication skills. This requires mature nurses who are comfortable with themselves, enjoy working with people, and are able to be self-reflective. As the nurse's role changes during the relationship, nurses must be able to handle this changing role and manage their own feelings as well as those of their clients.

Time

The time required to build relationships with patients runs counter to today's world of managed care. Peplau's theory only works if nurses have the time to establish rapport and move the relationship forward. For this reason, Peplau's theory is most often employed in long-term facilities (Thelander, 1997), case management settings (Forchuk & Brown, 1989), and outpatient therapy situations, including private practice (Lego, 1997).

Staff Support

Staff support with strong internal communication is required to discuss clinical work and resolve problems that may arise. This model makes great emotional demands on the nurse. Peplau herself recognized this need and the problems that can arise when such support is not available. Among Peplau's personal papers at Radcliffe College is an account of a sexual assault on a young student nurse by a patient whom Peplau had at one time treated. The student had done nothing wrong, yet was so shaken by the attack that she had kept the entire experience to herself and simply decided to leave nursing. Peplau encountered the girl immediately after the assault. In reflecting on the incident she wrote, "We must talk about problems. Anything that isn't talked about can't be tamed and understood, and anything that isn't understood can't be changed." This story had a positive ending. Peplau persuaded the nursing student to discuss her story with staff. It turned out that she was not alone. Others had similar experiences, and believing they must be somehow to blame, they were too upset and embarrassed to discuss their experiences. Once discussed, the staff members developed a strategy for dealing with this particular patient and were able to provide valuable support to each other (Peplau, personal communication).

CONCLUSION

Is there a future for Peplau's work? For more than 50 years, Peplau's model has provided a solid framework for guiding the nurse–patient relationship. Perhaps its greatest value is in offering us the realization of the power of the interpersonal relationship, and how we, as nurses, can use this valuable tool to enhance patient care, promote healing, and move forward as a profession.

REFERENCES

Belcher, J. V. R., & Fish, L. J. (2002). Interpersonal relations in nursing: Hildegard Peplau. In J. George (Ed.), *Nursing theories: The base for professional nursing practice* (5th ed). Englewood Cliffs, NJ: Prentice Hall.

Forchuk, C., & Brown, B. (1989). Establishing a nurse–client relationship. *Journal of Psychosocial Nursing & Mental Health Services, 27*(2), 30–34.

Howke, C., Brophy, G. H., Carey, E. T., Noll, J., Rasmussen, L., Searcy, B., & Stark, N. L. (2002). Hildegard Peplau: Psychodynamic nursing. In A. Marriner-Tomey & M. R. Alligood (Eds.), *Nursing theorists and their work* (4th ed., pp. 335–350). St. Louis: Mosby.

Lego, S. (1997). Top ten reasons why psychiatric nurses are a good resource. *Journal of the American Psychiatric Nurses Association, 3*(2), 35–39.

Miranda, J., Hohmann, A. A., Attkisson, C. C., & Larson, D. B. (Eds.). (1994). *Mental disorders in primary care.* San Francisco: Jossey-Bass.

Peplau, H. E. (1952). *Interpersonal relations in nursing.* New York: G. P. Putnam's Sons. (Reprinted, 1991, New York: Springer).

Peplau, H. E. (1964a). *Basic principles of patient counseling* (2nd ed.). Philadelphia: Smith, Kline & French Laboratories.

Peplau, H. E. (1964b, May). *The heart of nursing.* Keynote address at the New Brunswick Association of Registered Nurses Annual Meeting, Bathurst, New Brunswick, Canada. Schlesinger Library, Radcliffe Institute for Advanced Study, Harvard University, Peplau Collection, Carton 23, File 812.

Peplau, H. E. (1964c, October). *The nurse–patient relationship.* Paper presented at the Ohio State Nursing Association convention, Columbus, OH. Schlesinger Library, Radcliffe Institute for Advanced Study, Harvard University, Peplau Collection, Carton 39, file 1451, p. 3.

Peplau, H. E. (1975, November). *Reflections on a career in nursing*. Keynote address at the Nursing Alumni Association Annual Meeting at the Medical College of Georgia, Atlanta, GA.

Simpson, H. (1993). *Peplau's model in action*. London: MacMillan Education Ltd.

Thelander, B. (1997). The psychotherapy of Hildegard Peplau in the treatment of persons with serious mental illness. *Perspectives in Psychiatric Care & the Journal for Nurse Psychotherapists, 33*(3), 24–32.

CHAPTER 23

Development and Psychometric Analysis of the Cancer Rehabilitation Questionnaire

Patrice K. Nicholas
Jean D. Leuner
Tamara Hammer
Inge B. Corless

Over the past two decades, advances in cancer treatment have increased the number of cancer survivors and the time span of survivorship. At the same time, survivorship poses ongoing physical, psychological, functional, existential, economic, and social challenges (Leigh & Stovall, 1998). For many patients, cancer becomes a chronic illness that requires rehabilitation. Nearly 4% of the U.S. population (7.2 million) are adult survivors of a cancer diagnosis. Among survivors, 63% reported that 5 or more years had passed since diagnosis, and nearly 10% reported that it had been at least 25 years since their diagnosis (Hewitt, Breen, & Devesa, 1999).

In this era of increased survival rates, cancer survivors and oncology professionals are faced with a frustrating array of poorly understood functional, physical, and psychological problems (Reh, 1999). As a result of these developments, cancer rehabilitation and health-related quality of life are moving to the forefront of cancer-care research (Arnold, 1999; Dirksen, 1995; Gotay & Muaoka, 1998; Leigh & Stovall, 1998; Little, Paul, Jordens, & Sayers, 2002; National Cancer Institute, 2002; Nicholas et al., 2004; Vaughn & Meadows, 2002; Zebrack, 2000a, 2000b, 2003; Zebrack & Chesler, 2002; Zebrack & Zeltzer, 2003). Well-validated, reliable instruments are needed to quantify the multiplicity of early and late effects associated with cancer treatment and rehabilitation (Anderson & Burckhardt, 1999; Cella, Hahn, & Dineen, 2002; Cella & Tulsky, 1993; Nayfield, Ganz, Moinpour, & Cella, 1992; Ramfelt, Severinsson, & Lutzen, 2002; Watson, 1990). This chapter focuses on the theoretical background related to cancer rehabilitation and quality of life in the development of a new instrument, the Cancer Rehabilitation Questionnaire (CRQ), and provides an examination of the psychometric properties of the CRQ.

Issues of rehabilitation and quality of life have taken on greater significance for those affected by colorectal cancer. Recently, the National Cancer Policy Board (NCPB) and the Institute of Medicine (IOM) (2003) commissioned a report on quality care for cancer survivors. Among the issues identified in this report were cancer rehabilitation and quality of life. Population trends in aging and improved cancer survival are likely to result in increased cancer prevalence, but few studies on the burden of illness among cancer survivors are available (Yabroff et al., 2004). Because of the importance of rehabilitation and quality of life for individuals living with cancer, the present study was undertaken to examine these issues in patients with colorectal cancer.

BACKGROUND

Cancer rehabilitation is an emerging area of research across the trajectory of the cancer experience. Cancer rehabilitation is defined as ". . . a dynamic process directed toward thc goal of enabling persons to function at their maximum level within the limitations of their disease or disability in terms of their physical, mental, emotional, social, and economic potential" (Dudas 1984, p. 6). Early work in cancer rehabilitation focused primarily on acutely hospitalized patients, who often underwent physically disabling surgical procedures (Ganz, 1999). Dietz (1969) focused on adaptive cancer rehabilitation and formulated four related categories: preventive, restorative, supportive, and palliative. In later research, Ganz (1999) further developed the concept of cancer rehabilitation to encompass broad areas of human functioning, such as physical, psychological, social, and vocational activities. In a classic review, Watson (1990) suggested that cancer rehabilitation involves maximizing independence and dignity while reducing the extent to which cancer interferes with physical, psychosocial, and economic functioning.

Sabers et al. (1999) investigated the utility of a Cancer Adaptation Team to recognize and address rehabilitative needs of hospitalized oncology patients. The Cancer Adaptation Team consisted of a psychiatrist, a registered nurse, a physical therapist, an occupational therapist, a social worker, and a chaplain. The study demonstrated significant functional gains for cancer inpatients who received interdisciplinary rehabilitation services. A second study by Petersson et al. (2002) focused on rehabilitation efforts in newly diagnosed breast, gastrointestinal, and prostate cancer. In this study, two coping styles, "monitoring," or cognitive scanning, and "blunting," or cognitive avoidance, were studied. The authors found that the monitoring concept was useful in predicting successful cancer rehabilitation.

Despite the lack of consensus about the meaning and measurement of cancer rehabilitation, the concept will continue to evolve as cancer survival rates increase in the 21st century. The present study was undertaken to further explore cancer rehabilitation as well as quality of life in the colorectal cancer population, and to extend the measurement of the concept in this understudied population.

Although quality of life measurement is a frequent outcome measure in cancer clinical trials, numerous conceptual and operational definitions of the term exist. Ferrans (1990a, 1990b) defined quality of life as an individual's perception of well-being that stems from satisfaction or dissatisfaction with dimensions of life that are important to the individual. The dimensions that affect quality of life were further categorized as health and functioning, socioeconomic, psychological-spiritual, and family. Building on this definition, Grant et al. (1990) included the following broad set of attributes, or dimensions, of quality of life from their meta-analysis of this concept: psychological well-being, physical well-being, sequelae of disease and treatment, social and interpersonal well-being, and financial and material well-being.

Previous studies in the colorectal cancer population have indicated that colon cancer patients and rectal cancer patients may report differences in quality of life. In their study of quality of life and independence in activities of daily living of colorectal cancer patients undergoing surgery, Ulander, Jeppsson, and Grahn (1997) found a significant improvement in emotional functioning, appetite, and global quality of life at follow-up. Colon cancer patients had less pain and less constipation postoperatively than did those with rectal cancer. Sailer et al. (2002) later investigated health-related quality of life for two reconstructive methods following low anterior resection of the rectum. The findings indicated that patients who underwent coloanal J pouch reconstruction had better functional results and improved quality of life in the early months after surgery in comparison to those who received straight coloanal colostomies. In another study, Esnaola et al. (2002) investigated quality of life in patients with locally recurrent rectal cancer treated with resection or nonsurgical palliation. The study findings indicated that symptom management, including more aggressive pain management, may help improve post-treatment quality of life.

THEORETICAL FRAMEWORK

Cancer rehabilitation and quality of life are key components of the cancer experience. Cancer rehabilitation is viewed along a continuum from diagnosis through treatment and rehabilitation. Although cancer rehabilitation is viewed as an important aspect of cancer as a chronic illness, few studies have explored the concept, particularly in patients with colorectal cancer. In addition, instruments measuring cancer rehabilitation are lacking. Figure 23.1 displays the dimensions of cancer rehabilitation and quality of life. Both cancer rehabilitation and quality of life are influenced by the cancer experience and should be evaluated across the trajectory of illness. Some key dimensions overlap whereas others are unique. For example, both cancer rehabilitation and quality of life share dimensions related to the physical, psychological, and role/relationship, or family, areas. Cancer rehabilitation also addresses future orientation, whereas quality of life addresses distinct spiritual and socioeconomic aspects. The theoretical framework addressed the unique and overlapping nature of the concepts of cancer rehabilitation and quality of life. The development of the Cancer Rehabilitation Questionnaire was based on the theoretical framework and specific dimensions of cancer rehabilitation: physical, psychological, future orientation, and role/relationship.

METHOD

The study used a cross-sectional, descriptive design to examine the CRQ as a measure of cancer rehabilitation in a sample of colorectal cancer patients ($n = 103$) at a large northeastern U.S. cancer center. After Institutional Review Board (IRB) approval was obtained, 327 patients were selected from the tumor registry at the cancer center. The data were collected as part of a larger study to examine rehabilitation issues and quality of life in patients with colorectal cancer. A study questionnaire was sent to the patients along with an explanatory letter describing study

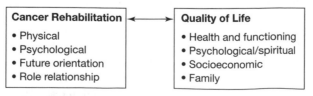

Figure 23.1 Relationship between cancer rehabilitation and quality of life.

procedures and addressing the risks and benefits of participating in a study. Of the 327 questionnaires mailed, 103 returned questionnaires were received from colorectal cancer patients, representing a 33% response rate.

Concurrently, data were collected from the medical record of each study participant. Data collected from the record included past medical history, primary site of cancer, evidence of metastatic sites at diagnosis, types of cancer, Duke staging at diagnosis, type of treatment received, the presence or absence of colostomy, and the goal of treatment (cure, control, or palliation).

Instruments

The data for this study were obtained using a demographic questionnaire, the Cancer Rehabilitation Questionnaire (CRQ), developed by the investigators, and the Ferrans and Powers Quality of Life Index (QLI) (Ferrans & Powers, 1985, 1992).

Cancer Rehabilitation Questionnaire

The Cancer Rehabilitation Questionnaire (CRQ) was developed by the investigators to measure the concept of cancer rehabilitation. After an extensive review of the literature on cancer rehabilitation (including CINAHL and Medline searches), a 34-item version of the CRQ was developed and pilot tested. Three oncology advanced-practice nurses established content validity. After further pilot testing, a 26-item version of the CRQ was developed.

In this study, subjects responded to 26 items on a 5-point Likert scale ranging from "strongly disagree" to "strongly agree." Total cancer rehabilitation scores were determined by summing the Likert scores from each item of the 26-item scale. The possible scores for the total CRQ range from 26 to 130. The instrument has four subscales: physical (8 items), psychological (5 items), future orientation (7 items), and role/relationship (6 items). The Likert scores of constituent items were summed to obtain scores for each of the four subscales. Negatively worded items were reversed for scoring. Higher scores indicated greater satisfaction with cancer rehabilitation issues. Items for the total CRQ and each of the subscales are displayed in Table 23.1.

Quality of Life Index

Quality of life was measured by the Quality of Life Index (QLI) developed by Ferrans and Powers (Ferrans, 1990a, 1990b; Ferrans & Powers, 1985, 1992). These authors defined quality of life as an individual's perception of well-being that stems from satisfaction or dissatisfaction with dimensions of life of importance to the individual. The domains of the QLI include health and functioning, socioeconomic, psychological/spiritual, and family.

The QLI has two sections that measure satisfaction with the items and the importance of the items. Respondents then rate each item on a 6-point Likert-type scale. Quality-of-life scores are calculated by adjusting satisfaction scores and importance scores, producing the highest score for items that have both high satisfaction and high importance responses.

Satisfaction is measured on the QLI through responses to 34 items on the 6-point Likert scale ranging from "very satisfied" to "very dissatisfied." The importance of each item to the individual is rated on a 6-point Likert-type scale ranging from "very important" to "very unimportant." The scores are calculated by weighing each satisfaction response with its corresponding importance. Individual item scores belonging to a given domain are summed for a domain score.

Table 23.1 Hierarchical Relationships Between the Global Construct of Cancer Rehabilitation, Four Major Domains and Specific Aspects of the Domain

Physical	Item
I am able to walk and move around comfortably despite my illness and treatment.	1
My illness and its treatment do not interfere with my energy level.	2
*My illness and its treatment cause pain.	3
My appetite is like it used to be.	4
*My bowel habits interfere with my activities of daily living.	5
I have been able to maintain or regain weight.	6
*I feel fatigue from the cancer and its treatment.	7
*I have difficulty fulfilling my daily responsibilities.	24
Psychological	
*My illness and its treatment make me feel anxious.	8
*I feel angry about having cancer.	10
My illness and its treatment have made spirituality more important in my life.	23
*I do not participate in the leisure activities that I used to.	25
*I have difficulty understanding the information that I receive for my healthcare providers about my cancer and its treatment.	26
Future Orientation	
I can think about the future because my illness and its treatment are under control.	9
My illness and its treatment have made me feel thankful for the future.	11
I am able to plan future activities.	16
I do not worry about health insurance.	18
*I am concerned about financial problems.	20
*I worry about losing my job in the future.	21
*My illness makes it difficult to seek a new job.	22
Role/Relationship	
My relationship with my family and/or friends has become closer.	12
*I need assistance for my family and/or friends to perform everyday activities (e.g., cooking, cleaning, dressing).	13
I feel comfortable talking with my family and/or friends about the future.	14
*My illness and its treatment interfere with my sexual functioning.	15
My illness and its treatment do not interfere with my ability to work (in or outside of the home).	17
I am able to talk about my illness and its treatment with my boss or co-workers.	19

*Negatively awarded items.

The domain scores are then summed for an overall quality-of-life score ranging from 0 to 30. The highest scores are produced by high-satisfaction/high-importance responses and the lowest are produced by high-dissatisfaction/low-importance responses.

RESULTS

Study Sample

Demographic Characteristics

Ages of the study participants ranged from 41 to 93 years (M = 66, SD = 10.64). Over 60% of the sample (63.5%; *n* = 65) were men, consistent with the data that males are more frequently diagnosed with colorectal cancer. Of those who responded to the question on ethnicity ($n = 71$), the ethnic representation included the following: Caucasian ($n = 65$), Latino ($n = 4$), and African American ($n = 2$).

Medical and Treatment Characteristics

The sample was evenly distributed with 48.5% ($n = 50$) of participants with colon cancer and 48.5% ($n = 50$) of participants with rectal cancer. Data for the location of cancer in three subjects were missing. For the majority of subjects (58.3%), the cancer was limited to a Duke's staging of 0 to 2. Thirty-three percent of survivors were initially classified with a Duke's staging of 3 to 6. At the time of diagnosis, 11.1% ($n = 11$) had metastases and 88.9% ($n = 88$) had no metastases. Fully 80.6% ($n = 83$) of the survivors were considered "healthy" by oncology healthcare professionals subsequent to therapy for cancer, although the mean carcinoembryonic antigen was 11.59. A large majority (97.1%) of study participants had received surgery. Other therapies were administered to the sample of patients with colorectal cancer, with 90.3% receiving intraoperative radiation, 55.3% receiving radiation, and 41.7% receiving chemotherapy.

Mean, Standard Deviations, and Ranges of Scores

The mean total score on the CRQ was 92.48, with a standard deviation of 18.15, and an actual range of 33 to 127 out of a possible range of 0 to 130.

Content Validity

Content analysis of the instrument was assessed by a panel of expert oncology nurse clinicians ($n = 3$) who evaluated the items for validity. Content validity for the CRQ was supported by a Content Validity Index of 0.90.

Internal Consistency Reliability

Internal consistency reliability was measured for the CRQ as a whole and for each subscale using Cronbach's alpha. Cronbach's alpha was 0.88 for the total CRQ. The psychological subscale showed the highest internal consistency, with a Cronbach's alpha of 0.85. For the physical subscale, the Cronbach's alpha was 0.82. Cronbach's alpha was 0.81 for the role/relationship subscale and 0.77 for the future-orientation subscale.

Test–Retest Reliability

Test–retest reliability was supported by retesting 19 subjects after a two-week interval. A correlation coefficient of 0.83 was obtained.

Construct Validity

In this study, a principal components factor-analysis (PCA) with orthogonal solution yielded four factors with eigenvalues greater than 1.0. There was a subject-to-item ratio of 4:1 for the procedure. The four factors with eigenvalues greater than 1.0 explained 55.8% of variance in the overall analysis. Factor I had an eigenvalue of 7.89 and explained 30.3% of the variance; factor II had an eigenvalue of 2.66 and explained an additional 10.2% of the variance; factor III had an eigenvalue of 2.2 and explained 8.5% of the variance. Lastly, factor IV had an eigenvalue of 1.78 and explained 6.8% of the variance. Typically, the cut-off eigenvalue used in factor analysis is 1.0 (Portney & Watkins, 2000).

Concurrent Validity

Concurrent validity was supported by correlations of 0.71 between scores on the CRQ and the Ferrans and Powers QLI.

Discriminant Validity

T-tests were calculated between colon and rectal cancer survivors for each of the four sub-scales and the total score on the CRQ. Significant differences were found, with rectal cancer survivors scoring lower than colon cancer survivors. Scores were significantly lower ($p < 0.005$) for rectal cancer survivors on the total CRQ and on several subscales. Specifically, rectal cancer survivors demonstrated significantly lower scores on the physical subscale ($p = 0.001$), the future-orientation scale ($p < 0.007$), and the role/relationship ($p < 0.03$) scale.

IMPLICATIONS FOR THEORY DEVELOPMENT AND INSTRUMENT DEVELOPMENT IN NURSING

In this study, the CRQ was found to possess the elements of a reliable and valid psychometric measure of cancer rehabilitation. The rehabilitation of cancer survivors is of great relevance and importance to nurses. Cancer rehabilitation is a complex, multifaceted, and somewhat abstract concept (Dudas, 1984; Dudas & Carlson, 1988; Mayer, 1992; Nicholas et al., 2004; Watson, 1990; Wyatt & Friedman, 1996), but this issue is critical to examine as more persons with cancer require rehabilitation. Therefore, a valid and reliable measure of rehabilitation such as the CRQ is needed so that nurses can more easily assess patient needs across the trajectory of the cancer experience.

The application of a theory-based framework to the development of an instrument such as the CRQ is important to theory development in nursing. Operationalizing the concept of cancer rehabilitation includes identifying symptoms that cause maximum distress and that reduce overall function, as well as quality of life. For example, research has suggested that targeted counseling by nurses is particularly effective in improving psychosocial and symptom-related distress in individuals living with cancer (Pedro, 2001). The CRQ provides a tool for clinical practice that may assist clinicians in targeting symptoms and evaluating the effect of nursing interventions.

More research into the effects of various therapies and approaches to cancer care are needed to promote cancer rehabilitation. Many interventions, including complementary and alternative therapies such as community-based fitness interventions, have been proposed in oncology practice. The establishment of a benchmark measure, such as the CRQ, may promote research that is focused on new interventions that support the cancer rehabilitation process.

Finally, instruments that measure baseline and post-treatment rehabilitation status are critical to assist patients who have undergone treatment across the cancer experience from initial diagnosis through rehabilitation. These measures may be useful to help patients make decisions about what is the best approach to treatment for them as individuals. Nurses must be cognizant of the need to address long-term needs of cancer survivors in clinical practice based on relevant theories and to include rehabilitation measures in the oncology population.

REFERENCES

Anderson, K. L., & Burckhardt, C. S. (1999). Conceptualization and measurement of quality of life as an outcome variable for health care intervention and research. *Journal of Advanced Nursing, 29*(2), 298–306.

Arnold, K. (1999). Survivorship group eyes future research goals. *Journal of the National Cancer Institute, 91*(7), 590–591.

Cella, D. F., & Tulsky, D. S. (1993). Quality of life in cancer: definition, purpose, and method of measurement. *Cancer Investigation, 11*(3), 327–336.

Cella, D., Hahn, E. A., & Dineen, K. (2002). Meaningful change in cancer-specific quality of life scores: Differences between improvement and worsening. *Quality of Life Research: An International Journal of Quality of Life Aspects of Treatment, Care & Rehabilitation, 11*(3), 207–221.

Dietz, J. H. (1969). Rehabilitation of the cancer patient. *Medical Clinics of North America, 53*(3), 607–634.

Dirksen, S. R. (1995). Search for meaning in long-term cancer survivors. *Journal of Advanced Nursing, 21*(4), 628–633.

Dudas, S. (1984). Rehabilitation concepts of nursing (continuing education). *Journal of Enterostomal Therapy, 11*(1), 6–15.

Dudas, S., & Carlson, C. E. (1988). Cancer rehabilitation. *Oncology Nursing Forum, 15*(2), 183–188.

Esnaola, N. F., Cantor, S. B., Johnson, M. L., Mirza, A. N., Miller, A. R., Curley, S. A., Crane, C. H., Cleeland, C. S., Janjan, N. A., & Skibber, J. M. (2002). Pain and quality of life after treatment inpatients with locally recurrent rectal cancer. *Journal of Clinical Oncology, 20*(21), 4361–4367.

Ferrans, C. E. (1990a). Development of a quality of life index for patients with cancer. *Oncology Nursing Forum, 17*(3 Suppl), 15–19.

Ferrans, C. E. (1990b). Quality of life: Conceptual issues. *Seminars in Oncology Nursing, 6*(4), 248–254.

Ferrans, C. E., & Powers, M. J. (1985). Quality of life index: Development and psychometric properties. *Advances in Nursing Science, 8*(1), 15–24.

Ferrans, C. E., & Powers, M. J. (1992). Psychometric assessment of the Quality of Life Index. *Research in Nursing & Health, 15*(1), 29–38.

Ferrell, B. R., Virani, R., Smith, S., Juarez, G. & National Cancer Policy Board and Institute of Medicine. (2003). The role of oncology nursing to ensure quality care for cancer survivors: A report commissioned by the National Cancer Policy Board and Institute of Medicine. *Oncology Nursing Forum, 30*(1), E1–E11.

Ganz, P. A. (1999). The status of cancer rehabilitation in the late 1990s. *Mayo Clinic Proceedings, 74*(9), 939–940.

Gotay, C. C., & Muraoka, M. Y. (1998). Quality of life in long-term survivors of adult-onset cancers. *Journal of the National Cancer Institute, 90*(9), 656–667.

Grant, M., Padilla, G. V., Ferrell, B. R., & Rhiner, M. (1990). Assessment of quality of life with a single instrument. *Seminars in Oncology Nursing, 6*(4), 260–270.

Hewitt, M., Breen, N., & Devesa, S. (1999). Cancer Prevalence and Survivorship Issues: Analyses of the 1992 National Health Interview Survey. *Journal of the National Cancer Institute, 91*(17), 480–486.

Leigh, A. S., & Stovall, E. L. (1998). Cancer survivorship: Quality for life. In C. R. King & P. S. Hinds (Eds.), *Quality of life from nursing and patient perspectives: Theory, research, practice.* Sudbury, MA: Jones and Bartlett.

Little, M., Paul, K., Jordens, C. F., & Sayers, E. J. (2002). Survivorship and discourses of identity. *Psycho-Oncology, 11*(2), 170–178.

Mayer, D. K. (1992). The health care implications of cancer rehabilitation in the twenty-first century. *Oncology Nursing Forum, 19*(1), 23–27.

National Cancer Institute. (2002). *Facing forward series: Life after cancer treatment.* Retrieved December 1, 2003, from http://www.cancer.gov/cancerinfo/life-after-treatment.

Nayfield, S. G., Ganz, P. A., Moinpour, C. M., & Cella, D. F. (1992). Report from a National Cancer Institute (USA) workshop on quality of life assessment in cancer clinical trials. *Quality of Life Research, 1*(3), 203–210.

Nicholas, P. K., Leuner, D. M., Hatfield, J., Corless, I. B., Marr, K. H., Mott, M., & Cross-Skinner, S. (In press, 2005). Instrument development and testing of the cancer rehabilitation questionnaire in patients with colorectal cancer. *Rehabilitation Nursing.*

Pedro, L. W. (2001). Quality of life for long-term survivors of cancer: Influencing variables. *Cancer Nursing, 24*(1), 1–11.

Petersson, L., Nordin, K., Glimelius, B., Brekkan, E., Sjoden, P., & Berglund, G. (2002). Differential effects of cancer rehabilitation depending on diagnosis and patients' cognitive coping style. *Psychosomatic Medicine, 64*(6), 971–980.

Portney, L. G., & Watkins, M. P. (2000). *Foundations of clinical research: Applications to practice* (2nd ed.). Norwalk, CT: Appleton & Lange.

Ramfelt, E., Severinsson, E., & Lutzen, K. (2002). Attempting to find meaning in illness to achieve emotional coherence: The experiences of patients with colorectal cancer. *Cancer Nursing, 25*(2), 141–149.

Sabers, S. R., Kokal, J. E., Girardi, J. C., Falk Philpott, C. L., Basford, J. R., Therneau, T. M., Schmidt, K. D., & Gamble, G. L. (1999). Evaluation of consultation-based rehabilitation for hospitalized cancer patients with functional impairment. *Mayo Clinic Proceedings, 74*(9), 855–861.

Sailer, M., Fuchs, K. H., Fein, M., & Thiede, A. (2002). Randomized clinical trial comparing quality of life after straight and pouch coloanal reconstruction. *British Journal of Surgery, 89*(9), 1108–1117.

Ulander, K., Jeppsson, B., & Grahn, G. (1997). Quality of life and independence in activities of daily living preoperatively and at follow-up in patients with colorectal cancer. *Support Care Cancer, 5*(5), 402–409.

Vaughn, D. J., & Meadows, A. T. (2002). Cancer survivorship research: The best is yet to come. *Journal of Clinical Oncology, 20*(4), 888–890.

Watson, P. G. (1990). Cancer rehabilitation. The evolution of a concept. *Cancer Nursing, 13*(1), 2–12.

Wyatt, G., & Friedman, L. L. (1996). Long-term female cancer survivors: quality of life issues and clinical implications. *Cancer Nursing, 19*(1), 1–7.

Yabroff, K. R., Lawrence, W. F., Clauser, S., Davis, W. W., & Brown, M. L. (2004). Burden of illness in cancer survivors: Findings from a population-based national sample. *Journal of the National Cancer Institute, 96*(17), 1322–1330.

Zebrack, B. J. (2000a). Cancer survivors and quality of life: a critical review of the literature. *Oncology Nursing Forum, 27*(9), 1395–1401.

Zebrack, B. J. (2000b). Cancer survivor identity and quality of life. *Cancer Practice, 8*(5), 238–242.

Zebrack, B. J. (2003). Reflections of a cancer survivor/research scientist. *Cancer, 97*(11), 2707–2709.

Zebrack, B. J., & Chesler, M. A. (2002). Quality of life in childhood cancer survivors. *Psycho-Oncology. Special Issue: Survivorship, 11*(2), 132–141.

Zebrack, B. J., & Zeltzer, L. K. (2003). Quality of life issues and cancer survivorship. *Current Problems in Cancer, 27*(4), 198–211.

Structuring Nursing Knowledge: A Priority for Creating Nursing's Future

Rozella M. Schlotfeldt

Nursing's future will be created only as the discipline underlying nursing practices is identified, structured, and continuously updated by systematic inquiry. The kinds of knowledge contained within the discipline are identified and an approach to its structure is proposed.

There can be little doubt that one of the highest priorities for creating an appropriate future for nursing is that of identifying, structuring, and continuously advancing the knowledge that underlies the practices of professionals in the field. That statement can be made because a consensus has not yet been attained concerning the subject matter that must be mastered by those who seek to practice general and specialized nursing. Surely by the beginning of the 21st century, nursing's body of knowledge will be identified, selected, verified, and agreed upon by qualified professionals in the field, effectively structured, and continuously updated to reflect newly discovered knowledge. Also, knowledge judged to be erroneous, inadequate, and outdated should be deleted. This knowledge will be derived from basic and clinical scientific research, both quantitative and qualitative, from philosophic and historical inquiries, and from evaluation research designed to establish valid criterion measures, devices, and approaches to establishing the efficacy and value of nursing's caring functions as they are relevant to the health, function, comfort, well-being, productivity, self-fulfillment, and happiness of human beings.

The thesis of this chapter is that only qualified professionals in the field, including general and specialist practitioners, educators, administrators, investigators, historians, philosophers, and theorists, should be given responsibility by the profession (however that is defined) to identify, verify, structure, and continuously update the extant content or subject matter that, at the minimum, should be included in the intellectual armamentaria of all professional nurses. This responsibility of the profession is essential to four functions: (a) the creation of comparable programs of study at the first professional degree level, (b) control of the profession's goals, mission, and accomplishments, (c) a valid procedure for licensing (not registering) all who qualify as professionals in the field, and (d) certification of bona fide nursing specialists.

Source: Rozella M. Schlotfeldt, Structuring Nursing Knowledge: A Priority for Creating Nursing's Future, *Nursing Science Quarterly,* 1(1) 1988, pp. 35–38, Sage Publications, Inc. Reprinted with permission.

NURSING AS A PROFESSION

Two major criteria must be fulfilled by any occupational group whose members earn and achieve the status of a profession, or more appropriately for nursing, a learned helping profession. First, a profession must have an institutionalized goal or social mission. Learned professions are valued by the societies whose members give them positive sanction for two major reasons: (a) the services learned professionals render are judged to be essential and beneficial for all members of society during particular times in their lives and (b) members of each learned profession have identified and come to a consensus about the knowledge that practitioners must master and use selectively, creatively, humanely, effectively, and ethically in providing those essential services. As a second criterion, each profession must support a cadre of investigators whose role is to continuously advance its knowledge with a view toward improving its practices.

The traditional learned professions have included the clergy, lawyers, and physicians. The clergy have been valued and supported because they are expected to be knowledgeable and skillful in providing spiritual comfort and well-being for all those who consult them. Lawyers are expected to master coded law and to apply their discipline fairly and skillfully in fulfilling the goal of preserving social harmony and justice. Physicians have been valued because knowledge of human ills and disabilities and their causes and knowledge of the means to eliminate, attenuate, or manage them and alleviate their noxious consequences are considered essential to the well-being of society. Are the caring functions and missions of nurses, namely, appraising and optimizing the health, function, comfort, independence, and potential of human beings, any less valued than spiritual comfort and well-being? Are they any less desirable than social harmony and justice? Are they any less important than finding causes for, diagnosing, and treating human ills?

Unfortunately, the caring functions typically provided by nurses were for too long considered to be mere extensions of the duties and obligations of wives and mothers, for which large amounts of professional knowledge were not considered essential (Reverby, 1987). Lay members of societies have typically not recognized, and nurses themselves have been remarkable tardy in identifying and organizing the several kinds of professional knowledge that are fundamental to executing the caring functions that nurses typically provide.

The essential and often crucial nature of nurses' caring functions in promoting the health and well-being of all human beings is finally being recognized by thinking people, including scholarly nurses. There is now general agreement (at least verbal agreement) that nursing's social mission is to appraise and assist human beings in their quest to optimize their health status, health assets, and health potential (Fawcett, 1983). Furthermore, general agreement exists that there is or should be a body of structured knowledge that professionals in the field agree represents the discipline that is functional to general and specialty nursing practices.

Nursing scholars have discussed, described, and characterized the discipline (Donaldson & Crowley, 1978), and in the recent past the American Association of Colleges of Nursing (1986) has reported findings from a "national effort to define the essential knowledge, practice, and values that the baccalaureate nurse should possess" (p. 1). Panel members expressed the belief that the essentials so delineated can be achieved within the traditional baccalaureate degree program in nursing and that the baccalaureate represents first-level professional preparation in nursing.

The efforts that have been made toward establishing the discipline represent significant steps toward achieving the goal of identifying, organizing, and achieving a consensus concerning the specific body of extant knowledge that underlies nursing practices. It must be noted, however, that there has not yet been a concerted effort to identify and obtain agreement about the currently available knowledge that is fundamental to nursing's growing number of declared specialties or even to obtain a consensus about the requisite knowledge and skills that define what nursing's specialties are. It must be recognized also that the subject matter that constitutes the discipline has not yet been identified and structured, and agreement has not been reached concerning appropriate and needed inclusions from qualified professionals in the field. This paper presents an approach to organizing the several kinds of knowledge contained within the discipline, a possible next step toward having qualified professionals select and structure the specific extant subject matter of the discipline about which agreement is needed.

Knowledge of the Discipline

Figure 24.1 shows the kinds of professional knowledge contained within the discipline, which is depicted as a large sphere having a permeable and expandable membrane (represented by the second sphere) to permit the continuous addition of newly discovered knowledge and the deletion of that found through systematic inquiry to be erroneous, inadequate, or irrelevant.

The largest segment of the sphere (*a*) represents nursing's scientific subject matter. Therein belongs all of nursing science (i.e., the verified facts, principles, and laws that have been discovered through scientific inquiry to be valid, relevant, and useful for nursing practice); included also are extant scientific theories that guide scientific investigations in nursing and those that have been proposed by scholarly nurses as promising explanations of phenomena that are of particular concern to nurses.

To date, much of nursing science has been discovered by basic scientists and subsequently found through empirical evidence and systematic study to be relevant. Nurse investigators have also been adding to nursing's scientific knowledge by testing the relevance and utility of theories generated by basic scientists in clinical nursing situations (Chinn, 1984). Few investigations have

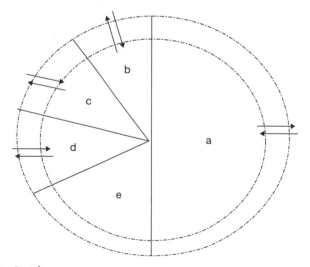

Figure 24.1 The Nursing Discipline.
(a) Nursing science; (b) nursing history; (c) nursing philosophy; (d) nursing strategies; (e) factors influencing human health. Arrows denote addition and deletion of knowledge. Person knowledge is excluded.

yet been reported that test scientific theories regarding human phenomena that are of particular concern to nurses but not to basic scientists (Silva, 1986). A plausible reason is that there is little agreement among nurses regarding the human phenomena that are of concern to nurses and how they should be characterized and classified and how knowledge of them should be advanced.

In general, nurses accept the notion that human beings are biopsychosocial beings (Engel, 1977). It is proposed here that the subjects nurses serve also exemplify assets of the human spirit of which relevant knowledge is inadequate. Those assets surely include human spirituality and other qualities of the human spirit, such as determination, verve, courage, beliefs, hope, and aspiration. Nurses surely hold responsibility for advancing knowledge of those health-seeking assets. In sum, human beings' health-seeking mechanisms and behaviors, beliefs, and propensities can be classified as biological, psychological (both emotional and cognitive), and sociocultural and as assets of the human spirit; all of them are directly relevant to the natural efforts by humans to seek and attain optimal health. Because so much scientific nursing knowledge remains to be discovered, it is safe to predict that nursing science will likely always represent the largest and most rapidly changing aspect of the discipline. Furthermore, nurses are increasingly recognizing the relevance of scientific knowledge from disciplines not traditionally judged to be relevant for nursing. Included, for example, are concepts, principles, and theories from economics, political science, administration and management, and computer science. The science fundamental to education has long been incorporated as an integral part of the discipline of nursing.

A second important segment of the sphere representing the nursing discipline is historical knowledge (*b*). Included is knowledge of the heritage of the occupation and the developing profession of nursing, including knowledge of people, circumstances, and events that have shaped that development. Included also is the history of nursing knowledge as it has been transmitted to generations of practitioners.

The third section of the sphere (*c*) represents philosophic nursing knowledge. Included are the profession's accepted values and codes of professional behavior. Included also should be the several philosophic theories that have been tested, found useful and relevant to nurses' work, and accepted as philosophic guides to practice. Illustrative are selected theories of value, justice and morality, and ethical theories. Because nurses are encountering increasing numbers of moral and ethical dilemmas and because nurses are increasingly manifesting interest in becoming scholars in the discipline of philosophy, it is predicted that nursing knowledge henceforth will include an increasing amount of tested and relevant philosophic knowledge that will be incorporated into the discipline.

The fourth section of the sphere (*d*) represents knowledge of nursing strategies, approaches, and technologies along with the scientific and artistic principles essential to their execution. Included also is knowledge of the prevailing healthcare system. Relationships between the goals and caring function of nurses and the goals and practice function of other health professionals in the existing healthcare system represent another important segment of the discipline.

Another significant segment of nursing's body of knowledge has always been knowledge of factors that influence the health status, health assets, and health potential of human beings, both favorably and unfavorably (*e*). Included is knowledge of biological, physical, and cognitive abilities with which people are naturally endowed and knowledge of environmental factors, economic and social circumstances, and changes associated with normal development, including the aging process. In the nursing perspective presented here, pathologies and medical diagnoses and treatments are factors that affect the health of human beings. Nurses must have adequate knowledge of these factors: such knowledge is an integral part of the discipline that must be mastered by nurse practitioners.

There is yet another kind of knowledge that is directly relevant to and essential to nursing practice. It is the knowledge that professionals must gain from relevant data concerning each person being served and then obtained through astute and perceptive observations. Personal knowledge of individuals and groups of persons is needed for nurses to respect the uniqueness of those for whom they provide exemplary services. For that reason, there can be no prescriptive nursing practice theories nor professional approaches to nursing care that are universally generalizable.

In summary, conceptualizing the discipline of nursing as an expandable and permeable sphere made up of segment of varying size provides an approach to classifying and organizing the several kinds of knowledge that constitute the nursing discipline. Such an approach demonstrates the vast and growing amounts of knowledge that professionals in the field must master and be able to use selectively, creatively, artistically, humanely, and skillfully to provide exemplary care.

Nursing should be recognized as a learned helping profession and a respected academic discipline. Surely nursing scholars will ensure the attainment of those goals by the beginning of the 21st century. Crucial to their attainment is identifying and attaining agreement about the human phenomena that are of particular concern to nurses, enhancing scholarly clinicians' involvement in generating promising relevant theories, and testing those theories as the means to discover knowledge through which to continuously improve nursing practices. Such an approach will ensure the availability of valid nursing knowledge in the 21st century and its currency during all centuries to come.

REFERENCES

American Association of College of Nursing. (1986). *Essentials of college and university education for professional nursing.* Washington, D.C.: Author:

Chinn, P. (1984). From the editor. *Advances in Nursing Science, 6*(2), ix.

Donaldson, S., & Crowley, D. (1978). The discipline of nursing. *Nursing Outlook, 26*, 113–120.

Engel, G. (1977). The need for a new medical model: A challenge for biomedicine. *Science, 196*, 129–136.

Fawcett, J. (1983). Hallmarks of success in nursing theory development. In P. Chinn (Ed.), *Advances in nursing theory development* (pp. 3–17). Rockwell, MD: Aspen.

Reverby, S. (1987). A caring dilemma: Womanhood and nursing in historical perspective. *Nursing Research, 36*, 5–11.

Silva, M. (1986). Research testing nursing theory: State of the art. *Advances in Nursing Science, 9*(1), 1–11.

CHAPTER 25

A World of No Boundaries

Margaret A. Newman

We have come a long way since the introduction of the World Wide Web. The Internet has diminished boundaries of physical space and time in a giant step toward a world of no boundaries. Views from outer space support this perspective. We experience nearly instantaneous communication in multiple directions around the world, without regard for time of day, and across barriers imposed by institutional structures. But these advances in globalization are not without ideological boundaries, in the world in general and in nursing in particular. The purpose of this article is to acknowledge the ways in which we create barriers to the understanding of nursing praxis and to recognize the connectedness of emerging nursing theories.

We have a tendency to dichotomize things. Even Florence Nightingale subtitled her classic treatise on nursing: *What It Is and What It Is Not*.[1] But Martha Rogers intuitively sensed the unitary nature of things.[2] Dialogue with her in the late sixties propelled consideration of health as a unitary concept. When she said that health and illness were simply expressions of the life process, my response was "oh, yes, opposite ends of the spectrum." No, she said. I contemplated her answer and with renewed fervor posed "then opposite sides of a coin." No, she said. Martha understood that opposites create boundaries and that there were no boundaries between health and illness. I had to give up my way of viewing things as opposites.

Ken Wilber led the way in pointing out that a world of opposites is a world of conflict and that a typical way of trying to solve the problem of opposites is to eradicate one of the opposites (e.g., disease).[3] It is difficult to let go of the categories (boundaries) imposed on life and health. Helpful, though, is the nature of rhythmic phenomena. It is possible to view body temperature, for instance, as fluctuating through highs and lows within a 24-hour period without labeling any of the measurements as pathological. The fluctuation represents a unitary pattern essential to life. Analogously one can begin to regard other so-called pathologies as fluctuations of the unitary process of health. Personal experience has taught me that health encompasses disease, and vice versa. It is strikingly clear that the old dichotomy between health and disease is no longer viable.

Wilber wrote:

> . . . we create a persistent alienation from ourselves, from others, and from the world by fracturing our present experience into different parts, separated by boundaries . . . each boundary we construct in our experience results in a limitation of our consciousness—a fragmentation, a conflict, a battle.[3(Preface)]

Source: Newman, M. A. (2003). A world of no boundaries. *Advances in Nursing Science, 26*(4), 240–245. Reprinted with permission from Lippincott, Williams & Wilkins.

That was the feeling I had while participating in some of the early nursing theory conferences in the late seventies and early eighties, a feeling that we were constructing boundaries between nursing theories, encouraging nurses to choose *one* and build their curriculum and practice on it. A competitive arena was created. Little attention was paid to the links between the theories. It was as if each stood alone. Since then, I have decried the boundaries imposed on nursing knowledge by conferences, organizations, and books that separate and isolate theorists of one persuasion from theorists of another, and also, that separate theorists and researchers from practitioners. Masson, a particularly wise practitioner, once wrote about her desire to be involved in research, her foray into the world of research conferences and journals, and her disappointment in not finding some practical information that could be of immediate use to her in practice.[4] The separation between theory, research, and practice has gone on far too long. The question for us today is how to go beyond the artificial barriers that separate them.

Things that we usually consider irreconcilable—the opposites—are like the crest and trough of a single wave; reality is not in the crest or the trough alone, but in the unity of one inseparable activity. Dividing lines (not boundaries) join and unite as well as divide and distinguish. Like light and dark, one cannot exist without the other.[3] Perhaps this is what was meant by Parse in her inclusion of paradox as important to nursing knowledge.[5] A line becomes a boundary when we forget that the inside coexists with the outside. We create boundaries where there are none and "these illusory boundaries, with the opposites they create, have become our impassioned battles."[3(p27)] A liberated person transcends opposites, like good and evil and life and death, moving to unity consciousness. According to Wilber, heaven is not all positives and no negatives, but no-opposites, ultimate reality as a union of opposites. At the highest level of consciousness, all opposites are reconciled.[6] Ultimate consciousness has been equated with love, which embraces all experience equally and unconditionally: pain as well as pleasure, failure as well as success, ugliness as well as beauty, disease as well as nondisease.

The convergence of various theories of nursing is becoming apparent. The crossover between theories of caring and the theory of health as expanding consciousness is remarkable.[7] Explication of the relationship between Watson's theory of caring and the science of unitary human beings has begun to illustrate the links between major perspectives of the discipline.[8] There is growing recognition that there are no real boundaries between nursing theories.

Within a unitary, transformative perspective, which Rogers introduced for nursing,[2] there are no boundaries. There are no boundaries between health and disease, between art and science, between research and practice, between nursing theory and nursing theory. In other fields, various approaches work under different circumstances, e.g., ice packs to prevent swelling immediately after an injury, with heat later on to facilitate the healing process. The same is true for nursing theories: some have more immediate relevance; others enlighten and transform for the long term. So what is the transcendent unity of theories of nursing?

Before addressing that question directly, I will mention briefly[2] other dichotomies that pervade the nursing literature and bear noting. First, the question of art and science.

There Is No Boundary Between Art and Science

Johnson, having done a thorough review of the literature on this subject, declared art and science as complementary.[9] Johnson's analysis of what she considers to be nursing art encompasses the nurse's ability to grasp meaning in patient encounters, to establish meaningful connection with the patient, to skillfully perform nursing activities, to rationally determine an appropriate course of action, and to morally conduct nursing practice. These dimensions—pattern recognition, connectedness, technical skill, rational action, and moral imperative—have been approached also as nursing science.[10] When the emphasis shifts to nursing practice (mutual process), there is no boundary between art and science.

Mitchell and Cody, advocates of Parse's human becoming school of thought, have questioned traditional boundaries between nursing art and nursing science.[11] They see art as a unitary experience that all-at-once is reflective and prereflective, rational and intuitive, and spanning all fields of knowledge. Watson, noted nursing philosopher-theorist, asserted the convergence of art and science in the caring-healing paradigm.[12] The art and science convergence has emerged as we have begun to let go of the separation of research and practice.

THERE IS NO BOUNDARY BETWEEN RESEARCH AND PRACTICE

Wilber reminded us that the scientific endeavors of naming and counting things have created a pervasive alienation and fragmentation of our world.[3] Abstractions transcended the concrete world, and another battle was launched between quantities and qualities. These classical boundaries (of classifications and measurements) were shattered as scientists began to explore the world of subatomic particles. They found that not only did these realities not fit the old physical laws, they couldn't even be located. The atom didn't exist as a separate entity but rather as "a set of *relationships* that reach outward to other things (emphasis added)."[3(p37)] It couldn't be located because it had no boundaries.

Reality is no longer a complex of distinct "things" but of interwoven aspects of multiple phenomena. Every entity interpenetrates every other entity. We are present in what we want to study; this interconnected web of relations reveals a network of inseparable patterns. One's sense of self envelops the All: ". . . there is no gap between you and your experiences . . . there is no gap between 'you' and the world which is experienced . . . there is no separate self."[3(p52)] This revolution in science brings us to where we are today in nursing knowledge—a world of no boundaries—and the awareness of no boundaries is unity consciousness. From a temporal perspective, reality is in the present—not what went before, or comes after: ". . . there is only now . . . the present is the only thing that has no end."[3(p59)] Being fully present in the experience of the present is the crux of unity consciousness and is requisite to nursing practice/research.

Wilber equated expanding consciousness with the dissolving of boundaries. We need to recognize that unity consciousness is entirely present now. It has no boundaries. It is omnipresent. It is everything we do, from washing dishes to reading the newspaper. It is not a future state; when we seek an experience of the future, we move away from present experience. Wilber suggested, "To move away from present experience implies that you and present experience are two different things . . . there is nothing but the present—no beginning, no end, nothing behind it, nothing in front of it."[3(pp153,158)] The past of memory and the future of anticipation are both seen as encompassed in the present. If we accept the omnipresence of all that there is, research regarding nursing practice must be centered in the "Now" of the moment, not looking back for causes or forward for predictions. Being fully in the present reveals insight and action. Cowling, a Rogerian theorist-researcher-practitioner, asserted that the purpose of nursing science is both action and theory, which occur simultaneously in the mutual process of pattern identification.[13]

In 1985, when Cowling, Vail, and I set out to develop a method of identifying pattern, we found ourselves engaged in a process much like practice.[14] It was research but it was also practice. Cowling went on to develop the unitary pattern appreciation models of practice and research,[15] and I took a stand that research into the nurse-client mutual process of patterning is not separate from practice.[10,14,16] It is praxis, a melding of theory, research, and practice. The response to my insistence that this type of research was practice ranged from definite rejection, based on the premise that the objectives of research and practice are distinctly different, to welcoming acceptance, as nursing researchers demonstrated that the hermeneutic, dialectic approach is at the heart of transformative nursing practice and contributes significantly to nursing knowledge.[17–19] Heron, known for his explications of cooperative inquiry, wrote:

> I participate in a unitive field of being-in-a-world . . . there is no gap between subject and object, between perceiver, perceiving and perceived, between consciousness and its content, . . . between form and process, between my being and my becoming.[20(p34)]

There Are No Boundaries Between Nursing Theories

Wilber asserted that different schools of thought "represent complementary approaches to different levels of the individual," and opposites are "complementary aspects of one and the same reality."[3(p23)] If we can let go of the boundaries we have constructed between nursing theories and examine the literature regarding the prevailing thematic concepts of the discipline, we will begin to experience unity consciousness, and all boundaries will disappear.

The process of emerging nursing knowledge is one of including and transcending that which has gone before. The literature supports the synthesis of caring and health with the underlying concepts of wholeness, pattern, mutual process, consciousness, transcendence, and transformation. The following statement, compiled from authors representing a variety of theoretical persuasions, illustrates the transcendent unity of the theories of nursing (quotation marks have been removed to facilitate the flow of meaning):

> The nursing mandate is to address the wholeness of the human being through caring, including a notion of health that spans all dimensions of life.[21] Health incorporates wellness, illness, well-being, and disease into a larger whole.[22] In the discipline statement, "caring in the human health experience," caring and health can be seen as dialectically related . . . they merge as the process of expanding consciousness.[17] Wholeness is the starting point with caring as the moral ideal.[23] Healing is not seeking a desired wholeness but rather is realizing an inherent wholeness.[24] Healing is the process of realizing one's pattern (wholeness).[25] Pattern is central to nursing; the theories of nursing focus on life's meanings.[26] Meaning and consciousness are constitutive of person–environment integration . . . life has transcendent meaning.[27] Transformation comes about in the process of pattern recognition through the dialectics of theory in action.[28] Nursing as mutual process is evidenced in dialogue, which is the interpenetrability of consciousness and uniqueness of meaning in nurse–patient encounters.[29] Nursing connects with deeply felt experience and meaning, has the capacity to step into another reality, to shift experience into a different realm.[30] There is a connection between self-transcendence and personal transformation relevant to expanding consciousness.[18] Consciousness is information in the form of pattern and meaning; expanding consciousness is seen in deepening meaning, insight, new ways of relating to self and others.[19]

Before leaving the focus on the discipline of nursing, I will add that there is no boundary between nursing and medicine. The acknowledgment of health as the pattern of the whole in nursing literature removes the boundary between nursing and medicine and requires a unitary perspective. This boundarylessness does not mean that there are no differences between the disciplines of nursing and medicine, but rather, as noted earlier, that they have a complementary relationship. Watson depicted nursing as the foreground and medicine as the background: "this new foreground becomes an integrating framework for the whole system."[23(p20)]

LETTING GO OF BOUNDARIES

Our nursing responsibility is to help patients let go of the artificial boundaries they have imposed on their lives and get in touch with the whole. The pattern is evolving to higher consciousness, but often one fights against it. For example, a woman who participated in one of my studies was imprisoned by the boundaries she had imposed on her life: bound by her obligations to her family, restricted and isolated from her own development as a person, feeling rejected by her children's choice of lifestyle, feeling alone and like a failure. She referred to herself as a "squirrel in a cage," a cage of self-imposed boundaries. What she needed to do was to let go of the boundaries and allow new relationships to evolve. The need is to let go and allow the pattern to unfold.

Others support the premise of no boundaries. According to Cowling: "all things are integral—what appears to be boundary is really artificial—there is no true local event in a world of integrality."[31(p2)] Watson placed emphasis on the relational aspects of nursing, connectedness, and consciousness: "Caring and healing are about relation, not separation, about meaning . . ."[23(p15)] Theorist Callista Roy referred to "the great gift of human consciousness" as the basis for human and environment transformations.[27(p9)] Philosopher Richard Tarnas asked "How can we participate in a transformative unfolding that would lead toward a more integral world?" and answered himself: by expanding our ways of knowing and creating a hermeneutics of trust instead of suspicion. "Knowledge becomes an act of love . . . we are an organ of the universe's self revelation."[32(p9)] He continued: ". . . it is a matter of experiencing, suffering through, the struggle of opposites within our consciousness," and ". . . in the spirit of Jung and Hegel, by suffering to the extreme under the great problem of opposites" to bring forth something new.[32(p10)] Letting go of boundaries between theories does not eliminate their substantive contribution; rather it facilitates a coherent presentation of the discipline.

What can be said about the discipline at this point? The literature supports the following dimensions:

☐ caring-healing within a unitary transformative perspective
☐ pattern as an inclusive, transcendent phenomenon that incorporates all that has gone before and vision of the future
☐ interconnected theories of unfolding meaning and insight as action potential

What can each of us do to let go of the boundaries we've constructed in our knowledge and practice? For starters, one has

☐ *to stand in the center of one's truth.* This admonition comes from Jose Arguelles, the Mayan scholar who predicted the harmonic convergence.[33] It is the primary task for everyone. It involves letting go of imposed, external values and allowing one's inner voice to emerge. To do so is to fulfill one's purpose in society.

☐ *to let go of rights and wrongs.* This basic dichotomy is pervasive in society. To let go of the boundary imposed by such a distinction is to allow oneself to reach out and love others who hold values contrary to one's own and to support their action potential.

☐ *to create a vision of a caring community from which transformation will follow.* A reminder may be indicated: Transformation occurs in far from equilibrium states through disruption at the intersection between order and chaos.

As I reach the conclusion of this effort to open our hearts and minds to the boundaryless nature of nursing knowledge, I feel a deep sense of "the world is too much with us." The world is ripe for transformation, and the profession of nursing is in a position to facilitate that transition. We must cease the binding conflict that exists in a struggle to protect false boundaries. As we explore a world of no boundaries, we will experience the compassion and creativity of unity consciousness.

REFERENCES

1. Nightingale F. *Notes on Nursing: What It Is, and What It Is Not.* Philadelphia: Lippincott; 1992 reproduction of 1859 First Edition.
2. Rogers M. E. *An Introduction to the Theoretical Basis of Nursing.* Philadelphia: Davis; 1970.
3. Wilber K. *No Boundary: Eastern and Western Approaches to Personal Growth.* Boulder, CO: Shambhala; 1981.
4. Masson V. Clinical scholarship and the pragmatic practitioner. *Nurs Outlook.* 1989;37:160.
5. Parse R. R. *Man-Living-Health: A Theory of Nursing.* New York: Wiley; 1981.
6. Bentov I. *Stalking the Wild Pendulum.* New York: Dutton; 1978.
7. Newman M. A. Caring in the human health experience. *Int J Hum Caring.* 2002;6(2):8–12.
8. Smith M. Caring and the science of unitary human beings. *Adv Nurs Sci.* 1999;21(4):14–28.
9. Johnson J. L. A dialectical examination of nursing art. *Adv Nurs Sci.* 1994;17(1):1–14.
10. Newman M. A. *Health as Expanding Consciousness.* 2nd ed. Sudbury, MA: Jones & Bartlett; 1994.
11. Mitchell G. J., Cody W. K. Ambiguous opportunity: Toiling for truth of nursing art and science. *Nurs Sci Q.* 2002;15(1):71–79.
12. Watson J. The theory of human caring: Retrospective and prospective. *Nurs Sci Q.* 1997;10(1):49–52.
13. Cowling W. R. A unitary-transformative nursing science: Potential for transcending dichotomies. *Nurs Sci Q.* 1999;12(2):132–135.
14. Newman M. A. Newman's theory of health as praxis. *Nurs Sci Q.* 1990;3(1):37–41.
15. Cowling W. R. Unitary pattern appreciation: The unitary science/practice of reaching for essence. In: Madrid M, ed. *Patterns of Rogerian Knowing.* Sudbury, MA: Jones & Bartlett; 1997.
16. Newman M. A. The research–practice relationship. Commentary: Research as practice. *Nurs Sci Q.* 1991;4(3):100–101.
17. Litchfield M. Practice wisdom. *Adv Nurs Sci.* 1999;22(2):62–73.
18. Neill J. Transcendence and transformation in the life patterns of women living with rheumatoid arthritis. *Adv Nurs Sci.* 2002;24(4):27–47.
19. Pharris M. D. Coming to know ourselves as community through nursing partnership with adolescents convicted of murder. *Adv Nurs Sci.* 2002;24(3):21–42.
20. Heron J. Spiritual inquiry as divine becoming. *ReVisions.* 2001;24(2):32–41.
21. Cody W. K. Lyrical language and nursing discourse: Can science be the tool of love? *Nurs Sci Q.* 2002;15(2):98–106.

22. Leddy S. K. Toward a complementary perspective on worldviews. *Nurs Sci Q.* 2000;13(3):225–229.
23. Watson J. *Postmodern Nursing and Beyond.* Edinburgh, Scotland: Churchill Livingstone; 1999.
24. Cowling W. R. Healing as appreciating wholeness. *Adv Nurs Sci.* 2000;22(3):16–32.
25. Smith M. C. Health, healing, and the myth of the hero journey. *Adv Nurs Sci.* 2002;24(4):1–13.
26. Dobratz M. C. The pattern of the becoming-self and dying. *Nurs Sci Q.* 2002;15(2):137–142.
27. Roy C. A theorist envisions the future and speaks to nursing administration. *Nurs Admin Q.* 1997;24(2):1–12.
28. Chow J. D. Interruption to research design: Substance-driven research. *Adv Nurs Sci.* 1999;22(2):39–48.
29. Bowers R., Moore K. N. Bakhtin, nursing narrative, and dialogical consciousness. *Adv Nurs Sci.* 1997;19(3):70–77.
30. Chinn P. L., Maeve K., Bostick C. Aesthetics and art of nursing. *Sch Inq Nurs Pract.* 1997;11(2):83–96.
31. Cowling W. R. President's message. *Rogerian Nurs Sci News.* 2000;12(4):2.
32. Tarnas R. Is the modern psyche undergoing a rite of passage? *ReVision.* 2002;24(3):2–10.
33. Arguelles J. *The Mayan Factor: Path Beyond Technology.* Santa Fe, NM: Bear & Company; 1987.

SECTION 3

ADVANCING THE PROFESSION

Karen A. Wolf

The history of nursing offers a window on society and the potential for dynamic change in health care. As noted in the first section of this text, the growth of American nursing has been forged by complex social, economic, and political forces. The tensions generated between the push to achieve professional status and the pull to meet societal needs have, in turn, at times resulted in contradictory goals. In this final section of the text, contributors reflect on nurses' quest to professionalize nursing. Professional hallmarks such as higher education, theory and knowledge development, ethical codes, and professional journals are a testament to nurses' perseverance and tenacity. Collectively, these authors suggest how the nursing ideas and actions of the past have helped to shape the present and have set into motion patterns for future changes in the profession.

The idea of nursing, historically rooted in the care for the sick and in the provision of nurturance for those vulnerable to ill health, is foundational to the profession. As noted throughout this book, the nature of nursing as a practice discipline is imbued with ideals of service and self-sacrifice. These ideals are at the root of nursing's most fundamental and persistent contradictions. The banner ideals of service in caring professions such as nursing have conflicted with efforts to achieve professional status. Professionalism speaks to both an individual's claim to expertise and to a recognition of the collective claim of professionals for social recognition. This underlying tension between the quest for professional autonomy and societal legitimacy and nurses' subservience to service ideals and institutional paternalism are highlighted in the first two chapters of this section. In Chapter 26, Karen Wolf describes a "slow march to professional practice." Drawing on the social history of nursing work, Wolf suggests that the ideology of professionalism has been a powerful means to push for change in nursing but an all too often illusive goal. As healthcare professionals and hospitals faced the challenges of war, nursing shortages, and economic turmoil, nursing's quest to professionalize often took a back seat to expedient labor-force development. Wolf suggests that, in the current climate of health care complexity and accountability, the ideology of professionalism serves as a legitimating framework for change. Despite institutional innovation, barriers to greater autonomy and recognition persist. By contrast, in Chapter 27 Melinda Jenkins showcases the efforts of nurses to practice autonomously in nursing centers. Jenkins reviews the historical development and current status of nurse-managed centers. Her chapter highlights how these environments foster nursing autonomy. She urges nurses to work together and with policy makers to advance the potential of nursing centers as a means to expand health care for the underserved and to support more autonomous nursing practice in community settings.

A prime event in the advancement of any profession is the initiation of a journal to communicate the ideals, knowledge, and skills of the discipline. The journalistic power team of Mason, Schorr, Flanagin, and Kennedy, provide a retrospective of the role of journals in shaping the nursing profession in Chapter 28. Their years of experience and knowledge as nurse–journalists provides a powerful perspective on the cultural hegemony of journals. As they note, the extraordinary variety of nursing journals has moved the nursing profession ahead, building a diverse and shared knowledge for practice and influencing the direction of education, theory, research, and policy.

A central question in nursing history has been, "Has nursing education driven change in practice or has it been nursing practice that has pushed the educational system to change?" Consideration of the many facets of this question begins with a look at the contentious debate over "entry into practice." In Chapter 29, Lucille Joel, educator and nurse leader, examines the lack of consensus and suggests that the nursing profession must come to an agreement about this issue in order to meet the future demands. The need for more educated healthcare providers is growing along with the complexity of healthcare system technologies, therapeutics, and regulations. Joel suggests that nursing look to other professions for models of change.

By contrast, Elizabeth Speakman, a leader in associate degree education, provides a compelling overview of the evolution of associate degree education in Chapter 30. She notes that associate degree graduates are the largest group in the healthcare workforce, but "like the elephant in the living room," there is little or no acknowledgment of their contribution to health care by nursing leaders. The history of associate degree education reflects an expedient approach to meeting labor force demands during nursing shortages. Speakman emphasizes the key role associate degree education has in helping people access nursing as a career. As she cites the economic, racial, and economic diversity of the associate degree nurse, Speakman challenges other educational routes to follow.

The expanding boundaries of practice and education are the topic of Chapter 31 by Joyce Pulici and Chapter 32 by Michael Carter. Offering a concise overview of the history of advanced practice, Pulcini asks the question, "Are the knowledge and skills of advanced practice today the basic skills of tomorrow?" Carter reviews the history of doctoral education in nursing, citing the variety of programs and titles that have emerged as doctoral education has evolved. Carter suggests that ambivalence toward doctoral education was due to the large numbers of "first generation doctorally prepared nurses educated in other fields." The development of doctoral education was spurred by faculty needs in baccalaureate degree and master's degree programs. Doctoral programs too often fell short in finding a balance between research and practice knowledge. The current debate about doctoral education is about the potential benefit of developing a clinical doctorate. This shift in focus reflects the growing power of advanced practice nursing and recognition of the need to better prepare nurses to be innovators and evaluators for clinical practice. Looking toward the future and suggesting that nursing should seek educational parity with other professions, Carter urges the nursing profession to support clinical doctorate program development as the basis for advanced practice.

Susan Gortner, in Chapter 33, reflects on the history of nursing knowledge development from the early days of research to the legitimization of nursing science. Her account richly details the early years, when nurse-centered research overpowered patient-centered research, to the present era of complex investigations across a variety of nursing domains and practice settings. As she acknowledges the social and political influences of the past and looks to the future, Gortner urges nurse researchers to forge ahead to address fundamental problems at the 'biobehavioral interface' and to strengthen collaboration with other disciplines.

In Chapter 34, Hollie Noveletsky makes the case for reflective practice. Addressing the idea that most practice knowledge is rooted in actual practice, she examines the role of reflective practice as an effective means to uncover and evaluate practice knowledge. She notes that the ideas and process of reflective practice will help nurses to better understand the knowledge emerging from the relational nature of nursing's paradigmatic constructs. Noveletsky urges that nursing education should support the development of "reflective nurses."

Another way to look at nursing knowledge development is to consider what domains receive our attention. Patricia Maher, lamenting professional nursing's move away from the spiritual emphasis of Nightingale, entreats nurses to reclaim spirituality in nursing practice. In Chapter 35, she suggests that nurses cannot truly understand suffering and the human condition without having a better understanding of spirituality. She notes that "the practice of nursing requires integrating two ways of knowing: one through revelation, reflection, and relationship and the other through the scientific method." Drawing on her own practice experience, Maher exemplifies the central role of spirituality in caring for and relieving suffering. She cautions nurses not to assume that spirituality can simply be integrated into practice as "content" or technique and argues for new approaches, such as reflective practice, and expanding nurses' spiritual, theological, and cultural understandings to discover a new language to reflect the spirituality in nursing practice.

In Chapter 36, Noreen Frisch examines the growth in interest and use of alternative and complementary modalities for health care as both a consumer trend and a growing trend in nursing and medicine. Frisch suggests that this "expansion" in therapeutic options is readily compatible with the disciplinary context of nursing. Frisch further illustrates the fit between nursing theory and alternative and complementary modalities by drawing on examples from nursing theorists such as Roy, Rogers, and Watson. She urges nurses not to treat these modalities as contextual techniques, but instead advises nurses to place them in context and document them within the nursing taxonomy.

In Chapter 37, John Twomey, a nurse ethicist, examines the history of the nursing codes of ethics. Twomey observes that the development of a code of ethics is consistent with the growth of a profession and that the ANA code has contributed substantially to knowledge development in the realm of ethics. The ANA code, according to Twomey, is critical because it "stakes the claim to the emergence of nursing as a scientific but humanistic health group that constantly strives to update its knowledge base and has rightfully taken its place with the nation's accepted healthcare leaders." Moving from the theory of ethics to an ethics action, in Chapter 38, Evelyn Quigley challenges the nursing profession to embrace the ethical imperative "to do no harm" and respond to the call to action to improve patient safety in health care. She highlights the complex regulatory and interdisciplinary imperatives and calls for nursing action leadership.

In the final two chapters, the question of how to effect change in health care is addressed. In Chapter 39, Brenda Navidjon and Jeanette Ives-Erickson tackle the recurring problem of nursing shortages and suggest that unlike previous shortages, the current shortage is more complex. They suggest that the global and structural nature of the current nursing shortage requires radical action and collaboration among nursing leaders in practice and education, healthcare executives, government, and the media.

This suggestion of improved collaboration between nursing and the larger society is heard again in the final chapter, Chapter 40, in which the locus of change shifts from nursing as a profession to the potential of nursing ideals to improve global health. In this final chapter, Beck returns to Nightingale's ideas of nursing and restates Nightingale's belief in the power of nursing to change the world. As Beck advocates for nurses to embrace the legacy of Nightingale's vision for nursing, she introduces the Nightingale Initiative for Global Health. This call to action for global health demonstrates the power of nursing ideals to guide humanity for the future of our planet.

As this section of the books comes to a close, we have come full circle from Nightingale's idea of nursing as a service in the 19th century to the current rebirth of interest in Nightingalc as an advocate for global health promotion. Such is the history of nursing ideas, dynamic and cyclical, seeking understanding aimed at easing human suffering and promoting health and developing our knowledge and skills with new insights and contextual applications. Nurses will continue to be challenged by the social condition of each new age to guide knowledge development through practice, education, and research. As the Global community of nurses grows the new challenge is for nurses to share, critique, and refine their disciplinary knowledge; and to work collectively with other disciplines and communities for health. As we look back at the history of nursing ideas, we can develop a great respect for the nursing legacy; and a hope for nurses's future contributions to global health. To paraphrase the late nursing scholar Jo Ann Ashley, "This I believe is the power of Nursing!" (Wolf, 1996).

REFERENCE

Wolf, K. A. (1996). *The Selected Writings of Jo Ann Ashley*. Boston: Jones & Bartlett, National League for Nursing Press.

CHAPTER 26

The Slow March to Professional Practice

Karen A. Wolf

> *Nurses do love nursing, but they want nursing to be, in so far as possible, a profession, and the things they stress when they talk about the economic conditions in which they work are apparently those things which other professional workers take for granted:*
> *Reasonable hours*
> *Adequate income*
> *Constructive leadership*
> *Opportunity for Growth*
>
> —Mae Burgess, 1928, p. 482

Nursing's quest for professionalism has shaped nursing education and practice, past and present, in the United States and abroad. The emergence of professional practice models over the past quarter century represents the latest in professionalizing trends. This effort by nurses and healthcare managers to restructure the workplace and nursing work highlights the evolution of nursing from a simple matter of tasks to the complexity of knowledge-based practice in rapidly changing healthcare organizations. The current healthcare environment is faced with a wide range of regulatory and financial pressures. These include demands to justify healthcare service outcomes, the drive to maintain biomedical and technological currency, and a recurrent nursing shortage. Looking back through nursing history, one can see that crises in the healthcare system create opportunities for nursing. Too often, nursing's responses to crises have not created outcomes that serve both the interests of the profession and the public. Today, as nurses once again find themselves in the midst of a crisis, there is an opportunity to renegotiate the organizational realities of health care and to advance the contribution of professional nursing to healthcare outcomes.

NURSING AS A PROFESSION: KEY IDEAS FOR INTEGRATION

What makes work "professional work"? Nursing has struggled with this question throughout its history. For most of the 20th century, nursing was considered a semiprofession or a profession-in-progress by sociologists (Bucher & Strauss, 1961; Etzioni, 1969). The attention that nursing leaders have given to professional development is manifest in the push for control over educational standards, efforts to develop a theory base for nursing practice, the growth of professional organizations and journals, and, more recently, the reorganization of nursing work within "professional nursing practice models." The nature of professional nursing work differs today than it did for the sacred three professions of medicine, law, and the clergy in 1900. The autonomous "solo" professional serving the public with expert knowledge and skill is now a rare phenomena. Few occupations can claim pure professional autonomy, because the reach of corporate and institutional control now dominates most sectors of the economy.

Autonomy, a hallmark of professionalism, can be differentiated into autonomy of decision making relative to the client and/or patient care and autonomy from the employing institution (Manthey, 1991). Autonomous practitioners are those who have direct lines of access to clients, who are responsible for their own practice decisions, and who are accountable to clients, peers, and professional organizations, as well as to the courts, for their conduct (Marram, Schlegel, & Bevis, 1974). The nursing profession has struggled with the idea of autonomy because most nurses are employed and subordinated to the authority of organizations such as hospitals (Wolf, 1993; Reverby, 1987; Ashley, 1976). The claim to autonomy with regard to the freedom to make decisions about patient care has advanced over the past few decades, fueled by the development of primary nursing models (Hegyvary, 1982). More recently, health services research studies have integrated the concept of nursing autonomy. For example, a recent study by Aiken and colleagues (2002) suggested that increasing nursing autonomy and control over the practice setting was associated with improved patient care outcomes.

Nursing can no longer be viewed as a subsidiary function of medicine that is proscribed by doctors orders; nursing care now reflects a patient-centered approach based on nursing theory and shaped by a "nursing process" of reasoning. Current legal and professional regulations legitimate this nurse-driven process of practice. The body of statutory and case law that governs nursing practice holds nurses accountable to a definition of practice that recognizes and codifies practice in accordance with current nursing knowledge and clinical practice standards. Accountability is inherent to autonomy. By definition, *accountability* calls for professionals to substantiate the reasons for their actions and to compare them with established standards (Merriam Webster, 1993). The demand for professional accountability has been spurred on by the health-outcomes movement and patient safety concerns.

Professionalism should and does benefit the public. However, professionalism also arises out of self-interest and provides a means by which occupational groups exert influence to advance their own interests in society. The interest may reflect a desire for greater societal power and/or an increase of rewards or benefits for the group. As such, the quest for professional status by nursing reflects an attempt to access and achieve mobility. Professionalism, by reflecting the underlying meritocratic values of our society, offers a rational system for distributing status and rewards.

Professionalization provides access to social mobility. According to Hughes (1971), there are two types of mobility. The first is the rise of the individual by entering an occupation of high prestige or by achieving special success in his or her profession. The second is the collective effort of an organized occupation to improve its place and increase its power in relation to other occupational groups. In the case of nursing, mobility has traditionally been measured against or referenced to other groups, such as physicians.

Since the 1970s, interest in "professionalizing" nursing work has emerged in healthcare organizations as a means to provide a substitute motivation for workers with blocked access to structures of mobility. The ideological draw of professionalism is that it offers the promise of higher status and control. A crucial issue that arises out of the trend to professionalize work is the struggle of workers, including nurses, to exercise control over the context (environment) and content of their work. The ability to exercise control, however tentative, appears to mediate individual and collective tensions that arise from the heightened expectations of a more educated nursing workforce. By "professionalizing" the workplace, management seeks to counter more traditional collective action, such as unionism. Educated to be "professionals" in colleges and universities, nurses now expect to exercise their knowledge and skills without organizational or bureaucratic constraint. The heightened expectations of nurses is a double-edged sword, offering a challenge to traditional hierarchical controls and opportunity for institutional enhancement.

As hospitals and other healthcare institutions confront the increasing complexity in health care, the application of professional knowledge and skills becomes essential to institutional functioning. That professional knowledge and skills serve institutional goals to solve institutional problems is now embraced by healthcare administrators as an asset, rather than a threat to traditional authority. Perrow (1972) observed in his classic treatise on bureaucracy that professionals, far from antithetical to institutional bureaucracy, are in fact readily harnessed to serve the needs and problems of organizations. Nurses have historically highlighted this phenomenon. More recently, other traditional professions (physicians, lawyers) have become "organizational professions." Yet, despite nurses' central role in healthcare services, they have struggled to develop, assert, and be recognized for their professional expertise. Imbued with managerialism, nursing work in hospitals has evidenced a professional paradox (Fourcher & Howard, 1981). The application of nursing knowledge and skill in managing patient care in hospitals has a long history of being subjugated to nursing and hospital administration. Nursing expertise has more often than not been invisible and undervalued, and autonomy of practice has been absent.

ROOTS OF NURSING CONTRADICTIONS

The concept and actual practice of nursing work has evolved dramatically over the past 100 years. But like many evolutionary paths, old or outdated conceptions of nursing persist. As a result, both popular and professional conceptions of nursing are riddled with contradictory views. Prior to Nightingale's reforms in England, nursing was largely women's work. Nursing was viewed as an extension of motherhood, midwifery, or religious duty. By the late 19th century women working as nurses began to fill a role in the administration of poverty. Because health care and nursing care of the sick was intertwined with poverty, caring for the sick was largely caring for the poor. Nursing was commonly carried out by impoverished women who worked as "nurses" in almshouses caring for the poor, the sick, and the destitute. These untrained able-bodied paupers worked for room and board. The harsh reality was that these nurses were viewed as part of the chaotic environments in which they worked. The Dickinsonian image of "Sary Gamp," a low-class drunkard and disheveled woman, was reflective of the persistent stigma that Nightingale sought to escape with the formal education of a higher class of women (Dean & Bolton, 1980; Williams, 1980).

Although some few nurses saw their work as a religious service, the role of religious values waned with the disintegration of church-based nursing orders with the rise of Protestantism in England. Hospitals, lacking the support of religious nursing orders, struggled to provide nursing care that was haphazard at best. Nurses lacked a systematic set of skills, a knowledge base, or training. Nightingale sought to modernize nursing by developing a trained nursing labor force composed of a higher class of women.

Nightingale also sought to link nursing education with the more formalized development of hospitals. Influenced by her experiences in the Crimean, Nightingale recognized that nursing care was the major determinant of hospital outcomes. A brilliant and politically astute woman, she took on nursing reformation with a passion born of her religious beliefs and desire to reform social expectations for women. Nightingale advanced her case for training nurses based on data. Nightingale contributed some of the earliest biostatistical data of hospital conditions and outcomes, drawing connections between the environments of care and the contribution of nurses (Dossey, 1999).

Despite Nightingale's innovative ideas to systematize the education of nurses, the origins of modern nursing were seeded with social constraints. Nightingale (1866) wrote to a friend that "the whole reform in nursing both at home and abroad has consisted of this: to take all power over the nursing out of the hands of men and put into the hands of one female trained head and making her responsible for every thing. . . ." Nightingale and her contemporaries purposely overlooked the traditions of men in nursing, such as the work of the Knights Templar (Bullough & Bullough, 1984). The concept of nursing discipline projected by Nightingale, as well as by nursing leaders in the 20th century, held nursing to conventional standards of female subservience within a hierarchy of a "moral" female authority. Nursing was embraced as a feminine endeavor that was to be the singular focus of the nurse's life. Imbued with inherent religious values, nursing was viewed as a selfless act, and the reward for nursing work was deemed intrinsic to the work itself. Nightingale, although a feminist and supporter of women's suffrage, struggled with contradictions of class and gender as she advanced her campaigns for nursing and health. Despite Nightingale's political opinions, modern nursing was reconceptualized as "a woman's calling," and hence doubly subordinated to the paternalism of society.

NURSING TAKES ROOT IN THE UNITED STATES

The universal traditions and nursing functions of caring for the sick have existed for centuries. The power of Nightingale's reforms to formalize and reshape nursing has been evident in their global reach. In the United States, as in many other countries, the importation of the Nightingale schools of nursing legitimated nursing work as an occupation for women. Hospital-based schools of nursing offered women access to education and the potential for employment, creating an option for a sustainable livelihood. Employment as a head nurse or private duty nurse was a welcome alternative to agrarian domesticity or mill work.

The demand for nursing grew in response to hospital growth. As industrialization spurred the growth of larger communities, hospitals proliferated and became a central feature of community life (Rosenberg, 1989). Social reformism was a major force because it spurred the development of both public health and hospital-based services to provide health care to the growing industrial labor force (Rosenberg, 1989; Starr, 1982). From 1875 to 1924, the number of hospitals grew from just over 170 to more than 7000 (Rosner, 1989). However, as noted by Stevens (1989), the central role that health care would take in American society was being shaped by the growing power of medicine. A benevolent paternalism pervaded the structure of healthcare services and harnessed the potential of nursing to support the role of medicine and hospitals (Ashley, 1976). By the early 1900s, the growth of hospitals in the United States generated an unprecedented demand for nurses. The growth of technology from basic advances such as x-rays and anesthesia fueled excitement in hospital investment. Physicians invested their money and technology into hospitals, securing power in their communities as well. Hospitals became a focal point of community life, and hospitals became both a symbol of the prosperity of a community and a focus for social reformism.

The thirst for a cheap and rapidly produced labor supply overshadowed concerns over standards of quality education. From 1900 to 1920, the nursing profession grew "from one in which there were more than 10 times as many physicians as nurses, to one in which there was less than one physician for every nurse" (Burgess, 1928, p. 43). As hospitals grew, schools of nursing were created to provide a labor force for the hospitals, often at the expense of inadequate education (Ashley, 1976). As Dock and Stewart (1938) noted in their history of nursing, "the excess of poor schools and poorly prepared nurses was attributed in large measure to the apprenticeship system that prevailed, with its overemphasis on practice service at the expense of education" (p. 183). Formal studies of nursing education, such as the Goldmark report (1923) and the Grading Committee Report of the National League for Nursing Education (1926), addressed the issue of raising standards for nursing education. Dock and Stewart (1938) suggested that despite the many recommendations for reform, "the system was too deeply rooted and the funds for putting nursing schools on a sound economic and education basis were simply not generally available" (p. 183). Despite forward movement with the establishment of university schools of nursing at Columbia, Yale, and Western Reserve, the push to establish college entrance as a requirement for practice was eclipsed by the hospital training schools. The fundamental professional goal to control the entry into the profession was overridden by hospitals' needs for a cheap labor supply.

The rapid expansion of a nursing labor force occurred with little regard for educational quality. Hospital administrators recognized the economic benefit of using student labor, and physicians began to appreciate the good nursing care offered by graduates of such training. But by the 1930s, concerns about overproduction of nurses emerged and was underscored by the Great Depression. A third of all hospital schools of nursing closed between 1929 and 1939. Nurses, no longer able to secure private duty work, sought employment in hospital wards for hourly or group nursing work. But as Reverby (1979) noted, hospitals were slow to hire graduates as staff nurses, despite admonishments by the nursing leaders and the American Nurses Association. Modified "grouped" private duty nursing efforts transitioned the development to staff nursing. The dire economic conditions of the Depression reshaped nursing work and healthcare services. Nursing shifted away from private freelance work to organized nursing services in hospitals and public health. As nursing became embedded in hospitals, the primacy of the nurse–patient relationship, a characteristic of private duty nursing, eroded, and the nurse became subordinated to the paternalism of the hospital (Dock & Stewart, 1938; Ashley, 1976).

THE CHANGING ORGANIZATION OF WORK

The organizational culture of hospitals, characterized by strong gender-based roles and a hierarchical authority structure, was fertile ground for the application of industrial management methods. The ideas of scientific management made an easy leap from factory floor to hospitals in the first half of the 20th century. Frederick Taylor, the architect of many scientific management ideas, was of a new breed of industrial engineers. His primary concerns were enhancing worker productivity and limiting the threats of unions in order to advance profit from capitalism. Scientific methods were intended to extract labor from workers at the shop-floor level by dividing work into discrete tasks to be done by individual workers. "Taylorism" spread to hospitals and was embraced by nursing leaders, and the quest for efficiency in hospital operations mirrored the factory push toward mechanistic functioning. The application of Taylor's scientific management methods to hospitals included division of labor, the task orientation of "functional nursing," and standardized and proscriptive "procedure manuals." Hospitals were in a unique position to max-imize the control and the execution of nursing work, because they were often both the diploma schools for training nurses and the employer. The hospital culture was able to secure the loyalty of nurses through both school ties and training (Wolf, 1993).

Management in hospitals emerged largely at the ward level. Mobility in nursing became tied to the management structure. Nursing leadership embraced managerialism, because it offered the potential for mobility and status recognition for women. Subordinated to physicians, nurses were unable to gain control over access to patients, use of technology, or application of knowledge. Nursing leader Isabel Stewart attempted to advance "scientific nursing," which she thought could be employed in conjunction with industrial methods for standardization and efficiency of hospital care to wrest control from hospitals. However, her academic approach to building a sci-entific basis for practice was viewed skeptically by nurses and never gained sufficient financial support (Reverby, 1987). Nurses continued to follow orders under a system where work concep-tion was clearly separate from execution.

That the adage "a nurse is a nurse is a nurse" was born in this period reflects the view that nurses were considered an interchangeable part of the hospital machine. Although many nurses preferred to work as private duty nurses, the changing economics of the Great Depression made this an unstable option by the 1930s (Reverby, 1999). As a result of application of scientific man-agement methods to nursing, patient care became fragmented, task oriented, and management fo-cused. Case-based nursing, rooted in the tradition of private duty nursing, fell victim to what was viewed as "progress." New models of care, such as group nursing and functional nursing, reflected the pooling of scarce nursing labor resources to meet the needs of the organization, not the patient.

Following World War II, team nursing became the common model of nursing care organi-zation. The team nursing concept was influenced by wartime experiences and the emerging hu-man relations school of management. The goal was to create a team of nursing care providers led by a professional nurse. Emphasis was placed on effective communication and delegation to en-hance team functioning. However, nursing shortages often resulted in team leaders struggling to provide care with inadequately trained staff. The result of the team approach was more a func-tional approach to care, with emphasis on task completion rather than patient care (Hegyvary, 1982). Because of tradition and nursing shortages, remnants of mechanistic task performance continued to permeate the work culture of hospitals and counter professionalization attempts. Nursing leader Lydia Hall, a fierce opponent of team nursing, challenged nursing to put its rhetoric of professionalism to the test of practice. She instituted a system of professional nurs-ing practice at the Loeb Center, Montefiore Medical Center, in New York City in 1963. The Loeb model of care emphasized nursing autonomy and accountability, giving the nurse responsibility for providing care and making care decisions for his or her patients during the full duration of their hospital stay (Hall, 1969). Her visionary efforts planted ideas for change; however, few hos-pitals adopted her model.

INSTABILITY IN THE NURSING LABOR FORCE

Despite the emphasis on efficiency and rationality in hospital management, the nursing labor force continued to be racked by instability. Recurrent nursing shortages during the 1940s and 1960s led to the policies that increased the production of more nurses and "short training" nurses in particular. These nursing shortages set the pattern for subsequent policy initiatives dominated by hospital interests (Grando, 1998). Hospital administrators and nursing leaders first encouraged licensed practical nurses and then associate degree nurses. In the midst of the shortages, attempts to fill nursing positions were like filling a leaking bucket. Nurses were clearly unhappy with work conditions and compensation. Shortages of nurses left team nurse leaders working alone as captains of understaffed nursing teams. While hospital nursing administrators struggled with the outflow of nurses, nursing educators struggled with the quest to professionalize nursing. The development of nursing knowledge and skills took on renewed urgency at mid-century. Nursing scholars such as Virginia Henderson (1966) sought to reclaim the primacy of the nurse–patient relationship and expand the focus of nursing care beyond efficiency to a process-oriented effectiveness.

The post–World War II period led to increased federal funding for nursing and health care. Along with the funding came a new closer scrutiny of hospital costs. As the federal government became more involved with funding hospital care, the drive to disentangle educational costs from nursing care costs took force.

By the late 1960s funding of nursing education began to move away from the hospital training schools to colleges and universities. Early doctoral programs (see Chapter 32) developed as hybrid degrees, between nursing and fields such as education, sociology, psychology, and biology. These graduate programs had as their primary focus the development of a pool of nursing educators. But within a few years, collegiate nursing education institutions expanded programs in nursing administration and clinical specialization. Graduate education became the primary incubator for nursing theory and the growth of professional knowledge and values.

By the 1970s, a culture of professionalism emerged in nursing, fueled by the growth of nursing scholarship. This resulted in a gap between nurses' expectations and the experiential reality of nursing work. This gap, or "reality shock" (Kramer, 1974), was evidenced by the rapid turnover in staff nursing and nurses' growing discontent. Despite the move to a more efficient hospital functioning, the nursing labor force continued to be racked by instability. Once again, nursing shortages led to the increased production of more nurses, in particular "short training" nurses. Hospital administrators and nursing leaders encouraged the addition of associate degree nurse production as a solution.

Nursing education, long tied to hospitals through the tradition of hospital diploma school, began to break free in the 1960s. The federal government took up more of the financial burden for nursing education. But as nursing education moved into colleges, the trade-off was the loss of nurses' loyalty to hospitals, a central characteristic of hospital-diploma-school nurses. While hospital administrators struggled with the outflow of nurses, the growth of college-based programs at the baccalaureate and associate degree levels infused nursing with a new drive for professional status. As the development of nursing knowledge and skills took on more status and legitimacy, the predominance of nursing management as the primary means of career mobility came to an end (Wolf, 1993).

MILITANCY ROCKS THE HOSPITAL BOAT

Discontent with the reality of nursing work reflected the changing values and expectations of nurses. With rising expectations of professionalism, nurses' desires for control over their work were influenced by the new social realities of women's employment. Nursing was no longer viewed as a transient occupation for women to keep them busy until they married. The growing careerism sharpened nurses' lenses to workplace realities. Turnover rates in hospitals reflected the discontent with working conditions and benefits. Nurses, college educated and empowered by the emerging women's movement, were no longer willing to bow to the paternalism of hospital administrators.

At various points in nursing history, nurses had discussed or attempted the use of collective action or unionism. The rate of nurses organizing for collective bargaining began to increase in the 1960s, but it was not until 1974, with the addition of amendments to the federal Taft-Hartley Act, that the potential impact of collective bargaining was realized (Foley, 1993). These amendments provided federal protection to nurses and other healthcare employees of nonprofit healthcare institutions with regard to the right to organize. The operational structure of the amendments emphasized that nurses were to be a separate and distinct bargaining unit.

The potential of the nursing labor force to be a catalyst for the unionization of the entire hospital labor force was clearly recognized by hospital administrators and "union busting" consultants. This, in turn, resulted in the idea of requiring hospital employees to organize into separate bargaining groups. Nurses were courted initially by professional nursing organizations, such as the ANA-affiliated state nursing organizations. Within a few years, more traditional industrial and trade unions, such as the United Auto Workers (UAW) and the American Federation of Teachers (AFT) joined efforts to organize nurses and other healthcare workers. The ANA-associated state nursing organizations were viewed as the lesser of two evils because the professionalism inherent in the nursing leadership tempered the militancy.

Hospital administrators explored a variety of means to fight the spread of hospital unionism (Kohles, 1994). Treating various types of hospital workers as contract workers was common, but this approach was neither cost nor outcome effective for nursing. Another approach was to create a new work culture and structure that would divide nurses from other hospital employees. This served a double purpose. First, it helped to insulate other hospital workers from nursing collective action. Second, it held the potential to curb the militancy. To effectively bridge the reality gap that had led to nurse militancy, nursing and hospital administrators needed to realistically grapple with the roots of nurses' frustration. The long-standing paternalism was no longer an effective means of controlling nurses.

Nursing is Not Alone: The National Crisis in the Quality of Work Life

By the late 1970s professionalism, long viewed as an unnecessary extravagance, was to become a mantra for nursing management. The growing belief that creating a more professional work climate could mitigate the potential for workplace militancy shaped efforts to restructure nursing work in hospitals. As hospital administrators and nursing grappled with what was perceived to be an issue of militancy versus professionalization, the issue was reflected in broader discussions of an emerging national crisis in workplace relations. Nationally, as concerns over decreases in worker productivity grew, labor experts debated the origins and solutions to worker discontent across a wide range of occupations and professions. The U.S. Department of Health, Education, & Welfare (1973) funded a study—"Work in America"—that asked the question: "What do workers want?" The study yielded the following answers: interesting work, enough help and equipment to get the job done, enough information to get the job done, enough authority to get the job done, good pay, opportunities to develop special abilities, job security, and the ability to see the results of one's work. National labor and management experts debated innovations such as worker control programs and work restructuring. However, the long-standing dominance of industrial labor skewed the perspective of labor experts who were slow to recognize the power and problems of the emerging service sector, and specifically the healthcare labor force.

By the mid-1970s, the nursing profession was in the midst of a collective feminist consciousness raising (Wolf, 1993). Nursing's perspective on nurses' discontent with their work held that the conditions nurses faced were unique and were often viewed within the context of gender and professionalism. Jo Ann Ashley (1996), a feminist nursing historian, offered the most vocal of the feminist perspectives. She described nurses' perceived powerlessness to change their situations as a consequence of their unique socialization as a female-gendered occupation and a result of the cultural barriers to the exercise of the power of nursing within paternalistic institutions.

Caught in a rapid current of cultural change, nursing and hospital administrators were pushed by nurses and pulled by larger social, economic, and political currents to face change in healthcare organizations. Collegiate nursing education, which had begun to embrace the notion of nurses as change agents, contributed to a new professional consciousness. The power to change nursing realities was slowly unleashed.

The unfreezing of hospital nursing to change was rapidly catalyzed as the potential threat of collective bargaining became evident to nursing and hospital industry management. Nurses, like workers in other industries and service sectors, wanted control over their work and a more equitable and open system of resource allocation and rewards. Control involved complex problems of achieving and sustaining authority and ensuring accountability for nursing practice. The potential scope of control ranged from specific day-to-day patient care decision making to participation in organizational governance, such as goal setting and finance (Witte, 1972; Siriani, 1984). Hospital decision making is typically viewed as hierarchical, with organizational control at the top and "bedside" or patient-care issues at the bottom. But in reality the arenas of decision making are overlapping and interconnected within hospital organizations.

PATIENT-CENTERED CARE AND THE EMERGENCE OF PRIMARY NURSING

As the workplace reforms movement moved forward in the 1970s, the desire for control over patient care took precedence in most organizations. This reflected the growing necessity for greater nursing decision making given the rapidly increasing complexity of the patient care. Chapter 10 of this text discusses the impact of technology on nursing work. The most influential development was primary nursing. According to Marram, Schlegal, and Bevis (1974), primary nursing was a developmental step in professional practice development that supported "the distribution of nursing so that the total care of an individual patient is the responsibility of one nurse, not many nurses" (p. 1). Many of the ideas inherent in primary nursing were previously noted by Lydia Hall (1969) at the Loeb Center. Influenced by the wave of quality in work life ideas in the contemporary management literature, primary nursing was invented as an approach to job redesign. This job-redesign approach had been applied successfully in industrial management in Europe and Japan. The primary nursing model offered hospital management a way to counter worker complaints about deskilling. The work of nursing was restructured and enlarged to make nurses accountable for the whole of patient care rather than just for specifics tasks. Primary nursing was also ideologically imbued with professionalism.

The association between primary nursing and enhanced professional orientation was noted in many studies beginning in the 1970s (Marram, Schlegal, & Bevis, 1974). Manthey (1980), an early proponent of primary nursing, noted that primary nursing reflected a philosophical commitment to decision making at the level of action. Primary nursing, drawing on professionalism, sought increased accountability by the nurse for patient care, a rational system of care provided by the nurse who is most knowledgeable about the patient, individualized and personalized patient care, and increased equality among nursing staff (Marram, Schlegal, & Bevis, 1974). To support the initiation of primary nursing, registered nurses had to be "reskilled," and hospitals sought to increase the staffing levels of registered nurses while decreasing the employment and roles of licensed practical nurses and nursing assistants. In most instances, this necessitated increased funding or significant reallocation of funds, made possible in the late 1970s by government and private support to hospitals.

Primary nursing provided a process by which patient-centered care could be individualized yet applied within a standardized nursing process. However unique each patient-care situation might be, the process of nursing judgment and discretion became predictable. The application of the nursing process as a method of solving nursing care problems became central to nursing education and practice in the 1970s. The development of professional nursing standards for care by the ANA further codified this process orientation. However, the growing complexity of patient care and the increasing body of nursing theory would soon shift nursing's emphasis to critical thinking.

Despite the shift in control over nursing education from hospitals to academic institutions, the reality was that most nursing graduates were going to be employed by hospitals. Nursing educators faced pressure to produce a product "nurse" that met the hospital labor market needs in terms of skill, as well as price.

As legal and regulatory pressures for greater accountability mounted, new demands for documentation shaped the day of hospital nurses. Nurses expressed a sense of being pushed into documentation at the expense of being pulled away from patient care. As one primary nurse noted, "Make sure your patient care is your priority, but don't forget your paperwork" (Wolf, 1993, p. 115). The strain of competing demands between the work of nursing and the documentation of the work emerged as a recurring theme underlying alienation and nurse dissatisfaction. As nurses grappled with the potential of primary nursing to provide rewards, the reality of the system's constraints and the contextual issues of organizational control became more apparent.

THE MISSING LINKS: SHARED GOVERNANCE AND RECOGNITION

The initiation of shared governance in healthcare institutions in the 1980s highlights an attempt to ease the tensions between administrative controls and professional work. Primary nursing, while restructuring nursing work, was quickly found to be limited in its scope. The work of nurses was embedded in the organizational context and was shaped by decisions that were often removed from their sphere of action. From staffing to equipment choice, these decisions often impacted patient care, leaving nurses frustrated, which compounded problems of turnover and militancy. Just as American industry struggled with the push to expand worker control without sacrificing managerial prerogatives, the push for workplace participation in decision making grew. Genuine participation was made difficult by the complex hospital authority structure, which kept nurses "trapped" between the dual hierarchies of medicine and the hospital administration.

The climb by nurses out from between these two systems of control generated both a threat and an opportunity for the reallocation of power in hospitals. Nursing leaders such as Manthey (1991) cautioned that in order for the reallocation of power to occur, a major change was required in the structure and operation of nursing departments. Change would require a major dismantling of the hospital hierarchy, beginning with the nursing departments. As Porter-O'Grady (2001) noted, "Implementing an empowered format such as shared governance means that the relationships, decisions, structures, and processes will be forever changed at every level of the system and that all the players in the organization will be different and behave differently as a result" (p. 5). The changes in patterns of communication and behaviors extended across relationships, not only nurse–nurse or nurse–patient, but also nurse–physician. Many physicians were initially ambivalent and threatened by shared governance (Wolf, 1993).

In the 1980s and 1990s, many hospitals moved toward flatter management structures in an effort to move toward shared governance. Work, previously viewed as a management prerogative, was typically distributed across the flattened structure to involve staff nurses as well as administrators in decision-making processes at the committee level. Nurse participation was concentrated at the committee level. A study by Jenkins (1988) observed that the expanded committee structure resulted in more time spent in meetings and an overall drop in hours per full-time employee. For example, Massachusetts General Hospital provides a wide range of committees in its governance structure, including such foci as patient-care quality, diversity, and staff recruitment (Erickson, 1996). Participation is based on an application; it is a selective process that draws from a pool of dedicated full- and part-time nursing staff who give generously of their time and expertise.

A parallel concern to expanded decision making has been the need to recognize nurses for their efforts (McCoy, 1999). Hospital nursing is complex and difficult work. Keeping experienced nurses at the bedside improves the quality of patient care and reduces recruitment and orientation costs. The challenge has been to find a way to reward nurses for a career in direct care rather than management. Career ladders typify the development of new reward systems. Career ladders provide a hierarchical system of rewarding professional behaviors, such as advanced education; scholarship; and contributions to the institution, such as committee work or clinical projects. This system provides the semblance of mobility by recognizing those nurses who choose to stay at the bedside. Given the recurrent stresses of nursing shortages, career ladders have provided another mechanism to attract and retain clinically expert nurses. The career ladder system has codified the job enlargement of the "professional nurse," while stimulating nurse productivity in a variety of areas, such as quality assurance, practice policy development, hospital public relations, and nurse recruitment (Wolf, 1993). However, the linking of remuneration with career ladder steps progression historically has been problematic for many hospitals. The hospital budget process and pressures to control nurse salaries has thwarted career ladder development efforts in some hospitals. Many senior nurses find themselves hitting the glass ceiling with new hires rapidly gaining more compensation. Healthcare organizations have also adopted nonmonetary systems of nurse recognition, such as the "professional nurse of the month" awards. These symbolic rewards, while recognizing clinical excellence, divert attention away from the concrete contextual realities of practice.

THE ATTRACTION OF MAGNET HOSPITALS

In the early 1980s, the American Academy of Nursing launched an effort to recognize hospitals for their ability to attract and retain nursing staff (Upenickes, 2003). The Magnet Hospital Program was launched based on a study that identified hospitals having low staff turnover, high nurse job satisfaction, and low staff nurse vacancy rates. The initial recognition went to some 41 hospitals. The results of the early magnet hospital studies highlighted the importance of organizational factors, such as participatory structures and processes, perceived autonomy of nurses, and empowering leadership (Scott et al., 1999). The characteristics of these hospitals paralleled many of the recommended changes of the quality of work life advocates. Policy reports by the Institute of Medicine (1981) and the National Commission on Nursing (1981) Report by the American Hospital Association gave added legitimacy to the move to restructure hospitals to better attract and retain nursing staff. Some 20 years after the initial magnet studies, a body of research has been collected to justify continuing support for the restructuring of systems of care. Current efforts focus on validating outcomes of care in magnet hospital systems, but a better understanding of the relationship between outcomes and nurses' autonomy is needed (Ritter-Teital, 2002; Havens & Aiken, 1999; Scott et al., 1999).

PROFESSIONAL NURSING AND NURSE STAFFING: CHICKEN OR EGG?

How well hospitals are able to sustain professional models is dependent on the political and economic climate of the healthcare market. Past nursing shortages generated greater leverage for nursing stakeholders. Yet as tensions in labor ease or are overcome by greater organizational pressure to contain or depress labor costs, the potential for backpedaling on professional nursing gains increases. Nursing has a greater potential to enhance quality outcomes by maximizing the use of professional expertise. As has been noted in recent studies, sustaining adequate nurse staffing may be one of the most important key factors in patient care outcomes (Cho et al., 2003; Aiken et al., 2002). Such research further underscores the importance of continuing professional models of development as they support the recruitment and retention of staff. For too long the value of nursing has been hidden in health care by data collection and information systems that give primacy to medicine. Emerging advances in nursing informatics will hopefully add to nursing's visibility and support continued vitality. A firm investment in professional models will also call for healthcare organizations to effectively match nursing education and talents with the complexity of the work. The corporatization of hospitals provides a relative opportunity for nursing to gain power in the healthcare organization. It is time for nursing to cease its dependence on the "good will" of institutions and to demand full participation in institutional policy making.

CONCLUSION

Throughout the history of nursing, professionalization has been a driving force for change. From the earliest innovations of Nightingale to the most recent nursing shortage, the work culture of nursing has been reshaped to meet the needs of society or managerial interests, often in the midst of crises. The slow march toward professional practice continues as models of nursing practice offer a powerful ideological hold. Nursing has been the influenced by ideas drawn from the sociology, management, and industry resulting in workplace reforms reframed within a "professional" lens. The power of professionalization has contributed significantly to the success of this reform, offering benefits to both healthcare institutions and nurses. However, nursing shortages remain. Challenging questions for the future include the following: To what extent are professional models of practice sustainable in the face of economic uncertainty? And can institutional control truly be ceded to nurses without a fundamental revolution in the overall restructuring of healthcare financing and service structure?

REFERENCES

Aiken, L. H., Clarke, S. P., Sloane, D. M., Sochalski, J., & Silber, J. H. (2002). Hospital nurse staffing and patient mortality, nurse burnout, and job satisfaction. *Journal of the American Medical Association, 288*, 1987–1993.

Ashley, J. (1976). *Hospitals, paternalism, and the role of the nurse.* New York: Columbia University Press.

Ashley, J. (1996). This I believe about power in nursing. In K. Wolf (Ed.), *Selected Readings of Jo Ann Ashley* (pp. 23–34). New York: NLN Press/Jones & Bartlett.

Bucher, R., & Strauss, A. (1961). Professions in progress. *American Journal of Sociology, 66*(4), 325–334.

Bullough, V., & Bullough, B. (1984). *The history, trends, and politics of nursing.* Norwalk, CT: Appleton Century Crofts.

Burgess, M. (1928). *Nurses, patients, and pocketbooks.* New York: Committee on the Grading of Nursing Schools.

Cho, S. H., Ketefian, S., Barkauskas, V. H., & Smith, D. G. (2003). The effects of nurse staffing on adverse events, morbidity, mortality, and medical costs. *Nursing Research, 52*, 71–79.

Dean, M., & Bolton, J. (1980). The administration of poverty and the development of nursing practice in nineteenth-century England. In C. Davies (Ed.), *Rewriting nursing history* (pp. 76–101). London: Croom Helm.

Dock, L., & Stewart, I. (1938). *A short history of nursing.* New York: G.P. Putnam's Sons.

Dossey, B. (1999). *Florence Nightingale: Mystic, visionary, healer.* Springhouse, PA: Springhouse Corporation.

Erickson, J. I. (1996). Our professional practice model. *MGH Patient Care Services, Caring Headlines, 2*(23).

Etzioni, A. (1969). *The semi-professions and their organization.* New York: Free Press.

Foley, M. (1993). The politics of collective bargaining. In D. Mason, S. Talbot, & J. Leavitt (Eds.), *Policy and politics for nurses* (2nd ed.) (pp. 282–302). Philadelphia: W.B. Saunders.

Fourcher, L., & Howard, M. (1981). Nursing and the managerial demiurge. *Social Science and Medicine, Part A, Medical Sociology, 15*(3 pt), 299–306.

Goldmark, J. (1923). *Nursing and nursing education in the U.S. Report of the Committee for the study of Nursing Education.* New York: MacMillan.

Grando, V. T. (1998). Making do with fewer nurses in the United States, 1945–1965. *Image: Journal of Nursing Scholarship, 30*(2), 147–149.

Hall, L. E. (1969). The Loeb Center for Nursing and Rehabilitation, Montefiore Medical Center, Bronx, New York. *International Journal of Nursing Studies, 16*, 215–230.

Havens, D., & Aiken, L. (1999). Shaping systems to promote desired outcomes: The magnet hospitals model. *Journal of Nursing Administration, 29*(2), 14–20.

Henderson, V. (1966). *The nature of nursing.* New York: MacMillan.

Hegyvary, S. T. (1982). *The change to primary nursing.* St. Louis: C.V. Mosby.

Hughes, C. E. (1971). *The sociological eye.* Chicago: Aldine.

Institute of Medicine (1981). *The study of nursing and nursing education.* Washington, DC: National Academy of Science Press.

Jenkins, J. (1988). A nursing governance and practice model: What are the costs? *Nursing Economics, 6*(6), 302–311.

Kohles, M. K. (1994). Commentary on union election activity in the health care industry. *Health Care Management Review, 19*(1), 18–27.

Kramer, M. (1974). *Reality shock: Why nurses leave nursing.* St. Louis: C.V. Mosby.

Manthey, M. (1980). *The practice of primary nursing.* Boston: Blackwell Scientific Publications.

Manthey, M. (1991). Delivery systems and practice models: A dynamic balance. *Nursing Management, 22*(1), 28–30.

Marram, G., Schlegel, M., & Bevis, E. O. (1974). *Primary nursing: A model for individualized care.* St. Louis: C.V. Mosby.

McCoy, J. M. (1999). Recognize, reward, retain. *Nursing Management, 30*(2), 41–43.

National League for Nursing Education (1926). *The grading committee report of the National League for Nursing Education.* New York: NLNE.

National Commission on Nursing. (1981). *Summary of public hearings.* Chicago, IL: The Hospital Research and Educational Trust.

Nightingale, F. (1866). Letter to Mary Jones. Cited on p. 25 in B. Abel-Smith, *A history of the nursing profession* (1960). London: Heinman.

Perrow, C. (1972). *Complex organizations: A critical essay.* Glenview, IL: Scott Foresman.

Porter-O'Grady, T. (2001). Is shared governance still relevant? *Journal of Nursing Administration, 31*(10), 467–473.

Reverby, S. (1979). The search for the hospital yardstick. In S. Reverby & D. Rosner (Eds.), *Health care in America* (pp. 206–225). Philadelphia: Temple University Press.

Reverby, S. (1987). *Ordered to care, the dilemma of American nursing, 1850–1945.* Cambridge: Cambridge University Press.

Reverby, S. (1999). Neither for the drawing room nor for the kitchen: Private duty nursing in Boston, 1873–1914, pp. 460–474. In J. Waltzer Leavitt (Ed.), *Women and health in America.* Madison, WI: University of Wisconsin Press.

Ritter-Teital, J. (2002). The impact of restructuring on professional nursing practice. *Journal of Nursing Administration, 32*(1), 31–41.

Rosenberg, C. (1989). Community and communities: The evolution of the American hospital. In D. Long & J. Golden (Eds.), *The American general hospital* (pp. 3–17). Ithaca: Cornell University Press.

Rosner, D. (1989). Doing well or doing good: The ambivalent focus of hospital administration. In D. Long & J. Golden (Eds.), *The American general hospital* (pp. 157–169). Ithaca: Cornell University Press.

Scott, J. G., Sochalski, J., & Aiken, L. (1999). Review of magnet hospital research: Findings and implications for professional nursing practice. *Journal of Nursing Administration, 29*(1), 9–19.

Siriani, C. (1984). Participation, opportunity, and equality: Towards a pluralist organization model. In F. Ficher & C. Siriani (Eds.), *Critical studies in organization & bureaucracy* (pp. 482–503). Philadelphia: Temple University Press.

Starr, P. (1982). *The social transformation of American medicine.* New York: Basic Books.

Stevens, R. (1989). *In Hospitals and in wealth. American Hospitals in the Twentieth Century.* New York, Basic Books.

Upenickes, V. (2003). Recruitment and retention strategies: A magnet hospital prevention model. *Nursing Economics, 21*(1), 7–13, 23.

Williams, K. (1980). From Sarah Gamp to Florence Nightingale: A critical study of hospital nursing systems from 1840 to 1897. In C. Davies (Ed.), *Rewriting nursing history* (pp. 41–75). London: Croom Helm.

Witte, J. (1972). *Democracy, authority and alienation in work.* Chicago: University of Chicago Press.

Wolf, K. A. (1993). *The professionalization of nursing work: The case of nursing at Mill City Medical Center.* Dissertation microfilms PUZ9322364. Ann Arbor: University of Michigan.

U.S. Department of Health, Education & Welfare (1973). *Work in America, HEW Report.* Cambridge: MIT Press.

C H A P T E R   2 7

Nursing Centers and the Autonomy of Nursing Work

Melinda L. Jenkins

Nurses comprise the largest group of healthcare professionals; they are highly trusted essential members of the healthcare team. Yet, direct access to nurses is extremely limited in the United States, due in large part to the funneling of nearly all third-party payments to physicians and hospitals, which employ the majority of the estimated 1.3 million nurses and nurse practitioners. Since the late 1980s, Medicaid and Medicare have paid nurse practitioners (NPs) directly, and additional federal contract monies have enabled modern nurse-managed centers to establish a position as valued alternatives in the healthcare marketplace. Most of the existing centers were initially intended to serve as learning laboratories to promote nursing and advanced practice nursing education and were funded by the Division of Nursing, U.S. Health Resources and Services Administration. In addition, a few nurse-managed centers began as Federally Qualified Rural or Public Housing Health Centers. Today, these nurse-managed centers aim to provide culturally appropriate primary health care to underserved populations and to integrate health promotion with acute and chronic disease care. This trend toward direct access to nursing services has accelerated as nurse entrepreneurs have begun to establish independent nursing practices funded by out-of-pocket and third-party payments. The purpose of this chapter is to review the historical development and current status of nurse-managed centers, to highlight how these environments foster nursing autonomy, and to suggest means for vibrant growth of autonomous nursing practice in community settings.

In the 20th century, several nurse entrepreneurs conducted groundbreaking autonomous work in their communities that continues to inspire present-day nursing centers. Lillian Wald, Margaret Sanger, and Mary Breckinridge were pioneers in providing direct access to what is now known as nurse-managed care. Each of these women sought to provide services to underserved populations with crucial gaps in primary health care. Though there is no evidence that they knew each other, they worked in a similar time, described in hindsight by social historian Paul Starr as the heyday of public health, before private health care became lucrative (Starr, 1982). They held in common their social consciousness and dedication to community health, their talent for garnering support and for financing their projects creatively, and their professional leadership that resulted in the creation of many influential and lasting institutions.

NURSE PIONEERS IN COMMUNITY-BASED PRACTICE

Lillian Wald

Lillian Wald, nurse and social reformer, left an imprint on health care at many levels. Her career in public health began in New York City in 1893 when she began to serve immigrant families who could not afford to pay for physician care. Although she was attending medical school at the time, she quit her studies to go into tenement houses on the Lower East Side to care for mothers and children facing public health problems such as poor sanitation, communicable diseases, and poor nutrition. At first there was no mechanism to fund this care, so the nurses providing it were themselves at risk for poverty.

With her colleague Mary Brewster, Wald founded the Visiting Nurses Service, which still exists today. Then, in 1895, they opened the Henry Street Settlement, a nurse-managed center that is still in operation under the auspices of the Pace University School of Nursing. By 1915, 100 Settlement nurses had made over 227,000 visits to more than 26,000 patients. Professing steadfast faith in her mission, she stated, "Never in all the years have we on Henry Street doubted the validity of our belief in the essential dignity of man and the obligations of each generation to do better for the oncoming generation" (Wald, 1934, p. 336). In addition to health services, the Henry Street Settlement provided nursing education, community education, youth groups, and a playhouse. It also served as the meeting place for what later became the National Association for the Advancement of Colored People (NAACP).

Wald also broke new ground for direct payment of organized home nursing care based on the projected savings due to the prevention of severe illness and death. In 1909, recognizing the real costs and value of nursing care, she designed an insurance program for the industrial policyholders of Metropolitan Life Insurance Company whereby visiting nurses received a steady income for their work. Nurse home visits to sick policyholders were quickly shown to reduce death benefits paid out nationwide. After a peak in 1931, the number of policyholders using the service dropped as the cost per visit rose. Undoubtedly, the movement of care into hospitals and an overall decrease in mortality contributed to the demise of the program in the 1950s (Buhler-Wilkerson, 1993).

Among Wald's great achievements was the establishment of the U.S. Children's Bureau, which eventually evolved into the current Bureau of Maternal-Child Health. In 1912, Wald was awarded a gold medal by the National Institute of Social Sciences for her efforts that led to this organization. That same year, she created the National District Nursing Service of the American Red Cross.

Another of her lasting innovations was the naming of *public health nursing*. According to Karen Buhler-Wilkerson (1993), "Wald claimed she chose the title 'public health nurse'" to place emphasis on the "community value of the Nurse whose work was built upon an understanding of the social and economic problems invariably accompanying patient's ills" (p. 1780). Wald became the first president of the National Organization for Public Health Nursing. In addition, her vision paved the way for the development of the school nurse role in New York City, with the placement of nurses in public schools.

Unfortunately, Wald's ideal of uniting care for sickness and health was thwarted in the 1920s due to contextual changes, including a perceived threat to physicians' and hospitals' incomes (Starr, 1982). In the face of this opposition, Buhler-Wilkerson (1993) maintains that "organized nursing was never able to create an institutional framework that would allow nurses to perform both preventive and curative activities" (p. 1783). Today's lack of payment for much preventive care, including that in nurse-managed centers, stems from policies that grew from the separation of population-based public health and individual private health care in the 1920s.

Margaret Sanger

A mother with three children of her own, Margaret Sanger earned a living as a public health nurse in New York City, caring mostly for obstetrical cases. Through her work, she came to know many women weary from childbearing. In 1912, she became acutely aware of the stress caused by unplanned parenthood when one of her patients on the Lower East Side self-induced an abortion and died (Lynaugh, 1991). Following this event, Sanger determined that, "no matter what it might cost, I was finished with palliatives and superficial cures; I was resolved to seek out the root of evil, to do something to change the destiny of mothers whose miseries were vast as the sky" (Sanger, 1938, p. 92). Thus, she sought to learn as much as she could about birth control in order to prevent similar occurrences.

In 1914, Sanger started a magazine, *Woman Rebel*, that provided information on contraception. Providing such information was illegal—according to the federal Comstock Law—and she was indicted on postal obscenity laws (Katz, 2002). Escaping to England, she persisted in her endeavor, directing the distribution of 100,000 copies of a pamphlet that contained explicit instructions on several methods of contraception.

When Sanger returned to the United States in 1915, the government dropped its case against her. In 1916, she and her sister Ethel opened the first birth control clinic in the United States in Brooklyn. After operating for nine days, the clinic was closed, and Sanger was arrested and imprisoned. However, as a result of her legal appeal, physicians were exempted from the Comstock Law if they prescribed contraceptive information for medical reasons. So, in 1923 Sanger opened another birth control clinic, this one run by a physician. Subsequently, in 1936 physicians also were exempted from the ban on importing birth control supplies.

Sanger utilized a variety of means for funding her efforts to provide women with birth control. Her marriage to a wealthy man and her ability to solicit funding from other private donors allowed her to maintain her activism. Eventually, though, she came to be seen as being too radical for the movement she had begun. For example, she examined the use of birth control to decrease genetic defects (NYU, 2002), a shocking concept at the time. Additionally, she opposed racism by providing birth control in Harlem with the help of W.E.B. DuBois (Planned Parenthood, 2000). Despite opposition from the Catholic Church, the family planning movement seeped into the mainstream, moving away from the feminist ideal of reproductive freedom and toward a moderate goal of family child spacing (Katz, 2002). In 1939, the American Birth Control League (founded by Sanger) merged with the Birth Control Clinical Research Bureau and became the present-day Planned Parenthood Federation of America (Katz, 2002).

In 1952, Sanger helped found the International Planned Parenthood Federation. In addition, throughout the 1950s she also arranged funding that contributed to the development of the birth control pill. In 1965, over 50 years after she first began her campaign, and just a few months before she died, the U.S. Supreme Court, in *Griswold v. Connecticut*, legalized birth control for married couples. The Court's decision is yet another example of how Sanger's work changed the life choices that are available for millions of women and families.

Mary Breckinridge

After suffering personal tragedy, including the death of one husband, a divorce from her second, and the loss of her two young children, Mary Breckinridge resolved to turn her attention to others, vowing "to work directly for little children now and always—because that is the work I can do best, in which my health and enthusiasm and happiness do not fail" (Breckinridge, 1972, p. 73). Trained in Britain as a midwife, Breckinridge was inspired by a visit to a poor, rural area in Scotland where care was provided by nurse-midwives. Back in the United States, she established a nurse-managed practice in Kentucky, where seven generations of her family were buried (Lester, 2000). Breckinridge justified her choice of location, stating, "Not only was there no reason why the Kentucky Mountains should not be chosen, but we had the best of all reasons for choosing them, namely their inaccessibility—I felt that if the work I had in mind could be done there, it could be duplicated anywhere else in the United States with less effort" (Breckinridge, 1972, p. 158). Surveying lay midwives in the area, she found them to be mostly elderly and self-taught, delivering an average of 19 babies a year and seldom providing prenatal care. Maternal and infant mortality in the area were high. In 1925, Breckinridge and two colleagues, Freida Caffin and Edna Rockstroh, established the Frontier Nursing Service (FNS) in Leslie County, Kentucky. Initially, the FNS was funded as a private philanthropy, and its outpost centers were built with contributions of supplies and labor from the local community (Lester, 2000). Nurse-midwives trained in England (there were no midwifery schools in the United States at the time) rode on horseback over hill and stream to provide prenatal care and to attend births at remote Appalachian homes. Respectful of the local people, they were soon asked to care for entire families. FNS service fees were based on the local standard of living; chickens and produce were common forms of payment. Families were charged a base $1.00 a year fee, plus $5.00 for the delivery of a baby (Allen, 2000).

The FNS and its nurses were quickly embraced by the community. A local man, Matt Gray, lauded their efforts, proclaiming, "Good to people, the nurses were, and there weren't no finer woman ever crossed the water than Mary Breckinridge was . . . She was more help to this country than any other person that ever been in" (Gray, 2000). In addition to their goodwill and compassion, the nurses offered their extensive nurse-midwifery skills, and, as a result, maternal and infant mortality rates dropped rapidly soon after the FNS was started and continued to remain low for the duration of its existence. Nearly 18,000 babies were delivered between 1925 and 1975, with only 11 maternal deaths (USDI, 2000).

As demand for FNS services increased, Breckinridge began collecting donations from all over the country, including cities such as Louisville, Lexington, Boston, New York, Chicago, Detroit, and Washington, D.C. Interested parties sometimes even formed committees to support the Service. Betty Lester, a nurse who worked with Breckinridge, recalled, ". . . she [Breckinridge] never once asked for money. She always told them what the conditions were and what we were doing, and money just came in" (Lester, 2000). Breckinridge used these outside funds to expand the FNS by building additional centers. The Hyden Hospital and Health Center was opened in 1928 in addition to six outpost nursing centers built between 1927 and 1930. Located in the rural backcountry of Leslie and Clay Counties, the centers were between 9 and 12 miles apart, serving approximately 70 square miles each; each center was under the supervision of a registered nurse-midwife. The total area served was about 700 square miles (USDI, 2000). Even during the Great Depression, when many people could not afford to donate to the FNS, Breckinridge and others continued to serve the community. One midwife remembered these times, reflecting, "We didn't close down, we just managed. Some of the nurses had to leave and some of us stayed and we didn't have any money but we were very happy. We had enough to eat and a bed to sleep on and our horses were taken care of" (Lester, 2000). The nurses continued to live meagerly into the 1940s, traveling by foot or horse to make house calls. They did not have a jeep until the late 1940s (USDI, 2000).

In 1939, when 11 British nurse-midwives were called back to England at the beginning of the Second World War, Breckinridge opened the first nurse-midwifery school in the United States, the Frontier Graduate School of Midwifery, in order to ensure that there were enough nurses to sustain the FNS. Today, the school also offers graduate education for family nurse practitioners. Demonstrating national professional leadership, the American College of Nurse Midwives was founded by FNS staff in 1929 (ANA, 2003). Currently, FNS-educated nurse midwives and family nurse practitioners are working all over the world.

THE EVOLVING CONTEXT OF HEALTH CARE

The entire context of American health care has changed since the 1920s when our esteemed foremothers worked. Because hospitals and physicians dominated the formation of healthcare policy and reimbursement in the United States, financial incentives for practice, education, and research have left nurses and public health services behind. Much of the health care formerly administered by nurses and families in homes and communities has been subordinated to the control of medicine and corporate health, transforming health care from a public service to a big business (Starr, 1982). Federal funding to hospitals and physicians has been a major mechanism for this evolution, increasing from the 1930s on, with a rapid acceleration after Medicare and Medicaid were established in 1965.

The number of hospitals increased dramatically from 178 in 1872 to 4013 in 1920. During this period of hospital growth, dispensaries and public health clinics similar to Wald's blossomed as public health moved "from the environment to the individual" (Starr, 1982, p. 192). But, as social historian Paul Starr (1982) relates,

. . . doctors fought against public treatment of the sick . . . and attempts by public health authorities to establish health centers to coordinate preventive and curative medical services. . . . The defense of private interests set one of the limits to the rational organization of medical care in America . . . [with the] artificial separation of diagnosis from treatment, and more generally of preventive from curative medicine. (p. 181, 196)

According to Starr (1982), the rise of medicine as a sovereign profession in the United States was based on five structural changes that occurred during the first half of the 20th century (pp. 229–231). First, physicians kept informal control of practice by developing specialization and hospital privileges. Second, state licensing laws were passed to control labor markets. Third, the "capital investment required for medical practice was socialized" (p. 230), in that hospitals, medical schools, research, diagnostic labs, and public health centers for diagnosis and referral to private physicians were subsidized by public funds. Fourth, "no organized buyers offset the market power of physicians . . . doctors could then set prices" (p. 231). And fifth, internal boundaries of authority were established within the medical profession, squelching all attempts at outside management. Starr (1982) explains, "Private medicine was sustained by the willingness of public institutions to assume part of its cost" (p. 231). A substantial, if nonfinancial, cost was the separation of prevention and cure that continues in large part today.

While medicine was consolidating its power, the nursing profession struggled with poorly standardized hospital training of nurses and the use of nursing students as cheap labor in hospitals. The supply of nurses has fluctuated between a perceived scarcity during World War I to an abundance of unemployed nurses during the Depression, and back to today's nursing shortage (Reverby, 1987). Private duty nurses, a potential pool for public health care, evaporated after the Depression due to competition from charity-funded public health nurses and cheaper, untrained health workers. As a remedy, nursing leaders focused on improving education, not practice. Following recommendations in the 1922 Goldmark report and the 1934 Grading Committee report, nursing education was slowly upgraded to the baccalaureate level in a process that continues today (Reverby, 1987). Currently, nursing education continues to lag behind medicine in finding solid financial footing, partly because the steady stream of public funding for graduate medical education that was built into Medicare is not available for baccalaureate or graduate nursing education (Aiken & Gwyther, 1995).

In the 1960s, community health centers, similar in philosophy to nursing centers, were established with the requirement of a *physician* director, with the notable exception of a few rural and public housing health centers. This model holds promise for the future of nurse-managed centers, as will be discussed. Direct reimbursement to NPs from Medicare and Medicaid has been available only since 1989; legal technicalities still prevent many NPs from readily obtaining public or private managed care reimbursement. A serious side effect of this reimbursement situation is a severe lack of data on NP care from large public databases (Sullivan-Marx & Mullinix, 1999).

Similarly, research dollars for nurses from the National Institutes of Health have comprised only a small fraction of the whole, as the cadre of doctorally prepared nurses has grown slowly over the years. Yet, in the face of severe funding and policy constraints, nurses' commitment to community needs has spurred the building of an estimated 250 or more nurse-managed centers across the country (Matherlee, 1999).

Data from the American Academy of Colleges of Nursing's 1998 survey of 119 nurse-managed centers associated with schools of nursing showed that while over half of the nursing centers were in urban areas, they were located in diverse settings including nursing schools, elementary or secondary schools, neighborhood/community or senior centers, school health centers, churches, shelters, store fronts, hospitals and mobile vans. The populations served by nurse-managed centers were diverse in terms of socio-cultural background and health care needs. Within this culturally diverse population, some 30% of the population was non-English speaking. The vulnerability of the population was demonstrated by age, as well as the presence of problems such as homelessness, chronic illness and disability, and violence. More than one third of the population served was over the age of 85; and, other reported indicators of vulnerability included: homelessness—19%; victims of abuse—14%; substance abuse—11%; mental illness—8%; HIV-positive status—2%; migrant status—6%; developmental disabilities or handicapped—5%; pre-term infants—3%; prisoners—2%. While there was often overlap among the categories, some 21% did not report falling into any of the previous categories. (Berlin cited in Matherlee, 1999, p. 5).

THE NURSING CENTERS OF TODAY

In 1979, shortly after nurse practitioner graduate programs began to flourish, the American Academy of Nursing (AACN) recognized the value of faculty practice for educators to keep clinical skills and to provide mentorship to students (Evans, Jenkins, & Buhler-Wilkerson, 2003). Consequently, several schools of nursing began to open nurse-managed centers: 63 were estimated to exist by the early 1980s. Since 1986, under a number of Nurse Education and Practice Improvement Amendments Acts, nursing centers have been funded as special projects by the Department of Health and Human Sciences Division of Nursing. In 1987, 9 nursing centers were funded; 13 were funded in 1988, 15 in 1990, 17 in 1992, and 41 in 1998 (Clear, Starbecker, & Kelly, 1999). O. Marie Henry, Chief of the Division of Nursing, emphasized that funding to schools of nursing would increase the number of learning laboratories for caring for culturally diverse, underserved populations (Henry, 1978; Barnum, 1991). By 1998, out of approximately 553 AACN teaching programs, 119 had nursing centers (Berlin, 1999). In a comprehensive survey done in 2005, the MAC counted 103 academic nurse-managed centers in 86 schools of nursing. Selected centers in operation today will be presented here.

University of Wisconsin-Milwaukee School of Nursing

In 1979, the University of Wisconsin-Milwaukee School of Nursing opened an academic nursing center on campus. The center provides health promotion, group counseling, and support services to about 1500 patients a year. In addition, the center created opportunities for nursing education and research programs (UWM, 2005). A second center, the Silver Spring Neighborhood Center, was opened in 1987 to provide primary health care in a public housing community in northwest Milwaukee. This nurse-managed center was one of the first schools to receive Division of Nursing funding. Three more centers, including one serving the homeless and a school-based center, were begun in the early 1990s, and a second Division of Nursing grant was awarded. Faculty leadership for the centers was provided by Dr. Sally Lundeen; Dr. Sandra Underwood; Dr. Joan Wilk; Barbara Friedbacher, RN, MS; Mary Jo Baisch, RN, MS; and Jean Bell-Calvin.

Funding for the centers now comes from patient reimbursements and a variety of targeted grants. Graduate and undergraduate students rotate through the centers for community-based clinical experience. Several years ago, researchers at these centers began to use standardized terms from the Omaha System of Nursing Classification to establish a customized database for recording nursing diagnoses, interventions, and outcomes from patient encounters (Martin & Scheet, 1992).

East Tennessee State University College of Nursing

The Mountain City Extended Hours Health Center, one of East Tennessee State University College of Nursing's nurse-managed centers, is a Federally Qualified Rural Health Center in the Appalachian Mountains. It has obtained funding from the Division of Nursing for its educational mission to integrate behavioral health care with managed primary care and to provide clinical mentorship for primary care NP students as well as BSN students (ESTU, 2000). The faculty has published data that compare 680 of their NP–patient encounters with results of the National Ambulatory Medical Care Survey, which documents mostly physician encounters (Moody, Smith, & Glenn, 1999). In accord with multiple studies finding that NPs provide more health education than physicians, the researchers documented that NPs in the East Tennessee nurse-managed center "were more likely to provide counseling . . . about nutrition, exercise . . . smoking cessation . . . weight reduction . . . and family planning" (Moody, Smith, & Glenn,

1999). The center clearly fills a need for health promotion in an underserved area. In 2004, it was approved as a Federally Qualified Health Center, making it eligible for enhanced Medicaid payments.

Michigan Academic Consortium

The Michigan Academic Consortium (MAC) consists of four state universities with a total of eight nurse-managed primary healthcare centers that are funded, in part, by the W. K. Kellogg Foundation. The cooperating schools and their centers are:

- ☐ Grand Valley State University
  - Herkimer Health Center: Serves a vulnerable population in downtown Grand Rapids
  - Campus Health Center: Provides primary care to students, faculty, staff, and their families.
- ☐ Michigan State University College of Nursing
  - Health Care Center: Serves veterans through a capitated care contract with the Veterans Administration (VA).
- ☐ The University of Michigan
  - Community Family Health Center: Serves a diverse population on the west side of Ann Arbor with strong community involvement.
  - North Campus Family Health Services: Serves a diverse international student population.
- ☐ Wayne State University
  - Primary Care Nursing Service: A 21-year-old nurse-managed center located in the Detroit Medical Center.
  - University Public School Teen Clinic: Serves the students, faculty, and parents of a middle school.
- ☐ A joint venture between Wayne State University and The University of Michigan.
  - Imani Family Health Center, located in Tried Stone Baptist Church, provides access to care in the Virginia Park neighborhood (MAC, 2005).

The MAC is under the able leadership of Joanne Pohl, PhD, RN, CS, University of Michigan; Jean Nagelkerk, PhD, RN, FNP-CS, Grand Valley State; Jeanette Klemczak, MSN, RN, Michigan State; Stephen Cavanagh, PhD, RN, Wayne State; and G. Elaine Beane, PhD, Michigan Public Health Institute. Up to 80% of the MAC's patients are uninsured.

Supported with funding from the Kellogg Foundation, the MAC commissioned a survey of all schools of nursing and found 184 academic nurse-managed centers operating in the United States (Sebastian et al., 2002). In December 2003, the MAC held a National Nursing Summit to convene approximately 60 leaders in the field in order to build consensus on issues facing nurse-managed centers and to set priorities for action. The summary report is available at http://clcgi.cl.msu.edu/~npgrant/npgrant101/(FINAL)Nursing%20Summit%20Rpt%207.pdf.

The overall goal of the summit was to increase the number of center–community partnerships. In a consensus process, the group recommended the creation of unifying mechanisms to coordinate efforts to ensure financial stability; to standardize data collection, policies, and procedures; to coordinate advocacy and marketing messages; and to promote the centers' role in clinical education. The summit group highlighted the vast potential for mutual assistance in a strong national alliance.

NATIONAL ORGANIZATION OF NURSE PRACTITIONER FACULTIES

The National Organization of Nurse Practitioner Faculties (NONPF) has taken a leadership role in advancing the case for nursing centers. Organized in 1980, NONPF's mission is "to provide leadership in promoting quality nurse practitioner education at the national and international levels" (NONPFb, 2001). Its membership of over 1100 overlaps with that of several other groups, including the leadership groups at the MAC National Nursing Summit and the National Nursing Centers Consortium. The Faculty Practice Committee of the NONPF is a forum for NP faculty involved in maintaining clinical excellence through practice. A special interest group for Academic Nursing Centers is made up of NP faculty in practices affiliated with their schools of nursing. NONPF defines faculty practice as follows:

> Faculty practice includes all aspects of the delivery of health care through the roles of clinician, educator, researcher, consultant, and administrator. Faculty practice activities within this framework encompass direct nursing services to individuals and groups, as well as technical assistance and consultation to individuals, families, groups, and communities. In addition to the provision of service, the practice provides opportunities for promotion, tenure, merit, and revenue generation. A distinguishing characteristic of faculty practice within the School of Nursing is the belief that teaching, research, practice, and service must be closely integrated to achieve excellence. Faculty practice provides the vehicle through which faculty implement these missions. There is an assumption that student practica and residencies as well as research opportunities for faculty and students are an established component of faculty practice. (NONPFa, 1996)

Recently, several NP faculty members of the NONPF were involved in a special project to enhance community health curriculum content by involving students in nurse-managed primary care centers.

NATIONAL NURSING CENTERS CONSORTIUM

The National Nursing Centers Consortium unites its members in the mission "To strengthen the capacity, growth and development of nurse-managed health centers to provide quality health care services to vulnerable populations and eliminate health disparities in underserved communities" (NNCC, 2002). NNCC was started in the 1990s as a regional consortium of nurse-managed centers, most of which are owned by Philadelphia-area schools of nursing; in 1999 its board of directors voted to reach out for national membership and influence. Regional members have benefited from steady funding from the Philadelphia-based Independence Foundation, which is now directing the implementation of computer-based administrative, scheduling, and patient health records in several of the original member centers.

NNCC has advocated for expansion of laws and regulations in Pennsylvania that affect advanced practice. For example, Pennsylvania NPs were readily reimbursed by Medicaid fee-for-service after federal mandates. But when the state shifted to Medicaid managed care under a federal waiver, the assigned managed care companies blocked NPs from being credentialed as primary care providers to receive direct capitation payment for the same patients they had served under fee for service (Jenkins, 2002). Unfortunately, the problem also carried over into the Children's Health Insurance Programs that were funded through managed care organizations. After much lobbying by the NNCC, in cooperation with a statewide alliance, Pennsylvania NPs are now recognized as primary care providers by select managed care plans, as they are in several states, including Tennessee, Oregon, Texas, New York, Delaware, and Arkansas (Matherlee, 1999).

NNCC has obtained targeted grant monies for community health and patient education projects implemented by various teams of its member centers. On the federal level, the NNCC has worked to obtain an exemption for nurse-managed centers affiliated with public universities, which, except for having no medical director, meet the requirements for Federally Qualified Health Centers (FQHC). FQHC funds are administered through the Bureau of Primary Health Care within the Health Resources and Services Administration. FQHC status is highly desirable due to annual federal grants that support care to uninsured patients and to current regulations that mandate per-visit reimbursement for patient care, even in capitated Medicaid managed care environments (HRSA, n.d.).

MONEY, MONEY, MONEY: OVERCOMING THE BARRIERS TO FUNDING NURSING CENTERS

It is well known that health care in the United States is driven by financial realities that depart extensively from the free-market capitalist ideals of supply and demand and quality-cost balancing. The "invisible hand" that supposedly balances supply and demand does not have much influence on health care (consider the longstanding nursing shortage that has substantially failed to push up nursing salaries or improve hospital and other nursing work environments). The flow of information to consumers on the quality and cost of health care is constrained by both the technical and the inaccessible nature of much of the information and by the fact that most healthcare costs that head for third-party reimbursement bypass consumers. Within this economically controlled context, change is very rarely driven by impersonal market forces; change must be driven by a much slower and more political regulatory process. Over the past 100 years, the traditions and turf protections inherent in professional licensing have slowed the ability of nurse practitioners to advance nursing practice in order to fully exercise their extensive graduate-level educations. Thus, the settings where NPs have the most autonomy, nurse-managed centers, have suffered as orphans without a reliable home in U.S. healthcare financing. From Lillian Wald's time to today, centers that have struggled and failed have done so in large part because of the lack of stable financing for the centers and their NP providers. Matherlee (1999) summarizes the problem, stating:

> Just as the old public health nursing model faced funding problems, the nursing center must piece together clinical service, teaching, grant, and other funding in order to establish and maintain itself. While the same is true for other safety-net providers, the nursing center faces some particular difficulties. The relative newness of the reshaped model, the difficulty of moving from subsidized to self-sustaining, and issues surrounding independent practice for nurses are major barriers. (p. 2)

In addition to opportunities for direct reimbursement for care of insured patients, funding for nurse-managed centers from the Division of Nursing, the NLN, the AACN, the Robert

Wood Johnson Foundation, the W. K. Kellogg Foundation, the John A. Hartford Foundation, and the Independence Foundation were identified in a report from the National Health Policy Forum. The National Health Policy Forum defines nurse-managed centers as follows (Lockhart, 1995):

1. A nurse occupies the chief management position
2. Accountability and responsibility for client care and professional practice remain with nursing staff
3. Nurses are the primary providers seen by clients visiting the center

The report is available at http://www.nhpf.org/pdfs_ib/IB746_NursCenter_9-13-99.pdf.

THE POTENTIAL FOR VIBRANT GROWTH IN THE FUTURE

The goal of nurse-managed centers is to provide appropriate primary health care for all. Yet, this goal falls short within the current U.S. healthcare financing and delivery structure. In a partial effort to fill gaps in health care for the more than 40 million uninsured Americans, a variety of "safety net" providers and funding mechanisms have emerged. FQHCs are among the most stable and best known of the lot. Including nurse-managed health centers in this publicly funded category could rapidly increase access to primary health care. To accomplish this, some nurse-managed centers, particularly those owned by private universities, would need to restructure their governance to a community-controlled board of directors.

From their beginning in the 1960s as Community Health Centers, FQHCs have grown to include migrant, homeless, and public housing health centers, and their appropriation has grown to $1.3 billion for over 3000 clinics in fiscal year 2002 (HRSA, n.d.). Annual federal grants are available to support care for uninsured patients and to enhance comprehensive primary healthcare services. In 2002, 9.6 million people used FQHCs; the majority of patients lived below the poverty level. A small fraction of America's uninsured, 3.9 million, was served by FQHCs. A total of 4803 physicians provided 19,220,237 encounters, and 2367 NPs and physician's assistants provided 6,657,449 encounters.

The HRSA describes the importance of FQHCs, stating, "CHCs [Community Health Centers—the predominant FQHC model] provide family-oriented primary and preventive health care services for people living in rural and urban medically underserved communities" (HRSA, n.d.). Like the nursing centers of Wald and Breckinridge, the CHCs exist in areas of need, where barriers (economic, geographic, or cultural) limit access to primary health care for a substantial portion of the population. Similarly, the work of the CHCs is tailored to the needs of the community. CHCs attend to social needs by providing health education, transportation, translation, links to welfare, Medicaid, mental health and substance abuse treatment, food subsidies, and related services.

Currently, CHCs and many nurse-managed centers are beginning to use electronic health records. These may sustain safety net funding by providing a wealth of data about populations served as well as the similarities and differences in outcomes of care. As part of this, NP–patient interventions and NP–student interactions must be documented and analyzed to determine the reach of nurse-managed centers. The MAC convened a second national consensus conference in December 2004 to select essential data elements to monitor quality improvement in the centers.

By virtue of their ownership of nursing centers, nurses have the opportunity to be included in the development of primary care informatics that is now being led by the National Alliance of Primary Care Informatics (Bates & Jenkins, 2004; NAPCI, 2003), a group that was incubated within the American Medical Informatics Association (AMIA, 2003). The spotlight on public health due to current events and worldwide disease outbreaks may also lead to increased opportunities for nursing centers.

A concerted effort is now required of leaders of nurse-managed centers to overcome internal competition and to advocate for solid, ongoing public funding to care for their underserved communities. Since 2000, the National Organization of Nurse Practitioner Faculties Academic Nursing Centers Special Interest Group has worked to identify areas to share ideas and resources. Relevant issues were addressed at the Michigan Summit on nurse-managed centers in December 2002, where a thoughtful, consensus-building conversation begged for a national coordinating body. The strengths of MAC and NNCC must be combined to move toward a perpetuating infrastructure for nurse managed centers. As Ben Franklin said on July 4, 1776, at the signing of the Declaration of Independence, "We must indeed all hang together, or, most assuredly, we shall all hang separately." For more than a century, nurses have shown the contributions of their community-based practices in uniting the work of prevention and cure. It is time to weld the model to a sustainable future.

REFERENCES

Aiken, L., & Gwyther, M. E. (1995). "Medicare funding of nurse education. The case for policy change." *JAMA* 273(19): 1528–1532.

Allen, S. E. (2000). Guide to the Frontier Nursing Oral History Project, University of Kentucky Libraries, Lexington, KY, 40506. http://digilib.kyvl.org/dynaweb/kyvldigs/fns/@Generic__BookTextView/183, accessed 10/24/03.

AMIA, American Medical Informatics Association (2003). http://www.amia.org, accessed 10/24/03.

ANA, American Nurses Association (2003). Hall of Fame. http://www.nursingworld.org/hof/brecmx.htm, accessed 10/24/03.

Barnum, B. (1991). "An interview with America's highest-ranking nurse, O. Marie Henry." *Nursing & Health Care 12*(1): 24–25.

Bates, D. W., & Jenkins, M. L. (2004). The National Alliance for Primary Care Informatics: Development and Current Status. *Informatics in Primary Care* 12:183.

Berlin, L. E. (1999). Academic nursing center survey by the American Association of Colleges of Nursing. In K. Matherlee, Washington, D.C., National Health Policy Forum. http://www.nhpf.org/pdfs_ib/IB746_NursCenter_9-13-99.pdf, accessed 10/24/03.

Breckinridge, M. (1972). *Wide neighborhoods: A story of the Frontier Nursing Service.* New York, Harper & Brothers.

Buhler-Wilkerson, K. (1993). "Bringing care to the people: Lillian Wald's legacy to public health nursing." *American Journal of Public Health 83*(12): 1778–1786.

Clear, J. B., Starbecker, M. & Kelly, D. W. (1999). Nursing centers and health promotion: A federal vantage point. *Community Health* 21(4): 3–4.

ESTU, East Tennessee State University College of Nursing (2000). Health and Primary Care in Appalachia, HRSA. http://bhpr.hrsa.gov/nursing/fy02grants/abstracts/D11/D11%20HP%2000168-03.htm, accessed 10/24/03.

Evans, L. K., Jenkins, M., & Buhler-Wilkerson, K. (2003). Academic nursing practice: Power nursing for the 21st century. In M. D. Mezey & D. O. McGovern, *Nurses, nurse practitioners: Evolution to advanced practice*. New York, Springer.

Gray, M. (2000). Frontier Nursing Service Oral History Project: Interview with Matt Gray, July 21, 1978, University of Kentucky Oral History Program, Lexington, KY, 40506. 2003. http://digilib.kyvl.org/dynaweb/oh/kukoral/2kukoh/78OH144/@Generic__BookView, accessed 6/21/04 through http://kdl.kyvl.org/cgi/t/text/text-idx?c=oralhist&tpl=kukohfns.tpl.

Henry, O. (1978). *Demonstration centers for nursing practice, education, and research.* American Public Health Association Annual Meeting, Los Angeles, CA.

HRSA, Health Resources and Services Administration, Bureau of Primary Health Care (no date). Community Health Centers. http://bphc.hrsa.gov/chc/, accessed 10/24/03.

Jenkins, M. (2002). Abbottsford community health center and Pennsylvania politics. In D. Mason & J. Levitt, *Policy and politics in nursing and health care*. Philadelphia, Saunders: 87–91.

Katz, E. (2002). Margaret Sanger biography, NYU. 2003. http://www.nyu.edu/projects/sanger/msbio.htm, accessed 10/24/03.

Lester, B. (2000). Frontier Nursing Service Oral History Project: Interview with Betty Lester, March 3, 1978, University of Kentucky Oral History Program, Lexington, KY, 40506. http://digilib.kyvl.org/dynaweb/oh/kukoral/2kukoh/78OH146/@Generic__BookView, accessed 6/21/04 through http://kdl.kyvl.org/cgi/t/text/text-idx?c=oralhist&tpl=kukohfns.tpl.

Lockhart, C. A. (1995). "Community nursing centers: An analysis of status and needs." *Nursing centers: The time is now*. New York, National League for Nursing.

Lynaugh, J. (1991). "The death of Sadie Sachs." *Nursing Research 40*(2): 124–125.

MAC, Michigan Academic Consortium (2003). Report of the national nursing summit addressing nurse-managed health centers. http://clcgi.cl.msu.edu/~npgrant/npgrant101/(FINAL)Nursing%20Summit%20Rpt%207.pdf, accessed 10/24/03.

MAC, Michigan Academic Consortium (2005). Nurse managed primary care. http://www.minursingcenters.org, accessed 5/24/05.

Martin, K. S., & Scheet, N. J. (1992). *The Omaha System: Applications for community health nursing.* Philadelphia, Saunders.

Matherlee, K. (1999). The Nursing Center in Concept and Practice: Delivery and Financing Issues in Serving Vulnerable People, National Health Policy Forum, 2021 K Street, NW, Suite 800, Washington, DC, 20052. http://www.nhpf.org/pdfs_ib/IB746_NursCenter_9-13-99.pdf, accessed 10/24/03.

Moody, N. B., Smith, S. P., & Glenn, L. L. (1999). "Client characteristics and practice patterns of nurse practitioners and physicians." *Nurse Practitioner 24*(3): 94–103.

NAPCI, National Alliance of Primary Care Informatics (2003). National Alliance of Primary Care Informatics. http://www.napci.org, accessed 10/24/03.

New York University (NYU) (2002). The Margaret Sanger papers project: biographical sketch. http://www.nyu.project/sanger/aboutms.htm, accessed 5/24/05.

NNCC, National Nursing Centers Consortium (2002). Vision, mission, and goals. http://www.nationalnursingcenters.com/NNCC_About/VMG/VisionMissionGoals.htm, accessed 10/24/03.

NONPFa, National Organization of Nurse Practitioner Faculties (1996). Faculty practice definitions. http://www.nonpf.com/fpdef.htm, accessed 10/24/03.

NONPFb, National Organization of Nurse Practitioner Faculties (2001). Overview. http://www.nonpf.com/over.htm, accessed 10/24/03.

Planned Parenthood Federation of America (2000). About us: Margaret Sanger. http://www.plannedparenthood.org/about/thisispp/sanger.html, accessed 10/24/03.

Reverby, S. M. (1987). *Ordered to care: The dilemma of American nursing, 1850–1945*. Cambridge, Cambridge University Press.

Sanger, M. (1938). *An autobiography*. New York, W.W. Norton.

Sebastian, J., Stanhope, M., McGuire, R., & Rayens, M. K. (2002). Development of an academic nurse-managed center survey and database, University of Kentucky College of Nursing. http://www.mc.uky.edu/nursing/research/faculty/Grants/sebastian1.html, accessed 10/24/03.

Starr, P. (1982). *The social transformation of American medicine: The rise of a sovereign profession and the making of a vast industry*. New York, Basic Books.

Sullivan-Marx, E. M., & Mullinix, C. (1999). "Payment for advanced practice nurses: Economic structures and systems." In M. Mezey, D. McGivern, & E. Sullivan-Marx, *Nurses, nurse practitioners: Evolution to advanced practice*. New York, Springer.

USDI, U.S. Department of Interior, National Register of Historic Places (2000). History of Frontier Nursing Service, Frontier Nursing Service. http://www.frontiernursing.org/history_of_fsn.htm, accessed 10/24/03.

UWM, School of Nursing, University of Wisconsin-Milwaukee (2005). Institute for Urban Health Partnerships: Service, The UWM Academic Community Nursing Centers. http://cfprod.imt.uwm.edu/nursing/community/urban_health_overview.cfm, accessed 5/24/05.

Wald, L. (1934). *Windows on Henry Street*. New York, Little Brown.

CHAPTER 28

The Power of the Written Word: The Influence of Nursing Journals

Diana J. Mason
Maureen Shawn Kennedy
Thelma Schorr
Annette Flanagin

As of June 2004, 532 nursing journals were listed in the Cumulative Index for Nursing and Allied Health Libraries (CINAHL). These journals have been instrumental in shaping the thinking and practice of individual nurses, stimulating important debates that arise as ideas evolve, and providing an interface between nursing and society.

The history of nursing journals provides a lens through which to understand the current state of these publications and the contemporary issues confronting most of them. The issues surounding what biomedical and nursing journals publish may be more contentious today than at any other time. How nursing and its journals respond to these issues will influence their credibility among nurses, other health professionals, and the public as sources of information and perspectives on nursing practice, education, and research.

Many of the examples in this chapter are from the *American Journal of Nursing (AJN)*, as three of the four authors have been editors at the journal. However, we also interviewed editors of other nursing journals and have included their observations and experiences as well.

PURPOSE OF A JOURNAL

Binger (1981) noted that journals are a symbol of professionalism and a vehicle for personal, interpersonal, and interdisciplinary communication. Professional journals exist to inform, educate, stimulate, and keep readers up-to-date on what is happening in their profession with regard to research, clinical advances, the political environment, and anything and everything that affects their practice. In nursing journals specifically, attention is paid to the broad healthcare landscape and to the relationships of the people and the forces within it.

Journals also provide an opportunity for individual practitioners to be heard on the issues of the day, to exchange reports on their experiences and expertise, and to have their accomplishments and leadership recognized. The periodical nature of journals encourages ongoing discussion of controversial issues and topics.

Journals are a source of ideas, providing an important vehicle for disseminating research, particularly for applied disciplines such as nursing. We live in a time of unprecedented new knowledge being generated by research from around the world. Some journals are sources for original research, whereas others focus on translating that research into practice—and some do both. For example, a long-standing practice in the last decades of the 20th century was to instill normal saline into a tracheostomy or endotracheal tube prior to suctioning patients to "loosen" secretions. However, research documenting that this practice actually increased patients' distress and put them at greater risk of pulmonary infections emerged in the late 1980s and early 1990s and was published in several nursing journals (Ackerman, Ecklund, & Abu-Jumah, 1996; Whitnack, 2000). How did this research find its way into practice? Faculty and clinicians who read research journals shared the results of primary studies with their students and colleagues. Those nurses who did not read the research journals may have learned about the studies and their implications for practice in journals that focus on helping nurses to develop evidence-based care. As the Internet makes finding information easier, online journals provide opportunities for any clinician to quickly discover advances in nursing and medical knowledge.

Finally, for faculty, publishing in the leading peer-reviewed journals provides the evidence of scholarship that is necessary for tenure and promotion. As with other health professions, the number of publications for nurses and interest in nursing research have increased.

EVOLUTION OF NURSING JOURNALS IN THE UNITED STATES

The proliferation of nursing journals from 5 in 1888 to over 500 today is an outgrowth of the specialization within nursing, the formation of general and specialty nursing societies, and the movement of nursing education into the university and the accompanying expectations for scholarly output by faculty. Also, there are business expectations for journals to achieve annual growth in revenues to support professional membership societies and meet competitive financial expectations of for-profit publishing companies.

The *American Journal of Nursing*

In 1899, members of Associated Alumnae of Trained Nurses of the United States (which became the American Nurses Association [ANA] in 1911) voted to establish a journal that nurses would own and operate—an arrangement that was unprecedented for the nursing journals that existed at the time. Individual nurses paid $100 for a share in the journal, providing the initial funding for the *American Journal of Nursing (AJN)*. These nurses were committed to creating a vehicle for communications for the organization's 4000 members.

The first issue of *AJN* was published in October 1900. It set the standard for itself and subsequent nursing journals, despite its inaugural editor's statement to the contrary: "The first issue of the *Journal* can hardly be taken as a criterion of what is to follow" (Palmer, 1900, p. 65). Nevertheless, it included:

☐ An editorial by its first editor, Sophia Palmer, who eventually left her position as director of the Rochester City Hospital to develop the journal. Palmer wrote:

It will be the aim of the editors to present month by month the most useful facts, the most progressive thought, and the latest news that the profession has to offer in the most attractive form that can be secured. (Palmer, 1900, p. 64)

☐ A discussion of the importance of legislation to nursing's future by nurse activist Lavinia Dock ("What We May Expect From the Law").
☐ Lillian Wald's description of the Henry Street Settlement House that she founded on the Lower East Side of Manhattan to provide nursing and social services to the poor immigrants in that community.
☐ An article on infant feeding by a physician who wrote:

The decision to abandon the mother's breast for an artificial food is fraught with the greatest importance to the infant. No matter how well the artificial food may be managed, the child's chances of survival are greatly lessened by the change. (Thistle, 1900, p. 22)

☐ A description of nurses' journey on the hospital ship *Maine* to South Africa during the Boer War.

Throughout its history, *AJN* has evolved, provoked, and informed nurses worldwide, although its primary audience continues to be registered nurses in the United States.

In 1953, the management of *AJN* recognized that there was a need for new journals in response to societal and professional trends, including the movement of nursing education into the university, and it launched five new journals over the next 30 years (*Nursing Research; Nursing Outlook; MCN, The American Journal of Maternal/Child Nursing;* and *Geriatric Nursing*). The ANA was the sole owner of the AJN Company. In 1996, it dissolved the company and sold most of its journals to other publishing companies. *AJN* was bought by the successor of its original publisher, the J. B. Lippincott Company, now Lippincott Williams & Wilkins (LWW), a subsidiary of Wolters Kluwer, a large multinational publishing conglomerate.

Nursing Research Journals

One of the most important new publications developed by the AJN Company arose from the U.S. government's commitment to support the education of nurses and to develop a cadre of doctoral-prepared nurses after World War II (Baer, 1987). These new nurse researchers needed a channel for publishing their work. In 1949, the AJN Company consulted with the American Association of Collegiate Schools of Nursing and its five sister organizations (ANA, National League for Nursing Education, National Organization of Public Health Nursing, National Association of Colored Graduate Nurses, and American Association of Industrial Nurses) to develop a plan for publishing the first journal devoted to nursing research, *Nursing Research,* which premiered in 1953.

The founders of *Nursing Research* wanted the journal to address more than nursing education. Although studies of nursing education and nurses dominated the journal in its early years, its pages mirrored the profession's changing interests and emphases. In 1956, Virginia Henderson (Henderson, 1956) wrote a guest editorial in the journal that challenged the profession to develop a body of research focused on nursing practice, but the pages of *Nursing Research* continued to reflect the profession's obsession with itself, publishing study after study about nurses rather than patients. Diers (2004) and others continued to push the issue of clinically relevant research through their speaking and writing. Eventually, *Nursing Research* began to reflect the profession's realization that clinical care was its raison d'etre. Over the years, *Nursing Research* became the gold standard for the profession's research journals. It also continues a mandate stimulated by Henderson to educate nurses about research through its publication of articles discussing research methodologies, announcements of research conferences, and opportunities for research funding.

In the 1970s, nurses' generation of research began to outpace the capacity of *Nursing Research,* and other nursing research journals were launched. Today, journals such as *Western Journal of Nursing Research,* the *Journal of Applied Nursing Research,* the *Journal of Nursing Scholarship,* and *Research in Nursing and Health* provide venues for disseminating nurses' research. But increasingly, nurse researchers are seeking interdisciplinary venues for publishing their work. Studies with nurses as principals or coinvestigators now appear regularly in the *Journal of the American Medical Association (JAMA)*, the *American Journal of Public Health*, and other medical and interdisciplinary publications. For example, in January 1960 no nurse authors were included in the bylines of 57 articles published in that month's *JAMA*. In January 1970, 3% (1 of 33) of the articles in *JAMA* had nurses as coauthors, such as one by Runyan and colleagues on a program for care of patients with chronic illness (Runyan, Phillips, Herring, & Campbell, 1970). In January 2000 and 2004, the number of articles with nurse authors had increased to 10% (3 of 29) and 16% (5 of 31), respectively.

Society and Specialty Journals

Binger (1981) reported that 40 new nursing journals were launched between 1964 and 1979, more than in any other 15-year period in the 20th century. The titles of these new journals reflected the profession's move toward specialization, for example, *Journal of Emergency Nursing, Journal of Gerontological Nursing, Journal of Neurosurgical Nursing, Cardiovascular Nursing, Journal of Enterostomal Therapy*, and *Nephrology Nurse*. Most of these specialty journals were affiliated with a specialty nursing professional society. In fact, one of the hallmarks of a successful nursing organization is the publication of a journal as a communication organ and member benefit (Palmer, 1900; Binger, 1981).

For nursing societies, journals provide a vehicle for nurses to publish specialty-specific research and clinical review articles. These society or specialty journals also provide forums for communicating association work and policies to their members, ascertaining members' views on issues, debating hot issues, and developing their members' clinical skills. The American Association of Critical Care Nurses has three journals for its members: *Critical Care Nursing*, which serves as the clinical journal for members; *Issues in Critical Care Nursing,* which targets advanced practice nurses in critical care; and the *American Journal of Critical Care*, which is an interdisciplinary journal that publishes research and other papers, with a nurse (Kathleen Dracup in 2005) and physician serving as coeditors. Some societies share an official journal with other organizations. For example, several of the regional nursing research societies (e.g., Eastern Nursing Research Society) use *Nursing Research* as their official journal and provide it as a member benefit. These society-owned journals are important benefits of membership and serve as major sources of revenue to support the membership-driven missions.

General nursing journals, such as *AJN*, *Nursing 2005*, and *RN*, provide nurses with broad-based views of nursing and health care. The specialty journals advance specialty practice and research, covering topics with depth that nurses need to advance their practice in their specialty.

International Nursing Journals

As nursing has advanced in other countries, most of the developed nations now have more than one nursing journal. *Nursing Standard* is the leading general nursing journal in England, being the official journal of the Royal College of Nursing (RCN). The RCN has its own publishing house and produces 11 other journals. The *Journal of Advanced Nursing* is another nursing journal developed in England. It was launched in 1974 to provide "an international medium for the publication of scholarly nursing papers and a means of documenting the ever growing body of nursing knowledge" (Smith, 1976, p. 1). It differed from many other nursing journals by encouraging the sharing of authorship with those in other healthcare disciplines. Although interdisciplinary authorship could occasionally be found in other nursing journals of the day, the *Journal of Advanced Nursing* deliberately sought to promote interdisciplinary collaboration (Smith, 1976).

Sigma Theta Tau International, the nursing honor society, has used its journal—formerly *Image*, now the *Journal of Nursing Scholarship*—as a forum for reaching nurses around the world. The International Council of Nurses (ICN) publishes the *International Nursing Review*. Both of these journals include original research as well as literature reviews, news, and opinion pieces.

Of course, as journals make their contents available online, nurses are able to access journals from around the world with greater ease. However, language remains a barrier to more cross-national reading. ICN now publishes Spanish and Japanese versions of the *International Nursing Review*. *Health SA Gesondheid*, the nursing journal of South Africa, publishes some articles in English and some in Afrikaans.

As nurses begin to access other nations' nursing journals, the opportunities for shared knowledge and experiences proliferate. For example, in February 2000 *AJN* published a paper on magnet hospitals by Aiken and colleagues from the University of Pennsylvania (Aiken, Havens, & Sloane, 2000a). The editors of *Nursing Standard* believed the paper to be an important one for exporting the concept to Great Britain. In March of that year, *Nursing Standard* reprinted Aiken's article, and the Royal College of Nursing has begun to develop a plan for using the magnet designation in England (Aiken, Havens, & Sloane, 2000b).

THE JOURNAL AS A REFLECTION OF THE TIMES

Professional journals serve as historical archives for the profession because they chronicle events, news, research, and the evolution of knowledge as it unfolds. Although history texts certainly serve this function, they do so from a "hindsight" point of view. Journals chronicle events as they unfold. From the first inklings of an emerging issue in a news story to a report of new research changing practice to an editorial perspective and discussion in letters to the editor, a journal provides a record of the time of publication and documents evolving knowledge in nursing and related disciplines and often predicts changes to come within the profession and in related healthcare professions in the context of broader world events (Schorr & Kennedy, 1999).

At the turn of the 19th century, for example, the focus in early U.S. journals such as *The Trained Nurse and Hospital Review* and *AJN* was on the nurse's comportment, the image of the nurse as intelligent and professional, and nursing's need to be regulated by nurses and not physicians—issues that are still relevant today. It is perhaps no coincidence that this move towards legitimacy for nursing occurred in the context of the women's suffrage movement, when the nation's women began to seek a voice of their own and an identity apart from their husbands. The voting rights issue was hotly debated in the minutes of association meetings and in letters to the editor that appeared in *AJN* (including one from President Theodore Roosevelt), although Sophia Palmer, *AJN*'s editor, refused to allow *AJN* to take an official position on the issue, despite the wrath of staff member Lavinia Dock, an ardent suffragette. Palmer explained that it was a "professional journal, devoted to the interests of nursing" and would remain neutral "on all other broad questions" (Palmer, 1908, p. 956).

The public health movement that began as part of a philanthropic movement at the turn of the 20th century and blossomed in the 1930s can be traced in the journals. In early journals, articles on nursing practice focused on care in the home (e.g., caring for patients with fever, setting up the sick room, the importance of hygiene and proper nutrition, teaching new mothers), because that was where most nurses worked in the early part of the 20th century. (Hospitals did not become large employers of nurses until the late 1930s.) As nurses began to be hired by city health agencies to manage emerging public health problems, journal content shifted to include public health articles on topics such as communicable diseases (mostly tuberculosis, trachoma, diphtheria, and typhoid) and reports on nurses providing care to families and children in a variety of settings, including reports of nurses in schools and factories and even "floating hospitals" in New York and Boston that provided infant care and education to indigent mothers (Perry, 1900).

The Pacific Coast Journal of Nursing, first published in 1904 by the California State Nurses Association, carried regular reports from local public health districts. It also addressed public policy, urging the passage of federal health insurance so that the working class and the poor could receive health care. From 1900 through the 1930s, *AJN* published letters and reports by nurses who wrote eloquently about their experiences as "district nurses." For example, Lillian Wald described her work developing the Henry Street Settlement (Wald, 1902); Lina Rogers wrote about her experience as the first school nurse in Wald's experiment and about placing nurses in schools (Rogers, 1903). Another article reported on Mary Breckinridge and the Frontier Nursing Service of traveling nurse midwives that she founded to serve Kentucky mothers (Breckinridge, 1927). Jane Delano, chief nurse of the American Red Cross, was a monthly contributor who wrote about various Red Cross activities, including those of the Red Cross Town and Country Nursing Service that served rural communities and which later evolved into the Bureau of Public Health Nursing (Delano, 1914). Other articles focused on nurses' activities and care practices surrounding communicable diseases and women's and infants' health, which have continued to be major public health concerns.

In the second half of the 20th century, although articles in U.S. nursing journals reflected the transition of large numbers of nurses into hospitals, public health issues remained a focus. Some of the same infectious diseases continued to receive attention in the pages of nursing journals, but different diseases began to emerge: polio in the 1940s and 1950s, venereal diseases, tuberculosis, and AIDS through the rest of the century. At the beginning of the 21st century, many journals carried articles about infectious agents that could be used as biological weapons, while continuing to cover tuberculosis and other infectious diseases that challenge the public's health.

In the 1950s, *AJN* covered the debate over extending Social Security to include health care (although the Medicare bill did not pass until 1965). Reports from the 1958 convention of the American Nurses Association included a resolution that made nursing the only healthcare profession to support the bill ("Resolution on health insurance," 1958; Blasingame, 1958; Schorr & Kennedy, 1999). Other leading articles reported on nurses setting up free clinics in impoverished areas and outreach programs in housing developments and later, independent nurse practices. In the late 1980s, many nursing journals published editorials criticizing a flawed proposal for non-nursing personnel to be educated and licensed by non-nurses to carry out nursing tasks delegated by physicians; these writings were influential in helping to defeat the plan. In the 1990s, many articles covered the movement for a national health insurance program and nursing's own solution, "Nursing's Agenda for Health Care Reform" (American Nurses Association, 1991). The need for better health care for the elderly and the poor has remained an important issue addressed in journals (Stotts & Deitrich, 2004).

As with public health nursing, the history of modern military nursing can also be traced in the pages of nursing journals. The first issue of *AJN* carried a report from a nurse on the hospital ship *Maine* as it sailed to South Africa in 1899 (Hibbard, 1900). During World War I, *AJN* carried monthly reports on nurse recruitment efforts from Jane Delano, who as head of the American Red Cross was charged with building up the nursing reserves for the U.S. Army and Navy Nurse Corps (Delano, 1914). Detailed letters from nurses "over there" filled the pages along with impassioned letters admonishing nurses who had not "answered the call." The *AJN* also chronicled two new nurse training programs: the Army School of Nursing and the Vassar Training Camp. The Vassar summer program provided academic preparation to college graduates on campus and placed them in an affiliated nursing school. Both of these programs brought nursing education standards to a new level (Schorr & Kennedy, 1999).

In the 1940s, *AJN* again documented the impact of war on the profession ("Army and Navy nurse corps bill," 1947). It provided extensive coverage of the passage of the Bolton Act (the Nurse Training Act of 1943), which provided millions of federal dollars for a national recruitment campaign and scholarships and stipends for the Cadet Nurse Corps, and created a federal Division of Nursing. Numerous letters and detailed reports from and about nurses overseas appeared in every issue of the journal, as well as debates on a proposed draft for nurses and testimony as to why nurses deserved to have rank in the Navy Nurse Corps (Delano, 1914).

Coverage in U.S. nursing journals in later wars, especially after the Korean War, was mostly related to nursing shortages created by military needs and military recruitment efforts. Although there certainly were some reports and letters detailing nurses' activities in combat areas, there was markedly less coverage, and it also appeared less frequently, perhaps reflecting the country's mixed feelings over the Vietnam War, the Gulf War, and the Iraq War (Schorr & Kennedy, 1999).

In the early years, nursing journals largely focused on issues and events that were of direct concern to nurses and the profession (e.g., education, licensure, clinical practice articles). Later, some expanded their editorial focus to include broader healthcare issues, although specialty journals and association publications largely kept a focus in keeping with their membership. After Palmer died in 1920, *AJN* broadened its focus to include comment and coverage of issues that affect those for whom nurses care, giving it much leeway in covering sociopolitical issues and events.

For example, *AJN* has covered human rights issues. In the late 1940s, reports documented the American Nurses Association's struggle in addressing its own internal race issues (Black nurses could not belong to many southern state associations; Georgia was the last state to admit Black nurses, not doing so until 1961 [Carnegie, 2000]). In the 1960s and 1970s, coverage of the influence of poverty on health and the right of all people to health care included articles about migrant workers and nurses participating in protest marches, including the famed March on Washington in 1963. Women's rights and issues about equal pay were dominant in *AJN* in the 1970s (Schorr & Kennedy, 1999).

A recent event that caused many journals to reflect on the world in which we live, regardless of their editorial mission, was the September 11, 2001 terrorist attacks. With few exceptions, most U.S.-based nursing journals noted the event, as did some nursing journals representing other countries, even if it was only a mention in an editorial or in a special acknowledgment. The *Journal of Emergency Nursing* devoted its cover, president's message (from the Emergency Nurses Association), editorial, and 20 pages of first-person accounts to the event in its October 2001 issue.

Three large general nursing journals, *AJN, Nursing,* and *RN Magazine*, provided extensive coverage of the event and its after effects, including concerns over other types of terrorism, such as bioterrorism. *RN Magazine* devoted an editorial to the event and had six pages in each of the last two issues of the year chronicling first-person accounts of the attacks. An article on bioterrorism appeared in each of the subsequent four issues. *Nursing* had an editorial on the attacks and carried pieces on bioterrorism in two later issues. *AJN* also devoted its editorial to the attacks, but because the journal's offices are housed in New York City, it also included eyewitness testimony from the editorial staff and on-the-scene interviews with nurses at emergency facilities. Subsequent issues included articles on nurses involved in both local and federal responses, a six-issue series on bioterrorism agents, and artwork by nurse/artist Charles Kaiman who witnessed the burning of the towers and made a stark woodcut print to cope with his experience (Kaiman, 2001). In addition, *AJN* devoted most of its September 2002 issue to an anniversary retrospective on the attacks, including an analysis of changes in our public health system, ongoing health problems resulting from the attacks, and a tribute to the nurses who died, as well as a "healing" watercolor by Kaiman (2002).

IMPACT OF NURSING JOURNALS

So what has been the impact of nursing journals on the profession and society? We consider this question in six areas: communication, development of the profession, advancement of the art and science of nursing, development of standards of practice, furthering nurses' education, and development and promotion of nursing leaders.

Communication

Schorr and Kennedy's (1999) *100 Years of American Nursing: Celebrating a Century of Caring* documents how *AJN* has served as a vehicle for communication within nursing. The early days of the journal included minutes from local, state, and national nurses' meetings. Although *AJN* no longer provides this official record of meetings, some society journals do include information on actions taken by their organization's board of directors, announcements of new initiatives sponsored by the organization, and opportunities for member involvement.

Suzanne Smith, editor of *Nurse Educator* and the *Journal of Nursing Administration*, reports that these journals are now able to connect readers and authors more directly: "Since we started publishing authors' email addresses, I am no longer the intermediary between authors and readers. Readers now talk directly to authors." (Personal communication with M. Kennedy, November 4, 2003). This has become a common practice among journals, which fosters more collegial interaction but removes the editor from some of the readers' interests and opinions. But she adds, "With long lead times between shipping materials to production and publication, my journals are not the place to have ongoing, timely debate on a topic."

A particularly important development is the extent to which nursing journals have served to inform the public about the work nurses do and nurses' perspectives on the profession, health, and health care. *AJN* is sent to journalists across the country every month, and they are increasingly seeking out nurses and information on nurses' work for their stories. However, few nursing journals have the resources to conduct the media outreach necessary to bring what they publish to the attention of journalists.

In February 2000, *AJN* published a study of family members' and health care professionals' responses to family members being present during emergency resuscitation and invasive procedures (Meyers, Eichhorn, Guzzetta, et al., 2000). In May 2001, it published additional data from this same study that reported on how patients responded to having family members present during these procedures (Eichhorn, Meyers, Guzzetta, et al., 2001). Working with a New York City-based public relations firm, *AJN* launched a media campaign to bring the issue to the attention of journalists, and many quickly saw the importance of these studies to the larger public. As a result, major news outlets ran stories on the research, many pointing out that the work was published in *AJN* and conducted by nurses who cared about the issue. Stories appeared "above the fold" on the front page of *USA Today* and in the *New York Times*, *Washington Post*, *LA Times*, *Newsweek*, and a host of other national and local community newspapers and news weeklies. Stories were aired on radio stations across the country and featured on many national and local television news programs, including CNN and ABC's *World News Tonight*. Shortly thereafter, the *New England Journal of Medicine* published a physician-authored commentary on the practice, referring to the research published in *AJN* (Tsai, 2002); the American Heart Association changed its Basic and Advanced Cardiac Life Support protocols to include consideration of family presence; and policies supporting the practice began to appear in a growing number of hospitals, demonstrating the potential power of nursing journals to shape health care in this country.

Development of the Profession

Nursing journals have also influenced nursing's development by providing a forum for discussion of important issues. For many years, articles published in *AJN, Nursing Outlook, Image,* and other journals debated whether nursing was a profession. These articles served to enable nurses to move beyond the question, concluding that it had every right to consider itself a profession.

The development of the nurse-practitioner movement aroused editorial passion from its inception. In the early 1960s, Loretta Ford, dean of the University of Colorado School of Nursing, and Henry Silver, a pediatrician on the faculty, instituted a program to prepare pediatric nurse practitioners to handle the primary care of well children in rural Colorado (Silver & Ford, 1967; Silver, Ford, & Stearly, 1967). The success of the program galvanized proponents of expanding the scope of nursing practice; however, it also incurred a rash of opposition among (1) those who said public health nurses had always carried out this role (e.g., Lillian Wald on Henry Street and the Frontier Nurses in rural Kentucky) (Kalish & Kalisch, 1978); (2) those who claimed that nurse practitioners were just "junior doctors" (Schorr & Kennedy, 1999); and (3) organized medicine (Mason, Vaccaro, & Fessler, 2000). Issues of boundaries, preparation, and remuneration still afford good opportunities for editorial discourse, but, by and large, the role of nurse practitioners is now accepted and appreciated—at least within the profession. In fact, many graduate nursing programs closed their clinical nurse specialist tracks and replaced them with nurse practitioner specialties, leaving some to commiserate that nursing has lost its "knowledge disseminators," because one of the major roles of clinical nurse specialists is staff development.

When the Institute of Medicine concluded that there was not enough solid research to document a relationship between nurse staffing and patient outcomes (Wunderlich, Sloan, & Davis, 1996), most nursing journals communicated this to its readers through editorials and news reports. Nurse researchers such as Linda Aiken, Peter Buerhaus, and colleagues responded to this challenge with well-designed studies (Aiken, Clarke, Sloane, Sochalski, & Silber, 2002; Needleman, Buerhaus, Mattke, Stewart, & Zelevinsky, 2002) that were published in leading medical journals and covered by most nursing journals. These studies were used by nurses across the country to push for state and federal legislation to improve nurse staffing in acute care facilities. Staffing is now on the agenda of many policy makers, with California being the first state to mandate minimum staffing ratios. Even as transmitters of research published elsewhere, nursing journals have enabled the nursing community to stay current on research that can aid their activism and advocacy for patients.

Advancement of the Art and Science of Nursing

Virginia Henderson's 1956 editorial in *Nursing Research* and subsequent publications by Donna Diers (2004) raised nurses' consciousness as to the profession's failure to meet its social obligation of advancing patient care through clinical research. They stimulated a movement for clinical research that is serving the profession well.

At the same time that nursing has worked to gain credibility within the scientific and biomedical communities, the expectations for rigor in science have increased at most of the nursing research journals. In turn, journals that are more clinically focused have sought to publish articles that reflect quantitative science. Many of the research journals and broader nursing journals, such as *Journal of Nursing Scholarship,* have debated the place of qualitative research in nursing. The profession has come to embrace qualitative methodologies as being important to the development of nursing science, and such research can be found in all nursing research journals.

This thrust for legitimacy in the scientific world has played out in nursing journals in another way. Nurse practitioner, author, and poet Cortney Davis (2003) has argued that nursing has diminished the place and value of nurses' narratives and art as ways of understanding nursing and nurses' work with people. Some journals offer a page or two for nurses' narratives, others do not. The *Journal of Emergency Nursing* has routinely published art on its cover. *AJN*, which began to use art on its cover in 2000, launched an Art of Nursing page that same year and publishes Reflections, a column for nurses' narrative writing, every month. *Nursing* and *RN* both publish nurses' narratives.

Patricia Benner's book, *From Novice to Expert* (1984), helped to transform how nursing journals viewed narratives. Subsequently, Benner published a series of nurses' narratives with interpretive commentaries in *AJN* in the 1990s. These narratives served to help nurses think differently about their work. Through Benner, nurses were helped to articulate the deeper work of nursing—whether helping patients to find meaning in their illness, the value of intuitive ways of knowing about patients by the expert nurse, or understanding the responses of a patient to a terminal diagnosis. These writings have supported a movement to use nurses' narratives for promotions on clinical ladders within institutions.

Development of Standards and Practice

Nursing journals provide a mechanism for enhancing nursing practice, whether by publishing original research or translating that research for the clinician. Consider the following three examples.

In the late 1960s and 1970s, a great deal of research on the care of premature infants appeared. *AJN* published articles detailing the new "high-tech" perinatal units and reported on the work of nurse researchers Mary Neal and Kathryn Barnard, who had published their studies in research journals, including *Nursing Research* (Barnard & Neal, 1977). Neal, working first at New York University and then at the University of Maryland, studied the effects of simulated rocking motion on the growth and development of premature infants using a small motorized hammock placed inside the incubator (Neal, 1968). Her findings showed that rocking was associated with increased weight gain and better scores on tests related to motor and sensory functioning. At about the same time, at the University of Washington in Seattle, Kathryn Barnard, a nurse studying infant sleep patterns, devised a mechanized rocking bed for incubators that also included a tape-recorded heartbeat (Barnard, 1973). Today, rocking chairs have become standard furniture in hospital nurseries and neonatal units, and parents and caregivers are encouraged to hold, talk to, and rock the tiny infants.

Journals disseminate models of care. The hospice movement in the United States was advanced by the publications of Florence Wald, former dean of the Yale School of Nursing, who was intensely interested in patients' quality of life, particularly of those who were terminally ill. "What people need most when they are dying," she wrote in the October 1975 issue of *AJN*, "is relief from distressing symptoms of disease, the security of a caring environment, sustained expert care, and assurance that they and their families will not be abandoned" (Craven & Wald, 1975, p. 1816). When she met Cicely Saunders, who had trained in nursing, social work, and medicine and who founded the hospice movement at St. Christopher's in London, Wald left her academic position to work and study with Saunders. On her return to Connecticut, she assembled a multidisciplinary team that established the first hospice in the United States and nourished the growth of the momentous movement that hospice is in this country today.

Today, clinical nursing journals are primary vehicles for the dissemination of evidence-based practice, and two journals emerged to push nursing forward on the social mandate to document the evidence: the *Online Journal of Nursing Knowledge Synthesis* and *Evidence-Based Nursing* (published in the United Kingdom), which were launched in 1996 and 1998, respectively. Most nursing journals have changed their policies and standards to promote evidence-based practice, which often challenges outdated practices. In the May 2002 issue of *AJN*, Crenshaw and Winslow reported on their study of excessive preoperative fasting times that patients endured despite guidelines issued by the American Society of Anesthesiologists to the contrary (few patients should be told to be "NPO after midnight") (Crenshaw & Winslow, 2002).

AJN's publication of the two family presence studies, discussed earlier, was followed by numerous discussions of the practice in other nursing journals and by a survey of critical care nurses about family presence in their institutions that was published in both the *Journal of*

Emergency Nursing and the *American Journal of Critical Care* (MacClean, Guzzetta, White, et al., 2003) along with an editorial refuting the primary arguments against the practice (Mason, 2003). The publication of the survey results generated additional media attention. Now, many nurses and patients and their families expect institutions to have policies and procedures in place permitting family presence.

Furthering Nurses' Education

As nursing moved into the university, issues related to the education of nurses were debated in nursing journals. For example, the education of nurse practitioners began in 1966 as a six-week training program. As nurse practitioners began to proliferate and demand greater independence and prescriptive power, their educational preparation became the topic of journal articles and editorials (Mason, Vaccaro, & Fessler, 2000). It quickly became apparent that the credibility and scope of practice of nurse practitioners were dependent on standardized educational requirements. Today, the standard for nurse practitioner education is master's level preparation, and most certifications for nurse practitioners require such an education for new practitioners.

Perhaps the longest standing educational issue that continues to be debated in nursing journals is the "entry into practice"—the minimal educational requirements for entry into professional nursing. The issue has perplexed the profession for decades, but discussions of the importance of nurses' education have spurred both creative approaches to nursing education (e.g., associate degree programs, second degree programs for people coming into nursing with a degree in another field, and external degree programs) as well as conflict. The nursing community is split on the issue, with associate degree nurses and programs seeing the promotion of the baccalaureate degree as disenfranchising of the majority of U.S. nurses; proponents of the baccalaureate seek differentiation in licensing ("More letters; entry into practice," 2003). Journals provide opportunities for discussion of the issues and options for promoting the education of nurses—even if the issue remains contentious.

Most nursing journals also promote the continuing education (CE) of nurses by publicizing CE programs and offering CE credits for their articles. This has been particularly important for those nurses who reside in states that mandate a minimum number of annual CE credits for license renewal and for nurses who are certified and seek to renew their certification without sitting for an exam.

Nursing journals also help their readers to think about what constitutes thoughtful and persuasive discourse. Former editor of *AJN* and *Nursing Outlook*, Edith P. Lewis, periodically wrote editorials about how to write clearly and precisely, decrying nurses' use of jargon and language that obscured rather than illuminated their thinking (Lewis, 1974).

In one instance, *AJN* published a letter that the editorial staff and some readers found to be inflammatory and offensive. The letter was written in response to a commentary by a Muslim American nurse (Baqi-Aziz, 2001) about her experience of discrimination at the hands of her fellow nurses. The debate among the editorial staff centered on whether to publish even an edited version of the letter that removed the most offensive language. Most of the staff believed that it set the wrong example for readers as to what *AJN* would consider for publication. However, a couple of the editors believed that the letter illustrated the extent to which the profession is not as culturally sensitive as it claims and thought the situation had to be uncovered if the profession was to address it. The final decision to publish the letter was made after one staff member recommended that an editorial accompany the letter. The editorial explained the journal's usual letters' policy, which normally would not permit consideration of such letters, and why this letter was published, challenged the profession to examine its assumption that nurses try to be sensitive to their patients' cultural differences, and encouraged readers to criticize ideas rather than the people who propose them.

Some journals have been started to raise the level of discourse on a particular topic. Barbara Brown, editor of *Nursing Administration Quarterly (NAQ)*, says she was asked by the Aspen publishing house what she thought was needed in a new journal. She said, "A journal like the *Harvard Business Review* or *Administrative Science Quarterly* that is topically focused, aimed at leaders in the field, and raises the knowledge in the field." Today, "the articles in NAQ are in the forefront of what leaders should be doing," says Brown (Personal communication with T. Schorr, October 2003).

Development and Promotion of Nursing Leaders

Nursing journals have long provided a forum for developing and promoting nurse leaders. When nurses publish in a journal with the reach of *AJN* or the select audience of *Orthopedic Nursing*, the authors become viewed by many readers as experts and are sought out for speaking, consultation, or additional writing.

For example, Margo McCaffrey coauthored an article with Fay Moss in *AJN* in 1967 entitled "Nursing Intervention for Bodily Pain," in which she described her belief that the nurse's role in pain management was much more than dispensing analgesics; and that nurses had to begin their care by accepting patients' reports of pain (McCaffrey & Moss, 1967). Her continued documentation of her observations and experiences in caring for patients with pain has contributed to her status as a recognized pain expert who consults and teaches internationally.

To cultivate nurses' ability to position their expertise in this way, many nursing journals offer writing workshops for novices. For more than 10 years, *AJN* partnered with the American Association of Critical-Care Nurses and other national nursing organizations on mentored writing fellowships. Members of the association who had no experience in writing for publication were paired with members who were experienced in writing. In 2003, *AJN* and AACN announced at their celebration of that year's fellows that almost all of the past 10 years' fellows had gone on to hold leadership positions within the organization, including serving as president and as mentors for other fellows. Becoming a published author can bolster a nurse's professional career, distinguishing the nurse from peers who do not have that experience.

Editing a nursing journal also provides leadership opportunities. Indeed, editors of nursing journals are "keepers of the flame" and, as such, have important responsibilities. The decision of what the journal should publish provides an editor with the ability to shape what issues the profession considers. The journal's editorial page provides a pulpit from which editors can challenge readers to think and act differently, alert them to issues discussed in the journal, and pose some ideas for nurses to consider, whether clinical, policy related, or some other focus.

Editor of *Curtin Calls* and former editor of *Nursing Management*, Leah Curtin is passionate about what she writes in an editorial: "To write a good editorial, you have to really, really care about whatever it is you're writing about." (Personal communication with T. Schorr, October 2003). And it shows. Her editorials are highly regarded within nursing. Readers expect her to provoke their thinking, usually with good humor.

Similarly, Gail Lenehan, the editor of the *Journal of Emergency Nursing,* reports that she is passionate about all of her editorials, although she is concerned that some of her editorials are not positive enough. She believes in using the editorial pulpit to bring about change on issues, for example, honoring courageous military nurses, making the case for SANE (sexual assault nurse examiners), decrying current government attempts to jeopardize overtime pay, and advocating for a nurse when her Canadian hospital attempted to force the nurse to be on the SARS response team or be fired (the nurse had refused because she was a single mother and lived with her immunosupressed mother) (Personal communication with M. Kennedy, November 2003).

IMPACT ON NURSING'S ROLE WITHIN SOCIETY

Nursing journals have also helped to promote nurses' involvement in the broader society, often encouraging community engagement and informed activism.

Oftentimes, nurses focus their activism on their own interests, perhaps for good reason. The battle for respect and recognition as an independent profession has required nurses to advocate on their own behalf. For example, who could be called a "trained nurse" was an important issue for early nursing leaders. Reports of shady hospital schools that took advantage of students for labor and did little to educate them spurred the move for a standardized curriculum for nursing schools and fueled the debate for registration to keep unqualified women from calling themselves nurses and to protect the public from unqualified practitioners (Birnbach, 1999).

Sophia Palmer, *AJN*'s first editor, was one of the organizing forces behind two early American nursing organizations (the American Society of Superintendents of Training Schools for Nurses and the Nurses' Associated Alumnae, which became the American Nurses Association). She was a staunch and unrelenting supporter of state registration, and her editorials bespoke her feelings. Almost every issue of the early journals carried discussion and letters surrounding the issue, and she aggressively campaigned for state licensing laws. When New York passed its law in 1903 and formed the State Board of Nurse Examiners, she was one of the five nurses appointed and was named the president—a reward, perhaps, for all her efforts (Christy, 1975).

Another example of nurses' advocacy playing out in the pages of nursing journals is that of the legendary Lillian Wald, a superb communicator in person, in letters, and in the many publications she authored. She was prolific, writing about her causes and achievements in *Trained Nurse and Hospital Review, Survey, AJN*, and *Public Health Nursing.* She also wrote two books: *House on Henry Street* (1915) and *Windows on Henry Street* (1934). She was politically astute, had friends with money and influence in high places, and knew how to channel their efforts for the public good. She also was a scrupulous executive, keeping detailed records that documented to the penny all that was spent on her Henry Street Settlement clients and on her continuing efforts to improve health care for the poor.

Wald worked throughout her life for programs and institutions that improved the public's health: the New York Visiting Nurse Service, the concept of public health nursing and the National Organization of Public Health Nursing, school nursing, industrial nursing, the United States Children's Bureau, and the introduction of social work into municipal hospitals. She was even instrumental in bringing down Tammany Hall, as reported in an "Editorial Comment" in the January 1902 *AJN*:

> . . . the public press commented . . . that the women of the Nursing Settlement on Henry Street had been largely influential in rousing the women of upper New York to a knowl-

edge of the terrible conditions that existed in the slum districts under Tammany rule. . . . nurses, for the first time, were given recognition as political reformers, a place that, in the future, they would fill with great honor.

Journal of Emergency Nursing editor Gail Lenehan believes that nursing journals have an advocacy role (Personal communication with M. Kennedy, November 2003). Her journal has published articles and editorials on needlestick safety and latex exposure. *Curtin Call* editor Leah Curtin believes that editors should help shape the profession. "Objectivity," she says, "is indifference—a sign that you don't really care. Everyone has biases—it is appropriate to let your readers know what your biases are" (Personal communication with T. Schorr, October 2003). Other editors, such as Suzanne Smith (*Nurse Educator* and *Journal of Nursing Administration*), do not embrace the advocacy role: "I do not like to read nursing editorials that take a stand on a controversial issue—let's say mandatory staffing. I feel it is undue influence and simply one person's opinion. There are at least two equally valid sides to most issues we face in nursing. I want the facts; I'll make up my own mind" (Personal communication with M. Kennedy, November 4, 2003).

As of 2004, two U.S. nursing journals were focused on health policy (*Policy Politics and Nursing Practice* and *Nursing Outlook*), and many other journals have regular policy columns, such as the *Journal of Nursing Scholarship*, *Pediatric Nursing*, and *AJN*, or include news reports of health policy issues as they unfold. This illustrates the profession's evolution with regard to political matters (Cohen, Mason, Kovner, et al., 1996) and the contemporary consensus that nurses must be active in shaping the important policy issues of the times. But not all readers want their nursing journals to address broader policy and political issues, as letters to the editor of *AJN* have pointed out from time to time, indicating a continued reluctance among some nurses to see political matters as both personal and professional.

In most nursing journals, one can find evidence of nurses' sense of social responsibility, whether through letters to the editor about wars, articles about their health missions to other countries and communities in need, or editorials that show readers the connections between their daily practice and what is going on in society.

CHALLENGES CONFRONTING TODAY'S NURSING JOURNALS

Today's nursing journals are confronting issues that range from the business of publishing to potential conflicts of interest that can taint the credibility of what is published.

Challenges of the Publishing World

Publishing is big business, and nursing journals are not exempt. The worldwide trend in business mergers and takeovers has created a publishing world dominated by only a few players. Elsevier is the largest biomedical publishing conglomerate in the world, owning familiar publishing labels such as Mosby, W. B. Saunders, and Harcourt. The second largest is Wolters Kluwer, which owns Lippincott Williams & Wilkins, the former Aspen Publishing Company, and Springhouse. Both of these companies are publicly traded and struggle to turn a low-profit business into one that can satisfy shareholders' demands for growth and profits. To remain viable, journals in contemporary publishing houses must balance revenues from advertising and subscriptions against the cost of producing and disseminating the journal. In addition, many journals owned by professional societies provide needed revenues that support the organization's missions and activities. Whether published for profit or to serve nonprofit owners, nursing journals must balance editorial quality and integrity against often competing demands to maintain a positive financial margin.

Curtin Call editor Leah Curtin expresses concerns that "the publishers have gotten a stranglehold on nursing journals, and selling ads with editorial that supports the advertisers' products has become more important than informing and educating readers" (Personal communication with T. Schorr, October 2003). This concern is not unique to nursing. The International Committee of Medical Journal Editors (ICMJE) has established guidelines calling for the separation of advertising and editorial content, but not all journals follow these guidelines (http://www. icmje.org). The profit motive of the publishing world has resulted in the proliferation of "controlled circulation" regional magazines that rely solely on advertising revenues (mostly recruitment ads) and that do not adhere to the ICMJE's guidelines. Because they are provided free to nurses, they are sometimes viewed by readers as substitutes for professional journals. Editors who oppose the mixing of advertising and editorial content must wage contentious battles to maintain this separation when other controlled circulation publications that do not have this divide compete for the same advertising dollars. This raises the following questions: What do nurses view as reliable sources of unbiased information? Will peer-reviewed journals that adhere to the ICMJE standards be able to survive the competition of free publications that do not? However, such free publications may be able to reach nurses who do not subscribe to or read for-fee nursing publications.

Society journals face some of the same pressures in that they must generate revenues for the parent association or at least break even. Sigma Theta Tau International, the National League for Nursing, and other national nursing organizations have publishing operations that expand their ability to generate non-dues revenues. Some societies realize that they do not have the expertise and resources of the larger publishing houses and will award contracts to commercial publishing companies to publish their journals, often arranging for profitable royalty payments to the society.

Impact of the Internet

The Internet presents challenges and opportunities for nursing journals. Most nursing journals have an online presence, ranging from the posting of tables of contents, abstracts, or summaries, and information for authors to complete searchable versions of each issue to online versions with additional Web-only content. Business issues of what is available, to whom, and at what cost, as well as recent moves to make reports of all government-funded research freely available, complicate this opportunity. Should journal subscribers be able to access the journal's contents online at no cost? If so, how will the online version be underwritten? For many publishers, online access has increased the cost of doing business. However, in order to compete, paid subscribers, society members, researchers, and other prospective users of journal content must be able to access the journal online.

Many journals offer subscribers or dues-paying members access to online versions of journals through the fees that they pay annually for subscription or membership or for an additional fee. For example, NursingCenter.com is a nursing portal for all of Lippincott Williams & Wilkins' nursing journals. The CE articles and select other articles are available for free (the user who wants the CE credits must pay for them), but most of the other content is available on a pay-per-view basis and through online databases of biomedical and nursing journals to which many health libraries subscribe.

The Internet has also stimulated the creation of a number of online-only nursing journals, the first being Sigma Theta Tau's *Online Journal of Nursing Knowledge Synthesis*, which was started by Jane Barnsteiner. Today, numerous online-only publications exist, such as the *Online Journal in Nursing* produced out of Kent State University's School of Nursing and accessed through the ANA's Web site, http://www.NursingWorld.org.

There has been a movement within the biomedical research community to make research available for free to everyone under an open-access model. For example, journals published by the Public Library of Science (PLoS) are available to all users free of charge, but authors are required to pay up to $1500 for the review and publication of their manuscripts. This is not a new idea. Open-access, peer-reviewed journals in the health sciences, in which readers/users do not pay for access and such access is available immediately (i.e., at the time of publication) were first available in the late 1980s and early 1990s (Meyers, 2004).

Publishing companies and professional societies have expressed concerns about the equitability of the author-pay model, especially for resource-poor authors; whether the true cost of peer review, editing, and publishing papers under this model has been accurately determined; and whether the journal-based revenue that supports professional societies can be replaced by some other means or whether the loss of such revenue will result in the dissolution of these societies (Meyers, 2004; Association of American Publishers, 2004; Held, 2003; Horton, 2003).

Governments are considering laws that would require the posting of all reports of government-funded research on online databases at the time of publication or soon thereafter (e.g., 6 months after publication). Government agencies and other large sponsors of biomedical research are requesting, and in some cases requiring, the posting of all reports of funded research on online databases at the time of publication or soon thereafter (e.g., 6 to 12 months after publication). The *Journal of Clinical Investigation (JCI)* has provided completely free access for all content to all users since 1996, with no barrier of any kind, and has moved its financing away from dependence on print subscriptions to greater reliance on author charges and other means. However, unlike some other open-access journals, *JCI* asks authors to transfer their copyright to its publisher, the American Society for Clinical Investigation (Hawley, 2003). BioMed Central, a commercial publisher, has more than 100 open-access journals, including 1 nursing journal, *BMC Nursing*. Authors pay publication fees ranging from $525 to $1500 (depending on the journal) and retain copyright of their works by granting BioMed Central a license to publish the article and identify itself as the original publisher.

Most open-access journals waive the publication fees for resource-poor authors. Many of these journals rely on a mix of financing; in addition to author fees, other sources of revenue include subscriptions to print versions, institutional memberships, advertising, and sponsorships. One of the first peer-reviewed journals to experiment with free access to content, the *BMJ* (*British Medical Journal*) decided in 2004 that it would discontinue online open access after 10 years because of the financial losses incurred due to declining institutional subscriptions to its print version, a major source of revenue for its owner, the British Medical Association (Delamothe & Smith, 2003). To address the demands of users spurred by the open-access movement, many journals now offer open-access to some of their online content either immediately or after a delay (e.g., 6 months); such access is free of charge, although some of these journals still require users to register.

Open-access publishing is a controversial development that is transforming traditional publishing models. As of July 2004, the Directory of Open Access Journals lists 1148 journals in its directory, including 119 general medical journals, 42 public health journals, and 9 nursing journals (Directory of Open Access Journals, 2004).

Nurses' use of the Internet has grown exponentially in recent years, but many still do not have access to the Internet in their immediate work environments (Pravikoff, Pierce, & Tanner, 2003), and nurses in developing countries may not even have computers or libraries. The future of print versions of nursing journals will likely follow in the footsteps of all print magazines. At present, it appears that people will want access to journals online and will use the Internet to search for answers to specific questions. But nurses seeking to remain current on both clinical matters and nursing issues may prefer print versions, which are sometimes more convenient to read. The challenge is how publishers can provide both without jeopardizing their economic position.

Impact of Peer Review

Most U.S. nursing journals claim to be peer reviewed. If they were not, faculty would not submit manuscripts to the journal, because tenure and promotion require peer-reviewed publications. But one journal's peer review may not be equivalent to another's.

The peer-review process was designed to ensure unbiased evaluations of manuscripts. The double-blind peer-review model requires that both the author and the reviewer remain anonymous to each other (often called an *anonymous review*). The assumption underlying this model is that such blinding will ensure that the reviewer is evaluating the manuscript on its own merits—not on the basis of who the author is. It is still the editor's decision as to whether to publish the manuscript, but these reviews provide the editor with expertise that he or she may not have.

Double-blind review is the norm in nursing and some other disciplines (e.g., psychology) and in other professional communities in which there is concern that objectivity cannot be maintained or that the culture does not encourage open criticism. Single-blind review is used more typically in medicine and other sciences. In single-blind review, reviewers' identities are masked but authors' identities are not. Research comparing the double-blind and single-blind models of peer review suggests that the quality of reviews is not improved with the double-blind model, that identities of authors may still be revealed in double-blind review, and that bias continues to enter into the reviews in both models (Weller, 2001).

Some biomedical journals are moving to unblinded, or open, peer review, in which case the author knows who the reviewer is, and the reviewer knows who the author is. To prevent the reviewer from feeling pressured not to criticize the work of an esteemed author, the *BMJ* has experimented with publishing both the original paper and the reviews online. Thus, the reviewers are motivated to demonstrate that they can provide a knowledgeable and fair critique of a manuscript. This model also supports the idea of providing analyses of researchers' works for other scholars' consideration, thus furthering the development of new thinking on a topic. In 2004, *Nursing Research* became the first nursing journal to move to unblinded peer reviews of select manuscripts, with the commitment to post the original manuscript and the reviews online.

Ethical Challenges

Authors who publish in nursing and other disciplines face a number of ethical dilemmas involving issues of author accountability and responsibility. Typical dilemmas include questions of who is an author and who is not, the order of authorship for multiauthor papers, appropriate use and citation of other authors' work, duplicate publication, and conflicts of interest. A number of resources are available to help nurse authors address these common concerns (Oermann, 2002; Flanagin, 1998; Jones & McClellan, 2000; International Committee of Medical Journal Editors [ICMJE], 2003). Nursing journal policies on authorship accountability and responsibility help to foster integrity among nurse authors, researchers, and academicians.

The key to each of these concerns is transparency. For example, only those who have contributed substantially to a work and who can take public responsibility for the work should be listed as authors; others should be listed in an acknowledgment (ICMJE, 2003; Blancett, 1991; Carpenito, 1993; Anderson, 1995; White, Coudret, & Goodwin, 1998). A paper that relies on the work of others (and there are few that do not) should always reference the previous work and properly quote and cite the reuse of any content (Lok, Chan, & Martinson, 2001; Ellenchild Pinch, 1999; Flanagin, 1993). Authors should also be careful to reference their own work that is related to the same overall research project or that is otherwise similar in nature; not doing so could result in duplicate publication (Blancett, Flanagin, & Young, 1995; Yarbro, 1995). Duplicate publication because of improper attribution to previously published related work has been a problem for journals in nursing and other fields (Blancett, Flanagin, & Young, 1995; King, McGuire, Longman, & Carroll-Johnson, 1997) and continues to be today (von Elm, Poglia, Alder, & Tramer, 2004).

Of growing concern within the biomedical publishing community, and even with the public at large, is the potential for outside interests to bias what is reported in journals. Deyo and colleagues (1997) reported in the *New England Journal of Medicine* that he and two other colleagues at the University of Washington published research on various topics and were attacked by special interest groups and companies that did not like their findings. In one case, a pharmaceutical company tried to prohibit publication of the results of a study it had funded that demonstrated its new drug was not better than an older drug in the treatment of thyroid disease. Subsequently, Bekelman and colleagues (2003) published a report in *JAMA* demonstrating that drug studies with negative findings were more likely to be published if they were not funded by pharmaceutical companies.

A number of studies have found that authors with financial interests may be biased in favor of those interests. As the business world increasingly pays for physicians and nurses to consult with them, speak about their products, or study their products, concern about the bias that underlies publications by these clinicians has grown within the biomedical community and the public (Rennie, Flanagin, & Glass, 1991; Cho, Shohara, Schissel, & Rennie, 2000).

Conflicts of interest are ubiquitous and should always be disclosed by authors (Flanagin, 1998; ICMJE, 2003; King, McGuire, Longman, & Carroll-Johnson, 1997; Mason, 2000; Erlen, 2000). Many nursing journals are beginning to require authors to disclose all financial interests they have in relation to their manuscripts (this includes, but is not limited to, funding for research, sponsorships, employment, paid consultancies, honoraria, royalties, stock ownership/options, patents, and payment for expert testimony). These disclosures are then published along with the author's affiliations so that readers can judge for themselves the potential for any influence of financial interests in the same way that readers are made aware of other sources of influence on an author that are usually apparent from the authors' professional or academic degrees and contact information (e.g., profession, specialty, institutional affiliation, location, etc.). Full disclosure of the contributions of authors, sources used, related works, and relevant financial interests is the key to managing some of the common dilemmas authors face when publishing in nursing and other journals.

Conclusion

Nursing journals have a long history of providing the profession and its members with information and perspectives that challenge current practice. They are essential for nurses' scientific, clinical, and professional development.

References

Ackerman, M. H., Ecklund, M. W., & Abu-Jumah, M. (1996). A review of normal saline instillation: Implications for practice. *Dimensions in Critical Care Nursing, 15*(1), 31–38.

Aiken, L., Havens, D. S., & Sloane, D. M. (2000a). The Magnet nursing services recognition program. *American Journal of Nursing, 100*(3), 26–35.

Aiken, L., Havens, D. S., & Sloane, D. M. (2000b). The Magnet nursing services recognition programme. *Nursing Standard, 14*(25), 41–47.

Aiken, L. H., Clarke, S. P., Sloane, D. M., Sochalski, J., & Silber, J. H. (2002). Hospital nurse staffing and patient mortality, nurse burnout, and job dissatisfaction. *Journal of the American Medical Association, 288*(16), 1987–1993.

American Nurses Association. (1991). *Agenda for healthcare reform.* Washington, D.C.: American Nurses Asssocation.

Anderson, C. A. (1995). Author—what does it mean to be one? *Nursing Outlook, 43*(5), 199–200.

Army and Navy Nurse Corps bill. (1947). *American Journal of Nursing, 47*(5), 349.

Association of American Publishers/Professional and Scholarly Publishing Division. (2004). *Copyright and public access to federally funded scientific research: The erroneous premise of open-access advocates and H.R. 2613.* Accessed June 22, 2005, from http://www.pspcentral.org/committees/executive/sabo/doc.

Baer, E. (1987). Nursing's social history: New insights, new solutions. *Journal of Nursing History, 2*(2), 3–5.

Baqi-Aziz, M. (2001). Where does she think she is? *American Journal of Nursing, 101*(11), 11.

Barnard, K. (1973). The effect of stimulation on the sleep behavior of the premature infant. *Communicating Nursing Research, 6,* 12–33.

Barnard, K., & Neal, M. (1977). Maternal-child nursing research: Review of the past and strategies for the future. *Nursing Research, 26*(3), 193–200.

Bekelman, J. E., Li, Y., & Gross, C. P. (2003). Scope and impact of financial conflicts of interest in biomedical research: A systematic review. *Journal of the American Medical Association,* 289(4), 454–465.

Benner, P. (1984). *From novice to expert.* Menlo Park, CA: Addison-Welsey.

Binger, J. L. (1981). The nursing journal—learning resource, professional symbol, and commodity. *Image: Journal of Nursing Scholarship, 13*(10), 67–70.

Birnbach, N. (1999). Registration. In T. Schorr & M. S. Kennedy (Eds.), *100 years of American nursing: Celebrating a century of caring* (pp. 17–19). Philadelphia: Lippincott.

Blancett, S. S. (1991). The ethics of writing and publishing. *Journal of Nursing Administration, 21*(5), 31–36.

Blancett, S. S., Flanagin, A., & Young, R. K. (1995). Duplicate publication in the nursing literature. *Image: Journal of Nursing Scholarship, 27*(1), 51–56.

Blasingame, F. J. (1958). The AMA position on health insurance for the aged. *American Journal of Nursing, 58*(9), 1273–1274.

Breckinridge, M. (1927). Foreword to *Enter, the nurse-midwife* by Edna Rockstroh. *American Journal of Nursing, 27*(3), 160–164.

Carnegie, M. E. (2000). *The path we tread: Blacks in nursing worldwide, 1854–1994.* New York: National League for Nursing Press.

Carpenito, L. J. (1993). Loose authorship. *Nursing Forum, 28*(2), 3–4.

Cho, M. K., Shohara, R., Schissel, A., & Rennie, D. (2000). Policies on faculty conflicts of interest at U.S. universities. *Journal of the American Medical Association, 284*(17), 2237–2238.

Christy, T. E. (1975). Portrait of a leader: Sophia Palmer. *Nursing Outlook, 23*(12), 47–52.

Cohen, S., Mason, D. J., Kovner, C., Leavitt, J., Pulcini, J., & Sochalski, J. (1996). Stages of nursing's political development: Where we've been and where we ought to go. *Nursing Outlook, 44*(6), 259–266.

Craven, J., & Wald, F. (1975). Hospice care for dying patients. *American Journal of Nursing, 75*(10), 1816–1822.

Crenshaw, J., & Winslow, E. (2002). Preoperative fasting: Old habits die hard. *American Journal of Nursing, 102*(5), 36–44.

Davis, C. (2003). Nursing humanities: The time has come. *American Journal of Nursing,* 103(2), 13.

Delamothe, T., & Smith, R. (2003). Paying for bmj.com. *British Medical Journal, 327*, 241–242. Accessed August 15, 2004, from http://www.bmj.com.

Delano, J. (1914). American Red Cross Nursing Service. *American Journal of Nursing, 14*(6), 441–443.

Deyo, R. A., Psaty, B. M., Simon, G., Wagner, E. H., & Omenn, G. S. (1997). The messenger under attack—intimidation of researchers by special interest groups. *New England Journal of Medicine, 336*(16), 1176–1180.

Diers, D. (2004). *Speaking of nursing: Narratives of practice, research, policy and the profession.* Sudbury, MA: Jones and Bartlett.

Directory of Open Access Journals. (2004). Lund University Libraries. Accessed July 16, 2004, from http://www.doaj.org.

Editorial Comment. (1902). *American Journal of Nursing, 2*(1), 301.

Eichhorn, D., Meyers, T., Guzzetta, C. E., et al. (2001). Family presence during invasive procedures and resuscitation: Hearing the voice of the patient. *American Journal of Nursing, 101*(5), 26–33.

Ellenchild Pinch, W. J. (1999). Misquoting and quoting out of context. *Advances in Nursing Science, 21*(4), vi.

Erlen, J. A. (2000). 'Conflicts of interest': An ethical dilemma for the nurse researcher. *Orthopedic Nursing, 19*(4), 74–77.

Flanagin, A. for the International Academy of Nursing Editors. (1993). Fraudulent publication. *Image: Journal of Nursing Scholarship, 25*(4), 359.

Flanagin, A. (1998). Ethical and legal considerations. In C. Iverson, A. Flanagin, & P. B. Fontanarosa, *American Medical Association manual of style* (9th ed) (pp. 87–172). Baltimore: Williams & Wilkins.

Hawley, J. B. (2003). The *JCI*'s commitment to excellence—and free access. *Journal of Clinical Investigations, 112*, 968–969.

Held, M. J. (2003). Proposed legislation supports an untested publishing model. *Journal of Cell Biology, 162*, 2.

Henderson, V. (1956). An overview of nursing research. *Nursing Research 6*(2), 61–68.

Hibbard, M. E. (1900). With the *Maine* to South Africa. *American Journal of Nursing, 1*(1), 1–7.

Horton, R. (2003). 21st-century biomedical journals: Failures and futures. *The Lancet, 362*, 93–95.

International Committee of Medical Journal Editors (ICMJE). (2003). Uniform requirements for manuscripts submitted to biomedical journals: Writing and editing for biomedical publication. Accessed July 20, 2004, from http://www.icmje.org.

Jones, A. H., & McLellan, F. (2000). *Ethical issues in biomedical publication.* Baltimore, MD: The Johns Hopkins University Press.

Kaiman, C. (2001). September 11, 2001. *American Journal of Nursing, 101*(11), 96.

Kaiman, C. (2002). Prince's Bay, a painting. *American Journal of Nursing, 102*(9), 25.

Kalisch, P., & Kalisch, B. (1978). *The advance of American nursing.* Boston: Little Brown and Company.

King, C. R., McGuire, D. B., Longman, A. J., & Carroll-Johnson, R. M. (1997). Peer review, authorship, ethics, and conflict of interest. *Image: Journal of Nursing Scholarship, 29*(2), 163–167.

Lewis, E. (1974). Pretentious prose. *Nursing Outlook, 22*(7), 431.

Lok, C. K., Chan, M. T., & Martinson, I. M. (2001). Risk factors for citation errors in peer-reviewed nursing journals. *Journal of Advanced Nursing, 34*(2), 223–229.

MacLean, S. L., Guzzetta, C. E., White, C., Fontaine, D., Eichhorn, D. J., Meyers, T. A., & Desy, P. (2003). Family presence during cardiopulmonary resuscitation and invasive procedures: Practices of critical care and emergency nurses. *American Journal of Critical Care, 12*(3), 246–257.

Mason, D. J. (2000). 'One pill makes you larger. . .': Don't be seduced by pharmaceutical companies. *American Journal of Nursing, 100*(12), 7.

Mason, D. J. (2003). Family presence: Evidence versus tradition. *American Journal of Critical Care, 12*(3), 190–192.

Mason, D. J., Vaccaro, K., & Fessler, M. B. (2000). Early views of nurse practitioners: A Medline search. *Clinical Excellence for Nurse Practitioners, 4*(3), 175–183.

McCaffrey, M., & Moss, F. (1967). Nursing interventions for bodily pain. *American Journal of Nursing, 67*(6), 1224–1227.

Meyers, B. (2004). *Open access: A matter for definition.* Wheat Ridge, CO: Society for Scholarly Publishing.

Meyers, T., Eichhorn, D., Guzzetta, C. E., et al. (2000). Family presence during invasive procedures and resuscitation: The experiences of family members, nurses, and physicians. *American Journal of Nursing, 100*(2), 32–42.

More letters; entry into practice. (2003). *American Journal of Nursing, 103*(3), 69–70.

Neal, M. (1968). Vestibular stimulation and developmental behavior of the small premature infant. *Nursing Research Reports, 3*(1), 1, 3–5.

Needleman, J., Buerhaus, P., Mattke, S., Stewart, M., & Zelevinsky, K. (2002). Nurse-staffing levels and the quality of care in hospitals. *New England Journal of Medicine, 346*(22), 1715–1722.

Oermann, M. H. (2002). *Writing for publication in nursing.* Philadelphia: Lippincott.

Palmer, S. (1900). The editor. *American Journal of Nursing, 1*(1), 64–66.

Palmer, S. (1908). Editorial comment. *American Journal of Nursing, 8*(12), 956.

Perry, C. (1900). Our floating hospitals. *American Journal of Nursing, 1*(2), 104–107.

Pravikoff, D. S., Pierce, S., & Tanner, A. (2003). Are nurses ready for evidence-based practice? *American Journal of Nursing, 103*(5), 95–96.

Rennie, D., Flanagin, A., & Glass, R. M. (1991). Conflicts of interest in the publication of science. *Journal of the American Medical Association, 266*(2), 266–267.

Resolution on health insurance for the disabled, retired, and aged. (1958). *American Journal of Nursing, 58*(7), 984.

Rogers, L. (1903). School nursing in New York City. *American Journal of Nursing, 3*(6), 448–450.

Runyan, J. W., Phillips, W. E., Herring, O., & Campbell, L. (1970). A program for the care of patients with chronic diseases. *Journal of the American Medical Association, 211*(3), 476–479.

Schorr, T., & Kennedy, M. S. (1999). *100 years of American nursing: Celebrating a century of caring.* Philadelphia: Lippincott Williams & Wilkins.

Silver, H., & Ford, L. (1967). Physicians' assistants. The pediatric nurse practitioner at Colorado. *American Journal of Nursing, 67*(7), 1443–1444.

Silver, H. K., Ford, L., & Stearly, S. G. (1967). A program to increase health care for children: The pediatric nurse practitioner program. *Pediatrics, 39*(5), 756–760.

Smith, F. P. (1976). Editorial. *Journal of Advanced Nursing, 1*(1), 1.

Stotts, N., & Deitrich, C. (2004). The challenge to come: The care of older adults. *American Journal of Nursing, 104*(8), 40–47.

Thistle, W. B. (1900). Infant feeding. *American Journal of Nursing, 1*(1), 22–28.

Tsai, E. (2002). Should family members be present during cardiopulmonary resuscitation? *New England Journal of Medicine, 346*, 1019–1021.

von Elm, E., Poglia, G., Walder, B., Tramer, M. R. (2004). Different patterns of duplicate publication: An analysis of articles used in systematic reviews. *JAMA, 291*(8), 974–980.

Wald, L. D. (1902). The nurses' settlement in New York. *American Journal of Nursing,* 2:568.

Wald, L. D. (1915). *The House on Henry Street.* New York: Henry Holt, Inc.

Wald, L. D. (1934). *Windows on Henry Street.* Boston: Little Brown and Company.

Weller, A. C. (2001). *Editorial peer review: Its strengths and weaknesses.* Medford, NJ: ASIST Monograph Series.

White, A. H., Coudret, N.A., & Goodwin, C. S. (1998). From authorship to contributorship. Promoting integrity in research publication. *Nurse Educator, 23*(6), 26–32.

Whitnack, J. (2000). Installation of normal saline during endotracheal suctioning: Effects on mixed venous oxygen saturation. *American Journal of Critical Care, 9*(1), 78–79.

Wunderlich, G. S., Sloan, F. A., and Davis, C. K. (Eds.), Institute of Medicine Committee on the Adequacy of Nurse Staffing in Hospitals and Nursing Homes. (1996). *Nursing staff in hospitals and nursing homes: Is it adequate?* Washington, D.C.: National Academy Press.

Yarbro, C. H. (1995). Duplicate publication: guidelines for nurse authors and editors. *Image: Journal of Nursing Scholarship, 27*(1), 57.

CHAPTER 29

Education for Entry into Nursing Practice: Revisited for the 21st Century

Lucille A. Joel

CURRENT REALITY

We are in the midst of another shortage. Though scholars say it is different, because history doesn't really repeat itself, there are lessons that should have been learned. The fact that the average age of the practicing nurse is older only complicates some recurring patterns.

There has been a renewed appreciation for the presence of the RN in health care. This attitude has been the result of public opinion fueled by the increased acuity and frailty of patients in hospitals, home care, and nursing homes. The American public has reason to fear for their safety and care, and nurses are seen as their advocates (Joel & Kelly, 2002). Employers are scurrying to rehire all the nurses that they let go during some of our more poorly thought out decisions on reengineering, reorganizing, and restructuring. And nurses are having second thoughts about working in an environment that is unsafe and stressful. The reality of too many patients to be therapeutic, assistive personnel who practice on our license regardless of their ability, mandatory overtime, violence, HIV/AIDS, Hepatitis C, multi-drug-resistant tuberculosis, latex allergy, and much more, cause us to fear for ourselves as much as our patients. In fact, only 75% of current license holders are working at jobs that require the RN credential.

The healthcare industry has traditionally ignored the advice of the nursing profession. Proof abounds.

From the Nursing Home Reform Acts of 1987, where the industry lobbied to have "licensed nurse" substituted for "registered nurse" in the bill, under the pretext that the existing shortage would make the recruitment of RNs to nursing home practice in sufficient numbers impossible (Kelly & Joel, 1999), to the lobbying from hospital interests to continue diploma school education, while other healthcare fields had long ago aspired to higher levels of education, to the continuing resistance to paying a differential salary to the BSN graduate. These are only some of the most cruelly divisive situations, and clearly show how nursing has been dominated by an external locus of control. An external locus has divided our strength, created internal unrest, and kept nursing straddling the fence between expedient educational programs and those that create professionalism.

Source: Joel, L. (May 31, 2002). "Education for Entry into Nursing Practice: Revisited for the 21st Century." Online Journal of Issues in Nursing. Vol. 7, No. 2, manuscript 4. Available: http://www.nursingworld.org/ojin/topic18/tpc18_4.htm. Reprinted with permission.

Even as we have strained to make our educational programs consumer friendly with flexible admission requirements, Internet courses, external degrees, and guaranteed articulation, our enrollments have declined and the age of our students has increased. Young people making primary occupational choices are willing to invest time and effort in a field that guarantees status and prestige. And they are not impressed with what nursing promises. Nursing has been much more suited to the mid-life or retirement decision makers, where practicality may be the motive and associate degree nursing education the logical choice. Even for these atypical students, choices are made with a new appreciation for moderation in living. It is the attitude of people who put work in perspective and have a healthy self-respect for their contribution.

AN ANALYTICAL FRAMEWORK

This picture of the work of nursing frustrates the use of the term professionalism. While the literature contains endless definitions of the characteristics of a profession, there seem to be three areas of agreement: the professions are service oriented, learned, and autonomous. Each of these characteristics allows for a broad range of interpretation. It helps to further consider these essential elements and identify the point beyond which compromise is impossible.

No one would debate nursing's service orientation, though as we compete for full status in liberal arts institutions, the applied science nature of nursing has often become a liability. The traditional sciences accord the highest priority to the creation and expansion of knowledge, often with little regard for its practical usefulness. This value is deeply entrenched in higher education and determines the faculty reward system and status of the discipline. Academic medicine has largely avoided this conflict by establishing educational programs outside of the liberal arts setting. The continuing commitment on the part of medicine to practice has contributed to the second-class status of physicians within the broader academic community. Simply put, society accords special privileges to professionals because of their service orientation, while the academe penalizes them for the same characteristic.

It is not quite enough to say that professions have a service orientation. That service orientation must be relevant to the times and carefully orchestrated to meet specific social needs. Orchestration includes assuring an adequate workforce for a timely service role. In designing their practice role, the professions must walk a fine line between directing the market and responding to it. If the service ceases to be relevant, timely, and efficacious, the field of work will gradually disappear. Nurse practitioners and physician's assistants were the social response to the physician shortage of the 1950s; the licensed practical nurse was society's response in earlier generations to the need for increased nursing manpower. And again in the late 1980s, the American Medical Association proposed the creation of a new occupation, the Registered Care Technologist, to compensate for the shortage of nurses.

A body of knowledge and skills unique to the discipline and a considerable educational investment distinguish the professions. The art of professions is cognitive artfulness. It consists of the ability to manipulate in the mind circumstances that have never been experienced and see relevancy between situations that on the surface have little in common.

Nursing has made impressive strides in demonstrating its cognitive artfulness and exclusiveness. The existence of a variety of grand and mid-range theories allows the design of distinctive systems of caring, each focused on the same end. The required presence of nursing theories and research in the curriculum, the emphasis on theory development in graduate programs, and the governmental presence of the National Institute of Nursing Research are all indicators of our growing intellectual substance.

Autonomy has two perspectives, the autonomy of the field of work and the autonomy of the individual. The public has recognized the unusual degree of knowledge and skill in professional practice and the need for professionals to proceed with their work relatively unencumbered. Conversely, unsafe practice can seriously jeopardize the public good. The traditional model of autonomy has undergone some modifications in recent years, with the responsibility to seek and respond to input from consumers, government, and other communities of interest significant to the profession. What has never been challenged is the fact that the credential to practice is awarded to an individual in recognition of a primary obligation to the recipient of service as opposed to any employer or third-party payer. This model nurtures the confidentiality and trust that have traditionally characterized the provider–client relationship and rewards the provider with work that has a great capacity for self-expression. Balance is guaranteed by the presence of adequate peer review mechanisms.

Yet we continue to be constrained by institutional policies in the care of our patients, reticent to monitor the practice of our peers, fearful of transgressing the territorial boundaries of other disciplines, comfortable in a dependency which is more familiar than the unknown, lacking assertiveness to demand what is rightfully ours, and sometimes inappropriately reliant on external regulation and the opinions of others. We resist many of the developmental patterns that have been common to all professional fields: recognition of the need for assisting categories of technical manpower, educational upgrading, and the application of the products of scientific investigation to practice.

THE GROWTH AND DEVELOPMENT OF PROFESSIONAL AREAS OF WORK

Nursing is currently involved in the same painful sequence of events experienced by other disciplines as they emerged to full professional status. As a class, the professions can trace their roots to social necessity and the call for pragmatic service. The status of a discipline is closely associated with the length and rigor of the education required for entry into practice. In contrast to nursing, the traditional professions of medicine, law, and the clergy were always clear about their areas of social concern. Perhaps for this reason, they have prepared for practice in a concentrated course of study following a preprofessional curriculum. In fact, most of their work in standardization focused on upgrading the preprofessional course of study and admission requirements. In 1900, high school graduation was not required to begin study in medical school. By 1938, three years of undergraduate education were necessary, and by 1969, 85% of medical schools required a bachelor's degree. Law schools have followed a similar pattern. Given this history, and the general social structure of the United States, it is understandable why these professions chose to serve their publics within an entrepreneurial model. Freedom in practice, the absence of an early history as an employee, and direct access to clients soundly established the autonomy of the field and the clarity of the role. The practical nature of the work and a model of service delivery that reinforced independence and autonomy allowed the intellectual nature of the discipline to escape scrutiny. The nature of the discipline was further reinforced by a mode of teaching soundly rooted in the case method and Socratic approach. Although the independent practice model of American law and medicine has witnessed an upheaval in recent years, its developmental periods were from these origins.

In many ways the development of nursing can be better contrasted with the fields of social work, teaching, and engineering. The limitations of this paper do not permit us to fully chart the development of these fields, but some general observations seem relevant. Early in its history, social work was characterized as a woman's profession. Social work emerged as a discrete field due to the increased complexity of life and the breakdown of some of the traditional resources available to people through the family. In a manner similar to nursing, social work became intellectually vulnerable by building advanced preparation around functional roles. In the case of social work, these roles were in public policy and administration. Clinical practice was not considered sophisticated in the early days of the field. Clinical practice grew in strength when social work officially selected sociology as its common base, as opposed to a psychological emphasis.

Social work labored under disadvantages that were even greater than those of nursing. Social work has grown simultaneously with the history of organizations, and social workers have historically been salaried. Social workers in some states were not regulated until very recently, and consequently did not have the boundaries of their practice established by government. It is only since 1999 that all states and the District of Columbia have had credentialing requirements for social work practice and title protection. Though the bachelor's degree is required for entry into practice, an advanced degree is standard for many positions (Stanfield & Hui, 2002). But despite this progress, the regulatory requirement for the presence of social workers in institutions is frequently no more than tokenism. In reality, social work as compared to nursing has experienced greater standardization of education and practice, but less support of government.

Elementary and secondary schoolteachers can also trace their heritage to a technical education, namely, within the normal school system. As the scientific base for teaching grew, the baccalaureate became the necessary credential for teachers. Minimum standards for practice were formalized through statutory requirements in a state and seniority in a school system, and advanced educational achievement were recognized in the workplace through the advocacy of strong collective bargaining programs. Regardless of critics of governmental regulation, a whole class of professionals has been allowed to direct their practice in the best interests of the clients they serve. And collective bargaining has allowed them to expand their educational base and control their work environment.

Engineering provides another useful comparison. Engineers emerged from the ranks of craftsmen as the sciences of mechanics, chemistry, and electricity became more theoretical and complex. It is only in the last 20 to 30 years that engineering programs incorporated more than a smattering of liberal education. When the scholarly nature of the discipline as an applied science began to grow, a technical level of worker surfaced that would function under the direction of the professional engineer. Engineering has moved to specialist preparation with the first university degree as opposed to maintaining commitment to the generalist as the entry into practice position.

In summary, as professional areas developed, they seemed to have a clear picture of the service they provide and the knowledge and skills necessary to meet that commitment. Preparing for practice has been the initial concern, with a more liberalizing education only being proposed once the discipline matures and has some control over standardization of educational requirements. In most established fields, liberalizing and broadening the perspective of the professional has been accomplished through a preprofessional curriculum. In disciplines that developed later, professional and general studies have paralleled one another. All of these disciplines maintain intense practice experiences within the educational program or through an extension of the educational program. The student teaching experience, residencies in medicine, moot court, the law clerkship or legal clinics, and the residency in social work all intend to socialize the neophyte into the field and provide a transition to professional accountability.

This tendency to move in the direction of higher levels of education is not exclusive to the disciplines reviewed. Many of the health professions have followed suit, including occupational and physiotherapists, speech and language pathologists and audiologists, genetic counselors, pharmacists (already moving to the PharmD), dieticians, and more (Wisconsin Area Health Education Center [AHEC], 2002).

AND FOR NURSING, THE PAST IS PROLOGUE

By witnessing this evidence from the progress of other professional fields, it is obvious that nursing has resisted the normal course of occupational development. More correctly, any progress towards educational standardization or upgrading could jeopardize a substantial workforce for the healthcare industry. It was to no one's benefit to accomplish these things, except nurses themselves.

Organized nursing has had a historical commitment to advancing the educational preparation for practice.

As entry into practice programs became more diversified with the introduction of the associate degree and the growth of community colleges, that agenda was modified to include the need to standardize and distinguish between levels of practice. The associate degree as a route to preparing for a career in nursing did not require extensive justification. Its cost-efficiency had been proven, and in many instances it served as the vehicle for preparing the bulk of the nursing workforce in days of declining diploma education. Associate degree nursing was a response to social and consumer need and provided the technical associate that so many other professions have birthed.

The changed scope of nursing practice, the intellectual growth of the discipline, and the increased demands of the service environment bring an ethical obligation to consider complementary changes in nursing education, to revisit the "entry" issue.

Today's healthcare delivery system challenges the nurse with increased technology, the mandate for cost-containment, a new consumerism and growing demand for self-care, diminished use of inpatient facilities, and the continual call for counseling and health education. More attention is directed to utilization review and quality assurance and the need for case coordination in vertically integrated systems. The requirement for highly sophisticated providers and more independent decision making is obvious. Given a supportive environment, the more educated practitioner will be the most cost-efficient. This means commitment to a longer and more demanding education than the baccalaureate degree. Moreover, the increased demand for nursing services, as evidenced by the growing presence of chronic illness and an aging population, sustains the case for associate degree education.

Partitioning the nursing workforce in this way addresses another issue of contention. Contrasting the nurse prepared at the graduate level to the associate degree nurse demonstrates a significant difference in competency, one that is obvious to nurses, and additionally to the consumer, the industry, and allied healthcare interests.

This proposal is admittedly vague and leaves many bigger questions. How would titling be handled?

Nurses have traditionally derived their identity from their statutory titles rather than their academic degrees. The result is possessiveness of the title "registered nurse" and reticence for any one group to relinquish continuing right to this title. There is the tendency to personalize the issue and to feel threatened by policy decisions that will only impact future generations. So be it. Accepting that this credential only signifies safety in practice and is based on role delineation studies that measure performance in the year following graduation; it is a minimal standard.

How would specialization be handled? Would an additional credential be awarded to signify specialty competence? Would the "entry into practice" credential allow for specialization? How would this affect workforce projections? Would the largest number of nurses be needed at the associate degree or the graduate level? How would this impact the licensed practical nurse, if at all?

Then there will be those nay-sayers who caution against instituting more change in the wake of the recent slow but steady recognition of advanced practice nurses by state legislatures and the federal government. To them I would say that nursing would always be a work in the process of "becoming."

Despite all of these potentially difficult questions, the time has come to face a reality from which we can run, but cannot hide. We are confronted with occupational decision makers who are demanding a feeling of fulfillment and personal expression from their work. Nursing has had difficulty keeping that promise.

REFERENCES

Joel, L. A., & Kelly, L. Y. (2002). *The nursing experience* (4th ed.). New York: McGraw-Hill.

Kelly, L. Y., & Joel, L. A. (1999). *Dimensions of professional nursing* (8th ed.). New York: McGraw-Hill.

Stanfield, P. S., & Hui, Y. H. (2002). *Introduction to the health professions* (4th ed.). Boston: Jones and Bartlett Publishers.

Wisconsin AHEC Health Careers Information Center (AHEC). (2002). Healthcare occupation. Retrieved March 11, 2002, from http://www.wihealthcareers.org.

CHAPTER 30

The Elephant in Our Living Room: Associate Degree Education in Nursing

Elizabeth Speakman

INTRODUCTION

Nursing education and practice are rooted deeply in the societal, political, and economic contexts of our times. The progress that the nursing profession has made over the past 100 years has been forged by wars, epidemics, and economic and social turmoil. Reexamination of such mile markers can help us to understand nursing's past and help us look toward the future. As the profession once again confronts a nursing shortage, policymakers and educators have renewed the debate over the future of nursing education. The majority of nurses today are associate degree graduates. Efforts aimed at ending the nursing shortage must take into account the central role associate degree education plays in increasing the nursing workforce. Debates over nursing education all too often ignore this "elephant in the living room."

It would be remiss to examine associate degree nursing education without being cognizant of its place in the history of American nursing. Nursing education at the associate degree (AD) level initially was conceived as a way to alleviate the nursing shortage that followed World War II. Although implemented as a solution to the immediate problem of the nursing shortage, associate degree education was conceptualized and designed to meet the growing complexity of the healthcare system. Today, the profession grapples with some of the same issues that overwhelmed it following World War II. The current nursing shortage poses a renewed challenge in light of increased healthcare demands by the public. As nurse leaders search for solutions to the current nursing shortage, it would behoove them to acknowledge the valuable role of associate degree nursing in resolving nursing shortages of the past.

EARLY NURSING EDUCATION

Historically, nursing and health care have had strong ties to American politics and the larger economy. Throughout the history of the United States, the harsh realities of race, class, and gender have been reflected in health care. Until the 20th century, only the wealthy elite had access to adequate health care. Furthermore, in its early history the nursing profession was subordinate to medicine, which was a male-dominated profession. Because of this, nursing and nursing education were constrained by the power of patriarchy. Except for Catholic religious orders, which prepared their members to care for the sick, most nursing was administered by women with no formal training or education. If they were educated, such education may have been offered through a lecture by a local physician.

In 1798, Dr. Seaman, the medical chief at New York Hospital, organized the first regular training school for nurses. It was not until almost a generation later, in 1850, that the next attempt to educate nurses took place, in obstetrical nursing (Donahue, 1996). This lack of formalized nurse training resulted in a profession that lacked organization and consistency.

However, efforts by socially prominent women to provide "nursing care" during the Civil War led to an understanding that adequate nursing training was needed: "The strange neglect of nursing in the United States was identified and the need of good nursing emphasized at a New Orleans meeting of the American Medical Association in 1869" (Donahue, 1996, p. 265).

Following the Civil War, the number of nurse training programs increased dramatically. However, the type and length of education varied, ranging from home school correspondence coursework to hospital-based training. Ironically, early chronicles show that the only primary consistency in nursing education was that physicians did the teaching. Although nursing had gained positive public awareness, it lacked the ability to self-govern and self-administer. In light of these problems, some institutions, such as Woman's Hospital of Philadelphia, and later the New England Hospital for Women and Children, attempted to create nursing programs that focused on the education of nurses rather than on the care of patients (Donahue, 1996).

Three schools—the Bellevue Training School in New York City; the Connecticut Training School in New Haven, Connecticut; and the Boston Training School in Boston, Massachusetts—had a major influence on shaping nursing and nursing education. In addition, women of societal influence had changed the public's view of nursing and made it a suitable profession for women. However, students who applied to the nursing programs often met the prejudice that marked society at the time. Most training programs had a quota, whereby one Jew and one black individual were admitted to each class, and in the South, blacks were excluded all together. Despite these barriers, in addition to the long hours and sleeping near the wards in order to be available at a moment's notice, competition for admission to nursing programs was fierce. According to Donahue (1996):

> Nursing care became the major product dispensed by the hospital. The real function of the school of nursing became not education but service. In addition, no policy for control of the numbers of nursing schools or the standards for admission and graduation was established or accepted.
>
> Consequently a proliferation of nursing schools occurred. The first decade of the twentieth century demonstrated a period of phenomenal growth, with the establishment of close to seven hundred new schools. All schools' functions were ultimately placed under the control and direction of hospital authorities. (p. 274)

NURSING IN THE 20TH CENTURY

To understand the challenges faced by nurse leaders in the early 20th century, it is essential to have an appreciation of the changes in health care that occurred between 1870 and 1910. Developments such as the germ theory, scientifically based treatments, and the advent of urbanization, industrialization, and immigration contributed to a rapid increase in the number of hospitals. This growth in the number of hospitals continued well into the 20th century. In 1873, there were 178 hospitals with 50,000 hospital beds in the United States; by 1909, census takers counted 4,359 hospitals with 421,065 beds (Rosenberg, 1987, as cited in Connolly, 1998).

As America entered the 20th century, the need for formal nursing education and training was recognized and accepted by both medicine and the nursing profession. Hospital administrators realized that a school of nursing offered the labor needed to run a hospital. The care provided by nurses in a hospital became an integral part of the care provided by that hospital. The recognition that nurses had a direct positive effect on in-patient health improved the public's perception of the nursing profession. However, the national proliferation of hospitals and the subsequent increase in the size of the nursing workforce became problematic for the nursing profession.

Reverby (1987) has noted that although many hospitals opened their own schools of nursing, what was advertised as an educational opportunity was more often than not an exploitive system of securing cheap labor. Formal instruction was scant; instead, nursing students were assigned to work under more senior student nurses. Nursing students, then known as *pupil nurses,* were paid small allowances and received room and board for a 12-hour workday, 6 days a week, 50 weeks a year. Obviously, the hospital benefited more from this system than the student nurse. After graduating from a hospital-based training program, a nurse's employment was unpredictable. Few nurses assumed leadership positions in nurse training schools or hospitals. Most left the hospital environment and sought private-duty positions in homes. In some cases, hospitals hired out pupil nurses to serve as private duty nurses with no supervision, and the hospitals reaped the income generated by their labor (Reverby, 1987).

By the end of the 19th century, the development of a formalized nursing education system was underway in the United States. Nursing leaders, through the Society of Superintendents of Training Schools for Nurses, were the driving force behind curriculum reform. They worked to develop high educational standards for schools of nursing by establishing universal admission requirements, developing a sound program of theory and practice, and improving working conditions for nurses (Donahue, 1996). Subsequently, the need to educate nurse leaders to assume supervision of the new and revised curriculum evolved. At Teachers College, Columbia University, an 8-month course on nursing economics was created. Mary Adelaide Nutting, the Superintendent of Nursing at John Hopkins Training School for Nurses, became the chair of the nursing economics program and became the first nursing professor in the United States (Donahue, 1996). This was an important event in nursing history. The establishment of nursing education in institutions of higher education allowed nurse educators to create and maintain the integrity of nursing curricula at a national level. It also showcased nursing education at Teachers College, Columbia University, which became renowned for its curriculum development and leadership within the profession of nursing. It seems only fitting that the emergence of technical (associate degree) nursing in the 1950s was a product of the curriculum revolution at Teachers College, Columbia University. Innovative ideas continued to flow from Teachers College; by the 1940s, the college had established its reputation as a pioneer in nursing education (Haase, 1990).

Despite these advances in nursing education, many nursing schools failed to self-regulate or self-govern. The curriculum and educational experience varied widely from program to program. This, in turn, led to instability and a profession that lacked control over entry into practice.

This trend had a twofold effect on the nursing profession. The first was an impetus to enact and employ standards for admission to nursing programs. The second was the implementation of registration programs to protect society from unqualified nurses. By 1923, all states required licensing for nursing graduates (Donahue, 1996).

NURSING DURING WORLD WAR I

Many advances in nursing education and practice were the result of military and wartime pressures. At the end of the 19th century, the Spanish American War highlighted the ill-preparedness of the Red Cross nursing service to meet the needs of the battlefield and the need for an organized military nursing corp. In 1898, the first military nurses served in army hospitals in lieu of hospital corpsmen, who lacked training and experience and whose unsanitary practices made them unqualified to care for the sick (Donahue, 1996). The successful contributions of army nurses during this conflict led to the Army Reorganization Bill (1901), which established a permanent Nurse Corp composed of fully trained hospital graduates (Donahue, 1996).

Just as World War I shaped the American military, so, too, did it leave an indelible mark on the nursing profession. As World War I expanded, the need for nurses raised concerns as to whether an adequate nursing workforce would be available at military and civilian posts.

In an attempt to increase the number of nurses, prominent hospital and medical leaders proposed an abbreviated nursing education program that would eliminate admission requirements and forgo licensing. Nurse leaders viewed this attempt at deregulation as a threat to nursing's fight for self-governance and self-control, which had begun at the beginning of the 20th century. In response to this threat, a group of nurse leaders formed the National Emergency Committee on Nursing to examine the proposals created by hospital administrators and to create a faster and more efficient way to train nurses. They were committed to upholding standards and to devising a training method that did not forgo the strong admission criteria and licensing that had been the hallmark of good nursing education. The committee asked schools of nursing to expand their dormitories and to increase the number of clinical sites and instructors in order to attract and train more nursing students. In addition, the Army School of Nursing in 1918 granted 9 months of credit to women with a previous college degree (Donahue, 1996).

What is significant is that this committee looked for solutions outside its usual boundaries. They looked to recruit nontraditional students by encouraging women who already had a college degree and who had an interest in nursing. The nursing program at Vassar College offered a curriculum that prepared nurses over a shortened 2 year, 3 month preparatory course (Donahue, 1996). The creation of this program was an important step in nursing education for two reasons. First, it attracted nontraditional students. Second, it provided a sound nursing educational program in an abbreviated time frame. Both of these characteristics are part of the framework of associate degree education, which was created 50 years later.

The period following World War I was marked by an increased focus on public health as the country faced waves of immigrants and new threats of communicable diseases. The nursing profession moved ahead as its tireless leaders worked to raise nursing to a higher level of professionalism. Curriculum evaluation and studies of nursing education proliferated, as did nursing-focused texts and other nursing publications. Wartime nursing education planted the seed for nursing education at the associate degree level.

NURSING AND WORLD WAR II

Prior to World War II, the U.S. government had very little involvement in the healthcare delivery system (Dillon, 1997). Health care was overwhelming private, and the government paid for only 20 percent of the nation's health care (Haase, 1990). Hospitals were either private or public and primarily cared for the poor (Haase, 1990). Nursing, for the most part, occurred in the home, and most often with affluent patrons. After World War I, American health care began to change. Hospitals began to see a decline in mortality and morbidity rates because of the care provided by nurses.

As the nation prepared for World War II, so, too, did nurse leaders. The formation of the Nursing Council on National Defense allowed professional nurse leaders to coordinate a national effort that would profoundly affect the course of nursing history (Haase, 1990). As the peace deteriorated, nurse leaders kept a careful watch on events. When America entered World War II, nursing leaders participated in the wartime plan. Isabel Stewart wanted nurses to be prepared by learning from the mistakes and profiting from the achievements of World War I. With this in mind, Stewart convened a committee to address the position nursing should take with respect to national defense (Donahue, 1996). By the time war was declared, this committee, now called the National Nursing Council for War Service, was formulating plans to:

☐ Conduct a national survey of registered nurses
☐ Determine the role of nurses in national defense
☐ Expand the facilities or existing accredited schools (an activity that served particularly useful during World War I)
☐ Examine the phenomenon of nurses leaving civilian agencies to enlist in the Army and Navy Nurse Corps (Donahue, 1996)

These efforts led to the creation of the United States Cadet Nurse Corps Legislation, which was introduced to Congress by Congresswoman Frances Payne Bolton. Known as the Bolton Act, this legislation sought to increase the enrollment of nursing students through a federal subsidy for programs that would prepare nurses in an accelerated time frame. The Bolton Act resulted in the creation of the U.S. Cadet Nurse Corps.

The U.S. Cadet Nurse Corps met the quotas established to meet the nation's needs, and a total of 179,000 nurses joined the Corps. The Corps were a remarkable success in the recruitment of nurses into the profession (Donahue, 1996). The U.S. Cadet Nurses Corps educated nurses in an abbreviated 30-month format and an additional 6-month practice assignment. Created to ease the nursing shortage, the Cadet Nurse Corps had the unintended effect of upgrading nursing schools nationwide (ASBN, 2003).

Professional nurses contributed to the war effort both abroad and at home. More than 65,000 nurses served during World War II; nearly half of the nation's active registered nurses volunteered for active military duty. This placed an unprecedented demand on the nursing profession at home. As nurses attempted to compensate for workforce losses due to the war effort, they began to work longer hours. In 1943, the American Hospital Association reported that 23 percent of the hospitals in the United States were forced to downsize because of the lack of nurses (Haase, 1990).

After World War II, the United States was stronger. The post-war American healthcare industry underwent unprecedented changes and experienced new growth spurred by prosperity and technological advances. Hospital construction increased under the 1946 Hill-Burton Bill, more than 200 new drugs were developed, new surgical and medical approaches to treatment evolved, and specialized medical care came to the fore (Haase, 1990). This generated new demands for hospital care and qualified nurses who could provide that care.

However, in the post-war period the number of nurses declined rapidly, which led to an unprecedented nursing shortage. Women, who had proven their capability in traditional male positions while men were away at war, now sought job opportunities outside of nursing. In addition, the emerging social trend of "domesticity" meant that many nurses were returning home to marry and start a family. This deterred many women from considering a career or attending school.

In addition, the nursing shortage became even more acute as business and industry prospered and workers were given the opportunity to enroll in business-sponsored hospital insurance plans. At the same time, the scope of health care was expanding. Americans were living longer. New attention was given to mental health and maternal/child health care and health care was shifting from the treatment of disease mortality to the treatment of chronic illnesses.

The shortage of nurses reached an all-time high of 65,000 in 1953, just as Americans were seeking new and improved services (Dillon, 1997). The nursing shortage caught the public's eye, and its focus turned to how nurses were educated (Haase, 1990).

THE TECHNICAL NURSE: THE CONCEPTION OF THE ASSOCIATE DEGREE PROGRAM

Mildred Montag is considered to be the progenitor of modern associate degree nursing education. Her vision of nursing education was influenced by such leaders as Nutting, Stewart, and McManus when she was a doctoral student and faculty member at Teachers College, Columbia University. She fondly credited the influence these women had on her professional development (M. Montag, personal communication, 1999). Montag examined the development of the U.S. Cadet Nurse Corps as a conceptual model for the technical nurse program, later known as the associate degree nursing program.

The advent of the technical program was conceived to meet the nagging nursing shortage that plagued the post–World War II period. Nursing education up to and during World War II maintained its deep roots in hospital-based programs.

After World War II, the number of community colleges increased rapidly. Community colleges were formed to provide returning GIs an opportunity to earn a college degree while staying in their home communities. President Truman, through the establishment of the Higher Education Commission and the signing of the Service Man's Readjustment Act of 1944 (GI Bill), sought to provide opportunities to returning soldiers by supporting their education at the government's expense. The Commission recognized that returning servicemen needed educational institutions that allowed them to attend to the needs of raising a young family.

The Commission's support of community colleges was probably the most important change in American education in the 20th century. Although junior colleges had been established earlier in the 20th century, the Commission's report proposed sweeping changes in higher education and looked to develop colleges and curricula that attested to the needs of a democracy. The Commission, chaired by George F. Zoo, a long-time advocate of junior colleges, proposed to double college attendance by 1960. Other goals included integrating vocational and liberal education with the extension of free public education, eliminating racial and religious discrimination in education, and revising the goals of graduate and professional school education to make them effective in training research specialists and technicians.

Truman agreed with the Commission's report and urged Congress to establish community colleges; expand adult education programs; and distribute federal aid through scholarships, fellowships, and grant aid in education (Truman Presidential Library, 1947).

Creating associate degree nursing programs at community colleges was a potentially effective way to meet the nursing shortage. Individuals who may not have been able to attend traditional baccalaureate or hospital-based programs because of family responsibilities were given access to higher education as commuting students.

As discussed earlier, nurse leaders were actively involved in the development of wartime nursing education. However, the post–World War II period held new challenges for nursing leaders as they attempted to meet the challenges of the nursing shortage. In 1945, a meeting was held at the U.S. Office of Education to explore the possibility of expanding the use of junior colleges to educate health professionals but nurse leaders were not invited to this meeting (Haase, 1990). Nurse leaders, having no desire to be left out, formed their own committee (National Nursing Council) to examine the development of nursing programs in junior colleges. A year before the publication of the Brown Report in 1947, this committee issued a position paper that called for moving nursing education from traditional hospital-based programs to institutions of higher education. Although this opinion was only that of the National League for Nursing Education Board, by 1950 the entire membership had adopted this stance (Haase, 1990).

Realizing that it was a fortuitous time to explore nursing education and the future of nursing, members of the council used funds provided by the Carnegie Foundation to engage Dr. Esther Lucile Brown, a social anthropologist, to determine society's needs for nursing and to establish recommendations for the future (Donahue, 1996; Haase, 1990).

Brown's report, *Nursing for the Future* (1948), proposed that the education of nurses be placed in universities and colleges, similar to how teachers were educated, and criticized hospital-based programs as inadequate and authoritarian (Haase, 1990). The Brown Report was viewed as an accurate assessment of the state of nursing education.

Following the Brown Report, the council approached the W.K. Kellogg Foundation for funding to help implement nursing education reforms. Although the W.K. Kellogg Foundation denied funding, it did support a five-day conference in Battle Creek, Michigan, in early 1949 to formulate a plan for how the Brown Report recommendations could be implemented. The Foundation also invited members of its educational advisory committee as well as prominent members of higher education, including key people from Teachers College, Columbia University, to the conference (Haase, 1990). The conference participants concluded that nursing was at a crucial turning point, and their findings became the impetus behind several planning meetings examining the implementation of nursing education at junior and community colleges.

The associate degree movement took form as the nation was faced with the reality that not enough young nurses were being educated or joining the nursing workforce to meet the nation's healthcare needs. Americans now viewed hospitals as essential institutions that provided health services that improved an individual's health and life expectancy. For the first time, the majority of children were being born in hospital settings rather than at home. Despite these advances, the traditional method of training nurses was outdated.

Traditional nursing education was structured in a rigid tradition that required students to live away from home. This, in turn, excluded a group of men and women who were interested in becoming nurses, but who had family and/or work responsibilities to manage as well. The discriminative criteria for admission up to this point did not help the profession of nursing. Traditional schools of nursing were often biased with regard to race, religion, gender, parental status, martial status, and geography. Nursing programs at junior or community colleges could offer nontraditional students the opportunity for a nursing career.

THE COMING OF AGE OF ASSOCIATE DEGREE EDUCATION

The growth of the community-college movement caught the attention of educators, policymakers, and nursing leaders. Montag, who is credited with the development of associate degree education, was strategically placed in time and place to serve as a catalyst. Montag's dissertation might simply have languished in a library had she not been a student at Columbia University during a critical period of policy debate about the future of nursing education (Hasse, 1990). Columbia University had always been at the cutting edge of nursing education. The university was noted for preparing nursing school superintendents and educators and for implementing the first doctoral program for nurses. Montag had the support of influential faculty members such as R. Louise McManus, director of the nursing program at Teachers College, Columbia University.

The foresight of McManus and other Teachers College faculty helped to translate Montag's ideas about a two-year nursing program into an entirely new nursing degree based on a community-college education. McManus enjoyed the friendship of many influential citizens. Mary Rockefeller, who sat on the board of the Bellevue School of Nursing, a formable school in its own right, called upon her friend Louise McManus to ask what she was planning on doing about the shortage of nurses. Because Teachers College had always been a leader, Rockefeller naturally believed that the faculty of Teachers College would have a plan to alleviate the nursing shortage. McManus believed that Teachers College should attempt to solve the nursing shortage and asked Rockefeller to finance a special project being conducted by one her doctoral students, Mildred Montag (M. Montag, personal communication, April 1999).

Mildred Montag began her dissertation research with an interest in vocational education. She had examined the Cadet Nursing Corps program and its success in providing a sound educational program in a short period of time. Montag's doctoral research and subsequent textbook changed the landscape of nursing education. She proposed a two-year program situated in the newly constructed community-college setting that would enable nurses to graduate with a college degree. Although often referred to as a terminal program, Montag frequently stated that a terminal program meant that the degree conferred a student with all the rights and privileges of a two-year college degree and that the degree itself was terminal, not the student's education or learning (M. Montag, personal communication, April 1999). The community-college degree provided the nursing profession with two opportunities: (1) the ability to offer nursing education in an environment that supported nontraditional students and (2) the ability to receive a college degree as a graduate nurse in a short period of time. This offered a true, sound solution to the post–World War II nursing shortage.

In January 1952, Teachers College launched the Cooperative Research Project in Junior and Community Colleges. The project was designed to create a new kind of worker—a college graduate who would be qualified to sit for the RN licensing examination in two years. The Cooperative Research Project was initially set up as a pilot program based on a model developed by nurse leaders during efforts to determine the nurse's role in World War II. It had proven to be a successful way to plan, develop, and evaluate nursing curricula. Schools that were interested completed a questionnaire, and project leaders made site visits to identify potential locations. Seven schools joined the project, which ran from 1952 to 1955 (Haase, 1990):

☐ Orange County Community College, Middletown, New York (1952)
☐ Fairleigh Dickinson University, Rutherford, New Jersey (1952)
☐ Henry Ford Community College, Dearborn, Michigan (1953)
☐ Weber College, Ogden, Utah (1953)
☐ Pasadena City College, Pasadena, California (1953)
☐ Virginia Intermont College, Bristol, Virginia (1954)
☐ Virginia State College, Norfolk Division, Norfolk, Virginia (1955)

The curriculum established by the Cooperative Research Project under Montag's guidance was patient centered, not disease oriented. The clinical rotations had a faculty member on the clinical unit and followed the broad fields that represented the everyday experiences of a nurse (Haase, 1990). The Cooperative Research Project staff provided summer workshops for faculty at each site and highlighted a new approach that included the fundamentals of nursing; the care of the mother and child, better known as maternal-child nursing; the psychosocial aspects of nursing; and the use of a college-based laboratory to supplement clinical rotations in healthcare facilities (Haase, 1990). The Cooperative Research Project, based on the doctoral research of Dr. Montag, gave birth to the associate degree nursing education program. From its beginnings, the National League for Nursing (NLN) supported and promoted nursing education at the associate-degree level. As a result of the NLN's leadership and guidance, a new worker emerged who would quickly become an integral part of nursing history and education (Fondiller, 2001). The expected increase in nursing school enrollments were supported by the development of new funding programs. And by the end of the first decade associate degree programs had expanded from the original 7 to 330 (Fondiller, 2001).

For more than two decades now, the majority of nurses have been educated in associate degree programs. Such programs continue to serve nontraditional students from diverse backgrounds. Associate degree programs have contributed to nursing's diversity. Graduates of such programs show strong performance on NCLEX/state board examinations and have high rates of employment.

Associate degree educators agree that nurses educated at the two-year level should continue their professional education. Students at the associate-degree level have always been encouraged, inspired, and challenged to seek baccalaureate and graduate education: "It is the professional responsibility of associate degree educators to facilitate the passage of students educated at the associate degree into baccalaureate programs and teach the value of lifelong learning" (Speakman, 2000, p. 3). But for many adult learners with family and social responsibilities, the two-year community college degree is accessible, affordable, and manageable with life's responsibilities.

Over the past 50 years of associate degree education, numerous attempts have been made to eliminate it as an option for the primary education of registered nurses. In 1965, the American Nurses Association endorsed a position paper that asserted that the minimum preparation for beginning professional practice should be at least a baccalaureate degree (Haase, 1990). More recently, similar attempts to adopt baccalaureate entry into practice have been promoted by the American Association of Nursing Executives (Bowcutt, 2005).

Despite these efforts, associate degree education has enriched the nursing profession by achieving the goal of promoting educational access for all students and by increasing the nursing labor force. "Registered nurses educated at the associate degree level not only mirror the nation's diversity but bring forth a myriad of experiences that allow them to become members of the health care team, responding effectively to the needs of those they serve" (Speakman, 2000, p. 3). The resilience of associate degree programs is rooted in their ability to provide a sound education in institutions of learning that support the diversity of adult learners. Many of these students may be returning to school after a long lapse of time, may have English as a second language, or may feel intimidated by major universities.

Excluding associate degree nurses from the professional arena will not only lead to a greater nursing shortage, but will also limit access to higher education to all Americans who choose it. Since 1952, associate degree programs have been a part of American nursing education. Supported by the National League for Nursing from its inception, associate degree programs provide individuals access to a college education by diminishing financial and/or personal barriers. If the nursing profession believes in the philosophy of inclusion, its leaders must embrace and find complementary relationships to include nurses educated at the associate-degree level.

Baccalaureate (BSN) programs that promote educational mobility to registered nurses in a supported environment will promote lifelong learning. BSN programs can be an effective vehicle to transform nursing practice and improve nurses' outcomes, as well as patient outcomes (Delaney & Piscopo, 2004). But, as emphasized by Edward O'Neill, Executive Director of the Pew Health Professions Committee, it behooves nurse educators and leaders to create smooth transitions between education and practice in order to meet the demands of nursing in the future (O'Neill & Coffman, 1998). Perhaps it is time to use the information from the margin to rethink the whole (Guinier, Fine, & Balin, 1997).

REFERENCES

Arkansas State Board of Nursing (ASBN). (2003). World War II Cadet Nurse Corp. *ASBN Update, 7*(4), 23–24.
Bowcutt, M. (2005). *Letters from the leadership. Voice of the leadership.* Chicago: American Association of Nurse Executives. Retrieved from http://www.aone.org.
Brown, E. L. (1948). *Nursing for the future.* New York: Russell Sage Press.
Connolly, C. A. (1998). Hampton, Nutting and Rival Gospels at the Johns Hopkins Hospital and Training Schools for Nurses, 1889–1906. *Image, 30*(1), 23–29.
Delaney, C., & Piscopo, B. (2004). RN-BSN programs: Associate degree and diploma nurses' perceptions of the benefits and barriers to returning to school. *Journal of Staff Development, 20*(4), 157–161.
Dillon, P. (1997). The future of associate degree nursing. *NLN Nursing and Health Care Perspectives on Community, 18*(1), 20–24.
Donahue, P. A. (1996). *Nursing: The finest art,* 2d ed. St. Louis: Mosby.
Fondiller, S. H. (2001). Nursing's pioneers in the associate degree movement. *NLN Nursing and Health Care Perspectives, 22*(4), 172–174.
Guinier, L., Fine, M., & Balin, J. (1997). *Becoming gentlemen: Women, law school and institutional change.* Boston: Beacon Press.
Haase, P. T. (1990). *The origins and rise of associate degree nursing education.* Durham, NC: Duke University Press.
O'Neill, E., & Coffman, J. (Eds.). (1998). *Strategies for the future of nursing: Changing roles, responsibilities and employment patterns of registered nurses.* San Francisco: Jossey-Bass.

Reverby, S. (1987). *Ordered to care: The dilemma of American nursing, 1850–1945.* Cambridge, MA: Cambridge University Press.

Speakman, E. (2000). The phenomenon of attachment between faculty and students and its effect on self-empowerment at an urban community college. Unpublished doctoral dissertation, Teachers College, Columbia University, New York.

Truman Presidential Museum and Library. (1947, December 15). Retrieved September 23, 2004, from http://www.trumanlibrary.org/publicpapers/index.

CHAPTER 31

Advanced Practice Nursing: Moving Beyond the Basics

Joyce Pulcini

According to the *American Heritage Dictionary* (1980), the term *advanced* means "ahead of contemporary thought or practice or at the highest level of difficulty." *Practice* is defined as "the exercise of an occupation or profession." *Nursing* has been defined as "The diagnosis and treatment of human responses to actual and potential health problems" (ANA, 1995).

Nursing has undergone many changes in the last century that have reshaped and expanded what is considered to be basic nursing. As nursing's role has evolved, so has its scope of practice. Many of today's nursing functions were originally within the realm of medicine or other disciplines. This metamorphosis has been part of the profession's gradual evolution and maturity over time.

Advanced practice nursing is defined by Hamric, Spross, and Hanson (2005) as "the application of an expanded range of practical, theoretical, and research-based competencies to phenomena experienced by patients within a specialized clinical area of the larger discipline of nursing" (p. 89). The term advanced practice nursing was coined to encompass four major roles within nursing: Clinical Nurse Specialist (CNS), Nurse Practitioner (NP), Certified Nurse Midwife (CNM), and Certified Registered Nurse Anesthetist (CRNA). The term distinguishes these nurses with "advanced" skills from those who practice as more traditional staff nurses and allows for a distinction between the nurse functioning at a more specialized level than the registered nurse. These roles also have been considered to be equally complex or at the same level of advanced practice. A common characteristic of these roles is the application of a greater breadth of knowledge and complexity of decision making to the problems of nursing care. Although each of these roles is distinct with regards to the specific areas of knowledge and skills that they draw on, they all require high levels of critical thinking, independence, and decision making.

Finally, the term advanced practice allowed for legislative changes to proceed with a minimum of confusion over how advanced practice and staff nurses differed. This distinction created opportunities for advanced practice nurses (APNs), but it also established a new class of nurse who seemed to some to be more privileged than their peers.

Each of these roles evolved a bit differently. The CNM evolved from the historical role of the midwife, who even today can be a non-nurse. The CRNA role evolved from the experiences of nurses in the Civil War who provided pain relief for soldiers (Hamric, Spross, & Hanson, 2005).

The CNS began to flourish in the 1950s and 1960s due to interest in promoting the highest level of nursing practice that coincided with the strong evolution of nursing theories and frameworks. This early CNS role had its roots in psychiatric nursing in the late 19th century and in specialist nursing roles in the early 1900s (Hamric, Spross, & Hanson, 2005). Initially, the CNS tended to work in hospitals or chronic care facilities caring for ill patients with specific health conditions. A major focus was the performance of indirect roles in nursing, such as consultation, research, staff education, and patient/family education. Although not exclusive, much of the practice was also directed toward care coordination or institutional management of care. This specialty practice often dealt with symptom management or diagnosis of responses to illness, rather than health promotion, and focused on a unique set of problems emanating from illness. CNSs are highly competent nurses with a specialty focus who effectively meet the needs of patients in an increasingly complex healthcare system.

However, as cost containment concerns became paramount and hospitals had to begin to cut costs in the 1980s, many of these CNS positions were eliminated even as staff nurses began to deal with sicker patients who had shorter stays in hospitals. In contrast, an increasing demand for nursing care in the community and long-term settings led to new opportunities for CNSs in home health care or specialized care for persons with HIV/AIDS or other chronic illnesses. At this time, CNSs began to function in community and long-term care settings as shortened hospital stays led to the discharge of patients "quicker and sicker" from hospitals or tertiary care facilities. In the past 10 years, the CNS has reemerged as an important component of patient care. The renewed interest in the CNS role has been fueled by regulatory and professional concerns. Pressures to demonstrate outcomes of care and to reduce risks such as patient injury or financial loss have generated a demand for the advanced practice knowledge and skills offered by the CNS (Heitkemper & Bond, 2004).

The NP role evolved from a shortage of primary care medical providers in underserved areas in the 1960s. Efforts to train NPs were spurred by progressive legislation of the Great Society era. As the federal government expanded financial access to care funded by Medicare, Medicaid, and community health center legislation, the need for more primary care providers became acute. The efforts to expand nursing practice were viewed by some in both medicine and nursing as a way for doctors to extend their care for patients using this new care provider.

This early concept of the NP role led many nurse educators to reject the idea of an advanced practice nurse and to close many avenues to university education. Thus, in the beginning years of NP role preparation, the majority of NP educational programs evolved outside of traditional nursing education in continuing education programs rather than in traditional master's programs. These early programs reflected the collaborative intent of nurses and more progressive doctors to create a new role for primary care practice. Through the NP role, the nurse's scope of practice expanded into realms that were previously only within the scope of medical practice, such as health assessment, medical diagnosis, and treatment of common and chronic illnesses. Most NPs functioned within the realm of primary care or generalist care, adding a strong health-promotion focus, while substituting for physicians who were not numerous enough to meet client needs. As the role has evolved, NPs have assumed greater responsibility in the management of more complex and chronic illnesses, and some have branched into specialty areas such as oncology, cardiology, or emergency care. When the NP role emerged, health promotion and disease prevention were being emphasized as an important component of primary care in all sectors of the healthcare system. As a result, NPs have a very strong foundation in direct patient care rather than in indirect nursing roles (Hamric & Hanson, 2003).

By the 1980s, the original community or public health focus of advanced practice was diluted as medical care became more individually focused and health financing failed to address public health needs. In this period, containment of healthcare costs was paramount in the minds of health policy makers, and the country was on the brink of replacing a public health focus with a system dominated by managed care. One exception was the community health CNS who continued to work in community settings such as Visiting Nurse Associations or home care agencies.

As more patients were discharged from the hospital due to shortened stays and prospective payment methodologies, the need for home care skyrocketed, and an entirely new sector of the healthcare system emerged. Cost-containment efforts of the 1980s were also a major force in the realignment of nursing roles. Diagnosis-related groups (DRGs) and cost-containment efforts led the public, insurers, and policy makers to demand more cost-efficient care. This changed the face of hospital nursing forever. Demands on nurses in in-patient settings increased exponentially. These developments led to nursing shortages and to periodic staffing crises, as were seen in 1989 and 2001.

Several occurrences led to fundamental changes in the mix of roles and the level of independence in nursing and to increasing difficulties in differentiating the various roles for nursing. An overarching factor was the women's movement, which reached its peak in the 1960s and 1970s, because it influenced the increased desire by nurses to have autonomy from other providers, such as physicians. This had a major effect on the nursing profession.

In the 1980s and 1990s, the NP role was viewed as a potentially cost-effective option to the growing need for healthcare services. It also received an enormous amount of attention in the public and professional press. Another important change was the increased movement of NPs into acute care and medical specialties from primary care settings. As NP education began to be housed in universities, the distinction between the NP and the CNS was blurred.

In the 1980s, the CNS role was seen as too costly by hospital administrations because of reduced reimbursements from Medicare and shrinking hospital budgets. Thus, many CNS positions were lost across the country as hospitals eliminated any position viewed as providing indirect care. Education for the CNS specialty suffered from a lack of consistency across programs and confusion over the definition of terms. Educational programs reflected this confusion by using the designations NP and CNS interchangeably or by creating blended roles. The blended role was intended to combine the best of both roles, but it also confused those credentialing or hiring these advanced practice nurses (Hanson & Hamric, 2003; Hamric, Spross, & Hanson, 2005). Currently, the predominant view is that the CNS and the NP role are distinct from one another and should have separate educational programs (Hanson & Hamric, 2003; NACNS, 2004).

Since the inception of advanced practice nursing, health policy and regulatory advances enabling practice have moved forward with unprecedented swiftness and congruity. These advanced practice roles seem to have captured the imagination and interests of nurses who want more independent decision making and relief from what has been an increasingly stressful hospital environment. Barriers to practice for advanced practice nurses have decreased greatly over the past 20 years as legislative reforms have swept the nation. Third-party reimbursement for services and legislation for prescriptive privileges are now almost universal for NPs, CNMs, and CRNAs. These regulatory reforms have been far-reaching and now have been adopted by virtually every state. (Pearson, 2004; Towers, 2004).

The role of advanced practice nurses has expanded well beyond initial expectations, and demands on practice continue to increase. For example, prescription writing now is virtually universal, and the types and breadth of prescribing has increased across all categories of NPs (Pulcini & Vampola, 2002; Pulcini, Vampola, & Levine, in press). These authors also speculate that practice barriers may be lowest in rural areas or other areas where there is a greater need for healthcare services.

EDUCATIONAL STANDARDS

Educational standards have evolved in different ways for each specialty. CNMs and CRNAs took the lead in establishing national standards for certification and program accreditation. The American Association of Nurse Anesthetists (AANA) established its own separate certification process in 1945 and an accreditation process in 1952 (AANA, 2004). The American College of Nurse Midwives (ACNM) established its certification process in 1971 and its own separate accreditation process in 1982 (ACNM, 2004). These efforts enabled these specialties to evolve with a consistency not seen in either NP or CNS educational programs, which expanded with less consistency and homogeneity.

Yet regulatory changes and reimbursement efforts for CNSs have lagged behind and are surrounded by controversy, such as whether prescribing should be part of the role (Lyons, 2004). Recently, CNSs have organized under the National Association of Clinical Nurse Specialists (NACNS) and have begun to standardize their education, regulations, and practice, publishing their landmark document, *Statement on Clinical Nurse Specialist Practice and Education* (2004).

Master's degree education preparation for NPs became the norm by the mid-1980s. Educational programs for NPs have become more congruent as a result of the National Organization of Nurse Practitioner Faculties' (NONPF) *Curriculum Guidelines and Program Standards* (1995), the *Domains and Competencies of Nurse Practitioner Practice* (2000), the *Criteria for Evaluation of Nurse Practitioner Programs* (2002a), and the *Nurse Practitioner Competencies in Specialty Areas* (2002b). As more NPs entered master's programs, the indirect-role (e.g., consultation, education, research) content in NP programs increased. Currently, more than 90% of NPs are master's prepared, and virtually all NPs are educated in graduate-level programs (Berlin, Stennett, & Bednash, 2004). The concept of the NP "tipped" in the mid-1990s, to use Malcolm Gladwell's (2000) term, and is now mainstream within nursing education. Currently, 330 graduate programs in nursing offer NP programs, with a total of 706 tracks, and 60% of master's program graduates are enrolled in NP programs (Berlin, Stennett, & Bednash, 2004).

A final factor to consider is the new master's entry option that is popular in nursing education today. This option, which allows a person with a non-nursing degree to earn a master's in nursing as an NP or CNS in two to three years, increased threefold in graduate nursing programs from 1990 to 2002 (AACN, 2003). This development is important because originally most advanced practice nurses had experience in nursing before entering the advanced roles.

THEORETICAL ISSUES AND CHALLENGES

This last shift has been an important factor in the current nursing environment. The key issue is that there are now entry level "advanced practice nurses." However, our understanding of "advanced" has not moved with this paradigm shift. What has occurred is that many of the skills involved in advanced practice roles have moved into the mainstream. Most new nurses see these distinct skills as basic rather than within "advanced practice." For example, many baccalaureate nursing programs now integrate physical assessment, pathophysiology, pharmacology, and health promotion, similar to advanced practice program curricula. Currently, the CNS, the CRNA, and the CNM are still viewed within the advanced practice role in the United States. But in many countries a clear precedent has been set for basic nurses to have the skills of the nurse-midwife.

Internationally, the advanced practice role is evolving in diverse ways depending on the historical, political, and social factors that have shaped the nursing role and educational programs in each country. The definition of advanced practice nursing being adopted by the International Council for Nurses (2002) is as follows:

> The Nurse Practitioner/Advanced Practice Nurse (NP/APN) is a registered nurse who has acquired the expert knowledge base, complex decision-making skills and clinical competencies for expanded practice, the characteristics of which are shaped by the context and/or country in which s/he is credentialed to practice. A Master's degree is recommended for entry level.

Many countries are beginning to develop advanced practice nursing programs. This role advancement is built on the strong role that nurses have in developing nations. The International Nurse Practitioner/Advanced Practice Nursing Network (INP/APNN), which is affiliated with the International Council for Nurses, has been instrumental in publishing definitions and scope and standards statements to guide nations in the development and expansion of advanced practice nursing. The challenge is to standardize practice definitions and educational standards while building and honoring the traditions of individual countries.

How do we, in 2004, reconceptualize the concept of "advanced practice," given the current state of nursing education for APNs both in the United States and internationally? Is our old concept of "advanced practice" out of date? Can we reconceptualize what we consider to be the skills necessary for entry into nursing practice? If we have been operating with an outdated definition of advanced practice, what are the skills or competencies of advanced practice nurses that can be expected on entry into the profession? Does one need a specified number of years of experience before being called "advanced," or are the skills that we once called "advanced" really mainstream or entry-level skills? If the latter is true, then we need to rethink the skills and competencies necessary for entry-level versus expert practice.

Grypdonck, Schuurmans, Gamel, and Goverde (2004) reconceptualize advanced practice nursing by making a distinction between nursing science and nursing practice. These authors point out that nursing science and nursing practice operate in different spheres and ways of thinking. For example, scientists base their decisions on the greatest possible degree of certainty, and clinicians deal with uncertainty every day. They say that expert advanced practice nurses effectively bridge that gap through their advanced education and practice experience. This is where the practice doctorate may really begin to fit into this complex continuum of advanced practice nurses (see Chapter 32 by Michael Carter).

In nursing, we have placed a great deal of weight on experience and position rather than on a specific level of knowledge. As we replace our current cadre of nurses with younger individuals, we would do best to see knowledge acquisition on a continuum, beginning with a set of basic practice skills and moving to expert practice that integrates scientific principles and research skills with ongoing teaching, mentoring, and expert consultation.

In the last 12 years, the cadre of generic master's programs or accelerated master's programs has grown threefold, and in many master's programs, these students comprise the majority of graduates. We must welcome these relatively young nurses into the fold of advanced practice nurses rather than exclude them and continue to operate in old ways.

In our reconceptualization of advanced practice, we might consider some way to recognize advanced practice through internships or other mechanisms of recognition. We may want to reconsider career ladders or Benner's levels of novice to expert practice. An expert advanced practice nurse should effectively use and incorporate research-based practice with a goal toward independent or collaborative research. Requirements for advanced practice nurses to precept, teach, or mentor newer nurses could be part of the certification credential. High-level skills such as consultation or clinical teaching require a body of expert knowledge and mastery of the content and are clearly in the realm of expert advanced practice nursing. Certification itself could be reframed to recognize entry-level versus expert practices, as was its original intent.

As we progress in redefining advanced practice, new technologies and knowledge, such as genetics and informatics, will increasingly enhance the patient-centered approach. Clinicians now are guided by state-of-the-art knowledge, which can be at the clinician's fingertips at any moment in practice through technology. In this new paradigm, the needs and demands of knowledgeable patients as well as scientific evidence-based guidelines will guide practice.

CONCLUSION

The nursing profession is now in a period of change, a paradigm shift. Nursing educators and policy makers must recognize this shift in order to plan for the future. As in the past, societal healthcare needs will shape the future direction of advanced practice nursing, and it will be up to our profession to change to meet those needs (Thompson & Watson, 2003). Our profession's ability to manage change and to move to a new conceptualization of advanced practice nursing will determine our success or failure in meeting societal needs. It is time to revisit even basic documents, such as the *Essentials of Master's Education for Advanced Practice Nursing* (AACN, 1996) and the *Essentials of Baccalaureate Education for Professional Nursing Practice* (AACN, 1998), which set the baseline definition of levels of nursing education. Our challenge now is to redefine "advanced" and recognize what is truly basic to all nursing practice.

REFERENCES

American Association of Colleges of Nursing. (1996). *The essentials of master's education for advanced practice nursing*. Washington, D.C.: Author.

American Association of Colleges of Nursing. (1998). *The essentials of baccalaureate education for professional nursing practice*. Washington, D.C.: Author.

American Association of Colleges of Nursing. (2003). *Accelerated programs: The fast-track to careers in nursing*. Available at http://www.aacn.nche.edu/Pulbications/issues/Aug02.htm.

American Association of Nurse Anesthetists, Council on Accreditation of Nurse Anesthesia Programs. (2004). *Introduction*. Available at http://www.aana.com/acreditation/.

American Heritage dictionary of the American language. (1980). Boston, MA: Houghton-Mifflin.

American College of Nurse Midwives, Division on Accreditation. (2004). *Division on accreditation*. Available at http://www.midwife.org/edu/education.cfm.

American Nurses Association. (1995). *Nursing's social policy statement*. Washington, D.C.: Author.

Berlin, L., Stennett, J., & Bednash, G. (2004). *Enrollment and graduations baccalaureate and graduate programs in nursing*. Washington, D.C.: American Association of Colleges of Nursing.

Gladwell, M. (2000). *The tipping point: How little things make a big difference.* Boston, MA: Little Brown Co.

Grypdonck, M., Schuurmans, M., Gamel, C., & Goverde, K. (2004). Uniting both worlds: Nursing science and advanced nursing practice. Presented at the International Nurse Practitioner/Advanced Practice Nursing Network Conference, Groningen, The Netherlands.

Hamric, A., & Hanson, C. (2003). Educating advanced practice nurses for practice reality. *Journal of Professional Nursing, 19*(5), 262–268.

Hamric, A., Spross, J., & Hanson, C. (2005). *Advanced practice nursing: An integrative approach.* St. Louis, MO: Elsevier Saunders.

Heitkemper, M., & Bond, E. (2004). Clinical nurse specialists: State of the profession and challenges ahead. *Clinical Nurse Specialist, 18*(3), 135–140.

International Council of Nurses. (2002). *Health Policy/Nurse Practitioner/Advanced Practice: Definitions and characteristics of the role.* Available at http://icn-apnetwork.org.

Lyons, B. (2004). The CNS regulatory quagmire: We need clarity about advanced nursing practice. *Clinical Nurse Specialist, 18*(1), 9–13.

National Association of Clinical Nurse Specialists. (2004). *Statement on clinical nurse specialist practice and education.* Harrisburg, PA: Author.

National Organization of Nurse Practitioner Faculties. (1995). *Advanced nursing practice curriculum guidelines and program standards for nurse practitioner education.* Washington, D.C.: Author.

National Organization of Nurse Practitioner Faculties. (2000). *Domains and competencies of nurse practitioner practice.* Washington, D.C.: Author.

National Organization of Nurse Practitioner Faculties. (2002a). *Criteria for evaluation of nurse practitioner programs.* Washington, D.C.: Author.

National Organization of Nurse Practitioner Faculties. (2002b). *Nurse practitioner competencies in specialty areas.* Washington, D.C.: Author.

Pearson, L. (2004). Sixteenth annual legislative update: How each state stands on legislative issues affecting advanced nursing practice. *The Nurse Practitioner, 29*(1), 26–51.

Pulcini, J., & Vampola, D. (2002). Tracking NP prescribing trends. *The Nurse Practitioner, 29*, 10.

Pulcini, J., Vampola, D., & Levine, J. (2005). NPACE nurse practitioner practice characteristics, salary, and benefits survey: 2003. *Clinical Excellence for Nurse Practitioners, 9*(1), 49–58.

Thompson, D., & Watson, R. (2003). Advanced practice nursing: What is it? *International Journal of Nursing Practice, 9*, 129–130.

Towers, J. (2004). Region one meeting of the American Academy of Nurse Practitioners, Portsmouth, NH, October 2004.

CHAPTER 3 2

The Evolution of Doctoral Education in Nursing

Michael Carter

INTRODUCTION

One of the most important aspects of any profession is the appropriate educational preparation of the leaders of the discipline. Almost without exception, the professions require that their leaders must hold doctoral degrees. The broad purposes of doctoral educational programs are to provide preparation that leads to careers in government, business, and industry, as well as academia (CAGS, 1990). Doctoral programs have been in existence since the Middle Ages, but it was during the 20th century that the United States saw a dramatic proliferation of doctoral educational programs in almost every academic field. The model of education that was created in the United States was built on earlier models from European universities. However, doctoral programs in the United States took on their own unique characteristics.

Nursing doctoral programs began in the latter part of the 20th century, after their development in most other fields. Perhaps this delay was because of nursing's unique history among the professions. Nursing in the United States began outside the mainstream of higher education and was located almost exclusively in hospitals. These hospitals, and the later universities where nursing educational programs moved, were controlled by administrative structures that are best described as highly paternalistic. These paternalistic organizations, in juxtaposition with the fact that most nurses were and still are women, may have delayed the profession from adopting doctoral degrees as the required credential for professional leadership. The profession adopted the master's degree early as the appropriate degree for leaders, and this may have been a disservice to the profession. Currently, nursing is far from having a unified approach to doctoral education.

The purpose of this chapter is to briefly discuss the history of doctoral education in general and nursing doctoral programs in particular. Clearly, this discussion is not exhaustive but is intended to provide an introduction to understanding doctoral education. Other, better historical overviews are available on the general topic of doctoral degrees (Harris, Troutt, & Andrews, 1980). This chapter also includes discussion of some of the controversies that are swirling about how doctoral degrees in nursing should be titled and structured and concludes with some ideas that may portend the future of nursing doctorates.

A BRIEF HISTORY OF DOCTORAL EDUCATION

The academic degrees that we see today are an outgrowth of the trade guilds and teaching guilds that flourished in Europe during the Middle Ages (DHEW, 1971). These early programs were often a product of the educational institutions that were either controlled or heavily dominated by the Catholic Church. Higher education was designed for the elite and certainly not for the general masses. Given this early tie with the Church, we can understand that many of the symbols, traditions, and rituals of the modern university emerged from the Church's influence on these schools. The doctoral gowns and hoods worn at graduation can be traced back to the garb worn by the priests.

The English word *doctor* comes from the Latin word *doctus,* the past participle of *docere,* which means "to teach" (*Webster's New Collegiate Dictionary*, 1979). Italian schools awarded formal doctoral degrees by 1219. This was the only degree offered by the schools, because they were preparing teachers. French schools used a slightly different approach and chose the name *masters,* from the Latin word *magister*, for their college graduates. Graduates from these schools were awarded the respective title and were admitted to the guild of teachers (Martin, 1989). Obtaining a degree meant that the graduate was fully qualified to serve as a teacher and did not need additional evaluation to begin this profession.

In the United States, the early colleges were established to prepare clergy and for the most part were built on the English and German systems of higher education. Harvard College was founded in 1636, and from that time until the Civil War, a little over 200 years later, the only degree that could be earned in the United States was the Bachelor of Arts. Alumni who paid fees were able to obtain the master's degree without further collegiate work. Scientists who wished to obtain additional education had to receive this training in Europe (DHEW, 1971).

Following the Civil War, American colleges began to change. Yale awarded the first PhDs in the United States in 1861 (Martin, 1989). For the first time, there was an emerging emphasis on graduate education and the underlying research that is a part of graduate education today. Many of the faculty had obtained their graduate degrees at German universities. The German graduate school model did not usually include required class attendance or examinations. Rather, students studied under the direction of a major professor, conducted an original piece of research, and were expected to successfully defend their work before the standing faculty of the university in order to be granted the degree. However, because graduate education was embedded in undergraduate colleges, graduate students in the United States were often required to earn grades and attend lectures.

In the latter half of the 1800s, several professional associations were formed to advance their respective professions. One of their early activities was to persuade state legislatures that the professional services offered by the various disciplines would be greatly improved by creating licensure or certification requirements. As a part of this effort, educational programs were developed that led to the professional doctorate, including the Doctor of Medicine (MD) and the Doctor of Dental Surgery (DDS). New medical schools began to offer limited instruction in allopathic or homeopathic medicine. Although offering a doctoral degree, most of these early schools were little more than diploma mills with few, if any, paid faculty, very limited instruction, and substantial reliance on clerkships with practicing physicians. By the late 1800s, there were many different types of professional schools, but there were no accreditation standards. Most had limited faculty and questionable curricula. Seldom were these programs more than a year in length, and admission depended more on the student's economic achievements than on the student's prior academic achievements (DHEW, 1971).

Efforts to standardize curricula began at the turn of the century and continued well into the 1900s. Calls went out to improve professional education as well as the quality of the PhD. By 1900, approximately 50 universities in the United States offered the PhD, but there was almost no quality control. At the best universities, the PhD was awarded after about two years of postbaccalaureate study. There were a number of calls to improve this situation. For example,

Abraham Flexner (1930) argued that the American universities had become misguided by their focus on preparing PhD graduates for practice and not for pure learning. He contended that this had diminished the quality of the education. His work in graduate education came on the heels of his work on the reform of allopathic medical education. By 1935, a fairly standardized model for PhD education was in place, and the emergence of various accrediting bodies ensured that quality standards were met. Many PhD programs were closed or merged because their quality did not meet emerging national standards.

Following World War II, a clear link developed between building the knowledge base for a specialized field and the award of the PhD in that field. For the first time, the U.S. government allocated funds to the building of the research needed to create new knowledge. A large portion of this new money was directed toward science as a part of the country's national defense efforts (Berelson, 1960).

In the early 1950s, a new debate emerged over whether the PhD should be the degree for the professions or whether the professions should use a professional degree such as the Doctor of Education (EdD), the Doctor of Business Administration (DBA), the Doctor of Public Health (DPH), or the Doctor of Nursing Science (DNSc). The professions believed that the PhD was the standard and was well understood and aspired toward that degree. Arts and sciences faculty believed that awarding a PhD with a specialty in the professions would diminish the degree. In general, the professions prevailed in this argument, and the PhD was selected as the appropriate degree. This degree did carry with it the concomitant requirement that the completion of a satisfactory piece of research was required for its award (Berelson, 1960).

Professions that wished to prepare their practitioners without this research requirement awarded a professional degree such as the Doctor of Osteopathy (DO), the Doctor of Medicine (MD), the Doctor of Dental Surgery (DDS), the Doctor of Dental Medicine (DMD), the Doctor of Pharmacy (PharmD), the Doctor of Veterinary Medicine (DVM), the Doctor of Optometry (OD), the Doctor of Chiropractic Medicine (DC), and the Doctor of Podiatric Medicine (DPM). These professional programs were not considered graduate programs because few of them required an undergraduate degree for admission and most did not build on undergraduate learning in a specific discipline to prepare for the profession (CAGS, 1966).

DOCTORAL PROGRAMS IN AND FOR NURSING

Stevenson and Woods (1986) identified four phases in nursing doctoral programs. Doctoral programs in nursing can be thought of as having four generations. The first phase was between 1900 and 1940, in which the Doctor of Education (EdD) or another functional degree was available. The second phase was between 1940 and 1960, when the degree could be obtained in a basic or social science discipline with no nursing content. The third phase was between 1960 and 1970, when a basic or social science PhD was available with a minor in nursing. The fourth phase began around 1970 with the rapid proliferation of the DNSc and nursing PhD programs.

The first research-focused doctoral programs in the United States were in various areas of science and did not seek to recruit nurses specifically. Nurses, as well as any other student, could be considered for admission if they possessed the necessary prerequisites. The problem was that few nurses at the beginning of the 20th century held an undergraduate degree. Basic nursing education was hospital based and did not award degrees.

The first doctoral programs that specifically recruited nurses were at Columbia University and New York University. These began in the 1920s and 1930s in education departments and were tailored to prepare nursing faculty. The programs awarded the PhD or EdD, but offered little, if any, coursework in nursing.

In the 1940s and 1950s, baccalaureate programs in nursing were created at a number of universities. Along with this move came important questions about the qualifications of the faculty. Faculty qualifications were a minor issue when the program was located in a hospital, but most universities held rather strict standards for faculty. Few nurses held baccalaureate degrees, and even fewer held master's degrees. Almost none held doctoral degrees, and the doctoral degree was the standard for university faculty positions.

This change in locus of nursing education gave rise to often acrimonious discussions among faculty at several schools of nursing about the need for doctoral education. These discussions often raised the following questions: Should the program of study be focused on the discipline of nursing or a science-related discipline? Should the degree not be in education, since most of the graduates would be educators? Would the master's degree not be sufficient, particularly if the focus of the master's degree was clinical nursing? If the new doctoral programs were to focus on nursing, from where would the faculty be drawn, as the number of nurses with doctorates in nursing was not sufficient for one school faculty let alone many schools?

Several schools did begin doctoral programs in nursing in the 1950s and 1960s. While the program at Teachers College continued in nursing education and nursing administration, the program at New York University reconfigured the curriculum to focus on nursing as the science of unitary humans (Rogers, 1966). Boston University designed the first program to deal with the clinical practice of nursing and created the Doctor of Nursing Science degree, with the first graduate in 1963. The University of California at San Francisco and the Catholic University of America followed Boston University's lead and established Doctor of Nursing Science programs shortly thereafter. The University of Pittsburgh created a PhD in clinical nursing around this same time. The University of Alabama at Birmingham developed a Doctor of Science in Nursing (DSN) shortly thereafter, and it was designed similarly to the DNSc (Kelly, 1978).

A serious problem remained, however, in that many of the key players concluded that nursing science was not of sufficient maturity to justify the PhD. Of course, no measure of scientific maturity was advocated. Perhaps this problem grew from the fact that most nurses with doctorates at this time had obtained their degrees in another discipline. Those disciplines had the appearance of maturity because they offered a doctorate. These nurses had not spent their doctoral study in nursing because such doctoral study was not widely available. Further, some of the writings of the period display a rather romantic and narrow view of what constituted science. Nursing research texts proposed that science was logical and orderly, when in practice this is seldom the case. Some called for nursing practice to be derived from science, and yet few scientists would argue that practice is derived from science (McManus, 1960).

Funds from the federal government helped a number of nurses to obtain doctoral degrees, which may have contributed to the continuing debate over whether the doctoral degree should be in nursing or a different field. In 1955, the United States Public Health Service started funding doctoral study through the federal Predoctoral Research Fellowship Program. Funds were awarded directly to the doctoral student, and several aspiring faculty members were able to fund their education through this mechanism. Between 1955 and 1970, 156 nurses were supported by Division of Nursing Fellowships (Grace, 1978). Almost none of these were in nursing.

Beginning in 1959, the Division of Nursing also funded the Faculty Research Development Grants Program. The purpose of these grants was to increase the research capabilities of faculty in graduate nursing programs by providing seed money. Eighteen institutions qualified for these grants between 1959 and 1968. Of these 18 programs, only 3 offered doctoral programs in nursing during the grant-funding period (1 PhD, 1 EdD, and 1 DNSc) (Martin, 1989).

In another attempt to increase the number of nurses with doctoral degrees, the Division of Nursing began to fund the Nurse Scientist Graduate Training Grants. The intent of this program was to build a cadre of nurses with doctoral degrees at universities and to increase the number of nursing doctoral programs. Funding was designed to assist nurses in obtaining doctoral degrees in fields that were viewed as "related" to nursing. These fields included such areas as sociology, psychology, anthropology, biology, and physiology, with the expectation that there would be coursework or a minor in nursing. Nine universities representing 34 different departments received these grants. Four of the 9 universities had doctoral programs in nursing at the time, but these were not eligible for receipt of this funding (Martin, 1989).

Beginning in the early 1970s, several new doctoral programs in nursing emerged. These new programs were most often in the older, more established schools of nursing. Growth continued through the 1980s and 1990s, with several new programs opening each year. The pace of new program development was often faster than the available faculty would have predicted would be the case. In 1970, there were 20 programs, but by 2000 there were 78 (AACN, 2002). Most of the research being conducted in these schools was done by students. Funding for nursing research in these schools was rare. The most common degree offered was the PhD, but several schools offered the DNSc or the DSN. Doctoral education in nursing became widely available throughout the United States during this time.

New approaches to delivery of the curriculum became available as well. Some schools offered a "summers option," in which courses were scheduled during the summer months when faculty in nursing schools who needed the doctoral degree could participate. Other schools offered weekend programs, and Web-based distance learning programs emerged as well. Interestingly, the rapid increase in the number of programs and the development of creative ways to deliver the curriculum did little to increase the number of graduates each year.

This rapid growth and creativity in curriculum delivery were partly responsible for the development of new standards for doctoral programs. The American Association of Colleges of Nursing created a set of quality indicators for research-focused doctoral programs in nursing (AACN, 1993). These indicators became the standard for evaluation of these programs.

The rapid proliferation of programs did not create a concomitant increase in the number of graduates. The new programs were small (averaging six graduates per year), and the length of time to obtain the degree continued to be long, primarily because of the number of part-time students. Even though the number of programs had increased from 20 to 78, there were only 200 more graduates in 1998 than in 1989, and most of that growth occurred prior to 1992 (AACN, 2003). Clearly, these research-focused doctoral programs could not be expected to meet the needs for nursing faculty because of the small numbers and the fact that all graduates did not assume faculty positions after graduation. Also, the median age of the graduates at completion of the doctorate was over 45 years.

CLINICAL DOCTORAL PROGRAMS

In 1979, the Frances Payne Bolton School of Nursing at Case Western Reserve University began a new approach to doctoral education in nursing (Standing & Kramer, 2003). Originally conceived as a first professional degree, the Doctor of Nursing (ND) was open to college graduates and prepared them to be nurses at a level similar to other health professional doctoral programs, such as medicine, veterinary medicine, dentistry, optometry, and others. The creation of this clinical program at the very time that nursing was struggling with building the research enterprise and research-focused doctorates was not accepted with universal agreement. Of some concern was how this program would be different from the DNSc. Up to this time, there had been the assumption that the PhD was to focus on scholarly research and the DNSc was to be the practice-oriented, clinical degree. Yet, studies had shown that the DNSc could not be distinguished from the PhD on the basis of admission standards, curriculum, or dissertation topics (Flaherty, 1989). For the first time, nursing had a doctoral degree that was open to non-nurses and that prepared the beginning clinician at the doctoral level.

Additional clinical doctoral programs were developed at Rush University, the University of Colorado, and the University of South Carolina. Today, most of these programs provide multiple entry points reflective of the diverse nature of nursing practice. Each of these programs prepare the clinician at the doctoral level to exert leadership in evidence-based practice, health policy, and management or education. These new programs created quite a stir, and one that the profession has yet to resolve. In 1963, when the first DNSc was awarded, the profession had assumed that the first clinical doctorate had arrived. But close inspection of the program showed that the DNSc curriculum required mastery within a field of knowledge and demonstrated ability to perform scholarly research—the very characteristics of the PhD (Standing & Kramer, 2003). The ND, on the other hand, focused exclusively on preparing a clinical leader, not a researcher.

The clinical doctoral programs to some extent reflected the tremendous changes that were taking place in the clinical practice of nursing. The early beginning of the nurse practitioner and clinical nurse specialist movements had taken place. New master's programs were opening each year, and the major thrust of these programs was on advanced nursing practice. State laws were changing, and advanced practice nurses were obtaining greatly expanded scopes of practice and prescriptive privileges. Most of these new master's programs were between 18 months and 2 years in length.

Concern among some faculty was building that the length and rigor of these master's programs needed to be improved and that the graduate should earn a doctorate. Yet, the doctorate needed to be focused in clinical practice. This position was consistent with the Council on Graduate Schools' position that "the professional doctor's degree should be the highest university award given in a particular field in recognition of completion of academic preparation for professional practice" (CAGS, 1966, p 3). The schools that created the ND programs were noted for their outstanding clinical master's programs. This new degree could be viewed as a logical extension of their programs.

Nursing educators have not universally accepted the ND program. As Standing and Kramer (2003) point out, reviews of nursing doctoral graduates published in the literature almost always ignore the graduates of such programs even though nearly 700 nurses hold this degree. The basis for ignoring or discounting these programs is not clear. The need for the clinical doctorate is clearly documented, and the demand for the scarce slots in these programs is also clear.

Recently, the University of Kentucky began a new clinical doctoral program, the Doctor of Nursing Practice (DNP). On close inspection, this program shares many of the same curricular components as the ND programs. An additional planning group has met for several years to build a consensus for the development of additional Doctor of Nursing Practice programs at senior universities. However, the distinctions between the Doctor of Nursing Practice and the Doctor of Nursing are far from clear.

FUTURE DOCTORAL EDUCATION

The future of research-based doctoral programs in nursing is not likely to be much different from the recent past. No mechanisms are in place to determine how many programs there should be or to enforce quality standards at these programs. The demand for nursing faculty in the future is acute, and this will likely drive the creation of many more programs. Nursing has not been susceptible to the requirement seen in other disciplines that the faculty should be engaged in funded research prior to offering a research degree. Most schools offering the nursing PhD cannot be considered research-intensive schools.

The decision of a school to offer the PhD versus the DNSc often has been primarily a political decision. The PhD is often governed by the rules of the graduate school in addition to the nursing school, and this may mean that approval would be more problematic. Some schools (such as the University of California at San Francisco, the University of Pennsylvania, and Indiana University) began their doctoral programs as DNSc programs and later converted them to the PhD. Only two schools have begun PhD programs and then added DNSc programs: the University of Tennessee Health Science Center and Johns Hopkins University. In general, faculty prefer the PhD, therefore it will likely continue to be the preferred degree in the future.

However, the world of clinical doctorates is quite different. The other major health professions have offered the clinical doctor's degree for a number of years. Pharmacy is the most recent profession to mandate the Doctor of Pharmacy (PharmD) as the single degree for professional practice. Nursing, the largest health profession, continues to prepare its beginning practitioners at less than the baccalaureate level. Attempts to alter this situation, even in light of important evidence of the value of higher education, have failed. What is emerging, however, is a de facto second license for nursing, the Advanced Practice license. This new license may accelerate the development of the clinical doctorate.

Nursing chose the master's degree as the minimum preparation for advanced practice. The master's degree in the United States has always been an unusual degree—more than the baccalaureate but less than the doctorate, and usually discipline specific. This degree is uncommon in the major health professions, at least as a professional degree. This degree designation is used for the Master of Public Health and the Master of Hospital Administration, but the other health professions use a nondegree, postdoctoral training period to prepare their specialists. Reasons as to why nursing adopted the master's degree are somewhat obscure, but are likely related to political considerations. Nursing's history of hospital-based education rather than degree-based education meant that much of nursing was left out of the advances in higher education during the 20th century. While medicine, dentistry, and to some extent, pharmacy were able to strengthen their educational programs within the university tradition, nursing was still knocking at the door. Few women were able to obtain college education until well after World War II. The idea that nursing should have a clinical doctoral degree similar to the other health fields would not have entered the minds of most academics, and certainly not most nurses, until recently.

Today, however, we see advanced practice nurses in roles that were unthinkable just a few years ago. Independent nursing practices in institutions and communities are making substantial changes in the way health care is delivered. The kind of education that these clinicians will need for the future cannot be achieved in today's master's programs. The future advanced practice nurses will need a minimum of a clinical doctoral degree and most likely will require substantial postdoctoral training in narrow specialties.

Not every school that currently offers the master's degree will have the faculty, clinical material, or other requisite resources to offer the clinical doctoral program. These programs are faculty intense, require interdisciplinary coursework with the other major health professions, and are costly to operate. Schools of nursing must have a substantial clinical practice operation to be able to mount such a program. These new programs will prepare highly competent clinicians for such roles as primary care provider for cross-site practice; midwifery practice that includes surgical abilities to perform cesarean sections; anesthesia providers to administer all forms of anesthesia, including intrathecal approaches; as well as national and international leaders in policy formulation, complex organizational administration, and master clinical teachers. These roles cannot be achieved by obtaining a research-focused doctoral degree, and certainly not by way of the master's degree.

CONCLUSION

Doctoral education in the United States underwent dramatic changes during the 20th century and will likely continue to evolve over the next century. Nurses were once educated outside the mainstream of higher education, but following World War II the locus of nursing education was moved to the university. This has brought with it the need for a faculty commensurate with that of the rest of the university. For the arts and sciences, that meant the PhD degree; for the professional schools, that has meant the clinical doctorate.

Nursing was a bit slow to embrace the idea that nursing faculty would need the research doctorate. But once the idea was adopted, many schools—some would argue too many schools—rapidly developed these programs. There is still a reluctance to move to the development of the clinical doctorate on a broad scale. The potential for this degree to alter the power and political relationships between nursing and other professions, however, is substantial.

The clinical doctorate can provide a skill and science base for the graduate that cannot be achieved in today's educational programs. This level of expertise will be critical as the nation focuses on improving patient care and the safety of the systems that deliver health care. Clearly, the clinical doctorate will bring with it a level of independent practice that cannot be achieved at less than the doctoral level. For the first time, nursing would have parity in educational preparation with other healthcare disciplines.

Nursing is the most comprehensive of all the health professions. Clinical practice demands of nursing clinicians an understanding of the human condition, the environments in which clients live, the systems of care delivery, and the political milieu of care. Preparation of clinical leaders fundamentally requires a doctoral degree. The time is now for the discipline to move to the clinical doctorate to complement the many substantial accomplishments that have taken place by the creation of the research-focused doctorates.

REFERENCES

American Association of Colleges of Nursing (AACN). (1993). *AACN position statement: Indicators of quality in doctoral programs in nursing*. Washington, D.C.: Author.

American Association of Colleges of Nursing (AACN). (2003). Indicators of quality in research-focused doctoral programs in nursing. *Journal of Professional Nursing, 18*(5), 289–294.

Berelson, B. (1960). *Graduate education in the United States.* New York: McGraw-Hill.

Council of Graduate Schools in the United States (CAGS). (1966). *The doctor's degree in professional fields. A statement by the Association of Graduate Schools and the Council of Graduate Schools in the United States.* Washington, D.C.: Author.

Council of Graduate Schools in the United States (CAGS). (1990). *The doctor of philosophy degree: A policy statement.* Washington, D.C.: Author.

Flaherty, M. J. (1989). The doctor of nursing science degree: Evolutionary and societal perspectives. In S. E. Hart (Ed.), *Doctoral education in nursing: History, process, and outcome* (pp. 17–31). New York: National League for Nursing.

Flexner, A. (1930). *Universities: American, English, German.* New York: Oxford University Press.

Grace, H. (1978). The research doctorate in nursing. In *Proceedings of the 1978 Forum on Doctoral Education in Nursing* (pp. 40–59). Chicago: Rush University.

Harris, J., Troutt, W., & Andrews, G. (1980). *The American doctorate in the context of new patterns in higher education.* Washington, D.C.: Council on Post Secondary Accreditation.

Kelly, J. (1978). The professional doctorate in nursing from the viewpoint of nursing service. In *Proceedings of the 1978 Forum on Doctoral Education in Nursing* (pp. 10–39). Chicago: Rush University.

Martin, E. J. (1989). The doctor of philosophy degree: Evolutionary and societal perspectives. In S. E. Hart (Ed.), *Doctoral education in nursing: History, process and outcome* (pp. 1–16). New York: National League for Nursing.

McManus, L. (1960). Doctoral education in nursing: A nurse educator responds. *Nursing Outlook, 8,* 543–546.

Rogers, M. (1966). Doctoral education in nursing. *Nursing Forum, 5*(2), 75–82.

Standing, T. S., & Kramer, F. M. (2003). The ND: Preparing nurses for clinical and educational leadership. *Reflections on nursing leadership, 29*(4), 35–37, 44.

Stevenson, J. S., & Woods, N. F. (1986). Nursing science and contemporary science: Emerging paradigms. In G. E. Sorensen (Ed.), *Setting the agenda for the year 2000: Knowledge development in nursing* (pp. 6–20). Kansas City, MO: American Academy of Nursing.

U.S. Department of Health, Education, and Welfare (DHEW). (1971). *Future directions of doctoral education for nurses.* (DHEW Publication No. (NIH) 72–82). Bethesda, MD: Author.

Webster's New Collegiate Dictionary. (1979). Springfield, MA: Merriam Webster.

CHAPTER 33

Knowledge Development in Nursing: Our Historical Roots and Future Opportunities

Susan R. Gortner

The historical development of American nursing research in the past century is traced, and projections for nursing in the 21st century are offered.

The purpose of this article is to provide an historical overview of nursing research in the past century and to offer projections on where our science will be headed in the 21st century. For the overview, a number of reviews were drawn upon[1–4] with reliance on the last citation, which surveyed published nursing literature from 1900 to 1975. In the last two decades, other analyses of published research have been carried out,[5–7] including an impressive first encyclopedia of nursing research.[8] Research agendas and priorities have been developed by the American Nurses Association Commission[9] and Cabinet on Nursing Research,[10] the Academy of Nursing Ad Hoc Group on Knowledge Generation,[11,12] and by consultant groups to the Division of Nursing's research program,[13,14] and to the former National Center for Nursing Research.[15] Recent research publications of the nursing schools at the University of California-Los Angeles (UCLA), University of California-San Francisco (UCSF), and the University of Maryland[16–18] were used to formulate contemporary research questions. As such, they are illustrative rather than representative. Projections for the 21st century have been drawn from the author's reflections on our science,[14,19–22] from Donaldson's seminal paper at the 25th anniversary of the American Academy of Nursing,[23] and from the latest research agenda of the National Institute of Nursing Research.[24] Comments will be made on how our practice has been affected through research, and where applications did not occur, when perhaps they should have. Examples will be from projects personally known to the author.

THE EARLY YEARS

Nursing practice and issues arising from practice have influenced research topics since the time of Nightingale.

Source: Reprinted from *Nursing Outlook*, 48(2), Susan R. Gortner, Knowledge Development in Nursing: Our Historical Roots and Future Opportunities, 60–67, copyright (2000), with permission from Elsevier.

While practice issues have varied since then, some early concerns regarding quality of care and qualified caregivers transcended the 19th and 20th centuries into the 21st century. It is no accident that the development of formal programs of nursing education was seen as the means to improve practice. Historical perspectives on nursing and nursing research may be depicted as follows: in the early 1900s, concern was for improvement of the public's health; major communicable diseases of childhood and adulthood were prevalent; maternal/child health had yet to benefit from prenatal care and improved obstetrical practices. Most surgery was done in the home. The literature in our professional journals addressed problems associated with tuberculosis, meningitis, scarlet fever, etc. In 1913, the committee on public health nursing of the National League for Nursing Education discussed its concern about infant mortality, prevention of blindness, and the problem of unlicensed midwives. The committee believed that the nursing profession should recognize its role in the prevention of unnecessary deaths among infants and in the prevention of unnecessary blindness, and that intelligent care of the sick must involve "some knowledge of the scientific approach to disease . . . causes and prevention. . . ."[4]

During the 1920s, the first case studies appeared; they were used both as a teaching tool for students and as a record of patient progress; nursing care plans for specific patient groups and procedures appeared (e.g., use of turpentine stupes), and continued until recently as a means to standardize and improve practice, medical as well as nursing. The case approach as a major research and teaching model in clinical nursing practice paralleled the use of case studies in medical practice and research. These case studies were used to describe unusual patient situations or symptoms and to report on the effects of nursing and medical therapies with groups of patients. According to personal interviews with the late Lucile Petry Leone,[a] the need for systematic evaluations of nursing procedures had its origins in the post-Depression years. The Depression forced the graduate nurse out of the home and into the hospital and, at the same time, the first postgraduate nursing programs began to develop.[4]

The war years prompted the collection of national data on nursing needs and resources (types, numbers, and uses of nurses). In the immediate postwar years, the federal government, assisted by professional nursing organizations and foundations, provided funds and staff to establish resources for nursing, one such being the Division of Nursing Resources of the United States Public Health Service created in 1948. Its staff carried out studies on nurse supply and distribution, job satisfaction and turnover, requirements for public health nursing services, personnel costs, and costs for collegiate nursing education. These studies were widely used throughout the United States, frequently in conjunction with federal staff consultation and training. A 5-year study of nursing functions and activities was begun by the American Nurses Association in 1950, resulting in functions, standards, and qualifications for practice,[25] as well as the publication *Twenty Thousand Nurses Tell Their Story*.[26] Also noteworthy during this time was the W. K. Kellogg Foundation Nursing Service Administration Research Project, in which faculty from 12 universities worked with Finer at the University of Chicago to determine needs for administrative science and skills in nursing.[27] Thus the period between 1930 and 1960 concentrated on the components of professional nursing practice and how best to secure them.

Focus on the organization and delivery of nursing services was given a boost when the Division of Nursing Resources initiated a small competitive research grant and fellowship program in 1955. Lucile Petry Leone, former director of the cadet nurse corps and then chief nurse officer and assistant surgeon general in the Public Health Service, convinced the surgeon general and the director of the National Institutes of Health to allocate $500,000 for grants and $125,000 for fellowships from the NIH budget. These programs were the precursors to the National Center for Nursing Research and the current National Institute for Nursing Research.[4] In 1952, the journal *Nursing Research* came into being; the first few issues contained a section entitled the "Research Reporter," in which areas suitable for research were noted; guest editorials emphasized the need for grassroots support of nursing research by hospitals, agencies, and schools. Lucile Petry Leone's editorial in the Fall 1955 issue summarized the types of studies needed in nursing, based on a staff paper she had prepared earlier. These types included studies of nursing care most essential to patient recovery; the nature of the therapeutic relationship; analysis and optimal use of nursing skills, and efforts to reduce staff turnover rates and student drop-out rates. Her thinking provided a visionary public platform for nursing research.[28]

Virginia Henderson's 1956 guest editorial noted that studies of the nurse outnumbered studies of practice 10 to 1, that more than half of the doctoral theses were carried out in the field of education, and the "responsibility for designing its methods is often cited as an essential characteristic of a profession. . . ."[29] Six years later, the first Nurse Scientist Graduate Training Grants were awarded to universities offering resources in one or more basic science departments for preparation through the doctorate. The first grant awards were to Boston University School of Nursing for training in biology, psychology, and sociology, and to the University of California School of Nursing for training in sociology. The next fiscal year, three additional grants were awarded, one to the UCLA School of Nursing for study in sociology; one to the University of Washington School of Nursing for graduate study in anthropology, microbiology, physiology, and sociology, and the third to Western Reserve University School of Nursing for study in biology, physiology, psychology, and sociology.[b] Subsequently, grants were made to schools of nursing at the University of Kansas, Teachers College–Columbia University, University of Pittsburgh, University of Arizona, University of Colorado, University of Illinois, and briefly, New York University (the grant program was terminated in 1975). Required interdepartmental seminars helped to define the boundaries of nursing science for the early grantees. It is not surprising that nurse scientist graduate training settings later developed into PhD programs in nursing.[22]

In the early 1960s, establishment of the American Nurses Foundation grants program helped to address the demand for more practice-related studies. The foundation published the priorities that would guide funding: effects of performance of nursing acts on the patient (i.e., nursing procedures and outcomes); effects on nursing of changing patterns of nursing care and changing health needs; and nursing in different process categories.[30]

Ellwynne Vreland, the first chief of the federal research branch, wrote Chief Nurse Officer Lucile Petry Leone in 1959 that studies were needed to further development of nursing theory by identifying the scientific content of nursing, by seeking and experimenting with new concepts of nursing (e.g., motivation—"finding out why nurses can 'bring back' patients who have given up and who fail to respond to careful medical treatment"), and by careful study of the nursing care given by expert practitioners (the specifics of expert nursing, etc.).[31]

Soon the specifics of expert nursing became apparent as several university schools of nursing undertook studies of the nursing process, patient responses to care, and behavioral phenomena. The Yale study of nursing effects on postoperative vomiting became widely cited because of its experimental design and findings suggesting that nurse counseling had a positive effect.[32] UCLA nursing investigators studied recovery stages from myocardial infarction[33] (interviews with cardiologists revealed no clear demarcation of stages appropriate for nursing detection), breastfeeding,[34] rooming-in,[35] and pain relief.[36] These became among the first practice-related studies to be published in the new journal, *Nursing Research*.

At UCSF, sociologists Strauss and Glaser combined talents with nurse investigator Quint to study hospital personnel's views on death and dying.[37] Quint's seminal study of the experiences of women and undergoing radical mastectomies[38] was to launch a scientific career that Donaldson has termed "pathfinding."[23] Studies at the University of Washington in the early 1960s focused on nursing services for psychiatric, tubercular, alcoholic, and maternity patients; variables included professional attitudes, activities, and accountability for patient care.[4] Batey's later expertise in research resource development was an outgrowth of her study with Julian of organizational patterns in psychiatric settings.[39] One of the earliest controlled attempts to document the effects of nursing intervention on the clinical progress of chronically ill adults was carried out by nursing investigators.[40]

At Presbyterian-University of Pennsylvania Medical Center, a project carried out between 1963 and 1967 in a special facility, the coronary care unit, demonstrated significant reductions in patient morbidity and mortality through continuous monitoring and prompt treatment by expert nurses.[41] This project had been supported by the fledgling research grant program of the Division of Nursing Resources; it was to become the model of coronary care nursing nationwide. It was also among the first reports of nursing research to be published in the *Journal of the American Medical Association*.

Thus the real thrust of nursing research began in the 1960s, a function of the vision of nursing leaders such as Lulu Wolf Hassenplug, Helen Nahm, Mary Tschudin, Hildegard Peplau, Virginia Henderson, Lucile Petry Leone, Ellwynne Vreeland, Faye Abdellah, and Jessie Scott, and the availability of public as well as private funds to support the studies and train nurses in research. I joined the division staff in 1966 to aid in the review of the Nurse Training Act of 1964, and in 1967 was appointed executive secretary to the Research in Patient Care Review Committee, the outside group of scientists charged with determining the scientific merit of research proposals submitted from throughout the United States. During my time as staff scientist and later as branch chief for research grants and fellowships, we attempted to nourish the growing enterprise of nursing research nationwide through staff consultation, conferences, research development grants, nurse scientist graduate training grants, and individual research fellowships. We publicized the grant programs,[42] urged scientific accountability for the profession[43] as a practice profession,[44] and early on attempted to show the contributions of research to patient care with a proposed classification, which named nursing research a "science of practice."[45]

To recapitulate, knowledge development in nursing began in earnest only 40 years ago, primarily in university schools of nursing where nurse scientist graduate training was ongoing in alliance with other disciplines, but also in medical centers such as the City of Hope, where Geraldine Padilla was director of research, at Luther Hospital in Eau Claire, Wisconsin, where Carol Lindeman was in charge, and at the Loeb Center for Nursing at Montefiore under the direction Gwenrose Alfano. The Loeb Center for Nursing, which demonstrated that cost-effective care could be rendered to elders in a nursing center, was not seen as an innovation until such practice innovations were publicized by the American Academy of Nursing. Why the lag in impact of this research?

Annual research conferences sponsored by the American Nurses Association and later by the regional nursing research societies provided forums for investigators to present their findings and learn the importance of public scrutiny.[4] The art of the critique developed gradually; communality and collegiality joined communication and publication as hallmarks of our research efforts, and greater sophistication among nursing's investigators and clinicians resulted in greater intradisciplinary and interdisciplinary collaboration.

THE TRANSITION YEARS

I have termed the period from 1965 to 1985 "transitional" because professional nursing took on major leadership activities to influence federal policy for nursing education and research. The American Nurses Association established a Commission on Research in 1971; the Council of Nurse Researchers was created in 1972. In a paper presented at the first program meeting of the council in 1973, I described the increasing concern that research financed by the federal government be related to major health priorities, stating that ". . . there is no mistaking the trend toward greater legislative specification of science in the health fields."[46] The scientist audience was urged to develop research priorities for nursing research.

In response, Lindeman undertook a Delphi survey of priorities in clinical nursing research through the Western Interstate Commission on Higher Education, with Division of Nursing support.[2] Respondents identified items on the quality of care, nursing role, nursing process, and the research process. Patient welfare concerns, particularly items related to nursing interventions to mitigate stress and pain, and to provide patient education and support to frail elders also were cited.[47]

When the late President Nixon impounded nurse training act, research, and fellowship funds in 1973, all federal support for fellowships and training grants was halted. The president was taken to court by a coalition of nursing organizations and forced to release the funds in 1974. The Division of Nursing held several invitational conferences on nurse scientist graduate training and doctoral personnel needs. Commission members traveled to Washington, D.C. in 1975 to meet with legislators and federal program staff, the first such contacts to be made by what was later to become the nursing research advocacy group. In my capacity as branch chief, I was asked to meet with commissioners to present program needs, vital information for program development and funding that had been embargoed as a result of closure of all public information offices in 1971. Although we could not publish grant and fellowship information, we could respond to requests for information about the programs. To their credit, grantees understood this constraint and found opportunities to request program information. Thus the commission was able to develop priorities for research training and research and set goals for accomplishing them including funding levels.[9]

Health science research training authorization was restored with the passage of the National Research Service Awards Act in 1974; two years later, primarily through Connie Holleran's efforts, the Division of Nursing research training programs were included.[48] Publication of a review of research grants awarded[1] was followed by two historical overviews of nursing research[2,3]; two new research journals, *Research in Nursing and Health* and *The Western Journal of Nursing Research* appeared in 1978. The 94th Congress specified $5 million for research projects in nursing and $1 million for research fellowships to be spent during 1977 and 1978, the first time funds for nursing research had been earmarked in the appropriation. Until then and since 1964, nursing research funds had been allocated along with nurse training act funds, although that act dealt exclusively with training to address the quality and quantity of professional nurses.[48]

This somewhat awkward allocation process and the difficulty health manpower legislation was experiencing in the 1970s led to open discussions by nurse scientists and educators regarding the need to locate the nursing research programs within the research environment of the National Institutes of Health. The discussions were frank and heated; well-respected deans worried that such a relocation would fracture federal nursing; others worried that nursing research could not mature if not nourished within the institute structure. Legislators were sympathetic and passed legislation (Public Law 99-158) authorizing a new center at the National Institutes of Health; it came into being in 1986 after a successful override of a presidential veto in main attributed to nurse scientist lobbying efforts, including the persuasive efforts of the entire membership of the American Heart Association Council on Cardiovascular Nursing which was meeting in Washington, D.C., at the time. Council Chairperson Marie Cowan adjourned us to go on the Hill. We did, and the entire California delegation was visited (including the senate office of then Senator Pete Wilson who voted to override the veto).

Coincidental with the establishment of the national center was the continuing work both of the American Nurses Association Cabinet on Nursing Research and the scientist group in the American Academy of Nursing. The cabinet published *Directions for Nursing Research: Toward the 21st Century* in 1985, setting goals, priorities, and strategies with dollar amounts to achieve them.[10] The next year the American Academy of Nursing held its annual meeting in Kansas City, with the program theme "Nursing in the Year 2000: Setting the Agenda for Knowledge Generation and Utilization." Stevenson and Woods provided a synthesis of the focus group priorities both for the new national center and also for research in the next two decades.[12] These specified fundamental knowledge development about clinical problems, followed by clinical therapeutics to test interventions, and increasing emphasis on health promotion, health status and functioning, on the family, and on vulnerable populations and age groups. Scientific knowledge synthesis was aided by the beginning of a series of annual reviews of nursing research under the direction of Werley and Fitzpatrick.

Oberst,[11] at the same Academy conference, provided a thoughtful insight for a possible Year 2000 research agenda:

> The heart of the problem may lie in the almost total absence of basic research into the nature of the phenomena we wish to influence. We know very little about patterns of fatigue and sleep or about the nature of immobility, confusion, or anorexia. We cannot expect to intervene to prevent or control a problem such as incontinence, for instance, without basic knowledge of the natural history of that condition in a variety of contexts.

Oberst also spoke to the extreme biophysical derangement associated with organ transplantation, microsurgery, and aggressive chemotherapy protocols, asking whether health providers know the short-term and long-term physical and psychologic effects of these events and their meaning for patients and families. This problem has continued to interest investigators. Mishel and Murdaugh studied an opportunistic sample of heart transplantation patients and families; this study is one of the finest examples of grounded theory methodology published.[49] Jenkins is among others studying the effects of aggressive protocols on quality of life.[18]

The transition years also saw the development of research on primary care and evaluation of nurse practitioner programs. Research was directed toward: (1) understanding the influence of structural variables on nurse practitioner performance (e.g., access to settings), (2) identifying personal and professional characteristics contributing to successful performance as a nurse practitioner, and (3) specifying the nature of clinical judgments used by nurse practitioners and physicians working collaboratively in patient care management to assign patients either to a nurse or to a physician and then reassign responsibilities as changes in health status occur. How do the management plans differ? This last question addresses the elusive nature of the nurse–patient encounter (the initial plan, examination, questioning, priority setting, treatment, and evaluation).[48] Ford and Silver evaluated the post-training activities of skilled pediatric nurses and found that these nurses could handle independently three-fourths of clinical visits in a rural station with high patient satisfaction regarding counseling and health monitoring.[50]

Lewis and Resnik evaluated the use of adult nurse practitioners at the University of Kansas medical clinic with similar findings.[51] To their disappointment, the program was discontinued after grant funding ceased. Veterans Administration (VA) South Hill Clinic in Los Angeles became the site of a second attempt to demonstrate the effectiveness of nurse practitioners in managing adult chronic conditions, this time those of veterans. Charles Lewis had just come to UCLA, Theresa Cheyovich was a visionary nursing chief at the Clinic, and I represented the "Feds" in the first interagency agreement signed by the VA with another federal agency. Two UCLA–trained PRIMEX nurses (UCLA was the original PRIMEX training site), one a former VA clinic nurse, undertook caseloads released by then 33 VA physicians, who had been painstakingly persuaded by Lewis to participate in the project. One nurse in particular was able to realize major changes in health status and outcomes of her veteran case load. Examining her encounters, we discovered she "contracted" with patients on a weekly basis, and used social persuasion and professional skills to bolster patient confidence in their own health management.[52] Further, the experiment was so successful that the VA proceeded thereafter to train and place nurse practitioners in many of its settings. Here is still another example of how nursing research has impacted practice.

NURSING RESEARCH BECOMES NURSING SCIENCE

What occurred also during this transition period was a shift in thinking from *research* to *science*, a recognition that what we had thought was nursing science was really research, the tool of science. Nursing science was depicted as a human science that had the additional requirement of intervention or clinical therapy. Nursing research was redefined "as the discrete and aggregated investigations that constitute the professions' modes and foci of inquiry . . ."[19] The phenomena of interest to nursing were already being documented through research to become tentative propositions about human health and illness, vulnerable population groups (the aged, the chronically ill, women, children, infants), and illness recovery processes and risk factors. The seminal essay by Donaldson and Crowley on "The Discipline of Nursing"[53] clarified our thinking on what might become our knowledge domains and syntax. Meleis' inaugural Helen Nahm lecture on nursing scholarship heralded both the scientific and theoretical developments that were to occur in the next two decades.[54] Clinical science was seen as focusing on human problems and treatment modalities; fundamental science was characterized as having no immediate utility but devoted to understanding basic processes across a wide variety of disciplines.[19]

The last period of knowledge development in this century witnessed an explosion of fundamental and clinical science activities in nursing. How these phenomena came about is described next.

NURSING SCIENCE COMES OF AGE

Our science came into maturity during the past decade and a half as a result of several factors. First, emphasis began to shift from discrete studies to aggregates of studies, the precursors of programs of research. This shift initially was encouraged by the Division of Nursing's Nursing Research Emphasis Grant Program, in which areas of concentration, such as vulnerable populations and health across the life span, were suggested as topics to be coupled with graduate education.[55] The program at UCSF concentrated on two of these areas and solicited proposals from faculty that would both extend knowledge and involve and excite graduate students; we were funded and renewed for 5 years. Second, schools of nursing began to recruit doctorally prepared faculty with excellent research preparation and programmatic interests that fit with concentrations of research within the school. University nursing schools featured "centers of excellence," in which faculty effort and talent were aggregated, acknowledging that selectivity was required to achieve excellence. Third, educational programs in many universities maintained sufficient stability that faculty time and effort could be redirected toward research. That is, curriculum revisions seemed to reach a plateau. Collaboration and colleagueship began to replace competitiveness and solo investigations. Fourth, external competition for research support increased as grant success was forthcoming from both public and private agencies; in the university systems, extramural support is one criterion for advancement up the faculty ranks. At UCSF initially, successful investigators received a bottle of champagne; later beer, and then soda sufficed. Fifth, arguments over appropriate methods, whether experimentation, description, and/or interpretation, waxed heatedly and then seemed to wane, as many of us put our energies into substantive activities, whether empirical investigations or philosophic musings, or both, as was the case with me. Sixth, scientists such as Lindsey, Cowan, Donaldson, Woods, Shaver, Brooten, Norbeck, and Dracup, to name but a few, took the brave step of becoming deans, thus reinforcing the science enterprise in their settings. With this momentum and influx of prepared scientist nurses, some of whom had been exposed to philosophers in their graduate programs, came debate about the nature of nursing science, what should be the prevailing worldview and research approach. We spent a great of time speaking and writing to empiricism, phenomenology (later hermeneutics), critical theory, and feminism, to name but a few. Post-positivists, of which I am one, were maligned for speaking to the components of "good science" such as credibility, reproducibility, and rigor.[22]

The knowledge development group at the American Academy of Nursing program meeting in 1986 attempted to draw a cease-fire between the received and perceived views of science, endorsing pluralism.[56] Meleis called for a "passion for substance" rather than a passion for method[57]; and I attempted to formulate a philosophy of science for nursing that would embrace values.[58] Notions about nursing research and its substantive activity also have been formulated throughout the years by Ellis,[59] Batey,[60] Barnard,[61] and Shaver.[62] The following represents but one definition of nursing science, drawing on Barnard[13,16] and Donaldson and Crowley[23]:

> Nursing science as a form of human science, has as its object of analysis the human organism, with particular reference to human response states in health and illness and health across the life span. Its aim is to generate a body of knowledge that can define patterns of behavior associated with normal and critical life events such as catastrophic illness; depict changes in health status and predict how these are brought about; and along with other scientific fields, determine the principles and laws governing life states and processes.[20]

In the decades of knowledge development documented in this review, nursing has identified with tasks and technology and has characterized itself as a compassionate human service; it has taken as its subject matter the ecology of human health and human responses to health illness. While these conceptualizations may appear sequential, based on historical literature, in reality they are concurrent.

The researchable components of human health across the life span comprise indicators of health status, biological and behavioral factors contributing to health and illness, culture, environment, and treatment outcomes. These components were displayed in the National Center for Nursing Research national nursing research agenda, developed after an invitational conference on research priorities in nursing science at which 50 nurse scientists were present.[15] To establish the agenda, priorities were selected on the basis of the existing knowledge base, opportunities, areas of low emphasis in other institutes, marketability, and available scientific personnel. These priorities were staged as follows: I—"HIV Positive Clients, Partners and Families" and "Prevention and Care of Low Birth Weight Infants"; II—"Long Term Care and Symptom Management and Information Systems"; and III—"Health Promotion" (in which the most critical issues for study are the fundamental psychosocial mechanisms underlying maintenance of health promotion behaviors . . .") and "Technology Dependency Across the Lifespan."[15]

Ten years later, the National Institute of Nursing Research (NINR) distributed a statement on strategic planning for the 21st century with this definition of research (not science!):

> Nursing research addresses the issues that examine the core of patients' and families' personal encounters with illness, treatment, disease prevention. NINR's primary activity is clinical research and most studies involve patients. The basic science is linked to patient problems.
> . . . Nursing research is essential in defining and confronting the compelling health and illness challenges of the 21st Century.[24]

These challenges include risk reduction, promotion of healthy lifestyles, enhanced quality of life for persons with chronic conditions, and care for persons at the end of life. These areas are familiar; they have remained persistent for more than 30 years. The National Institute for Nursing Research stated the following *scientific goals* for the next 5-year period:

1. Identify research opportunities that will achieve scientific distinction within the scientific and practice communities and within NIH as a result of their significant contributions to health:
   End of life/palliative care research
   Chronic illness experiences
   Quality of life and quality of care issues
   Health promotion and disease prevention
   Telehealth interventions
   Implications of generic advances
   Cultural and ethnic considerations to decrease health disparities
2. Identify future opportunities for high-quality cost-effective care for patients and contribute to the scientific base of nursing practice through research on:
   Chronic illness (arthritis, diabetes) and long-term care, including family care

Health promotion and risk behaviors
Cardiopulmonary health and critical care
Neurofunction and sensory conditions
Immune response and oncology
Reproductive and infant health

3. Communicate research findings
4. Enhance research training opportunities

These initiatives are already displayed in the research programs of many university schools of nursing. I reviewed the research publications from the schools of nursing at the UCLA,[16] UCSF,[17] and the University of Maryland[18] in preparation for the original presentation on which this article is based. The scientific topics in these settings include vulnerably populations, cardiovascular and other illnesses, symptom management, chronic pain, health promotion/illness prevention, risk reduction, quality of life, the family in health and illness, women's health, and nursing therapeutics (including intensive cardiac monitoring, coaching for recovery, and "kangaroo care"). As examples:

☐ Is pain relief universal or are there gender differences? (Miakowski & Levine, UCSF)
☐ Does an ischemia monitoring protocol result in improved patient outcomes? (Drew et al., UCSF)
☐ What is the relationship between daytime fatigue and sleep disturbance in women? (Lee, UCSF)
☐ Does a collaborative intervention (advanced practice nurses and community peer advisors) improve outcomes for cardiac elders? (Rankin, UCSF)
☐ What is the role of exercise in heart failure patients? (Dracup, Woo, Cowan, Vredevoe, Padilla, Doering, et al., UCLA)
☐ Can an intervention with low income adolescent mothers reduce HIV risk and improve health outcomes? (Koniak-Griffin, UCLA)
☐ What chromosomal abnormalities result from environmental toxins and affect reproductive health? (Robbins, UCLA)
☐ What is the quality of life experience of women with differing stages of lung cancer? (Sarna, UCLA)
☐ Can kangaroo care be as effective in ventilated infants as in premature infants? (Ludnington, University of Maryland)
☐ What are the effects of estrogen on platelet function after cerebral ischemia? (Kearney, University of Maryland)
☐ How do aggressive treatment modalities affect health status and quality of life? (Jenkins, University of Maryland)

In the study write-ups, investigators often revealed how their interests originated. Many investigators were and are advanced practice nurses. As such, they have credibility both as clinicians as well as scientists. Not surprisingly then, research findings have had an impact on practice by encouraging family sensitive care in several settings;[c] by enhancement of patient self-confidence and self-efficacy through coaching, counseling, and performance;[d] by advocating improved critical care heart monitoring procedures;[e] by early discharge of low-birth-weight infants;[f] and by sensory stimulation of the neonate, including skin-to-skin contact.[g] Whereas nursing investigators have not always received the publicity given medical investigation, this bias is changing slowly as more nurses are appointed and elected to public office and as more become members of scientific and governmental advisory groups. The media recognition awards given annually by the American Academy of Nursing also have been instrumental in raising the veil of public ignorance. Schorr and Kennedy's[63] splendid pictorial of 100 years of American nursing, just released, is a cause for celebration!

Where the areas of concentration some 20 years ago tended to reflect one dominant knowledge domain, for example, the psychosocial, now the biophysical, particularly biology and genetics, are reflected in the investigations noted above and elsewhere. This phenomenon may have been encouraged by the report of the National Center for Nursing Research biological task force, which stated: "the implications for the interface of nursing science with the biological sciences as a basis for research and its subsequent findings for practice are tremendous."[64] It also may be a natural development of better understanding that nursing problems cannot be solved within one knowledge domain; most involve multiple and complex factors.[20,21]

FUTURE OPPORTUNITIES

In preparing for this last section, I queried several colleagues throughout the United States to inquire where the future might lead us. Invariably, the response was: (1) to reexamine the impact of organizational structures on nursing effectiveness, (2) to continue to examine fundamental processes underlying human responses to health and illness, (3) to take the lead with family health, (4) to continue study of end-of-life and palliative care, and (5) to have an impact on health policy. I would add one more to which I would give considerable urgency: (6) to identify the biobehavioral factors (in epidemiologic terms, the host factors) that explain much of illness and associated behavior. These factors will frame why questions (e.g., why is it that personal recovery beliefs are such a powerful predictor of cardiac surgical outcomes along with the usual pathophysiologic markers?) that will bring our science into increasing respect within the greater medical science community at the National Institutes of Health and elsewhere.

Donaldson's "Breakthroughs in Nursing Research" given at the 25th Anniversary of the American Academy of Nursing in 1998, identified "pathfinders" who created a new realm of nursing research or reconceptualized an existing realm of nursing research.[23] Many were already working in the above areas 30 years ago. Noting that nursing has the "brilliance in family health," she encouraged us to know well the human genotype project, the environment as the social context for health, and to strengthen the bridge between public health and person/family health. To these I would add: strengthen collaboration (between nursing and other disciplines and within nursing) and continue to address fundamental problems at the biobehavioral interface.

Two additional opportunities need mentioning. Nursing has a proud heritage of safe and effective midwifery service that has affected health legislation for Medicaid and rural health but still has not removed barriers to hospital practice.[65] What may be needed here are collaborative teams of obstetrical fellows and midwives in some forward-thinking health science settings who will become "pacesetters" in collaborative practice.

Fagin's[66] guest editorial in *Nursing Outlook* on the changing burden of care brought on by managed care pleads with us in academia to *know* what it is like at the bedside. Without documentation of the effects of management on the burden of care, we may not save our workforce. Burden of care has been an issue for us and for housestaff throughout this century. To become clinically refreshed, I undertook a day of practice 20 years ago on a cardiovascular surgery unit.

I had forgotten what it was like to leave lunch half eaten in the staff room. What made this experience bearable was the professional support provided by my mentors, two cardiovascular clinical nurse specialists, with whom I collaborated in clinical research on cardiac surgery recovery.[h]

In conclusion, tribute is paid to readers who are pacesetters in clinics, hospitals, private practice, public health, and academia every day of their professional lives. Those of us now white-haired are grateful that you are where you are and are doing what you do. The future is really ours, as it was years ago!

ACKNOWLEDGMENT

I gratefully acknowledge the contribution of Rebecca Wilson-Loots, academic program analyst, Department of Family Health Care Nursing, University of California–San Francisco, for her assistance with the original paper.

NOTES

a. Lucille Petry Leone spent many hours with the author and the late Helen Nahm in the writing of the overview of nursing research. She died on Thanksgiving Day, 1999.
b. The first Doctor of Nursing Science program (in psychiatric nursing) was offered by Boston University; the next was at the University of California San Francisco. The first PhD program in nursing was begun by New York University, to be followed by the University of Pittsburgh.
c. Suzanne Feetham, Kathleen Dracup, and Catherine Gilliss are among the pioneers in family nursing research, along with Lorraine Wright of Canada, Sally Rankin, Maribelle Leavitt, and Kit Chesla are among others who have studied families in acute and chronic illness.
d. Louise Jenkins and Susan Gortner were among the first to employ self-efficacy as a variable in patient recovery; Sally Rankin, Diane Carroll, Mariead Hickey, Virginia Carrieri, and Marylin Dodd are among others who have studied self-efficacy in clinical populations.
e. Barbara Drew has been the pioneering investigator in this aspect of critical care nursing.
f. Eileen Hasselmeyer, Mary Neal, and Kathryn Barnard were the original pioneers in studies of neonate stimulation, followed by Anderson, Whalberg, and Lundington, among others.
g. Dorothy Brooten is credited for demonstrating the cost-effectiveness of low-birth-weight infants.
h. The author is indebted to Patricia Sparacino, cardiovascular surgery nurse specialist at the Medical Center, University of California–San Francisco, and Julie Shinn, clinical coordinator in cardiovascular surgical nursing at Stanford University Medical Center. Both are internationally known clinician/scholars and Academy members.

REFERENCES

1. Abdellah, F. B. Overview of nursing research 1955–1968. *Nursing Research* 1970;19:6–17, 239–52.
2. Lindeman, C. A. Delphi survey of priorities in nursing research. *Nursing Research* 1975;24:434–41.
3. DeTornyay, R. *Nursing research in the Bicentennial year*. Boulder, CO: Western Interstate Commission for Higher Education, 1976.
4. Gortner, S. R., Nahm, H. An overview of nursing research in the United States. *Nursing Research* 1977;26:10–32.
5. Brown, J. S., Tanner, C. A., Patrick, K. P. Nursing's search for scientific knowledge. *Nursing Research* 1983;32:29–32.
6. Jacobsen, B. S., Meininger, J. C. The designs and methods of published nursing research: 1956–1983. *Nursing Research* 1985;34:306–12.

7. Moody, L. E., Wilson, M. E., Smythe, K., Schwartz, R., Tittle, M., VanCort, M. L. Analysis of a decade of nursing practice research: 1977–1986. *Nursing Research* 1988;37:374–79.
8. Fitzpatrick, J. J., editor-in-chief. *Encyclopedia of nursing research*. New York: Springer, 1998.
9. American Nurses Association Commission on Nursing Research. *Nursing research: Toward a science of health care*. Priorities for research in nursing. Kansas City: American Nurses Association, 1976.
10. American Nurses Association Cabinet on Nursing Research. *Directions for nursing research: Toward the twenty-first century*. Kansas City: American Nurses Association, 1985.
11. Oberst, M. T. Nursing in the year 2000: Setting the agenda for knowledge generation and utilization. In Sorenson, G., editor. *Setting the agenda for the year 2000: Knowledge development in nursing*. Kansas City: American Academy of Nursing, 1986.
12. Stevenson, J. S., Woods, N. R. Strategies for the year 2000: Synthesis and projections. In Sorenson, G., editor. *Setting the agenda for the year 2000: Knowledge development in nursing*. Kansas City: American Academy of Nursing, 1986.
13. Barnard, K. E. Knowledge for practice: Directions for the future. *Nursing Research* 1980;29:208–12.
14. Gortner, S. R. Nursing research: Out of the past and into the future. *Nursing Research* 1980;29:204–7.
15. National Center for Nursing Research. *Report of the national nursing research agenda for the participants in the conference on research priorities in nursing science*, January 27–29, 1988 [unpublished]. Prepared by D. Bloch. Bethesda: National Center for Nursing Research; 1988.
16. *Research spanning the life cycle*. Vol 15. Los Angeles: University of California, Los Angeles School of Nursing, Fall 1998.
17. *The science of caring*. Vol. 11. San Francisco: University of California, San Francisco School of Nursing, Spring 1999.
18. *Advancing the science of nursing*. Vol 11. Baltimore: University of Maryland School of Nursing, 1997–1999.
19. Gortner, S. R. Nursing science in transition. *Nursing Research,* 1980;29:180–3.
20. Gortner, S. R. Knowledge development in a practice discipline: Philosophy and pragmatics. In Williams, C., editor. *Nursing research and policy formation: The case of prospective payment*. Kansas City: American Academy of Nursing, 1984.
21. Gortner, S. R., Schultz, P. R. Approaches to nursing science methods. *Image Journal of Nursing School* 1988;20:22–4.
22. Gortner, S. R. Historical development of doctoral programs: Shaping our expectations. *Journal of Professional Nursing* 1991;7:45–53.
23. Donaldson, S. Breakthrough in nursing research. Invited presentation. *Proceedings of the 25th Anniversary of the American Academy of Nursing*; 1998; Acapulco, Mexico.
24. Grady, P. Strategic planning for the 21st century. *Proceedings of the National Instituted for Nursing Research State of the Science Congress*; 1999 Sept. 16–18; Washington, D.C.
25. American Nurses Association. *Functions, standards and qualifications for practice*. New York: The Association, 1959.
26. Hughes, E. D. et al. *Twenty thousand nurses tell their story*. Philadelphia: JB Lippincott Co., 1958.
27. Finer, H. *Administration and the nursing services*. New York: Macmillan Company, 1952.
28. Leone, L. P. The ingredients of research. *Nursing Research* 1955;4:51.
29. Henderson, V. Research in nursing practice—When? *Nursing Research* 1956;4:99.
30. American Nurses Foundation. Research-pathway to future progress in nursing care. *Nursing Research* 1960;9:4–7.
31. Vreland, E. Memorandum to Lucile Petry Leone, chief nurse officer. *Some frontiers for nursing research*. February 1959.
32. Dumas, R. G., Leonard, R.C. The effect of nursing on the incidence of postoperative vomiting. *Nursing Research* 1963;12:12–5.
33. Coston, H. M. Myocardial infarction: Stages of recovery and nursing care. *Nursing Research* 1960; 9:178–84.

34. Disbrow, M. A. Any mother who really wants to nurse her baby can do so. *Nursing Forum* 1963;2: 39–48.
35. Ringholz, S., Morris, M. A test of some assumptions about rooming-in. *Nursing Research* 1961; 10:196–9.
36. Moss, F. T., Myer, B. The effects of nursing interaction upon pain relief in patients. *Nursing Research* 1966;15:303–6.
37. Glaser, B. G., Strauss, A. L. *Awareness of dying (Observation Series).* Chicago: Aldine Publishing Company, 1965.
38. Quint, J. *The nurse and the dying patient.* New York: Macmillan Company, 1967.
39. Batey, M., Julian, J. Staff perceptions of state psychiatric hospital goals. *Nursing Research* 1964;12: 89–92.
40. Little, D. E., Carnevali, D. Nurse specialist effect on tuberculosis: Report on a field experiment. *Nursing Research* 1967;16:321–6.
41. Meltzer, L. E., Pinneo, R., Ferrigan, M. M., Kitchell, J. R., Ipsen, J., Bearman, J. *Intensive coronary care: An analysis of the system and the acute phase of myocardial infarction.* New York: Charles Press, 1969.
42. Gortner, S. R. Research in nursing. The federal interest and grant program. *American Journal of Nursing* 1973;73:1052–3.
43. Gortner, S. R. Scientific accountability in nursing. *Nursing Outlook* 1974;22:764–8.
44. Gortner, S. R. Research for a practice profession. *Nursing Research* 1974;24:193–7.
45. Gortner, S. R., Bloch, D., Phillips, T. P. Contributions of nursing research to patient care. *Journal of Nursing Administration* 1976;6:22–8.
46. Gortner, S. R. *The relations of scientists with professional and sponsoring organizations and with society.* In Batey, M., editor. Issues in research: Social, professional, and methodological. Selected papers from the first American Nurses Association Council of Nurse Researchers program meeting. Kansas City: The Association, 1974.
47. Lindeman, C. A. Priorities in clinical nursing research. *Nursing Outlook* 1975;23:693–8.
48. Gortner, S. R. Trends and historical perspective. In Downs, F. S., Fleming, J. W., editors. *Issues in Nursing Research.* New York: Appleton-Century-Crofts, 1979.
49. Mishel, M., Murdaugh, C. Family adjustment to heart transplantation. *Nursing Research* 1987;36: 332–8.
50. Silver, H. K., Ford, L. C., Day, L. R. The pediatric nurse practitioner program: Expanding the role of the nurse to provide increased health care for children. *Journal of the American Medical Association* 1968;204:298–302.
51. Lewis, C. E., Resnik, B. A. Nurse clinics and progressive ambulatory patient care. *New England Medical Journal* 1967;277:1236–41.
52. Cheyovich, T. K., Lewis, C. E., Gortner, S. R. *The nurse practitioner in an adult outpatient clinic.* Washington, D.C.: Health Resources Administration. HEW Publication No (HRA) 76-29; 1976.
53. Donaldson, S., Crowley, D. The discipline of nursing. *Nursing Outlook* 1978;26:113–20.
54. Meleis, A. I. *The age of nursing scholarliness: Now is the time.* The inaugural Helen Nahm Research Lecture. San Francisco: University of California, San Francisco School of Nursing, 1980.
55. Holzemer, W. L., Gortner, S. R. Evaluation of the nursing research emphasis/grants for doctoral programs in nursing grant program 1979–1984. *Journal of Professional Nursing* 1988;4:381–6.
56. Stevenson, J. S., Woods, N. E. *Nursing science and contemporary science: Emerging paradigms.* In Sorenson, G., editor. Setting the agenda for the year 2000: Knowledge development in Nursing. Kansas City: American Academy of Nursing, 1986.
57. Meleis, A. I. ReVisions in knowledge development: A passion for substance. *Scholarly Inquiry Nursing Practice Institute Journal* 1987;1–19.
58. Gortner, S. R. Nursing values and science: Toward a science philosophy. *Image Journal of Nursing Scholarship* 1990;22:101–5.

59. Ellis, R. Values and vicissitudes of the scientist nurse. *Nursing Research* 1970;19:440–5.
60. Batey, M. Conceptualizing the research process. *Nursing Research* 1971;20:296–301.
61. Barnard, K. *The research cycle: Nursing, the profession, the discipline.* In Communicating Nursing Research. Vol. 15: Nursing science in perspective. Boulder: Western Interstate Commission for Higher Education, 1982.
62. Shaver, J. A biopsychosocial view of human health. *Nursing Outlook* 1985;33:187–91.
63. Schorr, T., Kennedy, M. S. *100 years of American nursing: Celebrating a century of caring.* Philadelphia: Lippincott Williams & Wilkins, 1999.
64. Hinshaw, A. S., Sigmon H. D., Lindsey, A. M. Interfacing nursing and biologic science. *Journal of Professional Nursing* 1991;7:264.
65. Diers, D., Burst, H. V. Effectiveness of policy related research: Nurse-midwifery as case study. *Image Journal of Nursing Scholarship* 1983;15:68–74.
66. Fagin, C. Nursing research and the erosion of care [guest editorial]. *Nursing Outlook* 1998;46:259–60.

CHAPTER 34

Reflective Practice: Empowering Nursing Knowledge

Hollie Noveletsky

Nursing's metaparadigm identifies the four constructs of person, health, environment, and nursing as the focus of concern for the discipline. Over the past decade, nursing has moved from debating competing theoretical frameworks towards an acceptance of multiple frameworks grounded within a humanistic-caring philosophy (Restrepo & Davis, 2003). Given the understanding of these constructs within a humanistic-caring philosophy, there is an appreciation that the implicit focus of concern for nursing is embedded within the interaction of the constructs and that the explicit manifestation of this interaction is contextually and temporally bound because "caring knowledge is socially embedded" (Benner, Tanner, & Chesla, 1996, p. 231). Socially embedded knowledge is influenced by culture, language, historical context, the evolutionary nature of the specific knowledge, and the collective culture of the cohort group of the practitioner(s) applying the knowledge (Benner et al., 1996). Reflective practice allows for the uncovering of these factors that impact the explicit manifestation of nursing within the human-health experience.

Reflective practice has gained significant attention in nursing education and practice over the past 20 years. Though the concept originated outside of nursing, it appears to offer the profession an avenue toward understanding and enhancing the interpersonal connections that represent the essence of nursing. This chapter will briefly review the development of the concept of reflective practice and its application within nursing. The philosophical fit between reflective practice and nursing knowledge development will be examined. In addition, the concept of reflective practice will be explored in relationship to nursing practice and education.

REFLECTIVE PRACTICE: WHAT IS IT?

Reflective practice is based on the concept of reflection developed by John Dewey in the early part of the 20th century. Dewey was a philosopher and educational theorist. He described *reflection* as the mental process of carefully and systematically examining the nature and basic assumptions of one's knowledge. The purpose of reflection, according to Dewey, was to gain a better understanding of situations that appeared obscure or uncertain. Through the process of questioning the basic tenets of one's knowledge, one can develop insight into the limitations of one's paradigm (Dewey, 1933). This insight, in turn, allows one to be more open to a broader understanding of an experience (Cotton, 2001; Teekman, 2000; Williams, 2001).

The concept of reflective practice was further influenced by the work of Donald Schon (1987) from the field of education. Schon noted that professionals from various fields of study were faced with two types of problems. The first type of problem was that of a technical nature and was solved readily "through the application of research-based theory and technique" (Schon, 1987, p. 3). The second type of problem was that of an uncertain nature in which various problems or situations arose that could not be resolved within the boundaries of technical knowledge. This type of problem required an awareness of the limitations of technical knowledge in addressing the complex, unique, or ill-defined situations that were often encountered in practice. Schon described this second type of problem as the "indeterminate zones of practice" (Schon, 1987, p. 6), where the professional must first identify the problem and then identify the type(s) of knowledge required to address the problem. Schon labeled the ability to address the problems that arose from the indeterminate zones of practice as "professional artistry" (Schon, 1987, p. 15). Professional artistry referred to the ability of expert practitioners to apply technical knowledge in creative and innovative ways or to recognize the need for new knowledge in order to address the uniqueness of the situation at hand.

Schon (1987) described reflection as the process through which one moved from being able to address purely technical problems to being able to address the more complex problems that arose within the indeterminate zones of practice. He held that although the novice could not be taught professional artistry, one could be coached through the use of reflection to develop an understanding of the complexities of practice. Schon identified two types of reflection: "reflection on action" (Schon, 1983, p. 278) and "reflection in action" (Schon, 1987, p. 26). Reflection on action was a retrospective analysis of an interaction, whereas reflection in action was a moment-by-moment appreciation of the variables impacting the interaction as they unfolded. Through reflection on action, one gained insight and understanding of the multiple factors that impacted practice. This insight allowed the novice to uncover the knowledge embedded in the "doing" within the contexts and constraints of practice. Schon referred to this knowledge as the "knowing in practice" (1987, p. 33). As the novice professional made explicit his or her knowing in practice, the novice began to grasp the complexities of practice and moved along the continuum from novice to expert. As the professional continued to develop a body of "knowing in practice," he or she became more insightful to the holistic nature of the interactions of practice. With this deeper understanding, the professional was better able to grasp the complexities of practice as they unfolded. Schon referred to the simultaneous processes of grasping the holism of practice while engaged in the act of practice as reflection in action and believed that it represented a more advanced level of reflection that signified expert practice.

REFLECTIVE PRACTICE AND NURSING KNOWLEDGE DEVELOPMENT

The process of moving from novice to expert has received significant attention in the nursing literature. Benner's (1984) work with expert nurses supports the works of Dewey and Schon. She found that expert nursing knowledge is informed by both the "limits of formal rules" (p. xix) and the "particular contingencies of a situation" (p. xx). Benner and her colleagues coined the term "reasoning-in-transition" (Benner, Hooper-Kyriakidis, & Stannard, 1999, p. 10) to describe a reflective process used by expert nurses to clarify "understanding and to resolve contradictions or confusions" (p. 10). Benner's reasoning-in-transition is similar to Schon's reflection in action, because both processes strive to clarify the uncertainty of action that arises in the indeterminate zones of practice and to expand knowledge for practice. Benner and her colleagues (1996) state that "scientific theories and information became knowledge and judgement only in the hands of skilled practitioners who have the opportunity to clarify, and extend general explanations through understanding particular situations" (p. 231). Reflective practice allows for the uncovering of knowledge embedded in practice and expands nursing knowledge.

The theory-practice gap has long been an issue of concern in nursing. Reflective practice has been identified as a possible means of bridging that gap (Duke & Appleton, 2000; Johns & Freshwater, 1998; Teekman, 2000). Parker (Fawcett, 2003) holds that practice is guided by theory and that theory is further developed by expert practice. She believes that theory is the first step in the spiral of theory–practice–theory, because theory shapes one's vision of an experience by identifying which concepts to examine. Through reflection on practice and reflection in practice, nurses can examine the truthfulness of knowledge within various contexts. Supporters of reflective practice believe that it allows for the development of tacit knowledge embedded in practice, the validation of knowledge for practice, and the identification of knowledge gaps within practice (Johns & Freshwater, 1998; Kim, 1999). Reflective practice allows for the innovative use of knowledge and the identification of the need for new knowledge as is required within the indeterminate zones of practice.

In addition, reflective practice offers nursing knowledge development a method of uncovering the implicit and explicit manifestations of nursing's metaparadigm. Johns (2003) notes that although the narratives used in reflection are subjective and contextually bound, identification of commonalities across various nursing reflections can uncover the broad range of manifestations of nursing within the human-health experience. Through reflection, nurses come to understand how caring is manifested within various clinical contexts (Schaefer, 2002). Reflection allows for discourse regarding the ontological, epistemological and ethical issues of caring within the human-health experience. This discourse, in turn, informs practice. As a result, a clearer understanding of what nursing care is and is not evolves. And as the contexts within which nurses interact with individuals in need change, so, too, will the philosophical issues that underpin the expression of nursing. This evolving discourse underscores Parker's theory–practice–theory spiral.

Practice

Benner and Wrubel (1989) argue "that caring as a moral art is primary" (p. xi) to the discipline of nursing. They state that the act of caring takes place within the "privileged place of nursing" (p. xi). This privileged place represents the intersection of a person with the health experience. It is manifested at times of health, illness, loss, and transition. These are the very personal and private experiences that nurses are allowed to witness in individuals' lives. Nursing within these privileged places is informed by science but guided by a philosophy of caring. The expert nurse realizes that the act of nursing within the human-health experience is more complex than can be delineated within a linear, scientific model (Benner & Wrubel, 1989; Watson, 1988). Therefore, a more holistic theory needs to be developed to bring to light and to guide expert nursing practice. Reflection can assist the nurse in uncovering and understanding the iterative, simultaneous, and unseen complexities of practice in order to develop tacit knowledge for practice and evolve toward expert nursing.

Reflective practice has been studied in a variety of clinical nursing settings, including transcultural (Fuller, 2003), administration (Johns, 2002), general medical/surgical (Teekman, 2000), oncology (Johns, 2002), and psychiatric nursing (Johns, 2002) settings. Researchers have found that by incorporating reflective practice into the clinical setting nurses develop an increased sense of self-awareness and understanding of the holistic nature of nursing (Johns, 2002). This self-awareness encompasses awareness of the client's, the nurse's, and the health care organization's values and the impact those values have on an interaction. There is greater awareness of the context of an interaction and its impact on an interaction. There is a recognition that the construct of differences of values and culture is universal to people and not particular to an individual. This recognition allows one to be open to acceptance of differences in all interactions versus seeing differences as a unique characteristic of a given situation (Fuller, 2003). This increased self-awareness allows the nurse to be more available to the patient, to be better able to meet the patient's needs, and to create more supportive environments for the provision of care (Fuller, 2003; Johns, 2002).

Teekman (2000) and Schmieding (1999) suggest that the incorporation of reflective practice into the clinical setting is empowering for nurses. Nurses are empowered through a greater understanding, deeper insight, and a reframing of problems as opportunities for growth and development. However, Johns (2002) warns that with the greater sense of self-awareness comes a potential for an increased sense of vulnerability. As the discrepancy between ideal and actual care becomes known and the constraints of context are made explicit, one may feel powerless. This potential underscores the importance of support and structure in the reflective process so that the nurse can process his or her evolving insights. Johns notes that the nurse must continually struggle to integrate the new knowledge gained from reflection into her or his existing paradigm. This struggle supports Parker's (Fawcett, 2003) belief in the theory–practice–theory spiral.

Some critics of reflective practice warn that it may represent a means of surveillance by the profession of the individual nurse (Gilbert, 2001). This could be accomplished through access to the private thoughts of the individual and guided discourse with expert nurses. In spite of this warning, Gilbert (2001) acknowledges that reflective practice appears to promote individual surveillance through self-managing of ethical issues and ensures safe and ethical nursing practice. Self-managing is achieved through "competing discourses of private (selfish) desire and public duty (selfless-obligation)" (Gilbert, 2001, p. 203).

Education

The concept of reflective practice has received a lot of attention in the field of nursing education (Chambers, 1999; Liimatainen, Poskiparta, Karhila, & Sjogren, 2001; Williams, 2001). In the nursing literature, the term *reflective practice* has been applied to a variety of processes. The common thread among the applications is that there is a dynamic interaction between an expert and a novice for the purpose of discovery within experience (Duke & Appleton, 2000; Johns, 2002). Pritzkau (1970) points out that dialogue provides the opportunity for a listener to draw out another's understanding of an experience in a new light. This new understanding comes from grasping the epistemological limitations of one's paradigm, which in turn allows for the transformation of understanding. This is achieved by explicating the juxtaposition of experience and thought within the constraints of context. Reflective dialogue allows the individual to see him- or herself as an agent of behavior who is influenced by his or her own history, knowledge, and context, but is not dominated by these factors. Thus, new understanding generates new actions, which in turn generates new understanding; knowledge, practice, and the individual evolve.

Reflection has been incorporated into a variety of models of nursing education. Across models and clinical settings, educators have found that reflection is a transformative (Duke & Appleton, 2000; Glaze, 2001, 2002; Liimantainen et al., 2001) and emanciptory (Glaze, 2001; Liimantainen et al., 2001) process. Students were noted to have increased awareness of the impact of societal constraints and of their own personal factors on the nature of an interaction (Glaze, 2001; Noveletsky-Rosenthal & Solomon, 2001). Reflection allowed students to appreciate the complexity of the holistic nature of nursing interactions, while maintaining a realistic understanding of the constraints of the context of the interactions (Chambers, 1999; Glaze, 2001). Chambers (1999) noted that reflection enabled the students to begin to develop a knowing in action that represented the movement along the continuum from novice to expert. The students recognized nursing as a creative activity, one that required innovative applications of knowledge to meet the demands of the individual situations. This recognition correlates with Schon's notion of the need for professional artistry within the indeterminate zones of practice.

Several factors have been identified as being essential to effectively incorporating reflection within a teaching framework. These include time (Glaze, 2002), support and structure (Glaze, 2002; Johns, 2002; Johns & Freshwater, 1998; Noveletsky-Rosenthal, 2001; Teekman, 2000), self-awareness (Freshwater, 2002), and trust (Noveletsky-Rosenthal, 2001). Time relates to the personal journey of the individual. Each person will evolve in his or her own way to reflect and incorporate new knowledge at his or her own pace. Support and structure refers to the power of critical dialogue to expand one's paradigm. Self-awareness underscores the need for the individual to be open to examining one's behaviors, beliefs, and values. And finally, trust is essential for the development of critical dialogue for the purpose of self-discovery.

One of the main concerns with the use of reflective practice as a model of education or professional development is the application of incongruent methods of evaluation of one's evolution in reflective capacity. Duke and Appleton (2000), in their review of the literature, note that attempts have been made to identify the individual components of reflection and to measure individuals' growth in reflective ability. However, the authors warn that these dimensions may represent an artificial fragmentation of a holistic construct. They argue that one's level of reflection or progress toward a greater depth of understanding should not be measured by quantitative measures. This point reinforces the basic assumptions concerning reflection. These assumptions are that the reflective process is a personal journey of self-discovery, it has no set starting point, the rate of development is individual, and there is no end point. Based upon these assumptions, measuring one's level of reflection and gains in insight appears to be inconsistent with the basic nature of the construct. A more holistic appreciation of the evolution of one's insight through the use of qualitative methods of inquiry may represent a more appropriate means of evaluating the reflective process.

FUTURE DIRECTIONS FOR REFLECTIVE PRACTICE IN NURSING

Theories inform our practice and at the same time constrict our vision and understanding of experience; and experience influences our theories (Fawcett, 2003; Watson, 1988). Dewey stated that "the nature of the problem fixes the end of thought, and the end controls the process of thinking" (Dewey, 1933, p. 15). The content of nursing knowledge is time and context dependent. As science evolves and paradigms shift, the content of knowledge changes. And although the process of knowledge development is less dependent on time and context, it is still dependent on paradigms. Reflective practice offers nurses a way of evaluating the type of knowledge necessary in the provision of care regardless of time, context, or paradigm. It is a means of evaluating both the process and content of knowledge development. Through reflection, nurses can evaluate the basic premises that guide their way of being in the world and interpretation of experience, including nursing care, in order to gain a fuller understanding of the world, another's experience, and the role of nursing in society. Change is an integral aspect of knowledge and practice (Parse, 2004). Through the use of reflection, nurses can learn to embrace change as an implicit characteristic of being and evolve nursing science and tacit knowledge to meet the ever-changing needs of society.

REFERENCES

Benner, P. (1984). *From Novice to Expert*. Menlo Park, CA: Addison-Wesley.

Benner, P. A., Hooper-Kyriakidis, P., & Stannard, D. (1999). *Clinical Wisdom and Interventions in Critical Care*. Philadelphia: W.B. Saunders.

Benner, P. A., Tanner, C. A., & Chesla, C. A. (1996). *Expertise in Nursing Practice*. New York: Springer.

Benner, P. A., & Wrubel, J. (1989). *The Primacy of Caring*. New York: Addison-Wesley.

Chambers, N. (1999). Close encounters: The use of critical reflective analysis as an evaluation tool in teaching and learning. *Journal of Advanced Nursing, 29*(4), 950–957.

Cotton, A. H. (2001). Private thoughts in public spheres: Issues in reflection and reflective practices in nursing. *Journal of Advanced Nursing, 36*(4), 512–519.

Dewey, J. (1933). *How We Think*. Lexington, MA: D.C. Heath & Co.

Duke, S., & Appleton, J. (2000). The use of reflection in a palliative care programme: A quantitative study of the development of reflective skills over an academic year. *Journal of Advanced Nursing, 32*(6), 1557–1568.

Fawcett, J. (2003). Theory and practice: A conversation with Marilyn E. Parker. *Nursing Science Quarterly, 16*(2), 131–136.

Freshwater, D. (2002). Guided reflection in the context of post-modern practice. In C. Johns (Ed.), *Guided Reflection: Advancing Practice* (pp. 225–238). Oxford: Blackwell.

Fuller, J. (2003). Intercultural health care as reflective negotiated practice. *Western Journal of Nursing Research, 25*(7), 781–797.

Gilbert, T. (2001). Reflective practice and clinical supervision: Meticulous rituals of the confessional. *Journal of Advanced Nursing, 36*(2), 199–205.

Glaze, J. E. (2001). Reflection as a transforming process: Student advanced nurse practitioners' experiences of developing reflective skills as part of an MSc programme. *Journal of Advanced Nursing, 34*(5), 639–647.

Glaze, J. E. (2002). Stages in coming to terms with reflection: Student advanced nurse practitioners' perceptions of their reflective journeys. *Journal of Advanced Nursing, 37*(3), 265–272.

Johns, C. (2002). *Guided Reflection: Advancing Practice*. Oxford: Blackwell.

Johns, C. (2003). Easing into the light. *International Journal for Human Caring, 7*(1), 49–55.

Johns, C., & Freshwater, D. (Eds.) (1998). *Transforming Nursing Through Reflective Practice*. Oxford: Blackwell.

Kim, H. S. (1999). Critical reflective inquiry for knowledge development in nursing practice. *Journal of Advanced Nursing, 29*(5), 1205–1212.

Liimatainen, L., Poskiparta, M., Karhila, P., & Sjogren, A. (2001). The development of reflective learning in the context of health counselling and health promotion during nurse education. *Journal of Advanced Nursing, 34*(5), 648–658.

Noveletsky-Rosenthal, H. T. (2001). Reflective practice. In A. J. Lowenstein & M. J. Bradshaw (Eds.), *Fuszard's Innovative Teaching Strategies in Nursing* (3rd ed.) (pp. 107–112). Gaithersburg, MD: Aspen.

Noveletsky-Rosenthal, H. T., & Solomon, K. (2001). Reflections on the use of Johns' model of structured reflection in nurse practitioner education. *International Journal of Human Caring, 5*(2), 21–26.

Parse, R. R. (2004). A human becoming teaching-learning model. *Nursing Science Quarterly, 17*(1), 33–35.

Pritzkau, P. T. (1970). *On Education for the Authentic.* Scranton, PA: International Textbook.

Restrepo, E., & Davis, L. (2003). Storytelling: Both art and therapeutic practice. *International Journal of Human Caring, 7*(1), 43–48.

Schaefer, K. M. (2002). Reflections on caring narratives: Enhancing patterns of knowing. *Nursing Education Perspectives, 23*(6), 286–293.

Schmieding, N. J. (1999). Reflective inquiry framework for nurse administrators. *Journal of Advanced Nursing, 30*(3), 631–639.

Schon, D. A. (1983). *The Reflective Practitioner.* New York: Basic Books.

Schon, D. A. (1987). *Educating the Reflective Practitioner: Toward a New Design for Teaching and Learning in Professions.* San Francisco: Jossey-Bass.

Teekman, B. (2000). Exploring reflective thinking in nursing practice. *Journal of Advanced Nursing, 31*(5), 1125–1135.

Watson, J. (1988). *Nursing: Human Science and Human Caring.* New York: National League for Nursing.

Williams, B. (2001). Developing critical reflection for professional practice through problem-based learning. *Journal of Advanced Nursing, 34*(1), 27–34.

CHAPTER 35

Reclaiming Spirituality in Nursing

Patricia Maher

INTRODUCTION

Nurses often experience an awareness of the spiritual dimension of their work yet feel uncertain how to integrate spirituality into care or define spirituality in practice. This has not always been the case. Florence Nightingale, the founder of modern nursing, saw nursing as spiritual work informed by science. She believed that spirituality was intrinsic to human nature, compatible with science, and the deepest source of human healing (Macrae, 1995). Despite a renewed interest in spirituality and a desire to better understand and recognize the spirituality embedded in practice, present day efforts to reintegrate spirituality into nursing care have met with little success. Nursing's theoretical paradigms have been unable to clarify the articulations of spirituality in practice, nursing education has not adequately prepared nurses to meet patients' spiritual needs, and nursing research has yet to explore the place of spirituality in healing. How then can nurses reclaim the spirituality that lies at the heart of the caring work that they do? It is essential to look back at the traditions of the profession to find insights and direction for future growth. It is important to identify barriers that have hindered the full expression of spirituality in nursing. It is crucial for every nurse to reflect on his or her practice with careful attention to moments of spiritual awareness and share those reflections with other nurses, for in that sharing the dimensions of a contemporary nursing spirituality will appear.

Nursing's quest for its spiritual roots is best undertaken with the knowledge that what is found will require interpretation in order to be relevant in the present time. Just as nursing has changed over the last two centuries, so, too, has spirituality. Contemporary spirituality is more detached from religious roots and more informed by secular, pluralistic, and individualistic orientations than was the case in Nightingale's time. The historical changes in the character of spirituality are described by Wuthnow (1999). Wuthnow documented an explosion of interest in spirituality and predicted that in the century to come, this interest will continue to mount, as will confusion and uncertainty regarding its nature. He suggested that there is no current model of spirituality that will move us towards realizing the deepest aspects of our lives and work, but proposed a practice-oriented spirituality as a way to proceed. Nursing as a practice-based profession is ideally suited for such a model.

I offer an example from my own practice of a seemingly ordinary moment of care that was filled with spiritual meaning. Charlie had been a hard-drinking and lonely man for most of his

417

life. He was orphaned at age 10 after his mother died during the flu epidemic of 1917, and he lived alone throughout his life, refusing to marry the woman he loved because he felt unworthy of her. I cared for Charlie at the end of his life, in his home. My visits were divided between evaluating and treating his many medical problems and listening to his stories about his barroom buddies, his unrequited love, and his travails in the healthcare system. A moment of spiritual significance arose during one of my home visits while I was checking his weight. I was helping Charlie to step onto the scale; he was weak and shaky and having a lot of trouble balancing. When the indicator settled on a number, I read it aloud because he was unable to see the scale, having become virtually blind from a recent stroke, "Seventy pounds Charlie." He took it philosophically, "I was never a big man, Patricia." But as he stepped off the scale he carefully looked in my direction, smiled, and asked, "Is it possible to feel good before you die?"

I had no answer then, but I have carried Charlie's question with me like a koan. A koan is a problem that requires the development of new ways of thinking that go beyond the rational mind and lead to the realization that you will not change the problem, rather the problem will change you (Remen, 1996). Over the years, I realized that Charlie was not really asking me a question as much as telling me that despite his dwindling weight, waning capacities, and imminent death, he was experiencing hope and the goodness of life. Charlie's smile was so much in contrast to my own feelings at that moment as I assessed his frailty and saw that his weight had plummeted. I now believe that Charlie felt good because of the compassion and companionship that he had received from his caregivers and because he had hope. Hope, in the sense of Vaclav Havel's (1990) definition, is "an orientation of the spirit, an orientation of the heart . . . not the conviction that something will turn out well but the certainty that something makes sense regardless of how it turns out (p. 181)."

My encounter with Charlie led me to identify two hallmarks of a spiritual exchange: the presence of hope and the surprise appearance of joy. I wonder about the nature of Charlie's hope. I believe that he tried to share his sense of feeling healed despite the clinical indicators that suggested that we were losing the battle for his life. I expect that he was also experiencing support and connection to others, connections that had eluded him in his earlier life. Then there was his joy. Noddings (1984) has suggested that "joy often accompanies a realization of our relatedness. It is the special affect that arises out of the receptivity of caring, and it represents a major reward for the one caring" (p. 132). Paradoxically, as Charlie received care, he began to give care, to his neighbor with whom he began to cook dinner, to his home health aide who was struggling with a personal problem, and to me with his offer of jokes and good humor. Charlie had not had many opportunities to either receive or to give care until the end of his life. Tillich (as cited in Noddings, 1984) has noted an additional source of joy: "the affirmation of one's essential being in spite of desires and anxieties creates joy . . . real joy is a severe matter; it is the happiness of a soul which is lifted above every circumstance. Joy is the emotional expression of the courageous yes to one's own true being" (p. 143–144). Charlie's hope and joy were well expressed; even now, many years later, I remember and can reexperience them. It was a gift of his spirit to me. Through that gift Charlie lives on in my thoughts, hopes, imagination, and work.

My experience with Charlie is not unique; accompanying patients through suffering often leads to the mysterious terrain of the spirit. Why is spirituality often revealed in the shadow of suffering? Younger (1995) has explained how suffering leads to alienation and disconnection from self and others as well as the loss of a sense of belonging in the world. She states that transcendence is "probably the most powerful way in which one is restored to connectedness and wholeness after an injury" (p. 61). Transcendence is an attribute of spirituality as is a sense of connectedness to self, others, the world, and for some but not all, a divine presence (Baldacchino

& Draper, 2001). Goddard (1995) describes spirituality as that which connects us to life, a dynamic transcending force that she has termed "integrative energy." Haase, Britt, Coward, Leidy, & Penn (1992) have asserted that spiritual connection is "richer than social support . . . a significant, shared, and meaningful personal relationship with another person, spiritual being, nature, or perhaps an aspect of one's inner self" (p. 146). Spirituality arises and comes into awareness through relationships and often in the face of suffering, it awakens and prepares the person for the possibility of healing through hope, connection, and sometimes joy. In this way, spirituality is much broader than religion and is pertinent to all people whether they are believers or nonbelievers. It is wrong to assume that if a person is not religious that spirituality should not be an important aspect of his or her care.

No one definition of spirituality has been accepted by nursing scholars (Brush & Daly, 2000; Goddard, 1995; Greasley, Chiu, & Gartland, 2001; Wright, 1998). The lack of an accepted definition has been an impediment to scholarship. To understand spirituality, two definitions are needed, the first to describe spirituality as a universal aspect of humanity and the second to depict spirituality as a field of study. A definition of spirituality as a dimension of the human person must include the notions of transcendence, connection, integration, and relationship. Hope and joy are hallmarks of its presence. Goddard (1995) suggested that spirituality is rightly thought of as "integrative energy." Spirituality is also a field of study. Schneiders (as cited in Rolheiser, 1999) defined spirituality as a discipline that "investigates spiritual experience in an interdisciplinary way, not only religious experience but also analogous experiences of ultimate meaning which have transcendent or life-integrating power" (p. 244).

Nurses investigate spiritual experiences through caring. There is no doubt that caring is a powerful means of knowing, but caring is also a complex, confounding, sometimes dangerous, and prophetic human endeavor. The discipline of nursing and the discipline of spirituality both require strong knowledge bases, a clear sense of the tradition of healing, spiritual maturity, and a rigorous but gentle means of reflection on practice.

HISTORICAL ROOTS

The relationship between nursing and spirituality has taken many forms over time. Before the 19th century, there was little besides spiritual care with which to heal. Within an overtly religious society, spiritual care was seen as a formidable and credible endeavor and people were suspicious of medical care for good reason. Ashley (1997), a nurse historian, reported that hospitals were places of poor sanitation and filth. Many women interested in nursing encountered societal prejudices that viewed nursing as disreputable. In order to avoid social disapproval, women joined religious orders in which healing was a vocation. This early involvement of religious orders was significant in shaping the relationship between spirituality and nursing (Webb, 2002).

Florence Nightingale was one of the first to bring spirituality and science together to improve the care of the sick. Nightingale gives a description of spirituality from *Suggestions for Thought*, "What do we mean by spirituality? Is it not feeling, as distinct from both intellect and from the affection of one human being to another? . . . feelings called forth by the consciousness of a presence of higher nature than human, unconnected with the material . . . this we are conscious is the highest capability of our nature" (as cited in Macrae, 2001, p. 21). According to Webb (2002), Nightingale envisioned nursing as mystical work similar to a religion; she believed that mystical experience, spiritual experience, was not found in withdrawal from the world but from action in it. According to Nightingale, the spiritual role of the nurse was not to pray that

God would act, but to act herself to reduce poverty and suffering and improve the health of others. Nightingale wrote:

> It did strike me as odd, sometimes, that we should pray to be delivered from plague, pestilence, and famine when all the common sewers ran into the Thames, and fevers haunted undrained land, and the districts which cholera would visit could be pointed out. I thought that cholera came that we might remove these causes, not pray that God would remove the cholera. (as cited in Macrae, 2001, p. 94)

She worked tirelessly to promote the science of nursing, reducing the death rate of soldiers in the Crimea on the basis of principles of hygiene and encouraging society to reduce the effects of poverty, which she saw as a source of illness and human suffering. According to Macrae (1996), Nightingale kept statistics throughout her life in order to understand principles of nursing, acknowledging no division between the statistical and the spiritual; she believed that statistics allowed people to see the world as God does. Nightingale was not afraid to question religious or spiritual ideas with science. She challenged the Biblical idea that poverty brings people closer to God when she saw in her statistical tables that, for the general population, poverty was correlated with crime, disease, and high mortality rates (Macrae, 2001, p. 30).

Nightingale was not alone in her struggle to understand the dimension of spirituality in care. Meehan (2003) studied the diaries of Irish nurses caring for soldiers during the Crimean War, the same war in which Nightingale made her reputation from 1854 to 1856. The diaries tell of a tradition called "careful nursing." One of the key features of this tradition was an attitude of "disinterested love" of patients. Meehan describes this as exemplified by great tenderness in patient care which disposed nurses to practice with affection, kindness, sympathy, humour and a bright and joyous spirits." (Meehan, 2003, p. 101). The diaries contain the insight that "disinterested love" is a necessary component of healing. The notion of "disinterested love" sought to go beyond a sentimental conception of care and to define the dimensions of compassion in healing, compassion that involved the healer's whole self—body, mind, and spirit. According to Tinder (1999), love/compassion is a necessary antecedent of hope.

Nurses in the early 20th century incorporated scientific knowledge into practice and revolutionized human caring. They did so in the face of sexism and institutional restraints. Although the status of physicians, who were mostly male, began to grow, similar improvements did not extend as fully to nurses, who were mostly women. Nurses were often taken for granted as inexpensive labor for the growing hospital industry, which participated in their training but exacted long hours in difficult conditions with poor pay (Ashley, 1997). Nurses' lack of power coexisted with a lack of value placed on care. Nursing care was characterized as unskilled women's work based not on intelligence, education, and skill, but on intuition and maternal instinct. Despite these restraints, nurses made a significant impact on hospital care. Ashley (1997) observed that "not until the profession of nursing became a reality did these institutions (hospitals) have a service to offer the sick that made them well" (p. 221). She concluded that "at the beginning of the 20th century nurses were the equals of physicians in their training and in their contributions to the health care of society. However they were not equal in the political and economic spheres of human activity and influence" (p. 224). The lack of political equality and its root cause, sexism, tilted health care toward a medical model based on science and away from a nursing model, which sought to synthesize care and compassion with science.

In the last decades of the 20th century, society began to come to terms with the limits of science and technology in addressing human illness. It was apparent that science had proven to be remarkable in curing many illnesses, but could not answer the many questions surrounding human suffering. Although there was a pressing need for an exchange between science and spirituality, communication had become difficult. The dichotomies of body/soul, faith/reason, and cure/care reflected the fractures that had developed between the scientific and the spiritual. Benson (1996) envisioned the rivalry between science and spirituality in terms of faith and reason:

> . . . for millennia, faith has enjoyed relevance to all the world's people, but when the West began to divide the mind/body spheres, sending faith and reason to opposite corners, faith did not appear to fare as well as reason because it became a private, personal matter and reason became a public, promotable good. (p. 171)

Spirituality moved from the public domain to the private domain as health care became more secular and science based. Furthermore, it became more complicated to talk about spirituality in public as American society became more religiously pluralistic. In an effort to be tolerant, spiritual and religious matters became personal matters removed from the public discourse of health care. Inadvertently, this led to silence and neglect. Spiritual care was commonly saved for the end of life when technology failed to offer more. It was administered by clergy or chaplains, "spiritual specialists" who spoke a different language, read different books, and thought within different paradigms of belief than the healthcare providers who stood with them at the bedside. Still, nurses in all areas of practice continued to share moments of spiritual significance with patients and longed for a way to think about their experiences. They believed that the role of the nurse went beyond calling the chaplain, but wondered how that role might be defined.

An interest in reclaiming the spirituality of care began to manifest itself in nurses' interest in holistic health. Nurses knew that technology did not substitute for attention, compassion, human touch, imagination, and hope. While caring for patients after illness, surgery, loss, disability, or a terminal diagnosis, nurses saw that they were on sacred ground, whether in the intensive care unit or in a patient's home. "After" can be an unknown, fearful, and foreign place. A person newly diagnosed must face the future in a body that has been newly labeled as diseased or disabled. It is the role of the nurse to accompany patients into this new territory with compassion, hope, and an ability to assist in their search for meaning. This entails a spiritual component of care that no nursing paradigm has yet captured.

As the 21st century dawns, there is a hunger for a return to caring, a realization that technology can wound as well as heal, and a suspicion that although nurses have gained much, something has been forgotten in the process. In caring for suffering people, nurses experience their own spirituality and the spirituality of those they care for in moments that are manifested by hope, compassion, the gratitude of recovery, the otherworldliness of death, and the surprise of joy. When nurses care, they bridge the chasm between science and spirituality.

NURSING INFORMED BY SPIRITUALITY: WHAT NURSES KNOW

Nurses know that the nurse–patient relationship is the starting and ending point of nursing care. It is from the vantage point of relationship that nurses understand the nature of nursing: its anthropology (what it means to be human), its epistemology (how nurses know), and its language (how nurses communicate what they know).

Nurses know that caring as a human response to suffering is a moral act and is the foundation of a nursing ethic. Stanley Hauerwas (as cited in Younger, 1995) noted that the primary moral role of nurses and physicians is to bind the suffering and the nonsuffering into the same community. In order to do this, patients must be freed from the isolation and alienation that result from suffering. Science can help to understand, prevent, and relieve suffering, but it cannot erase it altogether—the human work of caring is needed. The commitment to another that is predicated on the belief in an inherent dignity of every person is the first step in a therapeutic relationship. Science cannot substitute for that which is accomplished through relationship: transcendence from suffering and alleviation of alienation and isolation from others and from life itself.

Nurses know through caring. Although nursing's knowledge base encompasses many disciplines and is both art and science, nursing is a practice. The practice of nursing requires integrating two ways of knowing: one through revelation, reflection, and relationship and the other through scientific method, objectivity, and human reason. Nightingale described this melding of contemplation and action in the language of her time. The challenge for nurses today is to find a language that expresses nursing practice.

Nurses understand patients through a caring relationship and through caring a unique anthropology emerges. Nursing care calls into question an anthropology that envisions the human person as a whole consisting of physical, psychological, social, and spiritual dimensions. This framework does not meaningfully account for the connections within and between human persons. Neither does it address the scientific evidence that suggests that these dimensions do not exist separately; it is impossible to divide the mind and body, even for the purpose of analysis. Nurses know that human persons cannot exist without one another (love) and cannot survive without a community (justice). Otto (as cited in Baldacchino & Draper, 2001) defined the essence of spirituality as the numinous experience, a universal "idea of the Holy" unique to every individual. In this "complex feeling state of personal incompleteness," often triggered into awareness by a crisis, there is a "longingness to reach a higher power and find existential meaning" (Otto, as cited in Baldacchino & Draper, 2001, p. 836). Caring leads nurses to see humanity's inherent incompleteness (rather than wholeness) as a positive source of hope, love, justice, care, and ultimately healing. Goizueta (1995) wrote of a relational anthropology in which a person is not envisioned as whole, but seeks wholeness in relationship. A relational anthropology allows for a better understanding of the beneficial health effects of love, faith, hope, and community and a deeper appreciation of the etiologies of health problems that result from the deleterious effects of lack of care such as poverty, violence, and trauma.

Caring requires skill in forming relationships in order to understand the suffering of others. Communication with a suffering person requires dialogue that breaks the bonds of alienation. Freire (1999), a Brazilian educator, believed that dialogue becomes a relationship of trust when it is founded on love, humility, and faith. His description of liberating dialogue is of value to nurses; it is spiritual in nature in that it hopes to give birth to a person's voice, to return the person to community, to empower the person to create and transform circumstances, and to support the person's quest for love, connection, and justice. A dialogue is often accomplished when the nurse is silent, in the act of deep listening. According to Younger (1995),

There is a component of nursing assessment that is . . . a plan to be a silent responder, a dance partner who follows and then becomes a midwife to expression. And in paradoxical fashion, the following involved is actually leading. It leads the patient from the silence of alienation to the voice of connection. It is the privilege of those who care for the suffering to show them that they are not thereby excluded from the human community. (p. 71)

Nursing has a legacy of attention and commitment to the underserved. Since the time of Nightingale, nurses have believed that suffering should not be ignored and that caring is a powerful form of resistance to suffering. This global and particular commitment to the care of humanity is the core of nursing spirituality.

Barriers Separating the Disciplines of Nursing and Spirituality

The barriers that separate the disciplines of nursing and spirituality can be categorized into three areas. The first is the inadequacy of language to express spiritual concepts. The language of clinical communication, which is dominated by objective scientific terminology, is especially problematic. Second is the lack of theoretical paradigms that capture the concept of spirituality as a life-giving and integrating force that is essential for human healing. Third is the absence of content in religion and spirituality in nursing education.

Language

Communication about spirituality in nursing is made more difficult by the paucity of language to describe the spiritual aspect of human experience. Healing is usually spoken about in highly technological medical language, a language that patients are not well versed in. Patients' lack of understanding and inability to speak in the dominant language of care serves to create a distance between patient and provider and increase the alienation and sense of helplessness felt by those faced with an illness.

Nurses often find themselves in the role of interpreter. Every nurse has had the experience of standing by a patient during bedside rounds in which the patient listens to his or her condition being explained in medical terms, nods in agreement with the team of providers, only to turn back when left alone with the nurse and ask, "What did they say?" This question, often asked with expectancy, fear, and a wish for hope, requires a spiritual act on the part of the nurse. It necessitates an ability to look with the patient into the abyss and share what is seen so that the patient is brought with care and compassion into the reality of what has befallen him or her. Making meaning and expressing meaning are essential aspects of both spirituality and nursing. The spiritual aspects of caring can be hard to speak about, and it is at the bedside that nurses realize the deficiencies of language. How should nurses express the hope and the limitations of what they know in order to engage the patient in healing? Nursing needs to create a new language of healing to describe the intersections of the spirit with modern medicine, because it is there that nurses heal. Nurses need a language that is mystical, analytical, and prophetic, taking into account the importance and many meanings of silence.

Lack of Paradigms that Integrate Spirituality and Nursing

A renewed relationship between spirituality and nursing would require that spirituality be better recognized in the work that nurses do. Recognition of the spirituality inherent in nursing would deepen and refashion current frameworks of care. Reflective practice is a means of clarifying the boundaries and shared territories of nursing and spirituality. Only in reflection can boundaries be defined, debated, and redrawn. Reflection can take many forms; it can be meditative, collegial, casual, or academic. It can be expressed verbally, poetically, in art, or in formal presentations. Reflection on nursing care is the flip side of the practice of nursing care. Both sides are required to make a whole. Methods of reflection must be emphasized in the educational preparation of new nurses and in the continuing education of practicing nurses. When better methodologies for reflection are defined and integrated into practice, the spirituality of nursing, often hidden, will emerge.

Nursing Education

Although nurses integrate knowledge from many disciplines, theology and religion are usually not included. Nurses would benefit from courses that explore the intersections of nursing with theology, spirituality, and religious studies. Theology is of value to nursing practice in its potential to foster a better understanding of the relationship between faith and healing. Theology provides a way of knowing that is different from the scientific method and is based upon reflection on experience, meditation, and thoughtful consideration of wisdom traditions. Understanding ways in which healing has been envisioned and addressed by various religions over time would not only help nurses provide culturally competent care, it would also stimulate new thoughts on healing modalities and a fuller understanding of the human person. The study of theology and religion might also prepare the way for more reflective practice by suggesting methods of contemplation, attention, and silence.

CONCLUSION

The nursing profession stands at a juncture. Two roads can be seen: one leads to continued expertise in the management of technology, pharmaceuticals, and diagnostic and treatment modalities to improve patient care, the other turns back to reclaim the life-giving spiritual foundations of nursing, which are often at odds with the technological imperatives of health care. If nursing and spirituality are to resume their partnership, neither road will do. Nurses have come too far to turn back and their tradition is too rich to leave behind. So, a new way must be found. A renewed partnership between spirituality and nursing is not a matter of incorporating spirituality into nursing's existing paradigms, nor would the advances in science and technology fit into Nightingale's models of spirituality or the practice of "careful nursing" by the early Irish nurses. The new way requires that spirituality be better recognized in the work that contemporary nurses do. Recognition of the inherent spirituality of nursing will shed new light on the current paradigms of practice, transforming them. What has been hidden will emerge, and once it emerges, nursing practice will be made whole. Nursing and spirituality will once again become partners through the process of reflective practice. Unless nurses' understanding of nursing includes what is known scientifically and what is known through the revelation of caring for others, healing will not be advanced. The challenge of the 21st century rests in finding a way that allows spirituality to form a new and transforming relationship with nursing science and technology so that nursing spirituality will not simply be an intervention, but rather the very root and source of the practice itself. T.S. Eliot (1942) wrote that we shall not cease from exploration, and the end of all our exploring will be to arrive where we started and know the place for the first time. So it is in reflecting on spirituality in nursing, to undertake its discovery in our practice, is to celebrate what has always been there as source, sustenance, and inspiration, to see the daily seemingly ordinary tasks of caring as the work of creating a better world.

REFERENCES

Ashley, J. A. (1997). Myths and realities of apprenticeship in nursing. In K. A. Wolf (Ed.), *Jo Ann Ashley. Selected readings* (pp. 217–233). New York: NLN Press.

Baldacchino, D., & Draper, P. (2001). Spiritual coping strategies: A review of the nursing research literature. *Journal of Advanced Nursing, 34*(6), 833–841.

Benson, H. (1996). *Timeless healing. The power and biology of belief.* New York: Scribner Publishers.

Brush, B. L., & Daly, P. R. (2000). Assessing spirituality in primary care practice: Is there time? *Clinical Excellence for Nurse Practitioners, 4*(2), 67–71.

Eliot, T. S. (1942). *Four Quartets.* New York: Harcourt Brace.

Freire, P. (1999). *Pedagogy of the oppressed* (M. Bergman Ramos, Trans.). New York: The Continuum Publishing Co. (Original work published in 1970).

Goddard, N. C. (1995). Spirituality as integrative energy: A philosophical analysis as requisite precursor to holistic nursing practice. *Journal of Advanced Nursing, 22*(4), 808–815.

Goizueta, R. S. (1995). *Caminemos con Jesus. Toward a Hispanic/Latino theology of accompaniment.* New York: Maryknoll.

Greasley, P., Chiu, L. F., & Gartland, M. (2001). The concept of spiritual care in mental health nursing. *Journal of Advanced Nursing, 33*(5), 629–637.

Haase, J. E., Britt, T., Coward, D. D., Leidy, N. K., & Penn, P. E. (1992). Simultaneous concept analysis of spiritual perspective, hope, acceptance, and self-transcendence. *Image: the Journal of Nursing Scholarship, 24*, 141–147.

Havel, V. (1990). *Disturbing the peace* (P. Wilson, Trans.). New York: Random House. (Original work published in 1986).

Macrae, J. A. (1995). Nightingale's spiritual philosophy and it significance for modern nursing. *Image: Journal of Nursing Scholarship, 27*(1), 8–10.

Macrae, J. A. (1996). Florence Nightingale's spirituality. Paper presented at Harvard University Continuing Medical Education Program, *Spirituality and Healing*, Boston, MA.

Macrae, J. A. (2001). *Nursing as spiritual practice: A contemporary application of Florence Nightingale's views.* New York: Springer Publishing Co.

Meehan, T. C. (2003). Careful nursing: A model for contemporary nursing practice. *Journal of Advanced Nursing, 44*(1), 99–107.

Noddings, N. (1984). *Caring: A feminine approach to ethics and moral education.* Los Angeles: University of California Press.

Remen, R. N. (1996). *Kitchen table wisdom: Stories that heal.* New York: Riverhead Books.

Rolheiser, R. (1999). *The holy longing.* New York: Doubleday.

Tinder, G. (1999). *The fabric of hope. An essay.* Grand Rapids, MI: William B. Eerdmans Publishing Co.

Webb, V. (2002). *Florence Nightingale: The making of a radical theologian.* St. Louis, MO: Chalice Press.

Wright, K. B. (1998). Professional, ethical, and legal implications for spiritual care in nursing. *Image: The Journal of Nursing Scholarship, 30*(1), 81–83.

Wuthnow, R. (1999). *After heaven: Spirituality in America since the 1950s*. Los Angeles: University of California Press.

Younger, J. B. (1995). The alienation of the sufferer. *Advances in Nursing Science, 17*(4), 53–72.

C H A P T E R   3 6

Nursing as a Context for Alternative/Complementary Modalities

Noreen Cavan Frisch

NURSING AS A FRAMEWORK FOR ALTERNATIVE/COMPLEMENTARY MODALITIES

With nationwide interest in complementary health care, nurses have actively incorporated alternative/integrative modalities into their practice. Registered Nurses regularly attend continuing educational sessions on techniques such as acupressure, guided imagery, humor, massage, meditation, and therapeutic touch/healing touch. Review of continuing educational offerings advertised in holistic nursing newsletters and websites indicates that many nurses learn these techniques in sessions alongside other healthcare providers and are taught by non-nurses. In such situations, nurses may raise questions related to their legal scope of practice and the use of alternative/complementary modalities within professional nursing. When these techniques are taught by and practiced by individuals who are not nurses as well as by nurses, questions such as, "May a nurse practice guided imagery as an RN?" "May a nurse perform simple massage or therapeutic massage?" and "May a nurse practice therapeutic touch (TT) as a private, independent professional?" become critically important and not easily answered. While the practice of nursing is regulated by each state, ability to bring alternative/complementary modalities into a nursing context assists in defining the practice as part of professional nursing. When operating from a nursing perspective, nurses recognize that the ability to perform and use these techniques can be greatly enhanced when they integrate these techniques into the context of professional nursing. The purposes of this paper are to explore how a professional nursing context provides a discipline-specific direction to the practice of complementary/alternative modalities by adding qualities of assessment, reflection, and holism to the performance of the techniques, and to provide examples for nurses to incorporate alternative/complementary practices into care that is clearly identified as professional nursing.

Source: Frisch, N. (May 31, 2001). *Nursing as a Context for Alternative/Complementary Modalities.* Online Journal of Nursing. Vol. 6, No. 2, manuscript 2. Available: http://www.nursingworld.org/ojin/topic15/tpc15_2.htm. © 2001, Online Journal of Issues in Nursing. Article published May 31, 2001. Reprinted with permission.

ALTERNATIVE/COMPLEMENTARY MODALITIES

Alternative/Complementary modalities have been defined as treatment techniques whose goals are to evoke healing, taking into account the body–mind–spirit connection of every individual (Dossey, 1995). The use of the word 'alternative' became popular in the 1990s when holistic medicine was considered a new or emerging field. Then, 'alternative' medicine meant practices and healing techniques that were not generally taught in medical schools (Eisenberg et al., 1993), thus, alternative to the prevailing view.

The establishment and naming of the National Institutes of Health (NIH) Office of Alternative Medicine in 1992 reflected this definition. Over time, however, it became clear that such a definition was inadequate because many of the modalities were brought into medical school curricula, were taught as legitimate methods of care, and were incorporated in medical practice (Wetzel, Eisenberg, & Kaptchuk, 1998). Further, the use of the word 'alternative' implied that certain techniques were used instead of recommended biomedical treatments. The word 'complementary' gained popularity in the field, conveying the idea that the modalities or techniques could be used to complement and enhance the biomedical treatments. Thus, the branch of practice was renamed 'CAM,' complementary and alternative medicine, and when the NIH office was elevated to a center, it was also renamed as the National Center for Complementary and Alternative Medicine (NCCAM) (http://nccam.nih.gov). According to the current NCCAM factsheet, CAM refers to healing philosophies and approaches that Western medicine does not commonly use, accept, study, understand, or make available (NCCAM, 2001).

Many have implied that alternative care means holistic care; however, that notion has been justly criticized on the grounds that holism is defined more by the context of the care than by the actual treatment techniques employed (Saks, 1997).

Nursing, however, is an holistic approach at its essence. Review of every nursing theory in use today indicates that each of the theories define nursing by taking into account the whole person (George, 1995). Likely, it is because nursing is an holistic discipline that nurses have demonstrated great enthusiasm for the techniques and modalities associated with the field of complementary and alternative care as these techniques assist nurses to address the physical, mental, emotional, and spiritual dimensions of care. A study conducted in 1996 of nurses who defined themselves as 'holistic nurses' ($N = 708$) revealed that a majority of them defined their practice in relation to alternative/complementary modalities (Dossey, Frisch, Forker, & Lavin, 1998). Modalities most frequently used by these study respondents were: acupressure, aromatherapy, biofeedback, guided imagery, healing presence, humor, journaling, music therapy, meditation, relaxation, and therapeutic touch/healing touch.

For the purposes of this paper, alternative/complementary modalities refers to the techniques such as those listed above and practiced by nurses for the purpose of enhancing client healing. All of these techniques are immediately recognized as complementary/alternative and fit under the definition of NCCAM for CAM.

THE CONTEXT FOR PROFESSIONAL NURSING

There are two ways of thinking about nursing that underpin professional nursing practice and help nurses to understand and articulate a worldview. These are the nursing theories/conceptual models for practice and the current nursing taxonomies. Each of these approaches provide a unique and discipline-specific view of care, distinct from the care of other health professionals. Thus, alternative/complementary modalities performed from within a context of a nursing theory/ model take on meaning from within the theory as the modalities become part of purposeful action to achieve goals of care prescribed from within the theoretical point of view. Modalities performed and documented according to one of the standard taxonomies explicitly bring the modalities into the domain of nursing and make the performance of the technique part of nursing activities addressing a defined phenomena of concern. Each of these frameworks and their relationship to alternative/complementary modalities will be addressed below.

Nursing Theories/Conceptual Models

Nursing theory is the foundation of professional nursing practice (George, 1995). Theory articulates a worldview, suggesting how nurses interpret practice events and think about care. Each theory addresses the concepts of nursing's metaparadigm in a different way, exploring the relationships between and among the concepts of person, health, nurse, and environment. Theory-based practice is reflective practice—nursing is both providing care and thinking about care to ensure it is consistent with stated values and principles.

Modalities incorporated into practice from within a framework of nursing theory are given meaning from within the theory. Some of the modalities are compatible with the principles and concepts of specific nursing theories. In other cases, the theories themselves provide a mandate for a specific kind of nursing intervention. Nursing theory provides the language, concepts, and worldview to reflect on nursing care and on the use of alternative/complementary modalities. Several examples from selected nursing theories are discussed below.

The first example of use of alternative/complementary modalities and nursing theory will be drawn from the Modeling and Role-Modeling Theory of Erickson, Tomlin, and Swain (1984). The concepts of "Modeling" and "Role-Modeling" are central to the theory. Modeling is the process by which the nurse develops an image of the client's world, giving the nurse the ability to understand the world from the client's perspective, and Role-Modeling occurs when the nurse plans interventions to role-model health behaviors congruent with the client's worldview (Frisch & Bowman, 1995; Erickson et al., 1998) The theory is based on adaptation and through a specific assessment of adaptive potential, the Adaptive Potential Assessment Model (APAM), the nurse is guided to assess the client's strengths, areas of positive adaptation, and state of arousal (Bowman, 1997; Erickson & Swain, 1982). Professional nursing from within this framework requires that the nurse build a *model* of the client's world and from within that model the nurse must *role-model* health behaviors to assist the client to regain/attain health. Nursing care is planned only after discussion and mutually agreed-upon goals of care.

The concept of 'modeling' guides the nurse to specific modalities. When a nurse models the client's world, the nurse attempts to enter into the client's worldview. The nurse observes the client, and adapts his/her own timing and pacing to that of the client. If the client is in a state of excitement and breathing at a rapid rate, the nurse matches his/her breathing and actions to that of the client's. If the client is in a state of exhaustion, the nurse sits, is slow in movements, and paces him/herself to match the client's level of energy. If the client expresses anxiety and a desire to feel more calm, the nurse models the anxiety and, through conscious role-modeling, demonstrates for the client a means to slow breathing rate, relax, and take control of the anxiety first at the physical level and second at the cognitive, reflective level. The modalities of progressive relaxation, imagery, guided imagery, and hypnosis are techniques that are used to carry out the concepts of modeling and role-modeling. Thus, the techniques are used within the theory, not simply as modalities to help a client relax. The techniques become methods to carry out the basic principles of professional nursing practice. As integral to the theory, these techniques permit the nurse to assess the client within a holistic perspective, reflect and use the APAM model, plan care based on level of arousal according to the theory, and evaluate outcomes according to level of arousal and ability to self-regulate these feelings. The modalities, carried out by a professional nurse, have depth that is provided by a theoretical worldview and permit a sophisticated level of assessment.

Secondly, Roy's Theory of Adaptation will be explored. Central to this theory are the concepts of focal, contextual, and residual stimuli (Roy & Andrews, 1991). The focal stimuli are the conditions immediately confronting the client, the contextual are all other stimuli present, and the residual stimuli are those beliefs, attitudes, and conditions that have an indeterminate effect on the present condition. The nurse, operating from within this framework, assesses the stimuli and takes action to promote the client's adaptation in physiologic needs, self-concept, role function, and relations of interdependence nursing health and illness. Roy states that the "nurse acts as a regulatory force to modify stimuli affecting adaptation" (1980, p. 186).

Particularly with regard to contextual stimuli, there are several alternative/complementary modalities that permit the nurse to alter the stimuli and change unhealthy or noxious environmental stimuli to ones that are either neutral or wholesome.

Music therapy and aromatherapy are specific modalities that change the environment in which the client finds him/herself and are expressly designed to change the context of care from one that is deleterious to one that is supportive. These modalities can easily be seen as nursing activities promoting positive adaptation. Music therapy is a systematic application of music to produce relaxation and desired changes in emotions, behaviors, and physiology (Guzzetta, 2000), and aromatherapy is the use of essential oils to offer symptomatic relief or to enhance a sense of well-being (Buckle, 1998; Stevenson, 1994). Used from within Roy's Adaptation Model of Nursing, these two modalities take place within the nursing process and are interventions aimed at manipulating stimuli affecting client health. Given the use of the theory, the assessment of the need for the modality becomes part of reflective, holistic nursing care, and outcomes are interpreted from within the framework of adaptation, stimuli, stress, and a specific worldview.

Thirdly, there are several nursing theories that incorporate the concept of 'human energy field,' and 'environmental energy field,' specifically Rogers' Theory of Unitary Human Beings, Newman's Theory of Expanding Consciousness, and Parse's Theory of Human Becoming (Frisch, 2000). All energy-based modalities are congruent with these theories. While Therapeutic Touch (TT) is a modality developed and researched by nurses (Kreiger, 1979; Quinn, 1988; Straneva, 2000), other energy-based modalities such as Reiki and Healing Touch techniques are widely used by and taught to non-nurses. The theoretical frameworks for techniques involving human and environmental energy fields are nursing theories and the philosophies of Eastern traditions (Slater, 2000). For nurses engaged in energy-based techniques, bringing the techniques into a worldview of nursing permits the nurse to assess and practice with the benefit of reflection on the meaning of energy exchange and its effect on creating a reality for the nurse and client.

Lastly, in relation to Jean Watson's theory of Humancare, nurses will recognize that the most important aspect of all nursing activities are those actions that promote professional, compassionate, human-to-human interaction (Watson, 2000). For the theory of Humancare, the very basis of nursing is interaction and connection between two human beings. The modality of healing presence is a significant, important technique to provide trust and support and to initiate the caring encounter necessary for nursing to take place. Healing presence is one of the modalities stated frequently by holistic nurses in the survey of modalities used in nursing practice discussed above. Watson's theory elevates the importance of this nursing action to its rightful state in care—it is the prerequisite for any professional nursing activity. From within the worldview of the theory of Humancare, a nurse will identify presence as a very necessary nursing action. Presence is often described as 'being in the moment' (Dossey, 1995), or 'being with' rather than 'doing to' (Paterson & Zderad, 1976). There are three levels of presence defined for nursing practice: physical presence (being there), psychological presence (being with), and therapeutic presence as the nurse's reflectively relating to the client as whole being to whole being using all of his or her resources— body, mind, emotion, and spirit (McGivergin & Daubenmire, 1994). It is the final level, that of therapeutic presence, that fits best with the notion of Humancare. While many do not consciously think about healing presence as a modality, it requires skills of centering, openness, and intuition to employ for the good of client care. The theory of Humancare reminds nurses that healing presence *is* indeed a modality and one that has not received sufficient attention, development, and research as would be assumed, given how fundamental it is to the discipline.

Through examples from four distinct nursing theoretical frameworks, several complementary/ alternative modalities have been discussed as appropriate to incorporate into professional nursing. If one accepts the ideas that (1) professional nursing is based on theory and (2) that theory-based practice is reflective practice, the use of the modalities within theory becomes thoughtful and are considered as a means to understand and interpret a nurse's actions. Nursing theory provides a means to understand modalities and permits nurses to assess and incorporate new aspects of care into a larger, more holistic, and very professional, worldview.

Nursing Taxonomies of Nursing Practice

Taxonomies of nursing practice are the classification systems that provide frameworks for naming and documenting the phenomena of concern of professional nursing. The most widely known and used of these taxonomies is the NANDA Classification of Nursing Diagnoses (NANDA, 2001). Originally presented to the nursing community in the 1970s, the NANDA taxonomy is a statement of nursing problems and concerns. Over the years many nurses have worked within this (and other nursing diagnostic systems, for example, the Omaha and Saba systems) to identify and name all phenomena of concern to nursing. The current NANDA taxonomy lists over 150 nursing diagnoses, organized according to domains based on health patterns. Work presented at the last meeting of NANDA indicated that the nursing diagnostic taxonomy will include statements of problem, risk for problem, and opportunity or readiness to enhance a current condition (Jones et al., 2000). Thus, the current taxonomy of diagnoses presents a statement of conditions (both problems and opportunities to promote/enhance wellness) that have been identified by nurses as within the autonomous domain of nursing.

Newer taxonomies for nursing include the Nursing Interventions Classification (NIC), now in its third edition (McCloskey & Bulechek, 2000), and the Nursing Outcomes Classification (NOC), now in its second edition (Johnson, Maas, & Moorhead, 2000). These taxonomies list nursing activities that have been identified by nurses as actions they perform on behalf of patients/clients while providing direct and/or indirect care and measurable, core outcomes that are sensitive to nursing interventions. Taken together, the NANDA, NIC, and NOC provide as comprehensive a list as is available of the concerns, actions, and expected outcomes of nursing practice. These lists are remarkably useful for nurses using complementary/alternative modalities in practice.

Complementary modalities may be used by nurses and non-nurses alike; however, when used as part of nursing practice, the care should be documented in a nursing context.

While some modalities require additional certification and/or licensure in some states, (for example, massage therapy), most of the modalities used by nurses require a nursing license and documentation that makes clear that the care provided is within the scope of professional nursing practice. When a complementary/alternative modality is used to address a concern identified as a nursing diagnosis, the action becomes an identified nursing intervention planned to address/ remedy a nursing problem or concern. For example, when music therapy is provided to assist individuals obtain adequate sleep, the NANDA diagnosis of *disturbed sleep pattern* is the identified nursing problem and the intervention "*music therapy* as provided through tape recorded music at times of wakefulness" is a nursing intervention identified by the nursing community as within the domain of professional nurses. Likewise, when the nursing problem is *fear* related to undergoing medical diagnostic procedures (such as an MRI), and the nursing intervention is "*guided imagery* to assist the client with relaxation and distraction during the procedure," the problem, intervention, and outcome can be documented from within the taxonomic frameworks as nursing. To provide an example of a wellness-oriented nursing concern, when the nursing concern is *readiness to enhance spiritual well-being* related to a time in life when a client is examining his personal beliefs, values, and sense of future, the nursing intervention "*meditation facilitation* to focus awareness on an image or thought and to find a place of inner peace" is being used to address an identified nursing concern. A last example is the use of the intervention *Therapeutic Touch (TT)* as a technique to assist the client experiencing *impaired comfort related to severe itching*. The technique is being used to provide a nonpharmacologic treatment of a condition affecting the client's comfort and well-being. In each of these cases, the nursing activity is a complementary/alternative modality (music therapy, guided imagery, meditation, TT). Practice within the nursing context emphasizes that the modality is being used to address the human response to actual/potential health problems. Table 36.1 provides a summary of selected nursing diagnoses and interventions to indicate possible pairings of nursing concerns and actions.

When documented from a nursing framework, the nurse is making it clear that the modality is being used to address an issue that has been accepted by the nursing community as within the domain of nursing and within the phenomena of concern to professional nurses. Nurses documenting practice using these systems are accomplishing three important things: appropriate documentation of care, identification of work as within the scope of professional nursing, and building a body of knowledge for nurses on the use of specific interventions.

The taxonomies provide both a framework that helps nurses think in a holistic manner about what they are doing as nurses and increased justification for having a nurse perform the activities. The taxonomies themselves are atheoretical, meaning that they are not grounded in any of the nursing theories, they are simply a list of diagnoses, interventions, and outcomes. These diagnoses, interventions, and outcomes, however, can be used with nursing theory to guide the reflective interpretation of client conditions and selection of appropriate nursing interventions. Within the framework of nursing taxonomies, the alternative/complementary modalities become part of the nursing process—the documentation of nursing assessments, concerns, interventions, and outcomes.

Table 36.1 Selected Nursing Diagnoses and Nursing Interventions: Possible Pairings of Nursing Concerns and Complementary/Alternative Interventions

Nursing Diagnosis/Concern	Nursing Intervention(s)	Rationale
Impaired comfort	Acupressure, TT	To decrease perceived pain
Disturbed sleep pattern	Massage	To promote relaxation, rest
Social isolation	Animal-assisted therapy	To provide affection
Impaired coping	Humor	To facilitate appreciation of that which is funny, to relieve tensions
Hopelessness	Hope instillation	To promote a positive sense of the future
Spiritual distress	Spiritual support	To facilitate a sense of inner peace
Spiritual well-being	Spiritual growth facilitation	To support growth/reflection reexamination of values
Anxiety or fear	Guided imagery, relaxation therapy, biofeedback, calming techniques	To reduce sense of anxiety
Impaired communication	Art therapy	To facilitate expression

DISCUSSION

Alternative/complementary modalities are techniques used in healthcare practice to help clients achieve specific outcomes. Techniques, however, are just techniques, and can be used at the level of "doing things" without the reflection, thought, or interpersonal exchange required of and expected from professional nursing. Nurses are in an excellent position to adopt complementary/alternative modalities into practice that address assessed client needs and to use these techniques to achieve the goals of nursing. Use of theory and nursing classification systems help nurses use these complementary/alternative modalities professionally. Documentation of these techniques through either nursing theory or current nursing taxonomies makes the practice explicitly that of professional nursing. Care directed by nursing theory and/or care according to a standard nursing taxonomy is care that is generally regarded by the profession as within the domain of nursing. Thus, documentation of care from a nursing framework provides for practice which is recognizable as nursing and legally defensible as within nursing's scope of practice. Additionally, using modalities within nursing practice gives nurses an enhanced set of tools for practice—making the practice professional, whole, and client-centered.

REFERENCES

Bowman, S. (1997). *The APAM model: Flow chart.* Arcata, CA: Humboldt State University.

Buckle, J. (1998). Alternative/complementary therapies. Clinical aromatherapy and touch: complementary therapies for nursing practice. *Critical Care Nurse, 18*(5), 54–61.

Dossey, B. (1995). Holistic nursing practice. In B. Dossey, L. Keegan, & C. Guzzetta (Eds.), *Holistic Nursing: A Handbook for Practice* (3rd ed.) (pp. 5–25). Gaithersberg, MD: Aspen Publishers.

Dossey, B., Frisch, N., Forker, J., & Lavin, J. (1998). Evolving a blueprint for certification. *Journal of Holistic Nursing, 16*(1), 33–55.

Eisenberg, D. M., Kesler, R. C., Foster, C., Nortack, F. E., Calkins, D. R., & Delbanco, T. L. (1993). Unconventional medicine in the United States: Prevelence, costs, and patterns of use. *New England Journal of Medicine, 328*(supp), S246–S252.

Erickson, H. C., & Swain, M. A. (1982). A model for assessing potential adaptation to stress. *Research in Nursing and Health, 5,* 93–101.

Erickson, H. C., Tomlin, E., & Swain, M. W. (1984). *Modeling and Role-Modeling: A Theory and Paradigm for Nursing.* Lexington, SC: Pine Press.

Erickson, M. E., Caldwell-Gwin, J. A., Carr, L. A., Hamon, B. K., Hartman, K., Jarlsberg, C. R., Mc-Cormick, J., & Noone, K. W. (1998). Helen C. Erickson, Evelyn, M. Tomlin, Mary Ann Swain: Modeling and Role-Modeling. In A. Marriner Tomey & M. R. Alaligood (Eds.), *Nursing Theorists and Their Work* (4th ed.) (pp. 387–406). St. Louis: Mosby.

Frisch, N. (2000). Nursing theory in holistic nursing practice. In B. Dossey, L. Keegan, & C. Guzzetta (Eds.), *Holistic Nursing: A Handbook for Practice* (3rd ed.) (pp. 173–183). Gaithersburg, MD: Aspen Publishers.

Frisch, N., & Bowman, B. (1995). Helen C. Erickson, Evelyn M. Tomlin, & Mary Ann P. Swain. In J. George (Ed.), *Nursing Theories: The Base for Professional Practice* (4th ed.) (pp. 355–372). Norwalk, CT: Appleton & Lange.

George, J. (1995). *Nursing Theory: The Base for Professional Practice.* Stamford, CT: Appleton & Lange.

Guzzetta, C. (2000). Music therapy: Healing the melody of the soul. In B. Dossey, L. Keegan, & C. Guzzetta (Eds.), *Holistic Nursing: A Handbook for Practice* (3rd ed.) (pp. 585–610). Gaithersberg, MD: Aspen Publishers.

Johnson, M., Maas, M., & Moorhead, S. (2000). *Nursing Outcomes Classification (NOC)* (2nd ed.) St. Louis: Mosby.

Jones, D., Frisch, N., Gordon, M., Lunney, M., Krainovich-Miller, B., Stevenson, J., & Berry, D. (2000). White Paper: *Health promotion and wellness diagnosis.* Presented at the biannual meetings of the North American Nursing Diagnosis Association.

Krieger, D. (1979). *Therapeutic Touch: Using Your Hands to Help and to Heal.* New York: Prentice Hall.

McClosky, J. C., & Bulichek, G. M. (2000). *Nursing Interventions Classifications (NIC)* (3rd ed.). St. Louis: Mosby.

McGivergin, M., & Daubenmire, J. (1994). The essence of therapeutic presence. *Journal of Holistic Nursing, 12*(1), 65–81.

NANDA. (2001). *Nursing Diagnosis: Definitions and Classification, 2001–2002.* Philadelphia: Author.

NCCAM. (2001). Frequently asked questions: What is complementary and alternative medicine? *General Complementary and Alternative Medicine (CAM) Fact Sheets.* Retrieved May 15, 2001, from http://www.nccam.nih.gov/nccam/fcp/faq/index.html.

Paterson, J. G., & Zderad, T. (1976). *Humanistic Nursing.* New York: John Wiley & Sons.

Quinn, J. (1988). Building a body of knowledge: Research on therapeutic touch 1974–1986. *Journal of Holistic Nursing, 6*(1), 37–45.

Roy, C. (1980). The Roy Adaptation Model. In J. Riehl & C. Roy (Eds.), *Conceptual Models for Nursing Practice* (2nd ed.) (pp. 179–206). New York: Appleton-Century Crofts.

Roy, C., & Andrews, H. A. (1991). *The Roy Adaptation Model: The Definitive Statement.* Stamford, CT: Appleton & Lange.

Saks, M. (1997). Alternative therapies: Are they holistic? *Complementary Therapies in Nursing and Midwifery, 3*(1), 4–8.

Slater, V. (2000). Energetic Healing. In B. Dossey, L. Keegan, & C. Guzzetta (Eds.), *Holistic Nursing: A Handbook for Practice* (3rd ed.) (pp. 125–154). Gaithersburg, MD: Aspen Publishers.

Straneva, J. A. (2000). Therapeutic Touch coming of age. *Holistic Nursing Practice, 14*(3), 1–13.

Stevenson, C. J. (1994). The physiological effects of aromatherapy massage following cardiac surgery. *Complementary Therapies in Medicine, 2*(1), 27–35.

Watson, J. (2000). *Postmodern Nursing.* London: Churchill Livingstone.

Wetzel, M. S., Eisenberg, D. M., & Kaptachuk, T. J. (1998). Courses involving complementary and alternative medicine at U.S. Medical Schools. *JAMA, 280*(9), 784–787.

CHAPTER 37

The Role of Codes of Ethics in Nursing's Disciplinary Knowledge

John G. Twomey

Since the inception of modern nursing in the 19th century, considerable thought has been paid to the moral nature of the discipline. A cursory review of the writings of early leaders such as Nightingale highlights efforts to increase the numbers of qualified applicants into nursing. Although the call for "sober, honest, truthful, trustworthy applicants" (Dossey, 2000, p. 222) was based on an emotional desire to keep the ranks of the developing discipline free from scandal, it is now more accurate to describe the ethical core of nursing as being part of its intellectual heritage.

To fully appreciate the role of moral and ethical knowledge in nursing, it is necessary to examine the evolving development of ethics within the greater domain of disciplinary nursing knowledge. This examination requires a familiarity of how a distinct nursing ethic has emerged within the greater umbrella of bioethics. This historical occurrence cannot be fully comprehended without an appreciation of how the intellectual leaders of the discipline centered this development around an informal code of ethics for the profession that eventually became formalized into the current *Code of Ethics for Nurses* (American Nurses Association, 2001). Additionally, an ongoing issue within this profession of multiple subspecialty practices is whether a single code of ethics can serve a group of professionals with multiple interests and obligations that can pose intriguing individual moral challenges.

VIEWS OF ETHICS FOR NURSING

Founders' Views

Florence Nightingale, the intellectual matriarch of modern nursing, set strict standards of behavior for the women she recruited to her radical model of care. Her "modern" concept of nursing went beyond the traditional view of nursing that was inured with the notion that personal care was limited to the intimate. Generally, such care was delivered by the family or by those in society, usually women, who were forced to provide such intimate care for pay. These circumstances often were shameful for both caregiver and patient, for it meant that either had to leave the familiar bosom of the family and seek or provide services, through pecuniary means, that should have been given, not paid for (Rothman, 1990). Not surprisingly, premodern nursing, for pay, was considered in many societies to be on par with prostitution.

Nightingale's efforts often have been portrayed as persuading society, as well as the group of women recruited to her cause, to accept a notion of women who shared a devotion of intimate caring that divorced the emotion of caring from the physical. Nightingale's best-known works emphasize her drive to merge her strong belief in the emergent 19th century principles of public health and the scientific basis that such health was founded on with an interesting insistence on behavior that married military discipline with a fervor such as one could find in contemporary religious orders (Church, 1990).

It is not surprising that most accounts of Nightingale's views on moral behavior centered on her beliefs that nurses' personal behaviors were the most important part of the ethical role. Therefore, dress, decorum, and devotion were considered within the auspices of virtue and came to be how the public perceived how a professional nurse should be judged. But recent examination of Nightingale's correspondence suggests that she struggled to reconcile her public and private personas. Nightingale's much-touted public persona as a woman who sought to consolidate nursing's position through connections with powerful men has come into question. Widerquist (1992) has challenged F. B. Smith's widely accepted characterization of Nightingale's relationships as only being based on a need for power stating, " . . . they [her relationships] resulted not in a need for power, but from her idealized need for perfection and mutuality, i.e., sympathy, a quality of fellow feeling, with others before she was able to sustain a relationship" (p. 303). This interpretation may provide some evidence that although Nightingale seemed to prefer attention to rule in her nurses, she also viewed the perfect world as one based on virtues that included a spirituality that was embedded in an ethic of nursing care.

Nightingale's views almost completely dominated the vision of professional nursing that emigrated to the United States and elsewhere. Not until well into the 20th century did nursing practice based on her methods go much beyond education and practical nursing interventions. Subsequent American nursing leaders worked with little success to move nursing into modern professional reforms, such as control of entry into practice and nursing knowledge development, during the early genesis of nursing. However, they did confront the need to go beyond the concepts of duty and service as the core values of nursing. Early prominent American nurses such as Lavinia Dock and Annie Goodrich wrote persuasively of the need for nurses to go beyond etiquette in their practice. They called for nurses to recognize that the intimate nature of their practice was a basic ethical concept, and therefore a core value that necessitated more than superficial physical care (Hamilton, 1994). Hamilton (1994) argues that these beliefs ultimately were transformed into the concepts of compassion and caring. However, before they could become the core values of modern nursing, they needed to be separated from their original interpretations of being religious values. The development of ethical knowledge in nursing continually focused on virtues as well as principles. As will be discussed, the evolution of the current *Code of Ethics for Nurses* is a reflection of this intellectual tradition.

Views on Codes of Ethics

Early nursing leaders did not believe that ethical codes were necessary for the emerging profession. As has been noted, this was not from lack of interest in nurses' behaviors. In fact, leaders' attention focused heavily on nurses' behaviors, but their dictums to both their students and nurses under their direction focused on proper behavior when providing care, not of care directed by ethics. During much of the 20th century, the result was that nursing practice was rule bound in both scientific principles and professional behaviors. This devotion to policy was less the result of proven data, but rather emerged from the inability of nursing to successfully ingrain itself in the developing healthcare system its members as leaders rather than servants (Ashley, 1976).

Codes of ethics were not a primary part of the emergent health professions in the 19th century. The Hippocratic Oath offered a list of behaviors for healers. Historically, its use was limited to those who had knowledge of foreign languages and access to books. The Nightingale Pledge (http://www.accd.edu/sac/nursing/honors.html) offered a similar listing of virtuous behaviors. Some of these behaviors would appear in future nursing codes. Nightingale had no hand in writing the Nightingale Pledge, and she herself was famously opposed to external vehicles for guiding nursing behavior, such as licensure by government agencies. Finally, the lack of ethical codes for health professions during the 19th century reflected the absence of formal collective organizations. As professional organizations gained in size and power, their role in the development of ethical codes also increased.

Early American nursing leaders did address the issue of ethical codes, but found the argument for them to be unconvincing. Lavinia Dock and Annie Goodrich argued that ethical behavior was an essence of nursing and could be found within its practice of compassion and human interaction, not slavish devotion to rules. It is not surprising that Dock, with her experience at the Henry Street Settlement House, viewed nursing as a vibrant force that was attributable to the individual care that each nurse gave to her patients (Hamilton, 1994). Goodrich also rejected a code of ethics on the grounds that it took nurses away from compassion as a means and instead directed their efforts toward etiquette (Goodrich, 1932). Presumably, Goodrich did not agree with the code of ethics espoused by Isabel Hampton Robb (1900), as it was clearly a creed of etiquette.

A CODE OF ETHICS FOR NURSING

Ethical codes reflect a range of ethical theories and guidelines. Given the versions that have been presented to nurses, it is useful to consider how those who would use them should interpret the contents of such codes. Ethical guidelines are derived from bioethics. Bioethics draw on the knowledge and processes of ethics to examine health care; as such they apply to the moral behavior of any person performing actions because he or she has chosen to be a healthcare professional. It may or may not involve patients directly. *Nursing ethics* and *medical ethics* are subsets of bioethics that apply to those in the specific professions. All bioethical codes share many similar concepts.

Metaethics—Where Theories Live

The term *metaethics* refers to ethical theories that are applicable to bioethics. Two familiar broad ethical theories that most nurses recognize include deontology and utilitarianism (Beauchamp & Childress, 2001). *Deontology* grounds the ethical value of one's actions on the value of the act itself. If an act, like truth-telling, is good as a goal itself, then not adhering to that good is unethical. Therefore, telling a lie is unethical, even if it might ultimately provide a result that most reasonable people would define as good. *Utilitarianism* states that an act should be judged on how much good it produces. Contrast this view using the prior example.

A number of theories derive some of their base concepts from deontology and utilitarianism. These theories also fit under the metaethical framework. The most commonly recognized theory of bioethics is *principled theory*. Common concepts or principles such as patient autonomy, risk of harm, or provision of benefits have their base in principled theory. For example, the principle of autonomy has its theoretical underpinning in deontological thought. This thinking holds that a primary good is the respect for personhood, therefore all patients are given respect by allowing them to make fully informed decisions about their care. Principled theory is employed when those people making bioethical decisions weigh the varied principles to assess which principle is most applicable in a particular situation. This theory, though not perfect in its ability to answer all bioethical questions, became the most applied bioethical theory in Western medical culture in the latter half of the 20th century and continues to be an important part of contemporary bioethical discourse (Evans, 2000).

Recently, other theories have ascended in their contributions to ethical discussions, particularly in nursing ethics. *Communitarianism* is a framework of ethical thought that changes the locus of moral deliberation from the individual (as in the previously discussed theories) to the group within which the decision will be made. Therefore, the patient is recast from being an autonomous individual who is an isolated decision maker to one whose existence is made meaningful by being a member of a group. According to this theory, input from group members in decision making is just as important as that from the individual patient, because group members will be affected by the decision (Beauchamp & Childress, 2001).

Caring, or *contextual*, ethics provides a framework of ethical thought that grants insights into moral decision making that is appealing to many nurses. According to the theory of caring ethics, bioethical decisions are viewed through the prism of the relationship between the caregiver and the care recipient. Decisions are looked on as a means of maintaining the interdependent bond that a provider has with the patient (Noddings, 2003). Whereas principled theories tend to emphasize patient rights, caring and communitarian theories sees the individual as existing more within a nurturing role. This caring relationship places the provider on equal footing with the patient in the decision-making process.

The metaethical level of theories provides the basic reference point for any ethical consideration. It is important to recognize that this level is often unspoken when people put forward their beliefs in a moral discussion. When someone states, "I feel that we should do this because…" he or she is saying, "I believe this is an underlying core consideration." The core often lies within a broad theory. Such beliefs can also derive from other theoretical beliefs, such as religious theories on behavior, that often share the same values, such as the importance of providing justice to people.

For metaethical theories to be relevant to practice, their concepts need to be narrowed so that they can be applied to specific situations. The process of bringing theory to practice begins at the next level of analysis: descriptive ethics.

Descriptive Ethics—Where Codes Live

The descriptive level of ethical analysis is best understood as being juxtaposed between the metaethical (theory) level and the level below it, which is referred to as *normative* ethics, which can be likened to specific rules. *Descriptive ethics* provides broad descriptions of moral behaviors that are recognizable as coming from the theoretical frameworks already discussed. However, the guidelines that come from this level often have wide latitude and can be interpreted differently by the varied decision makers who use them, particularly when those decision makers approach the frameworks from different perspectives. For instance, both the nursing and medical codes of ethics have proscriptions from abandoning patients that are interpreted differently. Physicians, who have a legacy of operating their practices as businesses, are expected to continue to care for patients under many circumstances, but are allowed to refuse to care for patients who cannot pay them. By contrast, nurses, who come from a legacy of accepting patients who are assigned to them by their employers, have an ethic that only allows them to leave the care of a patient when another nurse will substitute and provide the needed care.

Descriptive ethics interpret the broad theories into understandable language so that the professions can adapt them to their professional needs. Therefore, the principle of justice, which states that people should be given what they deserve, is represented in the first provision of the *Code of Ethics for Nurses* (ANA, 2001), which states that nursing care is delivered without regard to economic status. Obviously, this statement is open to many interpretations, and how any individual nurse will abide by it depends on the specific professional situation. Indeed, this phrase within the first provision is not elaborated on further by the accompanying Interpretive Statement, whereas other pieces of the provision are interpreted in detail.

Descriptive ethical statements are heard widely when one is in professional training through formal and informal means of acculturation. New nurses are socialized through the use of such phrases as "to preserve confidentiality," "not to harm patients," "to make sure patients make informed decisions," and other slogans. When examined, such broad sayings provide little direction for the professional, for they are generally presented without context. In the reality of everyday practice, nurses and other healthcare professionals do share information without patients' permission, sometimes do inflict some harm when doing painful procedures, and may purposely allow patients to make decisions that are not fully informed because they agree with the patients' decisions.

However, descriptive ethics are important for several reasons. They provide the professions with valuable weapons in their efforts to win the public's trust and to legitimate the professions as forces in a society's health. The use of descriptive ethics helps the professions to maintain a dynamic legacy of continuous ethical thought by leaving open the predominant theories to interpretation in ways that the professions want their members to present themselves. For example, the current 2001 ANA *Code* contains phrases that can be traced back to the original code ratified by the membership over a half century ago. The current *Code* uses ethical referents that are well recognized by society and its members to draw attention to the newer, more modern and relevant interpretations that the profession needs in the 21st century (Daly, 1999).

Ethical codes also straddle the third level of ethical analysis—normative ethics. It is important to understand how such movement across the levels of analysis works to provide flexibility for professions as they address issues in their practice.

Normative Ethics—Where Codes Are Interpreted

Normative rules dominate our private and professional lives. They are seen in many forms, from civil regulations, such as traffic laws, to rules and regulations within our work settings. Normative rules can take the form of policies that govern professional practice, such as specifying which professionals can prepare drug preparations and which ones can administer them.

Professional standards of care also can be stated in normative fashion, for example, as evidenced by clinical pathways that dictate specific action given a patient scenario.

It is not difficult to recognize the form that normative ethics takes within the healthcare setting. Specific rules that limit accessibility to patient records, policies that define how much free care will be given to indigent clients, and other written guidelines exemplify normative ethics and display how broader forms of ethics are grounded in practice. Generally, clinicians are comfortable with normative ethical rules because they are easy to understand and can be amended when it appears that contemporary patient care dictates such changes. Consider informed consent policies in today's hospitals that dictate many more points within a stay where patients are asked to give permission for different procedures. The underlying concept of autonomy has a much stricter interpretation today than a generation ago when patients rarely were approached to give consent after signing a general consent form at the admitting office.

Ethical codes are not generally written at the normative level, but because members of professions seek specific guidelines, many professions provide interpretations of the descriptive ethics that codes reflect. As illustrated later in the chapter, the ANA *Code* provides a clear example of how a profession uses its professional code and adjunct policy statements to meet the needs of its members.

The Role of Codes

The existence of ethical codes for healthcare professionals is a relatively unquestioned phenomenon in current society. A listing of one Web site index of healthcare codes contains dozens of addresses, some of them being the base moral code of a given profession or professional subgroup, others providing interpretations of the individual code (http://ethics.iit.edu/codes/health.html). However, one simply cannot accept the premise that such codes exist because each health profession has such distinct ethical positions that they need to articulate them. Instead, codes must be seen as a vehicle for the legitimacy of a health profession itself.

Any group that claims to be a profession will exhibit a number of characteristics. The most common ones are claims to (1) a distinct body of knowledge, (2) control over the entry of members into the profession, and (3) a legitimacy and accountability of the professional group as it serves the needs of the society within which it exists. The latter is represented by the profession having leaders whose main responsibility is to help create an environment in which the profession can: (1) educate its members, (2) create knowledge through research that the profession can claim and pass on to its clinicians, and (3) participate in the policy process that society uses to negotiate relationships with the professions.

The means by which a profession accomplishes these tasks is through a leadership group. The collective action and influence of professional organizations are essential to the survival and advancement of a profession. Membership in a professional organization may be voluntary or mandatory. Whether or not a majority of the members have an active bond with the leadership organization, most professional organizations share the following features:

☐ Support through membership dues
☐ Some form of acceptance by government authorities as being a legitimate voice for its members
☐ A relationship with the institutions that prepare and employ its members

□ A governance model that allows participation by its members in its decision process
□ A permanent staff that conducts the daily business of the profession

The professional group has many challenges when trying to maintain the profession's recognized legitimacy, and an ethical code is often one of the tools it employs. Whereas one might assume that a code is simply the list of directions for a given professional, examination of any professional code provides evidence that part of being a professional in that given field is to accept the values that the group espouses. For example, the third provision of the current ANA *Code* states, "The nurse promotes, advocates for, and strives to protect the health, safety, and rights of the patient." Without fully deconstructing the statement, the main goal of this statement is to focus the reader on the object of the sentence, the patient. When this statement was written, the goal of the authors, which was accepted by the professional group, was to underscore that the nursing profession was primarily responsible to its patients, not employers nor third-party payers. In a time of complex professional relationships, the one person a patient can rely on is the (registered) nurse. This is a value that the profession wants the public to see that it strongly embraces.

Thus, it is essential to recognize that the code of nursing ethics is commissioned, accepted, and owned by the professional group. It reflects not just moral values, but also the ethical face that the professional wants to present to current society.

THE ANA CODE OF ETHICS

The current code of ethics for nursing was published in 2001. The development of this version of the code began at least 6 years earlier (Daly, 1999). The code's roots are embedded in a half-century of efforts at promulgating an ethical code. Early leaders of American nursing debated the need for a code of ethics for nurses, and early versions of nursing codes of ethics were proposed but not accepted (Fowler, 1999). In 1950, a formal *Code for Nurses* was accepted by the ANA (Fowler, 1992). During the next quarter century, this code was modified several times. For example, the ideas of etiquette and loyalty evolved over time into more professional concepts of professional autonomy and accountability (Scanlon & Glover, 1995). The code was again revised in 1969, and minor revisions occurred in 1976 and 1985 (Daly, 1999).

In 1995, the ANA called together a group of prominent nurse ethicists and asked them whether the 1985 version of the code needed further revision. When they replied affirmatively, the association appointed a Task Force of practicing and academic nurses to do a total revision of the *Code* (Daly, 1999). The group convened in 1997, and by the time Task Force was done and the current *Code* was accepted by the House of Delegates of the ANA in 2001, the *Code* had a new title and the 11 provisions of the 1985 *Code* had been reduced to 9. The Preface and the Interpretive Statements had all been rewritten, and an Afterword was added. The Task Force not only debated and rewrote multiple iterations of the new *Code*, but at every stage input was sought from interested parties, such as the state associations that make up the federal structure of the ANA, prominent nurse leaders in nursing education and practice, as well as subspecialty nursing organizations outside the ANA.

At one point, the adoption of the new *Code* was held up by debate and politics within the organization's House of Delegates. A temporary roadblock was generated by a deep schism between the state groups that formed this governance group over issues that the new *Code* addressed, particularly the role of the nurse in collective actions within employment settings. This dispute caused the *Code* to be sent back to the Task Force for further revision. As evidenced by this example, codes of ethics reflect more than the moral beliefs of the profession; they also are seen as powerful vehicles for professing the values of the profession—which are not always unanimous amongst the members of a given group.

Reading the Code

When anyone, nurse or layperson, reads the ANA *Code*, it is necessary to remember that it is a descriptive ethical document. This code is not unlike many other professional codes in that it attempts to voice the ethics and values of the profession. All professions have to go beyond the descriptive nature of their codes. These groups get to the normative level whereby their audiences can more easily understand the practicality of their code's messages in several different ways.

The ANA has long chosen to portray its ethical assertions through a three-level mechanism. The first level is the *Code*, with its nine provisions (see Box 37.1 on page 446). If you retrieve the *Code* online or acquire a copy of the ANA *Code* booklet, then you immediately have access to the accompanying Interpretive Statements, which offer more specific information to help to bridge the gap to the normative level. Provision 3, mentioned earlier, has six interpretive statements that begin to detail that the services that nurses provide to their patients include protection of sensitive information (3.1, 3.2) and extend to safeguarding the patient from impaired colleagues (3.6). If one reads any of those Interpretive Statements, it is clear that they are more specific than the parent provision, but that there is still a lot of latitude and room for interpretation within them.

The ANA also has a third category of statements, which are very normative, called Position Statements. These statements are policy statements that the organization promotes in several clinical and policy areas, including the areas of ethics and human rights. For example, the Position Statement on assisted suicide (http://www.nursingworld.org/readroom/position/ethics/et-suic.htm) begins with a strong declaration that nurses should not participate in acts aimed at helping patients end their lives prematurely through any means. However, another Position Statement on pain relief (http://www.nursingworld.org/readroom/position/ethics/etpain.htm) provides support for nurses to titrate narcotic pain relief to levels that might be lethal if the express goal of the act is to relieve pain, not cause death. The message is that individual nurses will never be able to ask their professional organization to completely answer all ethical questions. What will be found within the *Code*, the Interpretive Statements, and the Position Statements are mixes of ethical theory, professional values, and discussions of the competing issues within a given topic so that nurses can apply this guidance to their specific context.

As previously stated, the 2001 *Code* consists of nine provisions. The first three provisions describe the central nursing ethic as being that of the individual nurse providing care to patients. The first provision centers on social justice; the nurse is linked with providing care in an indiscriminate fashion, no matter the economic, racial, social, or value system of the patient he or she encounters. The second provision defines fidelity as a significant value of nursing, but it makes clear in no uncertain terms that the relationship most important to nurses is that with patients. The third provision focuses on the ethical duties of the nurse and specifies that protection of the patient is a major part of nursing. To fully understand these provisions, one must go to the individual Interpretive Statements. But if one stops momentarily to look closely at these introductory provisions, evident in these three statements of just 75 words, the professional organization puts forth a clear and cogent statement of philosophy. Nurses act without reflecting on the nature of their patient, they protect the patient, and, most importantly, they center their actions around a relational ethic that harkens back to the original nursing value of caring, which does not reduce the patient to just a body with an illness, but views the patient as a holistic being with complex needs that nurses can address (Bishop & Scudder, 1990).

The first three provisions also perform another task for the nursing profession. The 2001 *Code* is another step in the development of nursing's value system, particularly its beliefs about its own moral self. Earlier codes, formal and informal, moved from etiquette to duty. The emphases of such duties often were toward supposed colleagues, particularly physicians, who were actually superiors, if not employers. As social values changed, nursing's attention turned to values such as racial justice, and it shifted its loyalties in directions that allowed its members to focus on the objects of their care, the patient. The value of duty evolved into the concept of advocacy for the patient. But as bioethical views of the nurse–patient relationship moved away from the paternalism of the past, advocacy had to be modified. So a reading of the Interpretive Statements accompanying the first three provisions now holds language that emphasizes that coequal relationship between nurses and their patients. For example, Interpretive Statements 1.1 through 1.5 focus on issues of human dignity and describe the topic as accommodating issues as specific as pain relief and end-of-life care to such general issues as self-determination. Interpretive Statement 1.5 also notes that such respect extends to relations between all professionals, therefore placing nurses alongside all health colleagues in mutually supporting roles. This theme continues in Interpretive Statements 2.1 through 2.4. These statements play off the Provision's broad dictum that the nurse primarily serves the patient by recognizing that a practicing clinician has many claims to his or her time. The statements discuss how to identify and work with possible conflicts of interest and very pointedly note that any party to an ethical problem involving the nurse must have an equitable voice in a proposed solution.

Provision 3 reflects the historical threads that have made up the fabric of the ANA's ethical codes over the years. Over the years, many strong statements about confidentiality have been made at the Provision level. The Task Force working on the 2001 *Code* decided that many patient rights deserved the same level of protection as patient information, and Provision 3 addresses the need for nurses to also help to protect the autonomy of subjects in research as well as actively shield patients from impaired professionals or improper practice. Interpretive Statement 3.5 is the longest of the Interpretive Statements; it lays out a clear duty for the nurse to be a whistleblower, despite the acknowledged risks that acting in such a role places the nurse. This Interpretive Statement is written in such normative language that it could stand alone as a position statement on this topic.

In Provisions 4, 5, and 6, the *Code* shifts a bit as it addresses the nurse as a moral agent who has responsibilities of duty that provide good care in ways that go beyond direct patient care but that are truly within the venue of the profession. Provision 4 is very simple: Nursing care is delivered by nurses, and only nurses are responsible for nursing care that is delivered, even if that care comes from someone else. Anyone with the faintest familiarity with the history of professionalism in nursing knows that the profession has struggled to control a crucial piece of its discipline, that of entry into practice. The result is that not only are there multiple pathways of entry to the status of a registered nurse, much nursing care is and has been given by nonregistered nurses. All four of the Interpretive Statements in Provision 4 directly state that the ANA claims responsibility for maintaining the professional and ethical standards that define good nursing practice. In response to calls by other allied medical groups to be involved in providing semi-professional nursing care, Interpretive Statement 4.4 directly notes that nursing responsibilities can never be delegated, only specific nursing tasks, and only nurses can do that delegating. The ultimate responsibility for any nursing care is always owned by the nurses involved in that care, including those nurse administrators who provide the setting where care is given.

Provision 5 is a new and unique addition. For the first time in an *ANA Code of Ethics*, a statement that the individual nurse has moral worth is proclaimed in a provision. This represents the progression of nursing values through the years and shows that the profession feels comfortable in its development as a scientific discipline. As such, the profession can now more forthrightly assert its humanistic values, not just vis-à-vis the patient, but also as a part of the individual nurse's devotion to the profession, harkening back to the values of nursing's early leaders.

Provision 6 continues this theme of the nurse's responsibility for establishing the proper ethical milieu for the delivery of care, but what happens in this provision is evidence of the moral maturation of modern nursing, as the profession claims once and for all that nurses are not beholden to any other group to prepare the environment where they provide care nor will they take an ethical back seat to any profession in the overall moral milieu of the healthcare setting. A subtle shift occurs within Provision 6. Whereas the focus earlier in the *Code* is on the individual nurse, this provision begins to assign the broader responsibilities that the professional group wishes to claim. Although all of the first eight Provisions begin with the statement "The nurse . . . ," the latter part of the *Code* focuses more on the profession of nursing and the relationship of the individual nurse to the discipline.

The Interpretive Statements within Provision 6 begin to discuss the duties of the nurse that are not directly patient centered. Interpretive Statements 6.1 and 6.2 reiterate that the central virtues of the nursing profession cannot be imparted by the individual nurse without support. Therefore, the *Code* now addresses how the nursing profession must provide assistance to the nurse in ways that allow the nurse to practice in an ethically appropriate manner. The *Code* also makes it clear that the verb "to nurse" applies to the relationship of any nurse in any working relationship. So the nurse educators have duties to their students just as nurse administrators have responsibilities to the staff nurses under their authority. Consequently, staff nurses on a chronically understaffed unit have a moral responsibility to provide care that meets acceptable professional and ethical standards. If the usual pattern of care on the unit does not meet these standards, then the nurse administrator has at least equal responsibility to change the situation so that patients are treated safely and with respect.

Interpretive Statement 6.3 represents probably the most contentious issue that the profession currently faces. The topic of collective action rights and the role of the ANA in assisting nurses who choose to exercise those rights has rent the fabric of the professional organization within the past decade. Professional nurses have claimed the right to collective bargaining for over a half-century, with the ANA supporting this right by allowing each state unit to decide individually as to the level of involvement it will have in the matter. However, there is a sharp divide between those state nurses associations that reject this as a part of professional nursing and those that see it as an absolute good. This disagreement has escalated in recent years as a minority of registered nurses has come to believe that not only do nurses have a right to collective bargaining, but that professional nursing organizations should make representing nurses in collective bargaining a primary service. Despite the fact that the ANA has a stated goal and a defined subunit that addresses this issue, the disagreement over this issue has caused some state nurses associations to break away from the parent professional group and create their own group that does not accept the ANA's positions nor its code of ethics.

Therefore, Interpretive Statement 6.3 should be read as a policy statement from the ANA. It clearly supports the right to collective action and grounds that right within the duties of the registered nurse to ensure good patient care through the creation of a safe and nurturing environment as well within the right of the nurse to practice in a way so that the nurse is not continually morally degraded by having to work in substandard conditions. Between the lines is a belief that nurses deserve appropriate compensation and humane workloads. But because the definition of such terms is never clear-cut, and because the professional organization also must represent nurse executives and administrators, Provision 6.3 has language that matches the general descriptive tone of the overall *Code* and that leaves the topic of collective action somewhat understated.

The last three provisions of the *Code* should be read as disciplinary statements that continue to claim the place of nursing as a leader in healthcare policy and delivery. The profession, through the ANA, has made very determined efforts to place itself in the forefront of such efforts in the last quarter of the 20th century. Through documents such as *The Bill of Rights for Registered Nurses, Nursing's Social Policy Statement*, and the *Code*, the profession provides evidence of its leadership in providing ethical approaches to patient care (*Know Your Rights*, 2002).

Provisions 7 through 9 contain much material from past codes. Provision 7 synthesizes material from two of the provisions of the 1976 *Code* regarding nursing's duties to make ongoing contributions to the profession's body of knowledge. The Interpretive Statements of this provision try to balance the nursing profession's need for sophisticated knowledge through research and expert clinical experience without either shutting the staff nurse out of this dynamic role or by putting the onus on that same person to be "supernurse." Provision 7 reflects that the profession is moving forward and expects its members to make significant efforts toward disciplinary growth, even if by devoting oneself to personal professional growth at the bedside or just paying dues to the professional organization and attending local organizational meetings.

Provision 8 is a restatement of nursing's historical involvement in worldwide health. But the 2001 *Code* goes further and says that this commitment is made as a full partner with other health professions.

Provision 9, the final statement in the *Code*, is a self-reflective assertion that the ANA is the legitimate voice for the nation's registered nurses and that its current vehicles for portraying the face of nursing are well grounded. The three Interpretive Statements strongly declare that the association has done its job of providing a forum of debate that continues to provide a voice for the disparate viewpoints of the nation's largest group of healthcare providers. It also finishes laying out the case for the areas of interest in which nurses should have input. Interpretive Statement 9.4 stakes the claim that the professional organization rightfully speaks from valid nursing disciplinary interests when it engages in activities such as lobbying for changes in laws that affect patient health, such as domestic violence laws.

In summary, the *Code of Ethics for Nurses* is best read as a descriptive document that provides basic guidelines for ethical conduct of nurses engaged in patient care and professional growth. Its equal purpose, like that of other professional ethical codes, is to lay the groundwork for a claim to legitimacy for the profession as a respected group with equal moral standing within the nation's healthcare workforce.

Box 37.1 ANA Code of Ethics

The ANA House of Delegates approved these nine provisions of the new *Code of Ethics for Nurses* at its June 30, 2001 meeting in Washington, D.C. In July, 2001 the Congress of Nursing Practice and Economics voted to accepted the new language of the Interpretive Statements resulting in a fully approved revised *Code of Ethics for Nurses with Interpretive Statements.*

1. The nurse, in all professional relationships, practices with compassion and respect for the inherent dignity, worth and uniqueness of every individual, uniqueness of every individual, unrestricted by considerations of social or economic status, personal attributes, or the nature of health problems.
2. The nurse's primary commitment is to the patient, whether an individual, family, group, or community.
3. The nurse promotes, advocates for, and strives to protect the health, safety, and rights of the patient.
4. The nurse is responsible and accountable for individual nursing practice and determines the appropriate delegation of tasks consistent with the nurse's obligation to provide optimum patient care.
5. The nurse owes the same duties to self as to others, including the responsibility to preserve integrity and safety, to maintain competence, and to continue personal and professional growth.
6. The nurse participates in establishing, maintaining, and improving healthcare environments and conditions of employment conducive to the provision of quality health care and consistent with the values of the profession through individual and collective action.
7. The nurse participates in the advancement of the profession through contributions to practice, education, administration, and knowledge development.
8. The nurse collaborates with other health professionals and the public in promoting community, national, and international efforts to meet health needs.
9. The profession of nursing, as represented by associations and their members, is responsible for articulating nursing values, for maintaining the integrity of the profession and its practice, and for shaping social policy.

Reprinted with permission from American Nurses Association, Code of Ethics for Nurses with Interpretive Statements, © 2001 nursebooks.org, American Nurses Association, Silver Spring, MD.

ALTERNATIVE CODES

A continuing question nurses must consider is the need for alternative codes of ethics within the profession. It is certainly understandable when foreign nursing groups wish to state their own views on nursing ethical standards and develop their own codes that have limited applicability to American registered nurses (e.g., the Canadian Nurses Association and the International Council of Nurses). But many subspecialty nursing organizations in the United States have considered the issue of whether a code of ethics for their group would advance their agenda as well as the welfare of the patients they serve (Peterson & Potter, 2004).

It is debatable whether specialized registered nurses experience ethical issues differently than their colleagues in other areas. In a series of surveys across several nursing specializations, reports from nurses in different clinical specialties did not reflect striking differences between the ethical issues they experienced or how they were resolved. Instead, any differences could be predicted by the type of practice setting (Redman & Fry 1996, 1998a, 1998b). For example, pediatric nurses were concerned about child abuse (Butz, Redman, Fry, & Kolodner, 1998), whereas dialysis nurses reported the topic of ending treatment as a common ethical issue (Redman, Hill, & Fry, 1997).

Where specialty codes may have some contribution to an increased moral climate is when the descriptive level of the proposed code is minimized and the normative guidance to the specialty group and its outside audience is pronounced (Scanlon & Glover, 1995; Scanlon, 2000). An example of such a pathway is the program of the International Society of Nurses in Genetics (ISONG) (2004), which periodically prepares and releases position statements on discrete ethical issues that arise because of advances in genomic knowledge and subsequent impacts on genetic nursing practice, such as in the area of access to genetics services (ISONG) (2005).

CONCLUSION

Codes of ethics for health professionals provide guidance for conduct in patient encounters and justify the discipline's role as professional purveyors of care. The current ANA *Code of Ethics* represents a much needed upgrade of the profession's moral guidelines that strongly states the group's just place as the spokesman for its members. The *Code* stakes the claim to the emergence of nursing as a scientific but humanistic health group that constantly strives to update its knowledge base and has rightfully taken its place within the nation's accepted healthcare leaders. The nursing profession, guided by the *Code of Ethics*, maintains a pursuit of excellence in practice, research, and education. This is evidenced by the accomplishments of the National Institute of Nursing Research at the National Institutes of Health, as well as the many respected colleges of nursing and magnet hospital nursing organizations.

REFERENCES

American Nurses Association (ANA). (2001). *Code of Ethics for nurses with interpretive statement*s. Washington, D.C.: American Nurses Association.

Ashley, J. (1976). *Hospitals, paternalism, and the role of the nurse.* New York: Teachers College Press.

Beauchamp, T. L., & Childress, J. F. (2001). *Principles of biomedical ethics, 5th ed.* New York: Oxford University Press.

Bishop, A. & Scudder, J. (1990). *The practical, moral, and personal sense of nursing.* New York: SUNY Press.

Butz, A. M., Redman, B. K., Fry, S. T., & Kolodner, K. K. (1998). "Ethical conflicts experienced by certified pediatric nurse practitioners in ambulatory settings." *Journal of Pediatric Health Care, 12*(4): 183–90.

Canadian Nurses Association. *Code of Ethics for Registered Nurses.* Retrieved from http://www.cna-nurses. ca/pages/ethics/ethicsframe.htm.

Center for the Study of Ethics in the Professions. *Codes of Ethic online.* Retrieved from http://www.iit. edu/department/csep/ PublicWWW/codes/health.html.

Church, O. (1990). *Nightingalism: Its use and abuse in lunacy reform and the development of nursing in psychiatric care at the turn of the century.* In V. Bullough, B. Bullogh, & M. Stanton (Eds.), Florence Nightingale and her era: A collection of new scholarship (p 229–244). NY: Garland Publ., Inc.

Daly, B. J. (1999). "Ethics. Why a new code? Code for Nurses." *American Journal of Nursing, 99*(6): 64, 66.

Dossey, B. (2000). *Florence Nightingale: Mystic, visionary and reformer.* Philadelphia: Lippincott, Williams and Wilkins.

Evans, J. H. (2000). "A sociological account of the growth of principlism." *Hastings Center Report, 30*(5): 31–8.

Fowler, M. D. (1992). A chronicle of the evolution of the Code for Nurses. *Ethical dilemmas in contemporary nursing practice.* G. B. White, American Nurses's Association: 149–54.

Fowler, M. D. (1999). "Relic or resource? The code for nurses." *American Journal of Nursing, 99*(3): 56–7.

Goodrich, A. (1932). *The social and ethical significance of nursing: A series of lectures.* New York: Macmilan Company.

Hamilton, D. (1994). "Constructing the Mind of Nursing." *Nursing History Review II:* 3–28.

International Council of Nurses. *The ICN code of ethics for nurses.* Retrieved from http://www.icn.ch/icncode.pdf.

International Society of Nurses in Genetics (ISONG) (2005). Retrieved from http://www.ISONG.org.

Know Your Rights (2003). Retrieved from http://nursingworld.org/tan/novdec02/rights.htm.

Noddings, N. (2003). *Caring: A feminine approach to ethics and moral education.* Berkely: University of California Press.

Peterson, M., & Potter, R. L. (2004). "A proposal for a code of ethics for nurse practitioners." *Journal of the American Academy of Nurse Practitioners, 16*(3): 116–124.

Redman, B. K., & Fry, S. T. (1996). "Ethical conflicts reported by registered nurse/certified diabetes educators." *The Diabetes Educator, 22*(3): 219–24.

Redman, B., & Fry, S. (1998a). "Ethical conflicts reported by rehabilitation nurses." *Rehabilitation Nursing, 26*(4): 179–184.

Redman, B. K. & Fry, S. T. (1998b). "Ethical conflicts reported by registered certified diabetes educators: A replication." *Journal of Advanced Nursing, 28*(6): 1320–25.

Redman, B. K., Hill, M. A., & Fry, S. T. (1997). "Ethical conflicts reported by certified nephrology nurses (CNNs) practicing in dialysis settings." *American Nephrology Nurses Association Journal, 24*(1): 23–33.

Robb, I. H. (1900). *Nursing ethics for hospitals and private use.* Cleveland: E. D. Kloeckert Publishing.

Rothman, D. J. (1990). *The discovery of the asylum: Social order and disorder in the new republic, Rev. ed.* Boston: Little, Brown.

Scanlon, C. (2000). "A professional code of ethics provides guidance for genetic nusing practice. Material reprinted from this code with kind permission of American Nurses Publishing of the American Nurses Foundation/Association." *Nursing Ethics, 7*(3): 262–86.

Scanlon, C., & Glover, J. (1995). "A professional code of ethics: Providing a moral compass for turbulent times." *Oncology Nursing Forum, 22*(10): 1515–21.

Widerquist, J. G. (1990). Dearest Rev'd Mother. In Bullough, V., Bullough, B., & Stanton, M. (Eds.). *Florence Nightingale and her era. A collection of new scholarship*, p 288–308, NY: Garland Publ., Inc.

CHAPTER 38

Contributions of the Professional, Public, and Private Sectors in Promoting Patient Safety

Evelyn D. Quigley

Patient safety has become a national priority. The purpose of this article is to discuss the contributions of the professional, public, and private sectors regarding patient safety and to explore options in creating improved systems for this pressing issue. With the increased complexity of the healthcare system, workforce shortages, decreased reimbursement, and more demand for services, the imperative to find solutions for safer care is even more urgent. The pace of work has increased considerably, along with greater interdependence among healthcare professionals and in the various healthcare settings. This interdependent relationship calls for more frequent transfer of care from one professional to another, presenting frequent occasions for system failure and communication breakdown.

Additionally, due to the lack of integrated technology and appropriate decision support applications, steps to identify and reduce medical errors in healthcare have been impeded. Since the traditional reporting practice of healthcare settings has been to report one incident at a time, errors have been treated as singular incidents without regard to the frequency or intensity of impact. Due to malpractice and confidentiality concerns, the healthcare industry acknowledges that errors are generally underreported. Based on the unique response of individuals to medical treatment, medical errors can be difficult to recognize.

Strategies to create a safe care environment are being advanced from the professional, public, and private sectors. New safety standards will push healthcare institutions to be proactive rather than reactive in identifying and preventing potential sources of patient risk. How do healthcare organizations assist patients, families, and clinicians to deal with errors, failures, and accidents that result in harm? How do healthcare leaders cope with advocating open disclosure about errors and accidents in an industry that experiences negative publicity and high exposure to legal liability? An exploration of the contributions of various diverse constituencies will be conducted in pursuit of the potential for greater interaction with one another.

Source: Promoting Patient Safety. Online Journal of Issues in Nursing. Vol. 8, No. 3, manuscript 1. Available: www.nursing world.org/ojin/topic22/tpc22_htm. © 2003, Online Journal of Issues in Nursing. Article published September 30, 2003. Reprinted with permission.

RESPONSES BY PROFESSIONAL ASSOCIATIONS

American Nurses Association Response

While nursing has had patient safety as a primary focus, a coordinated and comprehensive system for patient safety has not existed. Various organizations have drawn attention to the need for the development and support of an integrated and comprehensive system that identifies and manages medical errors and rewards healthcare systems for positive outcomes. It was the American Nurses Association (ANA) Board of Directors that instituted the Nursing's Safety & Quality Initiative in 1994 (ANA, 1999). Given the fact that considerable restructuring was occurring in the healthcare industry, this multiphase initiative gave direction to the study of the impact of these changes on safety and quality of patient care as well as nursing. Numerous projects were launched from the investigation. Key focus was placed on educating registered nurses about "quality measurement, informing the public and purchasing/ regulating constituencies about safe, quality healthcare, and investigating research methods and data sources to empirically evaluate the safety and quality of patient care" (ANA, 1999, p. 1).

Of primary importance was the creation of a National Database of Nursing-Sensitive Quality Indicators (NDNQI). ANA defined nursing-sensitive quality indicators as "those indicators that capture care or its outcomes most affected by nursing care" (ANA, 1999, p. 4). In 1998, ANA funded the development of the national database for the nursing-sensitive quality indicators. The database was located at the Midwest Research Institute (MRI) in Kansas City, Missouri. The MRI and the University of Kansas School of Nursing jointly managed the database. The purpose of the NDNQI was to "promote and facilitate the standardization of information submitted by hospitals across the United States on nursing quality and patient outcomes" (ANA, 1999, p. 8). Hospitals have used the results from the database to make internal comparisons of their nursing quality and patient outcomes while also making comparisons of their performance with like organizations. Because healthcare organizations accredited by the Joint Accreditation of Healthcare Organization (JCAHO) are required to meet JCAHO 2002 staffing effectiveness standards, this database serves as an invaluable tool for nurse executives to effectively compare staffing patterns and methods with clinical outcomes (Runy, 2003). Presently, the NDNQI is housed at the University of Kansas School of Nursing with fiscal/legal support from the MRI and a participation of over 347 hospitals in 48 states and the District of Columbia.

Current studies validate the link between nurse staffing and outcomes of patient care. Aiken, Sean, Sloane, Sochalski, and Silber (2002) found links between high patient-to-nurse ratios, increased mortality rates among surgical patients, and the increased likelihood of nurse burnout and dissatisfaction. The study reported that mortality rates among surgical patients increased seven percent for every additional patient added to the average nurses' workload. The additional patient assignment contributed to a 23 percent increase in the odds of nurse burnout. Needleman, Buerhaus, Mattke, Stewart, and Zelevinsky (2002) concluded that a higher proportion of care provided by registered nurses and a greater number of hours of care by nurses per day are associated with positive patient care results. Some of the outcomes found were shorter lengths of stay, fewer urinary tract infections, and fewer cases of upper gastrointestinal bleeding for hospitalized patients.

American Medical Association Response

Another organization to study patient safety was the American Medical Association (AMA). By establishing the National Patient Safety Foundation in 1997, the AMA commissioned the Foundation to conduct a national survey to address patient safety issues in the healthcare environment (Harris & associates, 1997). The findings from the national telephone survey of 1513 respondents indicated that "the healthcare environment was perceived by the general public as 'moderately' safe" (Harris & associates, p. 3). The respondents stated that "carelessness or negligence on the part of healthcare professionals was the main cause of errors"; while, "the second most cited reason for medical errors was related to healthcare professionals being overworked, hurried and stressed" (Harris & associates, p. 5). It was noted that 95 percent of the respondents would report a medical mistake if they encountered one (Harris & associates). Recommendations were proposed for preventing medical mistakes. The major suggestions were to improve oversight of caregivers; ensure appropriate qualification and training of healthcare professionals; provide physician information to consumers; create an independent organization to examine the causes of medical mistakes; and increase the public's awareness of the issues surrounding errors (Harris & associates). Organizations may consider replicating this survey in order to have a greater understanding of their customer needs.

FIRST INSTITUTE OF MEDICINE REPORT AND RESPONSES

The most significant study that not only galvanized the healthcare industry but elevated the awareness of the public on patient safety was the Institute of Medicine (IOM) report on medical errors, entitled *To Err is Human: Building a Safer Health System* released in 1999 (Kohn, Corrigan, & Donaldson, 2000). The findings of the report produced a substantial media, public, congressional, and departmental response regarding concern for patients' health and safety.

According to the IOM report, in-hospital errors account for as many as 44,000 to 98,000 deaths each year in the United States. The IOM provided the following definition: "An error is defined as the failure of a planned action to be completed as intended (i.e., error of execution) or the use of a wrong plan to achieve an aim (i.e., error of planning)" (Kohn et al., 2000, p. 28). The study addressed errors in acute care hospitals but did not include data about care delivered in clinics, homes, rehabilitation centers, psychiatric facilities, or long-term care settings. It reported that in one year, more people die from medical errors than from breast cancer, AIDS, or motor vehicle accidents. Errors also caused injuries to patients; adverse events occurred in 3 to 4 percent of hospitalized patients, while 1 in 10 resulted in death. Errors occurred in virtually every hospital in the country. According to the study, medical errors were also costly. Total national costs were projected between $17 and $29 billion each year. Medication errors, which were among the most common errors, tacked on an additional $4700 to the average hospital bill each time they occurred. Most importantly, over half of all errors investigated were preventable. A major finding of the IOM report was that these errors occurred because of system failures rather than people problems; and preventing errors required designing safer systems of care (Kohn et al., 2000).

To help improve systems of care, the IOM report recommended a four-part plan for government and healthcare settings. The plan set forth the following recommendations:

☐ Establish a national center for patient safety
☐ Develop reporting systems to identify and learn from errors
☐ Raise standards for safety through regulatory and market forces
☐ Create safety systems in healthcare organizations at the care delivery level (Kohn et al., 2000, p. 6)

This first IOM report prompted considerable debate regarding the accuracy of the actual number of errors. Since the focus of the report was placed on errors occurring in hospitals, little is known regarding the number of errors or frequency of occurrence in home care, ambulatory care, nursing homes, or hospice settings. In addition, the report left the accountability for error management unclear by recommending both internal and external oversight. Porter-O'Grady and Malloch (2003) proposed that managing errors closest to the point of occurrence resulted in performance improvement, especially when a standardized national repository exists. In contrast, the authors indicated that external control reinforced a culture of blame.

On the other hand, the IOM report generated action from both the public and private sector. Within the public sector, President Clinton immediately ordered a government feasibility study. Based on the findings of the study in 2000, the President mandated that the IOM recommendations be implemented. Specifically, a 50 percent reduction in medical errors was to be achieved within the next five years. To further advance these directives, the President mandated that all 6000 hospitals participating in the Medicare program implement patient-safety initiatives, including medications and safety-oriented approaches (Kimmel & Sensmeier, 2002).

Agency for Healthcare Research and Quality Response

As described in the IOM report, a recommendation was made for the Agency for Healthcare Research and Quality (AHRQ) to create a Center for Patient Safety having accountability to the President and Congress (Kohn et al., 2000). To promote the patient safety agenda, the AHRQ received a $50 million grant to fund error-reduction research. It is interesting to note that the amount allocated by Congress for safety research in 2002 was less than half of 1 percent of the National Institute of Health budget for important medical research (Leape, Berwick, & Bates, 2002). The first effort of the AHRQ to investigate patient safety from an evidence-based medicine approach was published in a report titled *Making Healthcare Safer: A Critical Analysis of Patient Safety Practices* (Shojania, Duncan, McDonald, & Wachter, 2001). The report was a result of a commissioned group of 40 researchers, including experts in patient safety, evidence-based medicine, and various areas of clinical medicine, nursing, and pharmacy (Shojania, Duncan, McDonald, & Wachter, 2002). The research was conducted from a systemic approach addressing diseases and procedures. Results were reported by opportunities for safety improvement and for research. Evidence-based medical approaches were found to be as vital for advancing the patient safety agenda as were the advances proposed in the nonmedical field, such as bar-coding, simulation, and computerized physician order entry. The report called for greater emphasis on engaging the clinicians in the workplace to decrease risks attributed to care practices (Shojania et al., 2002).

The report received considerable attention. Some opposition surfaced regarding applying the principles of evidence-based medicine to patient safety practices. The method for the prioritizing of action items to improve patient safety were challenged and recommended for future research (Leape et al., 2002). However, there was agreement that the practice of anesthesia was an outstanding example of how a high level of safety could be achieved in healthcare. The success of this achievement was based on a broad range of changes in process, technological advances, training, and teamwork.

The Leapfrog Response

In addition to government agencies, the private sector also responded to the first IOM report. The Business Roundtable (BRT) formed a new program called "The Leapfrog Group," a coalition of Fortune 500 companies and other large private and public healthcare purchasers. Under Leapfrog, employers have agreed to base their purchase of healthcare on principles encouraging more stringent patient safety measures. These measures included computerized physician order entry, evidence-based hospital referral, and intensive care unit staffing by physicians trained in critical care medicine (Birkmeyer, Birkmeyer, Wennberg, & Young, 2000). There has been a positive response from the marketplace. Recently, the Leapfrog Group has been joined by JCAHO, increasing the original membership of 60 purchasers to more than 90 and now representing 25 million beneficiaries (Kimmel & Sensmeier, 2002).

Quality Interagency Coordination Task Force Response

The Quality Interagency Coordination Task Force (QuIC), which received direction from the President, reported more progress on the IOM recommendations. In order to consider all the important implications of medical errors, the QuIC proposed an expansion of the IOM's definition of medical errors. The QuIC defined an error as "the failure of a planned action to be completed as intended or the use of a wrong plan to achieve an aim. Errors can include problems in practice, products, procedures, and systems" (U.S. Department of Health and Human Services [U.S. DHHS], 2003b, p. 3435). The Center for the Medicare and Medicaid Services (CMS), an agency of the Department of Health and Human Services (U.S. DHHS), adopted the revised definition and published the results in the Federal Register (U.S. DHHS, 2003b). This expanded definition allowed for the identification of possible factors leading to errors, such as seclusion, restraints, equipment failures, and blood transfusions.

In the AHRQ evidence report, the term "error" was not included in the definition in order to minimize a negative connotation and because of the difficulties in specifying what constitutes a medical error. Rather, the authors defined a patient safety practice as a "type of process or structure whose application reduces the probability of adverse events resulting from exposure to the healthcare system across a range of diseases and procedures" (Shojania et al., 2002, p. 508).

For years, patient errors have primarily been addressed through malpractice litigation. Prior to the publication of the 1999 IOM report, the emphasis on having patients actively involved in error prevention was minimal. Organizations lack the processes to make the transition from a risk management environment of identification and discipline of individuals to a cooperative, system-based pursuit of improvement (Kohn et al., 2000). Because risk management is typically framed as a professional approach, organized medicine on one side, and the trial bar on the other, with patients the object of discussion and seldom involved in the process, the method for consistent patient involvement has not been designed (Sage, 2002). Forging stronger links with customer satisfaction and the clinical safety focus of the health system could be a start. In the review of several studies, Sage proposed that reducing lawsuits requires preventing errors and not just placating patients. Approaching legal aspects from a customer-focused perspective would not only control legal costs, but would also aid in conducting more reliable statistical analysis of medical practices in order to seek opportunities for improvement. With greater emphasis on advanced technology, "acting on the signals offered by patient complaints, therefore, can reduce both physician and interpersonal harm to patients" (Sage, 2002, p. 3004).

As was previously found in the AMA study, consumers offered several recommendations for preventing medical errors. Healthcare organizations are challenged to create innovative systems for engaging patients and their families in efforts to take action on steps following errors or on reporting near misses. Most recently, hospitals have endorsed polices and procedures to disclose such situations when they occur. However, a considerable amount of focus needs to be placed on moving from an adversarial, legal approach to a more inclusive, collaborative approach with the patient and family. Tools are available to assist healthcare organizations to assess their performance in this area. One such instrument, The Patient Safety Organizational Assessment Tool, developed by Wilson, provides a systematic method to evaluate current processes and systems and measure ongoing progress in establishing a safer environment (Sarudi, 2001).

SECOND IOM REPORT AND RESPONSE

In March 2001, the Committee on the Quality of Care in America produced the second IOM report, *Crossing the Quality Chasm: A New Health System for the 21st Century*. The focus of this IOM publication was a call for action to improve the nation's healthcare delivery system. With the aging of America, greater demand for services, and advanced technology and drugs, healthcare costs were increasing as resources were being overutilized. This report, like the first IOM report, repeatedly addressed patient safety problems with a major emphasis on redesign of the system. Six specification areas were recommended as significant when revamping the healthcare delivery model. These specification areas are: "patient safety, patient-centered care, efficiency, effectiveness, timeliness, and equity" (Committee on the Quality of Healthcare in America, 2001, p. 6).

Medicare Response

Again, the public sector responded when the CMS promulgated a new rule instructing hospitals to develop and implement quality assessment and improvement programs (QAIP) to identify patient safety issues and to decrease medical errors. The rule, Medicare Conditions of Participation (CoP), for hospitals went into effect on January of 2003 (U.S. DHHS, 2003a). U.S. DHHS Secretary Tommy G. Thompson said:

> This rule will encourage a greater emphasis on patient safety in hospitals. This serve as another step toward bringing improved patient safety, accountability and quality to the forefront of medical practice. Ultimately, we hope to create an environment where hospitals and other providers compete based on the quality of care that they provide to their patients. (U.S. DHHS, 2003a, p. 1)

Specifically, the QAIP of hospitals must reflect the complexity of the organization and services, be organizational-wide, focus on maximizing quality of care outcomes, and include preventative measures to promote patient safety. The expectation of the mandate is to ensure uniformity in quality standards for all Medicare-participating hospitals.

National Nursing Home Response

In November of 2002, CMS released nationwide data on quality measures of each nursing home in the United States. This national Nursing Home Quality Initiative (NHQI) was introduced to assure higher quality of care provided to Medicare and Medicaid beneficiaries. In addition to the previous reporting requirements, CMS contracted with the National Quality Forum (NQF) to develop 10 quality measures for consumers to compare the quality of nursing homes (NDHCRI, 2002). It is interesting to note that many of these indicators are descriptive of the nursing-sensitive indicators developed by the ANA. A comparable initiative requiring home health agencies to measure patient safety outcomes is expected to be announced by CMS in 2003 (U.S. DHHS, 2003a).

Joint Efforts

The demand for improvement in patient safety has been validated by the public, private, and regulatory sectors. Responding to the challenge offered by IOM, groups such as JCAHO, Leapfrog Group, AHRQ, and the Institute for Safe Medication Practice (ISMP) have all taken action to elevate the importance of patient safety and in some instances have points of intersection from their various recommendations. One such agreement was the need for greater education and training as it related to look alike/sound alike drugs. All addressed the big challenge of transforming the internal environment into a culture that embraced safety and delivered high reliability services. Additionally, transforming the external environment into a collective model of accountability was proposed to be equally challenging. With the recent alliance between JCAHO and the Leapfrog Group, healthcare leaders are faced with having to meet the new patient safety standards set by regulatory agencies and the marketplace.

JCAHO Response

Over the past years, JCAHO has answered the call by the IOM for greater accountability. One of the actions taken was to redesign the accreditation process. The direction of the revised process has been to concentrate on systemic recommendations and promote a nonprescriptive approach with the exception of sentinel review and reporting. JCAHO defined sentinel events as "unexpected occurrences involving death or serious physical or psychological injury, or risk thereof, which signal the need for immediate investigation or response" (Levy, 2001, p. 10). In 2001, JCAHO put into effect new standards requiring organizations to create a culture of safety; to implement a safety program with a specific visible administrative leader assigned the accountability for patient safety; and to disclose to patients the outcome of their care. Disclosure followed an earlier standard, when hospitals were required to report any incident of patient harm or death related to medical error, and to conduct an intensive review of the case. The methodology for analyzing these sentinel events was called a "root cause analysis" (RCA) and was grounded in industrial safety methodology (Kirkpatrick, 2003). The purpose of an RCA review was for hospitals to develop an action plan to ensure that the factors leading up to the sentinel event were resolved. Additionally, the JCAHO published the *Sentinel Event Alert*, which described actual cases and was intended to educate hospitals regarding errors that were occurring. The publication was also intended to stimulate a proactive stance so that organizations would examine their work processes and make the necessary changes. Levy (2001) indicated that perhaps the most controversial aspect of the redesigned approach by JCAHO is the requirement for healthcare givers to inform patients and their families when results of a procedure or action is not what was expected.

Based on a rigorous review of the reported sentinel events, the JCAHO in 2002 approved its first set of six National Patient Safety Goals (JCAHO, 2003b). These six goals with measurable objectives were intended to standardize the risk-reduction tactics used by healthcare organizations. Kirkpatrick (2003) indicated that by having organizations approach patient safety in a uniform way, JCAHO would be able to measure the effectiveness of setting key strategies. All hospitals will be required to comply with the six patient safety goals in future JCAHO surveys starting in 2003. "Failure to implement one or more of the recommendations (or acceptable alternatives) will result in a single special Type I recommendation" (JCAHO, 2003b, p. 2). The six key issues determined for compliance include accurate patient identification, effective communication, safe use of high-alert medication, elimination of wrong-site surgery, safe use of infusion pumps, and safe use of clinical alarms (Kirkpatrick, 2003). Each of the six standards and their implications for nursing practice will be described below.

NURSING'S ROLE

Nursing practice will influence all of the new standards on patient safety and outcomes of care. Nurses, by the very nature of their professional knowledge and skill, are critical resources to the organization. Nurses need to be given a strong and rightful place in decision making about issues relating to clinical practice. Nurses will affect patient safety in all healthcare settings. While the focus of the IOM study has been on acute care settings, nurses serve as the patient and family advocate no matter what setting of healthcare is required. With the advent of more procedures taking place in ambulatory settings, the potential for more injury to patients exists. Today, 65 percent of all surgical procedures do not involve a hospital stay (Lapetina & Armstrong, 2002). The intent of developing the nursing-sensitive indicators was to provide nurse executives with more definitive data to demonstrate the clear linkages between nursing interventions, staffing levels, and positive patient outcomes (ANA, 1999). The importance of advancing the nursing-sensitive quality measures for use in publicly available report cards cannot be over emphasized. As previously noted, the Nursing Home Quality Initiative mandated by the CMS is an example of the power of ANA's Nursing Safety & Quality Initiative of 1994.

Nurses will provide considerable leadership to the implementation of the JCAHO patient safety goals. The first standard, accuracy of patient identification, has two components. First, organizations are required to establish two patient identifiers, other than the patient room, such as patient's name, date of birth, or hospital identification number. The other component of this goal is to have a rigorous verification process followed on any surgical or invasive procedure to ensure correct patient, procedure, and site. Involving key stakeholders, such as nurses, in formalizing the two patient identifiers provides the opportunity for the organization to clearly establish indicators and measurement criteria at the same time. Standardizing the current (manual) process would increase understanding and support so hospitals could prepare for future bar coding technology.

Kirkpatrick (2003) stressed the fact that nurses needed to be more assertive when carrying out the second component of the identification requirement. Nurses need a routine method to ensure that the appropriate patient, the appropriate procedure, and the appropriate procedure site are verified in a consistent manner prior to the start of any surgical or other invasive procedure.

Nursing's role is critical in meeting the intent of the effective communication standard on orders and symbols, the second safety standard. This standard requires the accurate transcription of verbal and telephone orders, and the appropriate interpretation of difficult or unclear written orders. The relationship between the nurse and the provider giving the order contributes considerably to the success of this standard, since nurses are required to read back any verbal or telephone orders given. Kirkpatrick (2003) reported that hospitals would be required to formalize an approved abbreviation, acronym, and symbol listing, as well as to formalize a list of abbreviations that are not permitted, with clearly defined consequences for those not complying. The most controversial aspect of this standard is to define the consequences of noncompliance when physicians, nurses, and pharmacists are deviating from the organization policies and procedures.

Well-defined protocols developed by physicians, pharmacists, and nurses ensure safer use of high-alert medications. High-alert medications are those drugs which when misused have a "high risk of injury or death" (Cohen & Mandrack, 2002, p. 371). Because of their greater risk, special considerations are required when administering these drugs. Cohen and Mandrack (2002) reported that these high alert medications are packaged differently with visible warnings, stored differently so that they are separated from other medications, prescribed differently with standardized orders, and administered by requiring independent double-checking. Standardized protocols promote consistency of dosing calculation and methods of administration. Additionally, limiting the number of drug concentrations places additional control over medication errors. By standardizing the concentration of a medication, the dosing calculations are the same from one case to the other. Initiating protocols would not only provide direction for nurses in the administration of drugs, but also contribute to the development of educational tools and methods to verify consistency for patient and family education.

Previous reference was made to ensuring the correct identifier for the right patient. The major focus of the fourth safety standard is to eliminate wrong-site, wrong-patient, and wrong-procedure surgery. While the patient is very much involved with the process of site marking, another aspect of the standard is the verification process in the operating room. There are many similarities between the airline industry and surgical safety procedures. Airline safety processes include standardized procedures, checklists, explicit cross-checking, redundant checks, and a culture of equal accountability. Based on hundreds of little changes in work procedures, training, and system processes, aviation safety has established a strong safety culture (Leape et al., 2002).

Improving the safe use of infusion pumps is the fifth standard. The goal, specifically, requires infusion pumps to have a built-in protection from free-flowing fluids. Organizations can achieve this safety goal by involving nurses in the selection of products, setting minimum specifications for product evaluation, and defining the competencies required for nursing proficiency. Nursing education can schedule frequent educational skill development events to increase awareness of the safety features and ensure nursing proficiency through demonstration efforts. In addition, meeting this standard calls for a rigorous organizational maintenance program to serve as a check-and-balance system.

The sixth safety standard was designed to improve the effectiveness of clinical alarm systems. With the advanced technology, numerous alarms are available in patient care settings such as ventilator alarms, bed alarms, and pagers, to name a few. A major deterrent in meeting this standard is the potential to mute an alarm to create a quiet environment for the patient. To meet the intent of the sixth safety standard, organizations would need to validate that an active preventive maintenance program exists, and that the alarms are activated appropriately. Reviewers would call for evidence of compliance such as logs, records, usage, and training of healthcare workers. As was detailed in the fifth standard, organizations have the prerogative to define minimum specifications and educational requirements for their users. Nursing has an opportunity to work closely with other departments within the healthcare setting as purchasing decisions are made and maintenance programs are established.

Close attention to meeting the patient safety goals will be ongoing. JCAHO has announced its 2004 national patient goals. The new release reported that all of the 2003 goals will be continued with the addition of a new goal that will concentrate on reducing the risk of acquired infections in healthcare settings (JCAHO, 2003a).

Summary

There has been a convergence of thought among professional, private, and governmental healthcare decision makers that agree with the basic premise: patient safety will be a top priority agenda item for healthcare providers now and in the future. Various constituencies have contributed to the definition and detailed examination of the issues surrounding patient safety. In exploring the unique contributions of the major professional, public, and private groups, there are similarities and differences in the recommendations about the pathways to patient safety. All groups have validated the demand for improvement in patient safety. One agreement stated was the need for greater education and training as it related to look alike/sound alike drugs. Many of the constituencies addressed the big challenge of transforming the internal environment into a culture that embraced safety and delivered highly reliable services. Additionally, transforming the external environment into a collective model of accountability was proposed to be equally challenging.

The potential for these groups to interact with one another in order to create an even stronger infrastructure for patient safety is enormous. In fact, organizations that exemplify best practices in patient safety will be rewarded by the purchasers of health care and by accreditation agencies. Forging stronger links with the consumer is an untapped opportunity. Furthermore, linking consumer needs with the clinical safety focus of the healthcare system has the potential to decrease the risk of malpractice and enhance relationships. Nursing has a major role in providing leadership in the creation of solutions to advance patient safety standards.

References

Aiken, L. H., Clarke, S. P., Sloane, D. M., Sochalski, J., & Silber, J. H. (2002). Hospital nurse staffing and patient mortality, nurse burnout, and job dissatisfaction. *The Journal of the American Medical Association, 288*(16), 1987–1993.

American Nurses Association [ANA]. (1999). *Nursing facts: Nursing–sensitive quality indicators for acute care settings and ANA's safety & quality initiative.* Retrieved June 2, 2003, from www.nursingworld.org/readroom/fssafe99.htm.

Birkmeyer, J. D., Birkmeyer, C. M., Wennberg, D. E., & Young, M. P. (2000). *Leapfrog safety standards: Potential benefits of universal adoption* [Monograph]. Washington, D.C.: The Leapfrog Group.

Cohen, H., & Mandrack, M. M. (2002). Application of the 80/20 rule in safeguarding the high-alert medications. *Critical Care Nursing Clinics of North America, 14,* 369–374.

Committee on Quality of Healthcare in America, Institute of Medicine. (2001). *Crossing the quality chasm: A new health system for the 21st century.* Washington, D.C.: National Academy Press.

Harris, L., & associates. (1997). *Public opinion of patient safety issues: Research findings*. Commissioned for the National Patient Safety Foundation at the American Medical Association, September, 1997. Retrieved June 23, 2003, from www.npsf.org/download/1997survey.pdf.

Joint Commission on Accreditation of Healthcare Organizations. (2003a). *Joint Commission announces 2004 national patient safety goals*. Retrieved July 25, 2003, from www.jacho.org/news+room/news+release+archieves/nsg04.htm.

Joint Commission on Accreditation of Healthcare Organizations. (2003b). *Facts about patient safety*. Retrieved on June 6, 2003, from http://www.jcaho.org/accredited+organizations/patient+safety/facts+about+patient+safety.htm.

Kimmel, K. D., & Sensmeier, J. (2002). *A technological approach to enhancing patient safety* [Monograph]. Healthcare Information and Management Systems Society. 1–7.

Kirkpatrick, C. (2003). Safety first: The JCAHO introduces new patient safety goals. *NurseWeek, 4*(2), 19–20.

Kohn, L. T., Corrigan, J. M., & Donaldson, M. (Eds.). (2000). *To err is human: Building a safer health system*. Washington, D.C.: National Academy Press.

Lapetina, E. M., & Armstrong, E. M. (2002). Preventing errors in the outpatient setting: A tale of three states. *Health Affairs, 21*(4), 26–39.

Leape, L. L., Berwick, D. M., & Bates, D. W. (2002). What practices will most improve safety? Evidence-based medicine meets patient safety. *Journal of the American Medical Association, 288*(4), 501–507.

Levy, D. (2001). New standards enable nurses to shape patient policy. *NurseWeek, 2*(9), 10–11.

Needleman, J., Buerhaus, P., Mattke, S., Stewart, M., & Zelevinsky, K. (2002). Nurse-staffing levels and the quality of care in hospitals. *The New England Journal of Medicine, 346*(22), 1715–1722.

Porter-O'Grady, T., & Malloch, K. (2003). *Quantum Leadership: A textbook of new leadership*. Boston: Jones and Bartlett.

NDHCRI. (2002). Quality Counts: Nursing Home Quality Initiative. (2002). *Quality initiative to be conducted in nursing homes (ND-6SOW-O2-QP-32)* [Brochure]. North Dakota Healthcare Review, Inc.: Author.

Runy, L. A. (2003). Staffing effectiveness: A toolkit for JCAHO new standards. *Hospitals & Health Networks, 77*(3), 57–63.

Sage, W. M. (2002). Putting the patient in patient safety: Linking patient complaints and malpractice risk. *Journal of American Medical Association, 287*(22), 3003–3005.

Sarudi, R. (2001). Keeping patients safe. *Hospitals & Health Networks, 75*(4), 42–46.

Shojania, K. G., Duncan, B. W., McDonald, K. M., & Wachter, R. M. (Eds.). (2001). *Making health care safer:A Critical analysis of patient safety practices*. Evidence Report/Technology Assessment, No. 43. Prepared by the University of California at San Francisco-Stanford, Evidence-based Practice Center under contract No. 290-97-0013 for Agency for Healthcare Research and Quality; July 2001. Retrieved June 9, 2003, from www.ahcpr.gov/clinic/ptsafety/.

Shojania, K. G., Duncan., B. W., McDonald, K. M., & Wachter, R. M. (Eds.). (2002). Safe but sound: Patient safety meets evidence-based medicine. *Journal of the American Medical Association, 288*(4), 501–512.

U.S. Department of Health and Human Services. (2003a). *CMS issues final quality assessment and performance improvement conditions of participation for hospitals*. (Center for Medicare and Medicaid Services). Washington, D.C.

U.S. Department of Health and Human Services. (2003b). *Medicare and Medicaid Conditions of participation: Quality assessment and performance improvement*. (U.S. DHHS Publication No. 42 CFR Part 482). Washington D.C.: U.S. Government Printing Office.

CHAPTER 39

The Nursing Shortage:
Solutions for the Short and Long Term

Brenda Nevidjon
Jeanette Ives Erickson

Every article, speech, and interview about the nursing shortage notes that it is a different type of shortage than in the past. Some contributing factors remain the same, such as women having more choices for a career. Key differentiators from the previous two shortages are the aging of nurses, the general workforce shortages in ancillary professions and support labor, and the global nature of this shortage. In addition, the fundamental changes in how patients are cared for in a managed care environment are compounding the shortage. With decreased length of hospital stays and more acute care in the ambulatory and home settings, the need for experienced, highly skilled nurses is unmet. A numerical analysis may indicate enough current numbers, but the level of expertise may be the cause of the problem.

From an economic perspective, this shortage is being driven more by the supply side of the supply/demand equation than the demand side. Thus, this is a more complex shortage, which promises to worsen during the next decade as more nurses retire. Past economic solutions such as sign-on bonuses, relocation coverage, or new premium packages will have limited and temporary effects because they simply redistribute the supply of nurses, not increase it.

However, these solutions are already gaining in popularity again as evidenced by ads in local newspapers. The solutions to create a sustained improvement to the nursing shortage will need to be more radical than past shortages and must address many long-term issues.

In addition to the worsening nurse shortage is the shortage of other staff, including various allied health professionals, secretaries, and support staff. The shortages of other staff are adversely impacting nurses who have the most continuous and closest relationships with patients and their families. In the early 1990s, for cost-cutting reasons, there was an increased use of unlicensed assistive personnel. However, these models have failed due to increasing patient acuities, the concerns over medical errors, and the declining numbers of ancillary personnel.

Approximately one-third of the nursing workforce is over 50 years of age and the average age of full-time nursing faculty is 49 years. A study published in the July 2000 issue of *JAMA* predicts

Source: Nevidjon, B., & Erickson, J. (January 31, 2001). *The Nursing Shortage: Solutions for the Short and Long Term.* Online Journal of Issues in Nursing. Vol. 6, No. 1, manuscript 4. Available: http://www.nursingworld.org/ojin/topic14/tpc14_4.htm. © 2001. Online Journal of Issues in Nursing. Reprinted with permission.

that 40% of nurses by 2010 will be 50 years old or older (Buerhaus, 2000a). The challenge is for redesign of patient care delivery models that are built to support the practice of an older workforce. Nursing, a physically demanding profession, must address this challenge by initializing new technology into practice. Hospitals must support the aging nurse by offering flexibility in scheduling, increased time off, and sabbaticals.

In a Lexis/Nexis review of 6 months of news articles throughout the United States about the nursing shortage, every story noted the need for creative strategies. Disappointingly, few described any new interventions. The purpose of this article is to review several factors contributing to the shortage and present possible strategies to address them. The authors have chosen to review: trends in the general work environment, image of nursing, recruitment of students, retention of current nurses, and regulatory and policy issues. Solutions, some already underway in the United States, are highlighted. Primary nursing and patient focused care are discussed and a preferred model of care is described. We hope that this article will create a rapid communication of ideas to colleagues and stimulate others to build upon these ideas.

TRENDS TO CONSIDER

The general work environment in the United States is different than at the time of the last nursing shortage and needs to be taken into consideration when developing strategies to manage the shortage. There is blurring between what has been the traditional role of manager and the managed and between work and home. Rapid technological advances are changing the way in which work has been done. Organizations in all industries are dealing with a tight labor market and competing aggressively to hire the best and brightest. The following trends affect all work environments and provide a context in which the nursing shortage is evolving (Hymowitz, 2000; Lancaster, 1999; Shellenbarger, 1999).

- ☐ **Time over Money**—Employees today seek more personal time versus financial compensation.
- ☐ **Professional versus Personal Role**—Employees want to be active both at work and at home, not choosing between the two.
- ☐ **Rising Superclass of Employees**—As more employees opt for less stressful work/more personal time, a subgroup of employees, often characterized as more driven, are carrying the load of travel, relocation, and long hours.
- ☐ **Integration of Home and Work**—Employers are increasingly offering services to reduce the stress of managing professional and personal lives. These services include child and elder care, dry cleaning, house cleaning, on-site full service banking, and yard care.
- ☐ **GenX Entrepreneurs**—Employees in their twenties and thirties view the workplace differently, preferring greater autonomy and less bureaucracy. They are "loyal" to the work versus the employer. Thus, many are choosing independent work/freelancing, such as the temporary agencies in health care.
- ☐ **Collaborative Management**—Traditional models of administrative structures are also in flux with flattening of hierarchies and increased team structures. People who can create environments of teamwork and creativity are the definition of strong managers. No longer is top down control seen as desirable.

Given these trends, the following sections present the issues influencing the nursing shortage and describe potential solutions including efforts underway for addressing the shortage.

IMAGE

What the public thinks about nurses generally and what they specifically see or read in the media shape the current image of nurses. Annually, the nursing profession ranks very high as a trusted profession in the United States, above physicians and other healthcare workers. At the same time, the public is hearing about the stress nurses experience and the shortage of staff in hospitals; these reports prompt many to feel it is unsafe to leave family alone when hospitalized. There are images of striking nurses and headlines of layoffs and downsizing because of managed care. There are stories of nursing errors that have injured or killed patients, most recently in the *Chicago Tribune* (Berens, 2000a, 2000b, 2000c). These varied and conflicting images result in nursing appearing as an unstable, unpredictable, and high-risk career option. **Solution:** Nurses must become more of a voice in the press. With every article about the shortage of nurses, positive letters to the editor acknowledging the challenges of nursing and recognizing the rewards are needed. Negative, complaining letters perpetuate the image that nursing is not a good career choice.

Like other predominantly female professions, the public undervalues nursing. While the public indicates high trust of nurses, there is a lack of understanding about what nurses do. Often, the role of a nurse is defined in relation to the physician and may still carry the image of "handmaiden." This lowered status has implications for other indicators of the "value" of nursing to society: the funding provided for nursing education, the compensation nurses receive related to the responsibilities of the job, and the work environments that nurses endure. **Solution:** Central to this issue is the need to revise how nurses are valued. Initiatives at the local level can affect the compensation and work environment issues and will be addressed later. Increased funding for education needs both local and national attention as discussed later.

Nurses also shape the impression that others have about the profession. For instance, they may discourage children regarding nursing as a career choice. Nurses frequently report that they do not encourage their own children to consider nursing as a career. This is quite different than the message that doctors or lawyers give to children. In social settings, nurses may complain about their work or diminish their actions, rather than bragging about or promoting their contributions to individuals and organizations. **Solution:** As simple as it sounds, all nurses need to be aware of the way in which they discuss their work in public. Nurse executives can be helpful by starting an organizational campaign to educate their staff about how to communicate in social and community settings. Each nurse is the most important recruiter for an organization.

Currently, there is an opportunity for individual nurses and nursing organizations to recreate the public image of nursing, to help the community understand the importance of an adequate supply of well educated nurses, and to entice young people to consider the profession. **Solution:** Rather than having competing advertising campaigns for nurses, healthcare organizations could combine their resources and develop strategies to elevate the image of nursing. In a recent initiative, the University of Maryland School of Nursing has shown there is opportunity to partner with public relations firms to accomplish this. This school is partnering with Gilden Advertising, who is donating $1.2 million in cash, services, and in-kind gifts, to launch an integrated marketing plan to recruit more students into nursing (University of Maryland School of Nursing, 2000).

RECRUITMENT OF STUDENTS

For several years, enrollment in schools of nursing has been decreasing. According to the American Association of Colleges of Nursing's website (http://www.aacn.nche.edu), enrollments in bachelor's degree programs have declined for five years. The most recent data, for fall 1999, showed a 4.6% decline in enrollment and the decline occurred in every region. Enrollment also declined by 1.9% in master's degree programs but not uniformly across the regions.

Many reasons explain the continual decrease in enrollment in basic nursing programs. First and foremost is the fact that women have many choices today when selecting a post-high school education and career. Work conditions such as evening, night, and weekend shifts, or the exposure to contagious elements are cited as reasons that young people do not perceive nursing as a positive career choice.

The current nursing shortage has its roots in events of the 1990s. In the early 1990s, healthcare futurists were predicting a reduction in the number of hospital beds due to managed care penetration. Healthcare executives in all states watched the market changes in California in anticipation that capitation would be seen throughout the country. The nursing profession began to brace for an era of downsizing as hospitals were attempting to drive costs down by decreasing a patient's length of stay and adjusting their staffing models. A plan promoted by healthcare consultants was to reduce budgets by deploying assistive personnel where nurses once practiced. This resulted in layoffs of nurses in some parts of the country. The skill mix changes and movement of patients from acute care to home care or ambulatory settings forced many nurses to evaluate their personal decisions. Feeling devalued and disenfranchised, nurses left the profession of nursing. Thus, schools of nursing and prospective nursing student candidates were left with an impression that fewer nurses would be needed in the future.

A compounding factor in many nursing schools is the availability of nursing faculty. They, like nurses in healthcare delivery, are aging. Thus, for some schools, even if they could recruit more students, they may not have faculty to teach them. Similar issues contribute to the shortage of faculty: compensation, cost of advanced preparation, and work conditions. **Solution:** Are there ways in which the aging practicing nurse who can no longer manage the physical demands of the job can be used to educate new nurses? One concern about practicing nurses is that they do not have curriculum development and performance measurement skills. If this is a barrier for recruiting needed faculty, solutions should possible. New models of education are needed as acutely as new models of patient care delivery. Practice and education have a long history of not being aligned. Perhaps the conditions now exist to unite practice and education, to have each earnestly listen to the other, and to enable them to design solutions together.

Strategies to recruit students are needed for the long term since the predictions are for a worsening shortage over the next decade, but there are immediate interventions possible. Many efforts are underway to recruit high school students. **Solution:** In San Diego, six hospital systems have committed $1.3 million to support a program called, "Nurses Now," which will add faculty and additional student slots to San Diego University (Kucher, 2000). The *American Hospital Association News* reports that in Laredo, Texas, a hospital CEO worked with Texas A&M University to develop a four-year bachelor's program and is providing $425,000 in scholarships to local students over the next five years (Runy, 2000). In Morris County, New Jersey, the Board of Freeholders offered scholarships to students who agreed to work in a long-term care facility (Cichowski, 2000). The Dallas-Fort Worth Hospital Council raised $600,000 to expand student enrollment at local schools (Yednak, 2000). These are examples of various successful collaborative efforts among healthcare organizations, government, nursing associations, and nursing schools. Many more are happening at the local level.

Within the general student recruitment initiatives are efforts to reach minority students and young men. **Solutions:** Hodgman (1999) was project director of *Choose Nursing!*©, a state, privately, and federally funded project designed to recruit Boston public high school sophomores into a comprehensive two-year hospital program to foster and maintain their interest in nursing and prepare them to apply to collegiate nursing programs. Departments of nursing or specialty organizations could implement variations of this program. For instance, a local chapter of a national specialty organization could "adopt" a middle school or high school and establish an outreach program with students.

To ensure a continuous robust pool of nursing students, children must be reached earlier than high school. In fact, educators say that students often have their minds made up by fifth grade about desirable and undesirable careers. Thus, an early positive image of nursing for students is important.

Solution: One long-term strategy suggested by Ruth Kleinpell in *Nursing Spectrum Metro Edition* is that a new series of Cherry Ames stories reflecting society today might be inspirational to a new generation of girls and boys. Although this suggestion may be met with skepticism, think about the influence stories have on children, the influence the original Cherry Ames books had on so many. She notes that Harriet Forman, who has the copyright to some of the books and is an executive with Nursing Spectrum, is working on new stories (Kleinpell, 2000). For older readers, there are books of stories about nursing and nursing leaders. By working with middle and high school teachers, guidance counselors, and librarians, it is possible to introduce these books as resources. Nurses from a healthcare organization or a local chapter of a professional society could give these books as a gift. **Solution:** Current nursing students can be effective recruiters. Allentown's Cedar Crest College offers a four-credit course that requires students to make presentations in local schools, participate in elementary school clinics, update public libraries on nursing books, and create displays about nursing as a career (Wlazelek, 2000).

RETENTION OF NURSES

Retention of nurses begins with how the organization does or does not value the staff. Rhetoric not withstanding, most healthcare executives view staff as an expense and in times of financial constraint, as is currently the state, watch the personnel budget line very closely. It is key that executives reframe how they see staff, all staff. Rather than viewing staff as an expense, seeing them as any asset on the balance sheet will drive different decisions about the work environment. **Solution:** Healthcare executives, including nurse leaders, must learn new skills for valuing employees. The chief nursing executive in partnership with the head of human resources can facilitate the executive team's discussion of how they are valuing staff and how this is shown in the organization. The increasing union activity throughout the country is an indication that this discussion is needed.

Human resources in the form of registered nurses can arguably make or break an institution's image and competitive edge. Organizations that maintain a market advantage will be those who not only remain competitive from a cost structure, but who also attract and retain talent.

People determine organizational effectiveness and allow the organization to thrive in this competitive healthcare environment. Organizations that give attention to the employee market and understand what people are seeking from the work environment have a better chance to recruit and retain top talent, particularly given the current low unemployment. **Solution:** Identify what benefits would keep nurses in the profession and in a particular work setting. The best source is the nurses themselves, as discussed by Eulee Mead-Bennett and Ngozi Nkongho (1990). During the previous shortage, they interviewed staff nurses in several New York hospitals to learn what nurses saw as the causes of that nursing shortage and suggestions for alleviating it. Then, as today, they found that the following were areas needing short- and long-term solutions: autonomy, salaries, schedules, credibility gap, and professional respect.

In a more recent study, McNeese-Smith (1999) investigated staff nurse descriptions of job satisfaction and dissatisfaction. For the nurses in the study, salary and benefits were important but mentioned only briefly. A key finding was that the nurses in their study found satisfaction from direct care, yet their role was changing to be the organizer and coordinator of care. Another finding with implications for administrators was that those nurses who provide poor care, have a negative attitude, or are burned out create dissatisfaction for their coworkers. **Solution:** Administrators and educators must learn what the satisfiers are for staff. When roles are redefined, they must help staff identify new satisfiers. Human resource administrators must be responsive to the individuality of what is important to staff and create flexible and supportive policies and benefits.

Currently, there are critical needs for experienced nurses in the operating room, critical care, and neonatal care arenas. **Solution:** Hospitals are reintroducing intensive training programs for nurses in these specialties. This helps to retain nurses who are looking for a transfer opportunity as well as to recruit new staff. It also builds a career development path for staff. These training programs are not inexpensive, and nursing leaders must be prepared to justify the required budget. Given the cost of temporary staff, this should be a logical solution for the organization's leadership to endorse.

For at least two decades, the literature has promoted the notion that shared governance/shared leadership creates a more satisfying work environment. The research that has been done on magnet hospitals shows that organizational characteristics that attract and retain nurses include professional practice models for delivery of care with autonomy and responsibility for decision making. Participatory management, enhanced communication, and adequate staffing were relevant features of hospitals that nurses identified as good employers. While few hospitals have magnet status, the research remains relevant and applicable. **Solution:** Effective administrative structure, quality patient care, and investment in professional development of nurses are important. Staff must be involved in defining and developing the practice of care in the organization since they are the closest to the patient. This includes participation in the financial management of their unit.

MODELS OF CARE

One challenge for nursing will be to address the viability of primary nursing. While current perspectives and applications of primary nursing are absent from the literature, two editorials published in the *Journal of Professional Nursing* by Joyce Clifford of Beth Israel, Boston (1988) and Kathleen Andreoli of Rush Presbyterian/St.Lukes, Chicago (1992) remain valid. Clifford (1988) began her piece by challenging the statement that "Primary Nursing is dead." She argues that "Primary Nursing is alive and well." Why the confusion? She asserts that it is not always clearly understood that the development of primary nursing and a professional practice model comes from a strong philosophical commitment rather than merely from the understanding of a nurse–patient assignment method.

Clifford (1988) notes that time has shown that nurses will no longer accept the mere performance of tasks as their practice goal outcomes. Nor will they remain in systems that promote fragmented, uncoordinated care leading to dissatisfaction for everyone—the patient, the nurse, and the hospital. Instead, nurses seek opportunities to provide comprehensive, professional care through a system that allows for continuity of patient care as well as the opportunity for them to maximize their knowledge and skill. The change they made from a functional/team delivery system of care to a system that provides for a comprehensive, coordinated approach to patient care required the best prepared (i.e., the registered nurse) rather than the least prepared to be placed in the most direct and constant care relationship with patients and families. It is this relationship with patients that must be preserved for the future if a balance is to be struck between the goals of cost and quality in health care. This nurse–patient relationship is, of course, the underlying principle of primary nursing.

In the early 1990s, management consultants advocated for the development of a model called Patient Focused Care. However, for many, this model resulted in an increase of nursing aides and a decrease of professional nurses. Andreoli (1992) identifies the 1990s as the decade of ideal nursing skill mixes and delegation. Nurses must know what tasks are appropriate to "give away," how to manage the workload and be accountable for outcomes, and how to provide for the growth and development of non-RN caregivers and other support staff. Andreoli envisioned that this change would not come easily, and it hasn't. Nurses sometimes feel less valued when they must delegate tasks to a non-nurse. However, nursing can consider delegation, along with shared governance, as another form of empowerment.

Delegation, though, must be learned, practiced, evaluated, and improved. Delegation is an art, and the delegator must have an understanding of the essentials of management, chain of command, span of control, licensed versus unlicensed assistive personnel, nursing task versus professional responsibilities, liabilities, mentorship, evaluation, and continuous quality improvement. Andreoli stresses that in a successful delegation model, primary nurses will have time to give patients the benefit of their knowledge and skills. Tasks not requiring a nurse's educational preparation will be delegated to qualified assistive personnel. Nursing leadership must create an environment where delegation is supported and valued and positive outcomes are rewarded. The patient then is the winner with the best of both types of providers.

Numerous studies on delivery models and restructuring demonstrate that different staff mixes and approaches work in different settings. There isn't a "one size fits all" model. However, what must remain constant is the guarantee that every patient has a nurse.

An example of a futuristic model of care was developed at the Massachusetts General Hospital and presented as a Harvard Business School case study (1999). Similar to almost every other healthcare institution in America, this system of care delivery emerged after careful reflection on many factors: the local and national labor market, the changing profile of patients served, the nature of the workforce, and the systems or infrastructure that supported practice. The Massachusetts General Hospital Patient Care Delivery Model (Figure 39.1) was derived after

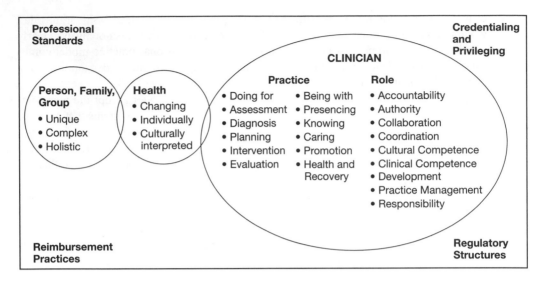

Figure 39.1 External Healthcare Environment.

careful development of vision, values, and long-range goals. In this model, vision, values, and goals converge to support the delivery of patient care. The model depicts the dynamic and therapeutic interaction that occurs between the professional care provider and the patient around issues of health and illness. The model reflects an open, evolving interactive system where there is continuous exchange occurring between the patient and the clinician (nurse, therapist, or social worker). The model also depicts the multiple internal and external forces that impact upon the patient's experience as well as the structures supporting the delivery of patient care.

The larger, important circle surrounding the core represents the interdisciplinary partnerships within the multiple settings where patient care is delivered. This is an important message for staff nurses who feel supported in their practice by all team members. While this is an example of one model that considered internal and external factors, it does reflect the elements that must be considered during this time of a structural shortage of healthcare workers.

Again, this shortage is different and most likely not cyclical in nature. In any model a balance must be struck between: (a) supply and demand, (b) quality and organizational effectiveness, (c) staff satisfaction, and (d) financial viability.

REGULATORY AND POLICY ISSUES

A number of regulatory and policy issues may also be exacerbating the shortage. These include state and federal law, regulation by accreditation/certification organizations, licensure and nursing practice acts, and requirements from reimbursement organizations, private organizations, and the government. Some issues are factors in causing nurses to leave the profession and others may be barriers for recruiting nurses. Specifically, in this section the authors look at: the complexity of documentation resulting from regulatory agencies; federal and state funding support to nursing programs; employment of foreign nurses; and the role of state Boards of Nursing.

In all sectors of patient care delivery, nurses complain about the amount and complexity of paperwork that has resulted from a multitude of actions by regulatory bodies and the reimbursement industry. Nurses find they are spending more time with paper than with patients. This dissatisfies nurses who want to have interaction with patients and families and may contribute to nurses leaving direct care positions, particularly in acute care settings. Although many believe that technology will solve this problem, those who are using electronic documentation systems report that they are not necessarily spending less time documenting. **Solution:** Within an organization, aggressive process improvement initiatives can help standardize and streamline documentation. Front-line staff should drive this process with consultation from internal experts in patient documentation, risk management, and reimbursement.

There is a clear need for an aggressive review of the federal and state support to nursing programs to increase the enrollment of students. Given the federal budget surplus, it is timely to expect increased support for schools of nursing and special scholarships to recruit students for basic and advanced nursing education.

Solution: As nursing organizations such as the American Nurses Association lobby for increased federal funding, individual nurses need to respond to the request for communication with their elected officials. Every nurse must become a vocal proponent of increased funding for nursing and educate their representatives that nursing is the necessary glue in health care. Grassroots lobbying efforts, such as those by the AIDS and breast cancer coalitions, have proven to be effective in increasing government support. **Solution:** Buerhaus (2000b) has suggested that the federal government create a commission to address the issue and attach funding to the recommendations. **Solution:** State level workgroups are underway in several states and some state legislatures have committed resources as noted above. More state level groups that unite nursing practice and education with state government will be needed. State nurses' associations can take a lead in initiating this work in states where it has not begun. Even if the state does not have a critical need today for more nurses, in the next few years all states will have this need.

A recruitment strategy that has been successful in the past and is being used again is the employment of foreign nurses. Hoping that this may be a solution, many are raising the question about reviewing federal policy regarding visas for foreign nurses. Currently, the federal policy is a barrier for recruitment of nurses from other countries. However, many countries, Canada for one, are also experiencing a shortage of nurses, and this strategy may not help. In fact, many are predicting that there is an emerging global shortage of nurses.

State Boards of Nursing also have an important contribution to make during this uncertain time regarding both the recruitment of nurses and retention of nurses. No doubt, there will be pressure to lower licensure standards to increase the number of graduate nurses. This would be a mistake as the Boards are responsible for protecting the public from unsafe, illegal, or unethical practice. During times of shortage and stress, the potential for unsafe practice may be heightened. However, Boards need to review their policies and procedures to determine whether those policies and procedures are contemporary or out-of-date and contributing to the nursing shortage. Another topic of great discussion is that of assistive personnel. As hospitals have increased their use of assistive personnel, many registered nurses have not been willing to remain on staff to supervise care of other providers. The Boards of Nursing define the scope of nursing practice and what can be delegated to others and should help to educate nurses about this issue. Also, rather than viewing delegation as promoting fragmentation of care, definition needs to be given as to how care can be enhanced by using the full capabilities of registered nurses. The American

Nurses Association's position statement on maintaining professional and legal standards during shortages is useful to read in this regard (ANA Board of Directors, 1992).

SUMMARY

There are 1.8 million nurses working primarily in hospitals. This is currently where the shortage is being felt or anticipated with the greatest concern, but all practice settings will ultimately be affected. There are a few quick fixes to the problem, but this shortage is structural in nature and requires short- and long-term strategies to mitigate the problem. In a Web search for "nursing shortage," the authors found over 18,000 sites. There is no lack of information and opinion about this evolving shortage. The authors have included below a brief list of websites that they found helpful.

As reviewed in this article, key factors contributing to this shortage are: the differences in the general work environment compared to past shortages, the ongoing struggle with the image of nursing, recruitment of new nurses, retention of current nurses, and regulatory and policy decisions that can be a barrier to recruitment or a cause of attrition of nurses. Models of care delivery are also discussed. There are solutions to enact for each of those factors and some are underway. In the short term, fiscal and marketing strategies may help. Changing the work environment will be necessary, however, for both the short and long term. Ultimately, it is the long-term solution of making the profession a desirable career choice that is essential. The good news is that nursing continues to be the most trusted and respected of all the healthcare professions. From a demand perspective, it is one of the fastest growing professions and thus offers a strong career opportunity for today's youth. The time is right for nursing's voice to be strong with the public, with healthcare system leaders, and with the government. With a strong united voice, nursing may be able to use this shortage as a catalyst for creating a solid foundation for the future of the profession.

Table 39.1 Recommended Websites Discussing the Nursing Shortage

American Nurses Association	http://nursingworld.org
Nurses for a Healthier Tomorrow	http://www.nursesource.org
Nursing Economics	http://www.ajj.com
The Forum on Health Care Leadership	http://www.healthcareforum.org
National League of Nursing	http://www.nln.org
Bureau of Labor Statistics	http://www.bls.gov
American Hospital Association	http://www.aha.org
American Organization of Nurse Executives	http://www.aone.org
American Association of Colleges of Nursing	http://aacn.nche.edu
Allnurses.com	http://allnurses.com
Nurse.com	http://nurse.com
HRLive	http://hrlive.com/reports/
Other Web sites:	
Specific state nurses' associations	
Nursing specialty organizations	

REFERENCES

American Nurses Association Board of Directors. (1992). Joint statement on maintaining professional and legal standards during a shortage of nursing personnel. Retrieved January 9, 2001, from http://www.nursingworld.org/readroom/position/joint/jtshort.htm.

Andreoli, K. G. (1992). Primary nursing for the 1990s and beyond. *Journal of Professional Nursing, 8*(4), 202.

Berens, M. (2000a, September 10). Nursing mistakes kill, injure thousands. *Chicago Tribune*, p. A1.

Berens, M. (2000b, September 11). Nursing accidents unleash silent killer. *Chicago Tribune*, p. A1.

Berens, M. (2000c, September 12). Problem nurses escape punishment. *Chicago Tribune*, p. A1.

Buerhaus, P. (2000a). Implications of an aging registered nurse workforce. *Journal of the American Medical Association, 283*(22), 2948–54.

Buerhaus, P. (2000b). A nursing shortage like none before. *Creative Nursing, 6*(2), 4–8.

Cichowski, J. (2000, September, 28). Tuition offered to attract nurses: Morris County Home is short of staff. *The Record*, Bergen County, NJ, p. L3.

Clifford, J. C. (1988, March–April). Will the professional practice model survive? *Journal of Professional Nursing, 4*(2), 77, 141.

Harvard Business School. (1999, March). *Case study: The patient care delivery model at the Massachusetts General Hospital*. Boston, MA, Unpublished.

Hodgman, E. (1999). High school students of color tell us what nursing and college mean to them. *Journal of Professional Nursing, 15*(2), 95–105.

Hymowitz, C. (2000, January 4). How can a manager encourage employees to take bold risks? *Wall Street Journal*, p. B1.

Kleinpell, R. M. (2000). Cherry was the apple of our eye. *Nursing Spectrum Metro Edition, 1*(2), 8–9.

Kucher, K. (2000, June 9). Six hospitals to help fund 'Nurses Now!': $1.3 million effort to boost graduates in the field. *The San Diego Union-Tribune*, p. B1.

Lancaster, H. (1999, December 21). A father goes to work and finds new ways make sense. *Wall Street Journal*, p. B1.

McNeese-Smith, D. (1999). A content analysis of staff nurse descriptions of job satisfaction and dissatisfaction. *Journal of Advanced Nursing, 29*(6), 1332–1341.

Mead-Bennett, E., & Nkongho, N. (1990). Staff suggestions on the nursing shortage. *Hospital Topics, 68*(4), 29–33.

Runy, L. A. (2000). Texas hospital tackles nurse shortage with novel long-, short-term solutions. *AHA News, 36*(20), 5.

Shellenbarger, S. (1999, December 29). For harried workers in the 21st century: Six trends to watch. *Wall Street Journal*, p. B1.

University of Maryland School of Nursing. (2000, October 16). Press Release: Gilden advertising donates $1.2 million to the University of Maryland School of Nursing.

Wlazelek, A. (2000, July17). Area hospitals blamed for shortage of nurses; workers say institutions have increased the workload and added to stress; fewer consider nursing careers. *The Morning Call*, Allentown, PA, p. B1.

Yednak, C. (2000, August 4). Hospitals offer nurses bonuses to recruit colleagues: Officials seek solutions to shortages that are growing with the Metroplex. *The Fort Worth Star-Telegram*, p. 1.

CHAPTER 40

Nightingale's Passion for Advocacy: Local to Global

Deva-Marie Beck

The farther away we get, the greater Nightingale appears. Each generation will undoubtedly see her in a different light and will discover new aspects of her life and character. But her influence will go on and we shall see more clearly that she belongs to no country or age or professional group, but to the world.

—Stewart & Austin, 1962, p. 119

REINTRODUCING NIGHTINGALE

Nightingale, the most well-known nurse in history, is famous for her contributions to the Crimean War, where she spent 21 exhausting months tending wounded and dying soldiers and was revered as the "lady with the lamp." Her small volume, *Notes on Nursing: What It Is and What It Is Not* (Nightingale, 1860), continues to be often quoted and is still used as a text in nursing education programs (Selanders, 1993). Nightingale also is acknowledged as being the founder of modern secular nursing because of her work to establish a formal nursing school in the 1870s and her close watch over her students (Dossey, 2000). These characterizations—a war-time heroine and a strict nursing educator who wrote a small book—form most of what has been known about Florence Nightingale. Because her accomplishments occurred more than 150 years ago, the contemporary relevance of Nightingale's work frequently is called into question. The stories about her severe sacrifice and her restrictive, demanding teaching techniques, as well as her Victorian-era text, are each seen as quaint, mostly outdated, or even detrimental to contemporary nursing practice (Dean, 1999).

However, these examples are only three tiny points taken from the much larger panorama of Nightingale's 50-year career. Beyond the decade of the 1850s and her own desk, her nursing school, and her country's war hospital, Nightingale took nursing much further still, to villages and towns across the world, to the halls of power and leadership, and to behind-the-scenes discussions that would shape the history of health care. Although she is famous for one book, she was a prolific writer, writing 20 other books, hundreds of monographs and articles, and thousands of letters well into the 1890s (McDonald, 2004). Together, her writings compose an opus of contributions not just to the evolving field of nursing, but also to related health disciplines, such as public health and hospital administration, that were rarely matched by any of her contemporaries, male or female, in any field (Dossey, 2000). Her tremendous body of work is just now becoming available to 21st-century readers (Dossey, 2000; McDonald, 2004; Dossey, Selanders, Beck, & Attewell, 2005).

The purpose of this chapter is to reintroduce this broader perspective of Florence Nightingale to the 21st-century nursing community and to focus on those aspects of her life, work, and insights that have not been well studied. In addition to being a battlefield nurse, a nursing author, and an educator, Nightingale was also a humanitarian, an environmentalist, an opinion molder, and a consummate change agent. She sought to create healthy communities around the world, across the British Empire, in Europe, the United States, Turkey, and even Japan (L. Selanders, personal communication, May 9, 2004). She saw her work as advocacy for the health of people and was keenly interested, even passionate, about the results. Because of the scope of her activities, she was, even in her own time, a well-respected, influential global citizen. She considered all of these activist approaches to be within the scope of her own nursing practice and distinguished between nursing the sick and *health-nursing*—a term she applied to all levels of health promotion activity, including local, regional, national, and global. She knew that even if she was working on a small, local project that her work could have broad, worldwide dimensions (Nightingale, 1893).

Many people and organizations from around the world still look to the Nightingale legacy for inspiration and guidance. This chapter describes a few of Nightingale's own lesser-known stories—as humanitarian, environmentalist, opinion molder, and change agent—and includes contemporary examples of nurses who have extended their practice to these arenas, acting locally and thinking globally. Nightingale's capstone 1893 essay, "Sick-Nursing and Health-Nursing," is reviewed to illustrate some of her comprehensive approaches to nursing and health.

As the relevance of Nightingale's perspectives to contemporary nursing scholarship is considered, nurses are encouraged to align themselves with Nightingale's example of global citizenship. One global effort that nurses can participate in is the Nightingale Initiative for Global Health (NIGH), an innovative project that incorporates many components of her exemplary leadership for nursing and the world (NIGH, 2005). The 21st-century world faces many major health concerns; wars and conflicts that inflict severe suffering; emerging epidemics; and environmental, economic, and climatic threats. Revisiting Nightingale's passion for health advocacy and the wider scope of her legacy provides a framework for nursing practice that is relevant to 21st-century health issues. If nursing's scope of practice could again incorporate Nightingale's wide range of competencies, the nursing profession would enter a new realm of service for the health of humanity, and, in return, would experience a profound level of fulfillment.

HER WORLDWIDE LEGACY

Although Nightingale was born into the rarified world of upper-class British aristocracy and lived most of her life in Britain, her legacy is remembered around the world. In London, Westminster Abbey is filled every year during a service convened on a date close to Nightingale's birthday in May. In this service, attended by more than 2000 nurses, midwives, health visitors, government ministers, and others, a lamp, symbolic of Nightingale herself, is passed down a procession of student nurses, representing the passage of knowledge from one nurse to another (Florence Nightingale Foundation, 2004). In the United States, the work of Nightingale has been commemorated since 2001 in Washington D.C. An election to the Episcopal Church Calendar of Lesser Feasts and Fasts established a tradition of services to honor her legacy and the nursing profession at the National Cathedral (Beck, 2005b). Across the globe, another present-day remembrance is the annual "lighting of the lamp," which is celebrated on Nightingale's birthday by nursing students at the School of Nursing at the Aga Khan University in Karachi, Pakistan (Aga Khan University School of Nursing, 2001).

Scholars celebrate Nightingale's work with renewed efforts at collection and study. In Canada, at the University of Guelph in Ontario, Lynn McDonald and colleagues have committed themselves to compiling Nightingale's complete works, including 14,000 letters from collections around the world, in a series of 16 volumes and on the Internet (McDonald, 2004).

The reverence for Nightingale's work extends across decades and continents. In India, Nightingale is widely acknowledged for her decades of service to the health of the Indian people. When she died, the great Indian leader, Mahatma Gandhi, then a young journalist, published a moving tribute describing the profound commitment of her life to humanity (Dossey, 2000). The life of Nightingale is taught in Japanese elementary school curricula, and she serves as a role model of near-icon status for Japanese schoolchildren. Japanese nurses understand her to be a spiritual icon who represents the strength needed to survive enormous hardship (Hiasma, 1996). In China, her name is remembered through a Florence Nightingale Medal, which is awarded each year to the nation's 10 best nurses.

Jean Henri Dunant, founder of the International Red Cross and the first Nobel Peace Prize recipient, credits his inspiration for his goal in life—to create a humanitarian organization to neutrally serve all wounded in battle, regardless of nationality—to Nightingale's example during the Crimean War (Dossey, 2000; Orange County Red Cross, 2004). At the entrance to the International Museum of the Red Cross and Red Crescent in Geneva, Switzerland, Nightingale is featured, along with Clara Barton, the American nurse who founded the American Red Cross, beside Dunant (International Museum of Red Cross and Red Crescent, 2004). These three are credited equally as the key initiators of a worldwide network to bring humanitarian relief to war-torn countries and the victims of natural disasters. In recognition of Nightingale's stature, the International Red Cross Florence Nightingale Medal is presented every second year by the International Committee of the Red Cross (Red Cross Society of China, 2004). This medal, which recognizes the humanitarian efforts of nurses, has been presented to hundreds of Red Cross and Red Crescent nurses from around the world (International Committee of the Red Cross, 2004).

In Istanbul, Turkey, the Scutari Barracks, where Nightingale served during the Crimean War, still stands as a Turkish First Army Base. Nightingale is the only Western woman in history to be revered, even today, across the Islamic world (Waddy, 1980), because of her willingness to attend equally the wounds of the Turkish Muslim soldiers as well as the British Christian soldiers at Scutari. She is commemorated as the "lady of the lamp" by the Florence Nightingale College of Nursing at the University of Istanbul, which educates undergraduate clinicians and graduate-level nursing scholars (Petenkin, 1996), and the Red Crescent School of Nursing features a costumed "Nightingale" in a ceremony of "Nurses Through the Ages" from ancient to modern times (Beck, 2005b).

In 1996, Florence Nightingale and other nurses were honored at a United Nations Summit for the first time. The setting was Istanbul (Constantinople in Nightingale's time), the host city for "Habitat II"—the United Nations Human Settlements Conference. Here, representatives of governments and of civil society from around the world convened to discuss the challenges inherent to human habitats—from the smallest village to the megalopolis. To highlight the connections between health and nursing's contributions to the conditions found in human dwellings, the United Nations International NGO (nongovernmental organization) Health Caucus cosponsored

"An International Tribute to Florence Nightingale at Scutari" with the Turkish First Army and the Wellness Foundation from North America (Beck, 2005b).

NURSES AS HUMANITARIANS

Because the casualties of the Crimean War were well published and because Nightingale's contributions there as a civilian humanitarian were so unusual, the Crimea became the backdrop of her fame. She was widely honored for her tireless devotion to the British soldiers (Selanders, 1993). In addition to providing exemplary bedside care in the Crimea, she maintained leadership, diplomatic, administrative, and policy roles. Although she was concerned with providing excellent care for "her soldiers" and seeing to their intake of nutrition, their pain, their rest, and their wounds, she also addressed their welfare in other matters, such as their isolation, their fear of death, their economic circumstances, and other social issues that often centered around gambling and prostitution (Dossey, 2000).

In its time, the Crimean War was like the Vietnam War in the 20th century, a conflict where popular concern for its grave consequences reached highly intense proportions. In this case, the British people were worried over the number of casualties and the causes of those casualties (Goldie, 1987).

When Nightingale arrived at the Scutari Barracks near the Crimean battlefields, she faced the severe challenges of human and environmental degradation. Sanitation was nonexistent, and thousands of men were dying of wounds infected from the overwhelming filth. Soldiers were regarded as expendable cannon fodder, because human and social rights were only for the privileged few. Faced with these problems, Nightingale implemented solutions grounded in her vision of nursing and health and reduced the Crimean wounded death rate from 45% to some 3% in less than 6 months (Dossey, 2000). At Scutari, Nightingale was acting locally for a global need.

A contemporary example of humanitarian nursing endeavors is the work of Joyce Murray, a professor at Atlanta's Emory University and president of the National League for Nurses. Her work in Africa as a nursing educator and director of the Carter Center Ethiopia Public Health Initiative has exposed her to a very different healthcare environment. At one point, war with neighboring Eritrea disrupted the initiative, but the ongoing challenges are even more basic. The initiative's top concerns are infant diarrhea, malnutrition, malaria, and HIV/AIDS, all of which are potential killers. Murray oversees the initiative's mission to develop health materials for use in training staff for 500 facilities that have been established to bring health care to rural Ethiopians, who comprise 85% of the population. Poor roads make it time consuming to take students into villages for hands-on training. Although the program's students can be taught in English, health education must ultimately be provided across a country in which 87 languages or dialects are spoken. "We will [soon] be evaluating the program's impact in more detail," Murray describes, "but we already know two areas that need more attention: mental health, particularly in families who've lost parents or husbands to HIV/AIDS and a CD-ROM-based means of continuing the education of graduating students, so they can become more effective teachers and keep up with new training materials being developed" (Carter Center, 2003).

NURSES AS ENVIRONMENTALISTS

In 1874, Nightingale drew upon her many years of exposure to the concerns about health in the British colony of India to write a 1600-word "letter to the editor" to the *Illustrated London News* entitled "Irrigation and Means of Transit in India." This text illuminates Nightingale's deep understanding of the connections between health and the environment. Her remarks anticipated the concerns of contemporary environmentalists who look to interrelated issues of sustainable development. Nightingale addressed a number of key issues affecting the health of Indians, including environmental degradation due to land overuse, lack of remedial investment in wasted land, and the resulting poverty and starvation of millions of Indian people—"one fifth of the human race—our fellow countrymen and countrywomen" (Nightingale, 1874).

In 1878 and 1879, after years of watching the British government's continued neglect and abusive treatment of the people of India, Nightingale became outraged at further abuses that led directly to deepening drought and famine. She decided to take her voice to the people in a series of several popular magazine articles. In these pieces, Nightingale illustrated her familiarity with health and environmental issues, such as deforestation, that would result in severe devastation, injuries, and death during the monsoon season (Dossey, 2000). Nightingale called into question the harsh realities of the economic policies that increased the suffering of the people, *"Now*, the money-lender and the agriculturalist are no longer allies, but enemies. They no longer have a common interest. Indebtedness is no longer a common transaction; it is a bondage" (Nightingale, 1879, p. 568).

Contemporary environmental activism by nurses is illustrated by the work of Meg Jordan. She, like Nightingale, uses her media and advocacy skills to be an effective environmental activist focused on improving health. Jordan travels the world to seek out botanical healing remedies in remote places. She then reports her findings on a syndicated radio show she cohosts called "Global Medicine Hunter" and provides her listeners with accurate reporting about best practices in traditional healing modalities (Jordan, 2004).

Eleanor Schuster and Hollie Shaner are two other examples of nurses who have injected environmental activism into their nursing practice. Their work is highlighted and reviewed on the Web site of the Nightingale Institute for Health and the Environment (NIHE) (Nightingale Institute for Health and the Environment, 2004). As a nursing environmentalist, Schuster has authored many articles on environmental issues for nursing journals, including "Earth caring" for the September 1990 issue of *Advances in Nursing Science* and "Greening the curriculum, feminine process in education" in the October 1993 issue of the *Journal of Nursing Education.* She has provided leadership to the profession, as evidenced by her authorship of a chapter on the environment for the *AHNA Core Curriculum for Holistic Nursing* (Dossey, 1997) and by her contributions as coeditor of *Exploring our Environmental Connections*, published by the National League for Nurses (1994). Shaner's writings have focused on environmental concerns arising from healthcare settings and their implications for nurses. She has written on such topics as pollution in hospital waste management, recycling strategies for nurses in the workplace, community health environmental issues, and Florence Nightingale's legacy for environmental activism and nursing practice. Many of Shaner's articles are available on the NIHE's Web site. This site also maintains an extensive catalog of resources, including books, videos, and a "Pollution Prevention Kit for Nurses" (NIHE, 2004).

Margaret (Peggy) Burkhardt is nurse practitioner and prolific author whose advocacy for the environment has focused on the relationship between nature and healing. Burkhardt has published several articles on healing and nature (Burkhardt, 1993, 1994, 2000, 2002) and seeks to explore avenues—both for her readers and for herself—to develop more conscious connections with the Earth. Further, she explains that studies of ecology and spirituality are often similar in that they espouse a theme of this connectedness. Because all things are connected, Burkhardt believes that our health and the health of the Earth are intimately connected, too (Burkhardt & Nagai-Jacobson, 1994, 1997, 2000, 2002). Her work reflects what Florence Nightingale herself profoundly experienced at the age of 17 while sitting out in nature, under the shade of her favorite tree. Remembering the moment later in her diary, Nightingale described how the experience was her "call from God" to seek and find a way to serve humanity as a nurse (Dossey, 2000). To further develop these ideas for contemporary nursing practice, Burkhardt gives national and international conference presentations and convenes experiential workshops and retreats. In these ways, Burkhardt assists nurses and others to explore their own relationships with nature and to develop greater consciousness of nature as both home and healer.

NIGHTINGALE AS OPINION MOLDER: LESSONS FOR NURSING

Nightingale had an affinity for influencing public awareness, as evidenced in the discussion of her work for environmental improvements in India. Throughout her career, she would use the media resources of her day to share her views on key issues related to human health at local, regional, and national levels. In her 1893 essay "Sick-Nursing and Health-Nursing," she remarked on the significance of this approach, reminding her readers that "you must form public opinion. . . . Officials will only do what you make them. *You*, the public, must make them do what you want" (Nightingale, 2005, p. 292). Nightingale was well placed to offer this strategy, based on her many years of effort to influence public opinion through letters to the editor, networking, and correspondence with journalists and other public opinion makers. Yet, during many periods of her life Nightingale shunned publicity and hesitated to allow her name to be used in support of causes. She did not accept overt leadership positions, but worked behind the scenes, allowing those who worked with her to take the credit. Although naturally quite reclusive, she also was working within the constraints of her times. Women, with the exception of the Queen of England, were not allowed to speak at Parliament. To influence her causes, Nightingale had to utilize "referent power," working with others in private and through others' public offices and external influence (Dossey, 2000; Selanders, 2001).

Although the 21st century is very different from the 19th in many dramatic ways, this similarity remains. Nightingale's example of quiet endeavors still profoundly impacts nursing's current approach to the molding of public opinion. As Buresh and Gordon (2000) address this issue in their comprehensive book, *From Silence to Voice: What Nurses Know and Must Communicate to the Public,* nurses have, for the most part, been conditioned to remain silent about what they see and to remain silent about what they have accomplished.

Despite the fact that the discipline of medicine has had no such constraints, nursing has shied away from making its work and the value of that work visible to the public. Buresh and Gordon (2000) also note the irony that the largest and most-respected healthcare profession "has been shown to be vastly under-represented in news coverage. . . . virtually missing from health reportage" (p. 2). According to their findings, "practically everyone has had more of a public voice on health and health care than nurses" (p. 2). They posit that this is a "disturbing discovery," with "far-reaching implications" for health and for the nursing profession itself.

A contemporary example of a nurse who is focused on using media "to inform, challenge, and enrich" the nursing profession is Diana Mason, the Editor-in-Chief of the *American Journal of Nursing* (*AJN*), the oldest and largest nursing journal in the world (see Chapter 28). Mason notes that the "work that nurses do—the work of caring—has the ability to transform our healthcare system," but she is "frustrated that nursing care is often invisible or taken for granted by the public" and is "determined that this caring be made visible" (Roberts, 2004). In addition to her writing, Mason also hosts a radio show called "Healthstyles," a weekly hour on WBAI-Pacifica Radio in New York City. In an interview featured on the Medhunters Web site, Mason discusses the many values of media work by nurses: "Media presence is huge in New York. I think the radio show, in particular, showed me what is possible in the use of media as a health promotion tool" and "I consider the radio program my community health practice. We deal with issues that make a difference to the public, such as teaching people how to fill out a healthcare proxy form or select a managed care plan. We were the first media outlet I know of to discuss the politics of AIDS and the resurgence of tuberculosis." Mason also uses her media resources to address difficult subjects that are painful *and* integral to the practice of nursing. For example, she cites an *AJN* article penned by Michelle Baqi-Aziz. This piece "exposed the prejudice that Muslim nurses face [and] subsequent letters were sharply divided and—at times—angry. Issues such as these provoke strong feelings, and some nurses feel these issues are too political. Nurses need to realize, however, that such issues affect them and that hearing both sides of an issue is vital in formulating a response" (Roberts, 2004).

Media, communication, and advocacy skills are essential elements for the promotion of health and the active support of the nursing profession in the 21st century. Multiple communication channels exist, including Web sites, e-mail, local radio talk shows, books, magazines, newsletters/nurseletters, and newspapers. The "products" of nurse communication range from formal health education to human-interest stories. Throughout the United States, local cable television channels continue to seek neighborhood involvement in their programming. In these settings, nurses, nursing students, and educators should be encouraged and trained to create, produce, and air their ideas for the value of health and health advocacy. "Nurse power" in the media for the promotion of health and humanity is in keeping with Nightingale's vision and is an essential tool of activism.

Nurses as Change Agents

Nightingale was a consummate change agent throughout her career. In the Crimea, in addition to caring for wounded and dying soldiers, she worked proactively to change the severe conditions they faced, many of which were caused by the neglect of British military strategists rather than from the effects of war itself. After her return from the Crimea, she spent more than three decades advocating for changes in health policies and their implementation, not only for Great Britain but also for the Indian subcontinent, Canada, Australia, and New Zealand. She took an expert consultative role in support of the British Army throughout the world and also advised Union Army leaders during the American Civil War. Nightingale effected significant changes in many sectors: hospital design, military provision, economic strategies for the poor, several areas of education, community development, agriculture, land-use and transport planning, concern for cultural diversity, and the development of statistical data to support improvement in health outcomes (Dossey, 2000; Keith, 1988; Nightingale, 1863; Seymer, 1954).

Nightingale initiated dialogue with experts in many fields and took leadership roles in policy-level initiatives (Simpson, 1977). In 1863, after consulting with Sir George Grey about their mutual concern for high mortality rates among native children who attended 142 English schools in Ceylon, Australia, Natal, the West Coast of Africa, and British North America, she generated detailed statistical analyses comparing adults and children and their illnesses and causes of death in hospital and home settings (Nightingale, 1863). Her interdisciplinary review not only described the factors involved, such as physical, social, and economic problems, but also reflected an acute understanding of the sensitivity for the emotional stress that people endure when they undergo drastic changes in their lifestyle (Nightingale, 1863; Beck, 2002).

In her efforts to effect change and policies, Nightingale was the consummate networker, writing to leaders at all levels of government, to policy makers, philanthropists, journalists, inventors, clergy, and educators, as well as to a wide circle of accomplished friends and family. Acting at the level of what would be identified today as a health minister, she served as consultant to many powerful leaders, including Queen Victoria, several prime ministers, regional governors, secretaries of war and state, commanders-in-chief, and five Indian viceroys, briefing them on her recommendations. She used the power of her networks to accomplish her objectives for changes needed for the health of humanity (Dossey, 2000; McDonald, 2004).

Contemporary nurses around the world continue to be inspired to influence policy in the tradition of Nightingale. Australian nurse Audrey Kinnear, a public health nurse and a senior policy officer in the health policy section of the Aboriginal and Torres Strait Islander Commission in Australia, has used a similar nursing perspective and her Aboriginal roots to be a change agent to heal her nation, her people, and herself. She was born into the "stolen generation" of Australian Aboriginal children removed by force from their parents, victims of federal policies that touched six generations prior to 1970. Kinnear has spoken out in response to recent national government denials that the long-term practice of removing Aboriginal children was a substantial wounding of the people involved and the national psyche. Kinnear testified before federal officials and cochaired the Australia-wide "National Sorry Day," which followed her testimony in May 2002. "I was born in a traditional Aboriginal community on my traditional lands, " Kinnear testified, "I was forcibly removed at the age of four years. . . . We've had so much stolen from us" (Australian Broadcasting Corporation, 2004). Even though there has been no official "apology" from the government, Kinnear has noted that these endeavors were healing experiences.

"Telling my story to the inquiry resurfaced a lot of that pain and gave me an opportunity to shed some of it. National Sorry Day helped us [all the citizens of Australia] to close some of the wounds again. It was people-initiated—Australians wanted to recognize and understand and grieve with us. Our nation needed to weep because of the dark history of Australia, so that we could move forward. Thanks to that process . . . Our people aren't victims any more' " (Kinnear, as cited in Lean, 1998).

NIGHTINGALE'S BROAD SCOPE OF NURSING PRACTICE

In 1893, Florence Nightingale published her last major comprehensive essay, "Sick-Nursing and Health-Nursing." This work contains insights she gleaned over her 50-year career on a wide variety of issues related to human health and well-being and reflects the broad scope of nursing practice she established with her work (Beck, 2005a). As she had done for her best-selling *Notes on Nursing: What It Is and What It Is Not,* Nightingale wrote her 1893 essay for a general audience. "Sick-Nursing and Health-Nursing" was submitted by the British Royal Commission to the Chicago World's Fair, which was also called the Columbian Exposition. The Exposition convened the first-ever official international convocation honoring the contributions of women to humanity. In her essay, Nightingale recognized the World's Fair as a new development that promised broader collaborations, and she envisioned a "future, which I shall not see, for I am old, may a better way [toward health] be opened!" (Nightingale, 2005, p. 296).

In distinguishing between "sick-nursing" and "health-nursing," Nightingale (2004) described the domain of "health-nursing" as those actions aimed at helping people to be healthy and to stay healthy—a far more significant approach than "sick-nursing." To this end, she asked the pertinent question, "What is health?" and gave a timeless answer, "Health is not only to be well, but to use well every power we have" (Nightingale, 2005, p. 289). Although she expected that this work would reach a wide audience of general readers, Nightingale (2005) also planned to reach policy makers. Examples of this focus include her note that "upon womankind, the national health, as far as the household goes, depends" (p. 288) and that "How to keep the baby in health [is] certainly the most important function to make a healthy nation" (p. 289).

Her 1893 essay also anticipated relevant contemporary health issues, noting that "everything comes before health," and that human beings are inclined "not [to] look after health, but after sickness" (Nightingale, 2005, p. 288). Additionally, she worried about those profiting from disease. She already had witnessed the trend toward profits being more important than providing a caring service—the usury of patients as consumers of costly care and the usury of nurses and student nurses as cheap labor. Nightingale strongly voiced her concern that these self-serving priorities were "the enemy of health" (p. 296).

Emphasizing the significance of caring to healing, Nightingale (2005) celebrated the work of the nurse at the bedside. While it may be that the "physician prescribes" the "vital force" for healing support, it is the "nurse [who] supplies it" (p. 289). She contended that a nurse's care is so valuable that it is the very thing on which "physicians or surgeons, must depend" (p. 289) for their own successes or failures. Nightingale realized that nurses also needed to care for themselves and for each other in order to sustain their contributions. Wherever nursing services might be provided, Nightingale knew that nurses' sustained ability to provide excellent practice would deteriorate if the "espirit de corps" between caregivers was lost, and she also noted the significance of "fostering that bond of sympathy" between nursing colleagues (Nightingale, 2005, p. 293).

At the end of the 19th century, Nightingale (2005) was concerned that the health systems that she had helped to initiate decades earlier would become "stereotyped" into structures that could not grow and evolve, noting that "no system can endure that does not march" (p. 295). Although she acknowledged the need for proper clinical experience, a strong knowledge base, and well-respected nursing administrative policies, Nightingale maintained that the most significant assurance of quality nursing came from within nurses themselves. She urged her readers to address the rewards and challenges their own practice issued by continuing to ask themselves what their "calling" is—such that the highest spirit, ethics, and integrity of nursing could be maintained (Nightingale, 2005).

NIGHTINGALE'S TOP PRIORITY

Nightingale saw health and the significant promotion of health as a top priority for nursing practice and for humanity. During Nightingale's time, the profession of nursing was developing its identity—distinctly separate from the domestic roles women normally brought to their homes and families—but it was unclear what its scope would be. More than a century has passed since Nightingale penned her 1893 essay calling for the priority of health and for nursing to remain open to possibilities and change. She, herself, had lived into her own possibilities.

Messias (2001) argues that nursing has lost track of this key Nightingale premise and urges nurses again to challenge the underlying assumptions that would value sickness-treatment approaches over those that promote health. Advocating for the reclamation of "health," she calls nurses to see beyond their currently defined boundaries and to regain Nightingale's premise that nurses can have a major, larger role in the health of humanity. In a related concern about limitations, Rush (1997) notes that nurses have been conditioned to limit the majority of their health promotion practice to the *micro* level of individual health. Rush attributes this trend to theories and models such as Pender's (1987) health promotion model that assumes that individual patients and their behaviors are the targets of nursing's health promotion efforts. Rafael (1999) notes that this specialization and focus on individuals has also been by political default. Nurses have repeatedly had to fight turf battles to stay in the larger health promotion arena and have lost ground in recent decades. Regrettably, this focus on the sickness and health of individuals has become the dominant "lens" for nursing practice since Nightingale's time.

One of the key opportunities that Nightingale saw for nurses was their role as health educators and their potential to collaborate with other educators. In her correspondence, Nightingale writes of her belief in the importance of education to health: "Oh teach health, teach health, teach health, to rich and poor, to the educated, and, if there be any uneducated, oh teach it all the more: to men—to women especially—to mothers, to young mothers especially . . . . for the health of their children comes before Greek and grammar" (Nightingale, as cited in McDonald, 1998, p. 275).

Throughout her career, Nightingale developed health programs, oversaw their implementation, and conducted research to determine if her ideas and applications could be used for the improvement of human health. However, she never accomplished these projects alone. She always worked in collaboration with others, including educators and other academics; local, regional, and national leaders; physical and social scientists; mathematicians; sanitation engineers; urban planners and builders; philanthropists; clergy; planners and implementors of health policy; communicators; writers; inventors; and citizen-activists (Dossey, 2000).

Reflecting this approach in contemporary terms, Fitzpatrick (2001, p. 215) calls for nurses to "be prepared to set aside traditional discipline concerns [studying and practicing in isolation] and engage in creative dialogue with members of other professional groups." Koerner (2001) envisions a similar expansion of nursing's healthcare horizons. She calls for nursing's contemporary agenda to include "concern for the whole world [that] supersede[s] individual needs and goals" and collaborations with other disciplines that result in a "synergy through sharing and pooling of resources and activities toward common ends" (p. 20). The benefit of collaboration is promoted by Messias (2001, p. 10), who argues that "forging collaborative partnerships and fostering bridges" is "one way nurses can link global values with local action." She also notes that "nurses can adopt a global framework by working toward the empowerment of women" and cites examples of "fostering community health partnerships with women's groups, women's networks, and community health workers" (Messias, 2001, p.11).

Building a Nursing Network
for Humanitarianism and Health

With the major health concerns faced by the world today, Nightingale's passion for health advocacy and global citizenship to inform and inspire 21st-century nurses to move into the wider scope of their Nightingale legacy. Recalling Nightingale's prolific (she wrote 14,000 letters) letter-writing approach to networking—both locally and globally—about health concerns, Dossey (2001) has wondered, "What would Florence have done if she had had fax machines, email, the Internet and satellite uplink?" As if in response to this question, and to incorporate all of the ways discussed in this chapter in which nurses can support humanity's health, the Nightingale Initiative for Global Health (NIGH) was created in 2004. The NIGH seeks to lay an innovative foundation on which to achieve a healthy world and to support relevant, contemporary, globally conscious nursing practices (Dossey et al., 2005). The NIGH seeks to encourage nurses and others to discuss, plan, and implement approaches that directly connect their professional development with Nightingale's legacy for a wider scope of nursing practice. To accomplish this vision, the NIGH has identified a series of goals that should be accomplished by 2020 (NIGH, 2005):

- ☐ To build a grassroots movement among nurses, healthcare workers, educators, and other global citizens—from every country and community—who will work together to inform, educate, and mobilize public opinion throughout the world towards the adoption of health as the universal priority of the United Nations and its Member States
- ☐ To use communications, media, preforming arts, and promotional tools for advocacy to these ends
- ☐ To identify, share, and actively encourage 'approaches that work' to create a healthy world
- ☐ To contribute positive solutions to the worldwide nursing shortage

Further, the NIGH is developing a series of interrelated strategies that can be used to mobilize efforts and advance policy. This includes the preparation of two UN General Assembly Resolutions to be voted on in 2007 (NIGH, 2005):

- ☐ The United Nations International Year of the Nurse in 2010 (the centennial of Nightingale's death)
- ☐ The United Nations Decade for a Healthy World, 2010–2020 (the bicentennial of Nightingale's birth)

The NIGH supports empowering nurses around the world to act as leaders of a grassroots global campaign to circulate "The Nightingale Declaration for Our Healthy World" as a universal signature campaign to be organized between 2005 and 2007. (The draft text of this Declaration is provided in Box 40.1 on page 484.) This grassroots action will inform national leaders about the opinions of their citizens. It also will further establish sites and contact persons for a network of regional NIGH Communities around the world and will help to create a network of NIGH resources. The first international conference of NIGH is proposed to take place in Nairobi, Kenya as early as 2005. This meeting will focus on global health issues in the African context and will specifically address advocacy and media skill-building of nurses and nursing students from around the world. The intent is to support their return to their home countries with the knowledge, communication, and leadership skills to support change. In addition, the NIGH will encourage the development and implementation of similar educational programs around the world, employing a range of media, including on-site workshops and a major Web-based presence.

The NIGH idea was birthed in November 2003 through discussions among four Nightingale scholars who have focused their research on revisiting primary Nightingale documents and interpreting them for contemporary relevance. These scholars, Barbara Dossey, Louise Selanders, Deva-Marie Beck, and Alex Attewell, also collaborated with several colleagues with extensive experience in nursing education and in international media and development fields, as well as business, education, and medicine. Although such a range of knowledge and experiences is a good way to birth such ideas, the creators of the NIGH are also clear that the only way the NIGH can successfully grow and be sustained is through the enthusiastic participation of many people with a variety of talents and disciplines across the globe. The success of this effort requires intensive networking around the world to encourage the formation of NIGH "Communities." The essential requirement is a commitment to the ideals of Nightingale's humanitarian work for health and a willingness to work toward the goals of the NIGH. To support these efforts, a Web site has been launched (http://www.NIGHCommunities.org), and this site will provide regular updates regarding the NIGH's global progress.

Today, despite the enormity of the world's health problems, more people than ever before are becoming aware of their own calling to do something positive. More sectors are involved, and more citizen-activists look to accomplish what they can, both as individuals and in collectives. The growing importance of NGOs such as Greenpeace and Amnesty International has given concerned citizens a voice (Crosby, 1998). Although the world's problems have not been totally solved through these efforts, human consciousness on these issues and their potential solutions have increased dramatically. Pesut (1999) suggests that nurses could well look to joining these efforts, making significant contributions toward the improved health of humanity from nursing's unique perspectives and experiences.

As bioethicist Benatar (1998) aptly remarked: "despair should not eclipse hope" and "hope is oxygen of the human spirit." It is essential for us to remember that "imaginative, global thinking and visionary actions" can "have major long term advantages for humankind" (p. 295). People have, throughout history, been able to envision better lives and to find significant ways to implement those visions.

Nightingale was one of those people. Characteristic of the nursing perspective, she said, "look for the ideal, but put it into the actual" (Nightingale, 2005, p. 295). To address the seemingly insurmountable problems she saw in her own lifetime, Nightingale followed her own sense of "calling," and saw health as "not only to be well, but to use well, every power" she had to use.

Box 40.1 Nightingale Declaration

"The Nightingale Declaration for Our Healthy World" is intended to be circulated and signed by millions of nurses, other healthcare workers and caregivers, and the public across the world between 2005 and 2007, in advance of the proposed United Nations General Assembly Resolutions for an International Year of the Nurse in 2010 and a United Nations Decade for a Healthy World, 2010–2020.

We, the nurses, health workers, and caregivers of the world, as peoples of the United Nations and citizens of its Member States, hereby dedicate ourselves to the accomplishment of a healthy world by the year 2020. We declare our willingness to unite in a program of action, sharing information and solutions to resolve problems and improve conditions—locally, nationally, and globally—in order to achieve health for all humanity. We further resolve to adopt personal practices and to implement public policies in our communities and nations, making this goal for the year 2020 achievable and inevitable, beginning today in our own lives, in the life of our nations and in the world at large. (Dossey et al., 2005)

Nurses—from all specialties and perspectives—can also focus their collective visions—from Nightingale's legacy for us—to sustain the health and the well-being of our species and to secure a vibrant future for our children and for all future generations.

REFERENCES

Aga Khan University School of Nursing. (2001). *Candlelighting service.* Available at http://www.akdn. org/agency/college_nursing.html.

Australian Broadcasting Corporation. (2004). *No stolen generation.* Available at http://www.abc.net. au/7.30/stories/s115691.htm.

Beck, D. M. (2002). *Florence Nightingale's 1893 'Sick-nursing and Health-nursing': Weaving a tapestry of positive health determinants for personal, community and global wellness.* Ann Arbor, MI: UMI Dissertation Services.

Beck, D. M. (2005a). Sick-nursing and health-nursing: Nightingale establishes our broad scope of practice in 1893. In B. M. Dossey, L. C. Selanders, D. M. Beck, & A. Attewell (Eds.), *Florence Nightingale Today: Healing, Leadership, Global Action.* Silver Spring, MD: Nursesbooks.org.

Beck, D. M. (2005b). Tributes to Nightingale's legacy: International celebrations to honor nursing. In B. M. Dossey, L. C. Selanders, D. M. Beck, & A. Attewell (Eds.), *Florence Nightingale Today: Healing, Leadership, Global Action.* Silver Spring, MD: Nursesbooks.org.

Benatar, S. R. (1998). Global disparities in health and human rights: A critical commentary. *American Journal of Public Health, 88*(2), 295–300.

Buresh, B., & Gordon, S. (2000*). From silence to voice: What nurses know and must communicate to the public.* Ottawa: Canadian Nurses Association.

Burkhardt, M. A. (1993). Characteristics of spirituality in the lives of women in a rural Appalachian community. *Journal of Transcultural Nursing, 4*(2), 19–23.

Burkhardt, M. A. (1994). Environmental connections and reawakened spirit. In E. A. Schuster & C. L. Brown (Eds.), *Exploring Our Environmental Connections* (pp. 287–306). New York: National League for Nursing.

Burkhardt, M. A. (2000). Healing relationships with nature. *Complementary Therapies in Nursing & Midwifery, 6*(1), 35–40.

Burkhardt, M. A. (2002). Healing relationships with nature. *The British Naturopathic Journal, 19*(1), 9–14. (Reprinted with permission from *Complementary Therapies in Nursing & Midwifery*).

Burkhardt, M. A., & Nagai-Jacobson, M. G. (1994). Reawakening spirit in clinical practice. *Journal of Holistic Nursing, 12*(1), 9–21.

Burkhardt, M. A., & Nagai-Jacobson, M. G. (1997). Spirituality and healing. In B. M. Dossey (Ed.), *AHNA Core Curriculum* (Chapter 6). Gaithersburg, MD: Aspen Publishers, Inc.

Burkhardt, M. A., & Nagai-Jacobson, M. G. (2000). Spirituality and health. In B. M. Dossey, L. Keegan, & C. Guzzetta (Eds.), *Holistic Nursing Practice: A Handbook for Practice* (3rd Ed.) (pp. 91–121). Gaithersburg, MD: Aspen Publishers.

Burkhardt, M. A., & Nagai-Jacobson, M. G. (2002). *Spirituality: Living Our Connectedness.* Albany, NY: Delmar Publishers.

Carter Center. (2003). *New director a quick study in Ethiopian health needs.* Available at http://www. cartercenter.org/doc1544.htm.

Crosby, B. C. (1998). *Leadership for global citizenship: Building transnational community.* Thousand Oaks, CA: Sage.

Dean, M. (1999, May 15). On leaving Nightingale behind. *Lancet, 353*(9165:1685).

Dossey, B. M. (1997). *Core Curriculum for Holistic Nursing.* Sudbury, MA: Jones & Bartlett.

Dossey, B. M. (2000). *Florence Nightingale: Mystic, Visionary, Healer.* Springhouse, PA: Springhouse.

Dossey, B. M. (2001, August 12). Keynote address presented at the "First Inaugural Florence Nightingale Commemorative Service," Washington National Cathedral, Washington, D.C.

Dossey, B. M., Selanders, L. C., Beck, D. M., & Attewell, A. (2005). *Florence Nightingale Today: Healing, Leadership, Global Action.* Silver Spring, MD: Nursesbooks.org.

Fitzpatrick, J. J. (2001). Interdisciplinary education for nursing. In N. L. Chaska (Ed*.), The Nursing Profession: Tomorrow and Beyond* (pp. 211–217). Thousand Oaks, CA: Sage.

Florence Nightingale Foundation. (2004). *Commemoration service.* Available at http://www.florence-nightingale-foundation.org.uk.

Goldie, S. M. (1987). *I Have Done My Duty: Florence Nightingale in the Crimean War: 1854–1856.* Manchester, UK: Manchester University Press.

Hiasma, K. K. (1996). Florence Nightingale's influence on the development and professionalism of modern nursing in Japan. *Nursing Outlook, 44*(6), 284–288.

International Committee of the Red Cross. (2004). *Florence Nightingale Medal.* Available at http://www.icrc.org/Web/Eng/siteeng0.nsf/html/funds_medals?OpenDocument.

International Museum of Red Cross and Red Crescent. (2004). *Discover the fascinating history of the world's first humanitarian organisation!* Available at http://www.micr.org.

Jordan, M. (2004). *Global Medicine Hunter.* Available at http://megjordan.com/meet.html.

Keith, J. M. (1988). Florence Nightingale: Statistician and consultant epidemiologist. *International Nursing Review, 35*(5), 147–149.

Koerner, J. (2001). Nightingale II: Nursing in the new millennium. In N. L. Chaska (Ed.), *The Nursing Profession: Tomorrow and Beyond* (pp. 17–27). Thousand Oaks, CA: Sage.

Lean, M. (1998). *Building bridges across the divides.* Available at http://www.forachange.co.uk/index.php?stoid=88.

McDonald, L. (1998). Florence Nightingale: Passionate statistician. *Journal of Holistic Nursing, 16*(2), 267–277.

McDonald, L. (2004). *Collected Works of Florence Nightingale: Introduction to the Project.* Available at http://www.sociology.uoguelph.ca/fnightingale/Introduction.

Messias, D. K. H. (2001). Globalization, nursing, and "Health for All." *Journal of Nursing Scholarship, 33*(1), 9–11.

Nightingale, F. (1860). *Notes on Nursing: What It Is and What It Is Not.* London: Harrison.

Nightingale, F. (1863). Sanitary statistics of native colonial schools and hospitals. *Proceedings, Annual Meeting National Association for the Promotion of Social Science* (pp. 473–489). London: National Association for the Promotion of Social Science.

Nightingale, F. (1874, August). Irrigation and means of transit in India. *The Illustrated London News.*

Nightingale, F. (1879, September). A missionary health officer in India. *Good Words,* 635–640.

Nightingale, F. (1893). Sick-nursing and health-nursing. In A. Burdett-Coutts (Ed.), *Woman's Mission: A Series of Congress papers of the Philanthropic Work of Women by Eminent Writers* (pp. 184–205). London: Sampson, Low, Marston.

Nightingale, F. (2005). Sick-nursing and health-nursing. In B. M. Dossey, L. C. Selanders, D. M. Beck, & A. Atewell, *Florence Nightingale Today: Healing, Leadership, Global Action.* Silver Spring, MD: Nursesbooks.org.

Nightingale Initiative for Global Health (NIGH). (2005). Available at http://www.NIGHCommunities.org.

NIHE. (2004). *Pollution Prevention Kit for Nurses.* Available at http://www.nihe.org.

Orange County Red Cross. (2004). *A Brief History of the Red Cross.* Available at http://www.informatics.org/redcross/history.html.

Pender, N. J. (1987). *Health Promotion in Nursing Practice* (2nd ed.). Norwalk, CT: Appleton & Lange.

Pesut, D. J. (1999). Millennium issues and nursing leadership. *Nursing Outlook, 47*(6), 242.

Petenkin, C. (1996, June 4). *Windows of wellness.* Keynote address presented at the International Tribute to Florence Nightingale, U.N. Human Settlements Summit, Scutari, Istanbul.

Rafael, A. R. F. (1999). The politics of health promotion: Influences on public health promoting nursing practice in Ontario, Canada from Nightingale to the nineties. *Advances in Nursing Science, 22*(1), 23–39.

Red Cross Society of China. (2004). *Health and Care.* Available at http://www.chineseredcross.org.cn/english/project/Rescue_3.htm.

Roberts, K. (2004). *The new AJN: Editor-in Chief Diana Mason.* Available at http://www.medhunters.com/articles/theNewAJN.html.

Rush, K. L. (1997). Health promotion ideology and nursing education. *Journal of Advanced Nursing, 25,* 1292–1298.

Schuster, E. A., & Brown, L. C. (Eds.). (1994). *Exploring Our Environmental Connections.* New York: National League for Nursing.

Selanders, L. C. (1993). *Florence Nightingale: An Environmental Adaptation Theory.* Newbury Park, CA: Sage.

Selanders, L. C. (2001). Florence Nightingale and the transvisionary leadership paradigm. *Nursing Leadership Forum, 6*(1), 12–16.

Seymer, L. R. (Ed.). (1954). *Selected Works of Florence Nightingale.* New York: Macmillan.

Simpson, D. (1977). Florence Nightingale by her god-daughter. *Nursing Times, 73*(5), 50–51.

Stewart, I. M., & Austin, A. L. (1962). *A History of Nursing: From Ancient to Modern Times: A Worldview* (5th ed.). New York: G. P. Putnam's Sons.

Waddy, C. (1980). *Women in Muslim History.* London. Longman Group.

Index

Brown, Lucille, 15
Brown Report (1947), 369
Buerhaus, Peter, 342
Bureau of Maternal-Child Health, 320
Bureau of Public Health Nursing, 338
Burgess, Mae, 305
Burgess, May Ayers, 10
Burkhardt, Margaret, 477–478
Business Roundtable, 453
Butterfield, Patricia, 106

C
Cadet Nurse Corps, 60, 339, 367, 370
Caffin, Freida, 322
California State Nurses Association, 338
Canada, 36, 73
Cancer, colorectal, 277–279
Cancer rehabilitation
  background of, 278–279
  definition of, 278
  overview of, 277–278
  theoretical framework of, 279
Cancer Rehabilitation Questionnaire (CRQ),
    279–283
Cancer rehabilitation study
  implications of, 283–284
  methodology for, 279–281
  results of, 281–283
Cardiovascular drugs, 241
Cardiovascular Nursing, 336
Caribbean, 185–186
Caring
  community health nursing and, 90
  as critical thread, 3
  empowered, 20
  explanation of, 194, 422–423
  machine technologies and, 122–124
  as nursing function, 288, 422, 481
  theoretical work on, 19–20
Carper, Barbara, 139, 140, 143, 146, 147, 151,
    178, 185
Case Western Reserve University, 387–388, 395
Cavanagh, Stephen, 326
Certified nurse midwives (CNM). *See also*
    Advance practice nursing
  educational standards for, 378
  historical background of, 375
  reimbursement for, 377

Certified registered nurse anesthetist (CRNA).
    See also Advance practice nursing
  educational standards for, 378
  historical background of, 375
  reimbursement for, 377
Chaotic families, 222
Cheyovich, Theresa, 399
Children, 73, 74
Children with chronic disabilities
  encouraging support use for parents of,
    228–229
  family adaptation and, 221–224
  overview of, 217–218
  parent coping factors and, 218–221
  social support for patents of, 224–228
Chopoorian, Teresa, 102
Christy, Teresa, 17
Chronic disabilities
  children with, 217–229 (*See also* Children
    with chronic disabilities)
  as family crisis, 217–218
Chronic grief, 207–208
City of Hope, 396
Civil Rights Act of 1964, 61
Civil Rights Movement, 61
Civil War, 5, 8, 57–58, 364, 375
Cleland, Virginia, 16
Clergy, 213
Cleveland Council of Black Nurses (CCBN), 65
Clinical Assessment of Confusion (CAC-A), 255,
    256
Clinical doctoral programs, 387–389
Clinical nurse specialist (CNS). *See also*
    Advance practice nursing
  community health, 377
  educational standards for, 378
  historical background of, 375–376
  role of, 377
Clinton, Bill, 452
Code of Ethics for Nurses (American Nurses
    Association)
  background of, 435, 436, 441–442
  discussion of, 439–441, 447
  provisions of, 442–446
Codes of ethics. *See also* Ethics
  background of, 435, 436
  descriptive ethics and, 438–439
  metaethics and, 437–438

Self-esteem, 24, 27, 28
Seneca Falls Convention, 8
Sentinel Event Alert (Joint Accreditation of
        Healthcare Organization), 455
Service Man's Readjustment Act of 1944 (GI
        Bill), 368
Sexual assault, 73–74
Sexual assault nurse examiners (SANE),
        346
Sexual harassment, 39–40
Sexually transmitted infections (STIs), 74
Shaner, Hollie, 477
Sigma Theta Tau International, 348
Silver, Henry, 341
Silver Spring Neighborhood Center, 325
Single-blind review, 350
Smith, Suzanne, 347
Smith-Rosenberg, C., 7
Social Policy Statement (American Nurses
        Association), 88
Social Reform Club, 69
Social support. *See also* Support groups
    encouraging use of, 228–229
    family adaptation and, 224–227
    parent perceptions of, 226–227
    types of, 225–226
Social work profession, 360
Sociopolitical knowing
    essential elements of, 148
    explanation of, 147–148, 185
Spanish American War, 366
Spirituality
    definition of, 151–152, 419
    historical roots of, 419–421
    language barriers and, 423
    nursing education and, 424
    nursing informed by, 421–423
    in nursing practice, 152–153, 432
    overview of, 417–419
    as personal knowing, 153–154
    prayer and, 206
    relationship between nursing and, 424–425
Stanton, Anthony, 8
Stanton, Elizabeth Cady, 8
Starr, Paul, 323
State Boards of Nursing, 468, 469
*Statement on Clinical Nurse Specialist Practice
        and Education* (National Association of
        Clinical Nurse Specialists), 378

Status contradiction
    gender as, 37–38
    reconciling, 38–39
Stereotypes, 15
Storytelling, 179–180
Stress, 218, 227
Structural adjustment policies (SAPs), 72, 75
Structuralized families, 222
Submission-aggression syndrome, 24
Suffrage movement. *See* Voting rights; Women's
        rights
Superintendents' Society (American Society of
        Superintendents of Training Schools
        for Nurses of the United States and
        Canada), 10, 11, 59
Support groups
    bereavement, 212
    encouraging use of, 228–229
    for parents of children with chronic
        disabilities, 227–228

T
Taft-Hartley Act of 1947, 16
Taylor, Frederick, 309
Taylor, Telford, 193
T-Double BCX Model of Family Adjustment and
        Adaptation, 222
Teachers College (Columbia University), 9–10,
        309, 320, 363–365, 369, 370, 385, 386
Team nursing, 310
Technology, 3, 121. *See also* Internet
Telenursing, 114
Terrorism, 340
Theoria: Journal of Nursing Theory, 169
Therapeutic touch, 432
Thompson, Tommy G., 63, 454
Thoms, Adah Belle Samuels, 11
*To Err is Human: Building a Safer Health
        System* (Institute of Medicine), 451
Torres, Gertrude, 102
The Trained Nurse and Hospital Review, 337
Training programs. *See* Nursing education
Transcultural nursing
    advantages of, 52
    explanation of, 51–52
    function of, 53–54, 69
Transpersonal caring-healing model, 105
Truth, Sojourner, 5, 8, 12, 58
Truth-telling, 195